New Insights into Amyotrophic Lateral Sclerosis

New Insights into
Amyotrophic Lateral Sclerosis

Edited by **Lisa Rowe**

hayle
medical

New York

Published by Hayle Medical,
30 West, 37th Street, Suite 612,
New York, NY 10018, USA
www.haylemedical.com

New Insights into Amyotrophic Lateral Sclerosis
Edited by Lisa Rowe

International Standard Book Number: 978-1-63241-296-6 (Hardback)

Printed in the United States of America.

Contents

Permissions

List of Contributors

Preface

Amyotrophic Lateral Sclerosis (ALS) continues to be one of the mysterious diseases of 21st century, even though ample amount of research; both pre-clinical and clinical, has been conducted during the past few years. Significant attempts have been made for the progress of pathophysiological models and understanding the underlying pathology, and with new instruments in genetics and transgenic techniques, the goal of finding a durable cure has come into scope. On the contrary, most pharmacological trials have remained unsuccessful in depicting an advantage for ALS patients. In this book, readers will find a compilation of state-of-the-art examination of human genetics in ALS, molecular basis of disease development and clinical manifestations, and new investigation principles in the area of electrophysiology. An overview about all relevant pharmacological trials in ALS patients is also included, while the book ends with a discourse on present developments and future trends in ALS research.

The information contained in this book is the result of intensive hard work done by researchers in this field. All due efforts have been made to make this book serve as a complete guiding source for students and researchers. The topics in this book have been comprehensively explained to help readers understand the growing trends in the field.

I would like to thank the entire group of writers who made sincere efforts in this book and my family who supported me in my efforts of working on this book. I take this opportunity to thank all those who have been a guiding force throughout my life.

Editor

Part 1

Cellular Pathophysiology, the Immune System and Stem Cell Strategies

Innate Immunity in ALS

John D. Lee[1], Jia Y. Lee[1], Stephen M. Taylor[1],
Peter G. Noakes[1, 2] and Trent M. Woodruff[1]
[1]*School of Biomedical Sciences,*
[2]*Queensland Brain Institute, University of Queensland,*
Australia

1. Introduction

Amyotrophic Lateral Sclerosis (ALS), also known as Lou Gehrig's disease, is the most common form of motor neuron disease. It is a debilitating, late onset neurodegenerative disorder that is characterized by the progressive death of upper and α-motor neurons within the central nervous system (CNS) (Bruijn and Cleveland, 1996). This results in symptoms of muscle weakness and atrophy of skeletal muscles, leading to paralysis and eventual death due to failure of respiratory muscles (Cozzolino et al., 2008). ALS has a prevalence of approximately 1~2 per 100,000 worldwide with males being more susceptible than females (1.3 ~ 1.6: 1) (Strong, 2003, Woodruff et al., 2008b, Worms, 2001). The majority of ALS cases (~90%) are thought to be sporadic with unknown aetiology and no robust environmental risk factors, with the remaining 10% being familial ALS. Of this 10%, approximately 20% have been linked to dominant mis-sense point mutations in the Copper/Zinc superoxide dismutase 1 (SOD1) gene which results in a gain of unidentified deleterious properties (Rosen et al., 1993). The two aetiologies of ALS (i.e. sporadic and familial) are indistinguishable on the basis of their clinical and pathological features, including progressive muscle weakness, atrophy and spasticity, each of which reflects the degeneration and death of upper and α-motor neurons (Boillee et al., 2006). The mechanisms leading to ALS are still unclear but theories have suggested that glutamate excitoxicity, oxidative stress, protein aggregation, mitochondrial dysfunction, cytoskeletal abnormalities and neuro-inflammation may all play a role (Bruijn et al., 2004). The present chapter will review the role of innate immune system, in particular the complement system, during the disease progression of ALS. It will review evidence for an involvement of the innate immune Toll-like receptor (TLR) system and receptor for advanced glycosylation and products (RAGE) in ALS patients and animal models of ALS. It will also comprehensively evaluate the role of the innate immune complement cascade in this disease. Finally, the future therapeutic possibilities for ALS, aimed at targeting components of the innate immune system will be discussed. We provide compelling evidence for specific inhibitors of complement C5a receptors as novel treatment strategies for ALS.

2. Innate immunity in neurodegenerative disease

Innate immunity is an evolutionary ancient system that provides the host with immediately available defence mechanisms. It is a rapid and coordinated cascade of reactions by host cells to protect them against foreign pathogens and insults (Akira et al., 2001, Nguyen et al., 2004). Until recently, the CNS was considered to be immunologically privileged because of its inability to mount an immune response and process antigens. Recent studies have revealed that immune surveillance and differentiation between self and non-self does take place in the CNS, where glial cells, including microglia, astrocytes and oligodendrocytes, act as CNS immune effector cells (Hanisch et al., 2008, Lehnardt, 2010, Ricklin et al., 2010).

The role of innate immune system in the CNS is mainly to provide protection to the neurons from foreign pathogens and injurious stimuli, and to maintain CNS homeostasis. It is also required for tissue modelling during development and following injury (Benard et al., 2008, Mastellos et al., 2005, Rahpeymai et al., 2006, Stevens et al., 2007). However sustained chronic inflammation might be harmful for neuronal integrity and may result in cellular dysfunction which triggers neurodegeneration. There is increasing evidence that suggests an involvement of the innate immune system in the development of neuro-inflammation which may drive the progression of many neurodegenerative diseases including ALS. Two major constituents of innate immune system are the TLRs and the complement cascade, each of which are described below.

3. Toll-like receptors (TLRs) and receptor for advanced glycosylation end products (RAGE) in ALS

TLRs are a large family of evolutionarily conserved transmembrane glycoproteins that initiate immune responses for host defence upon activation. These receptors are pattern recognition receptors that recognise pathogen-associated molecular patterns (PAMPs) from diverse organisms including bacteria, viruses, fungi and parasites (Liew et al., 2005). TLRs are expressed in various cell types in the CNS including microglia, astrocytes, oligodendrocytes and neurons (Aravalli et al., 2007, Bowman et al., 2003, Olson and Miller, 2004, Tang et al., 2007). This pathway has recently been implicated in the pathogenesis of ALS. Increased levels of TLRs (TLR1, TLR2, TLR5, TLR7 and TLR9) have been observed in mutant SOD1 mice as compared to controls (Letiembre et al., 2009) and mutant SOD1 expression in ALS has been suggested to facilitate microglial neurotoxic inflammatory responses via TLR2 (Liu et al., 2009). In addition, it has recently been shown that mutant SOD1 binds to CD14, which is a co-receptor of TLR2 and TLR4, and that microglial activation mediated by mutant SOD1 (G93A) can be attenuated using TLR2, TLR4 and CD14 blocking antibodies (Zhao et al., 2010). The involvement of TLR signalling in the pathogenesis of ALS is also supported by up-regulation of TLR2 and TLR4 mRNA and protein in the ALS patients, compared to control spinal cords. The increased expression level of TLR2 and TLR4 was shown on microglia and reactive astrocytes respectively (Casula et al., 2011). This suggests that TLRs could play a role in the progressive degeneration of motor neurons in ALS and indicates that the innate immune system is important in sensing neuronal injury and driving the progression of this disease.

In absence of pathogens, TLR signalling can also be activated via molecules called damage associated molecular patterns (DAMPs) including the high mobility group box 1 (HMGB1) protein released by injured tissues (Bianchi and Manfredi, 2009). HMGB1 is a nearly ubiquitous chromatin component that can regulate transcription of different sets of genes, including pro-inflammatory genes (Bianchi and Manfredi, 2009, Mouri et al., 2008). It can also be released passively by necrotic cells and actively secreted by stimulated monocytes/macrophages and astrocytes, which then bind to RAGE, TLR2 and TLR4. (Andersson et al., 2008, Hreggvidsdottir et al., 2009, Parker et al., 2004, Scaffidi et al., 2002). Therefore, HMGB1 can act as a potent pro-inflammatory cytokine-like mediator, thus contributing to amplification of the inflammatory response (Bianchi and Manfredi, 2007, Hreggvidsdottir et al., 2009). HMGB1-RAGE signalling has also been implicated in the progression of ALS where there was a significant increase in HMGB1 mRNA expression in ALS patient spinal cords when compared to normal individuals (Casula et al., 2011). The increased expression of HMGB1 was expressed by activated microglia and astrocytes in the spinal cord (Casula et al., 2011). Interestingly, there were no significant changes in RAGE mRNA expression in 12 ALS patients when compared to 6 controls. This observation could be due to the loss of motor neurons expressing RAGE in ALS patients, thus reducing the endogenous pool of RAGE mRNA. This same study also demonstrated that there is an increased expression of RAGE on astrocytes and microglia when compared to controls (Casula et al., 2011). Furthermore, serum soluble RAGE (sRAGE) levels were decreased in the serum of ALS patients when compared to normal individuals, where sRAGE is known to be a possible modulator of inflammation in several diseases (Ilzecka, 2009). Hence it is possible that low sRAGE levels may accelerate the neurodegeneration and could be a risk factor in ALS. This suggests that TLR/RAGE signalling may play a role in the disease progression of ALS, by activating microglia and astrocytes in the vicinity of motor neuron death. Targeting TLRs and RAGE may therefore be a novel therapeutic strategy to treat degenerative neuronal loss occurring in ALS.

4. The complement system in the CNS

The complement system is a key component of the innate immune system, which participates in the recognition, trafficking and elimination of pathogens and unwanted host materials. The complement system is an enzymatic cascade consisting of more than 30 plasma proteins and glycoproteins, and either soluble or membrane-bound receptors (Guo and Ward, 2005). Complement activation participates in host defence against pathogens primarily by cytotoxic and cytolytic activity through triggering formation of the membrane attack complex (MAC or C5b-9) on the target cell membrane (van Beek et al., 2003). It is activated via three major pathways: the classical, alternative, and lectin pathways; it is also activated by a recently identified fourth, extrinsic protease pathway (Huber-Lang et al., 2006, Thoman et al., 1984) (Figure 1).

The classical pathway is primarily activated in response to the recognition molecule C1q binding to antigen-antibody complexes such as immunoglobins (IgG and IgM) and pentraxins (such as C-reactive protein) bound to their targets (Ricklin et al., 2010, Woodruff et al., 2010). C1q may also bind directly to pathogen surfaces and to non-pathogen surfaces such as beta-amyloid and liposomes (Jiang et al., 1994, Marjan et al., 1994). The alternative pathway is activated by foreign surfaces which amplifies the slow spontaneous hydrolysis of C3 which leads to the formation of C3 convertases (Pangburn et al., 1981, Ricklin et al., 2010), whereas lectin pathway is initiated following the binding of mannose-binding lectin to carbohydrate groups on the surfaces of some pathogens (Woodruff et al., 2010). The activation of each of these pathways results in assembly of C3 and C5 convertase enzymes which cleave their respective inactive complement factors C3 and C5 into their active fragments C3a, C3b, C5a and C5b. This leads to the formation of MAC through the non-enzymatic assembly of C5b with complement factors C6-C9, forming C5b-9 on the cell membrane, which creates a transmembrane pore, ultimately leading to cell lysis (Podack et al., 1982). A recently identified fourth extrinsic pathway involves direct cleavage of complement 3 (C3) and complement 5 (C5) into C3a/C3b and C5a/C5b by proteolytic enzymes (serine proteases) such as kallikrein, thrombin and cell-derived proteases (Huber-Lang et al., 2002, Huber-Lang et al., 2006). As a result, synthesis of C5 by local inflammatory cells can produce C5a via cleavage of C5 with cell derived proteases, even when devoid of the complement cascade precursor, C3 (Huber-Lang et al., 2006). This pathway may provide a source of complement activation factors in the absence of upstream complement activation, and in a local tissue environment such as the CNS (Woodruff et al., 2010).

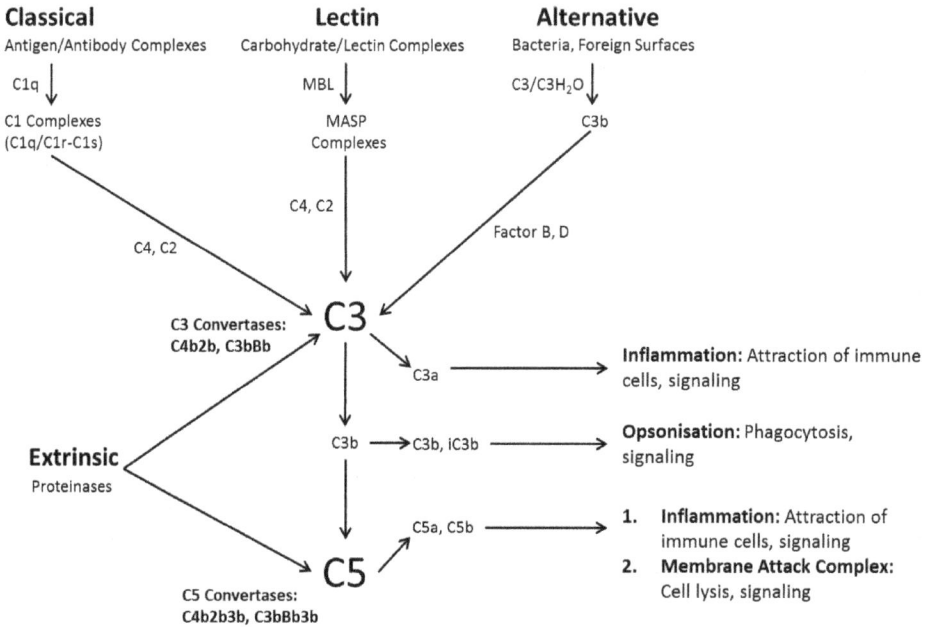

Fig. 1. Complement Cascade: Complement is part of the innate immune system and can be activated via four different pathways: the classical pathway, an antigen-antibody complex; the alternative pathway, activated by bacteria and foreign surfaces; the lectin pathway activated by mannose binding lectin; and recently discovered extrinsic protease pathway involving direct cleavage of C3 and C5. Each pathway converges at C3 and leads to a common terminal point which involves the formation of the cytolytic membrane attack complex (MAC) leading to cell lysis. Formation of pro-inflammatory anaphylatoxins C3a and C5a induces glial chemotaxis, generation of superoxide radicals and release of inflammatory mediators. C3b and iC3b facilitates phagocytosis by opsonising foreign pathogens.

The primary function of complement activation is to provide a rapid response to infection and injury by initiating the production of opsonins C1q and C3b to opsonise pathogens, the production of the pro-inflammatory anaphylatoxins C3a and C5a to recruit immune and inflammatory cells through ligand-receptor interactions with their corresponding receptors, C3aR and CD88, and the formation of cytolytic MAC, which ultimately leads to the destruction of invading organisms by cell apoptosis/necrosis (Liszewski et al., 1996).

C5a is considered to be the most potent inflammatory molecule generated upon complement activation and exhibits a broad range of functions. C5a exerts its effect through two high affinity receptors, the classical C5aR (CD88), and the C5a-like receptor 2 (C5L2/GPR77). The main C5a receptor, CD88 is a member of the rhodopsin family of seven transmembrane domain receptors coupled to the hetero-metric G proteins of the Gi subtype: pertussis toxin-sensitive $G_{\alpha i2}$, $G_{\alpha i3}$ or pertussis toxin-insensitive $G_{\alpha 16}$ (Amatruda et al., 1993, Johswich and Klos, 2007, Rollins et al., 1991). Cellular activation of CD88 involves intracellular calcium mobilization and activation of different signaling pathways including phosphatidylinositol-3-kinase/Akt (PI3Kγ; Perianayagam et al., 2002), Ras/B-Raf/mitogen-activated protein kinase (MAPK)/extracellular signal-related kinase (ERK) (Buhl et al., 1994), phospholipase A_2, phospholipase D (Cockcroft, 1992, Mullmann et al., 1990), protein kinase C (PKC; Buhl et al., 1994), p21-activated kinases, Rac GTPases (Huang et al., 1998), signal transducers and activators of transcription, sphingosine kinase (Melendez and Ibrahim, 2004) and NF-κB (Kastl et al., 2006). It is widely expressed on variety of cells and tissues, and its activation is known to have pro-inflammatory functions such as chemotaxis, degranulation, superoxide production, and release of proteases, eicosanoids, cytokines and chemokines from inflammatory cells (Gomez-Cambronero et al., 2007, Melendez and Ibrahim, 2004, Torres and Forman, 1999, Tsai et al., 2004).

The recently discovered C5a receptor, C5L2 has the conventional G-protein coupled receptor structure but it is not coupled to intracellular G-protein activated signaling pathways (Bamberg et al., 2010, Okinaga et al., 2003). Binding of C5a to C5L2 failed to induce intracellular calcium mobilization, extracellular signal-related kinase phosphorylation or receptor internalization, by contrast to CD88 (Cain and Monk, 2002, Okinaga et al., 2003). This has led to the proposal that C5L2 may act as a decoy anaphylatoxin receptor by regulating the availability of C5a to CD88, or by forming oligomers with CD88 to interrupt C5a-CD88 signaling (Rabiet et al., 2007). Although the mechanisms underlying C5L2 activation are still unknown, several recent studies in C5L2 knockout mice have showed greater response to C5a, a greater influx of inflammatory cells and a greater release of IL-6 and TNF-α compared to the wild-type mice (Rabiet et al., 2007). This suggests that C5a signaling via C5L2 may exert anti- inflammatory functions which buffer the effects of the inflammatory C5a-CD88 signaling pathway (Rabiet et al., 2007). Furthermore, studies have shown that C5L2 may function as an intracellular receptor, which becomes activated only after ligand binds to CD88. It was suggested that C5L2 negatively modulates C5a-CD88 signaling and limits the signaling capacity of C5a via its interaction with CD88 and β-arrestins (Bamberg et al., 2010, Van Lith et al., 2009). Any role for C5L2 in neurodegenerative diseases has yet to be properly elucidated.

Although the CNS does not receive the same composition of circulating complement factors synthesised in the liver by hepatocytes, due to the blood brain barrier (BBB), many studies have revealed that the CNS contains components of complement cascade, where they are expressed by astrocytes, microglia, oligodendrocytes and neurons (Barnum, 1995, Gasque et al., 1997, Nataf et al., 2001, O'Barr et al., 2001). Similar to the peripheral system, the role of complement activation within the CNS is thought to primarily protect the neurons from foreign pathogens through activation of inflammatory and immune cascades by surrounding glial cells. In addition to their immune surveillance functions, recent studies have shown that complement molecules also have a role in adaptive immune response, nervous system development, regeneration and regulating CNS homeostasis by clearing cellular debris and also eliminating excess synapses (i.e. synaptic pruning) (Stevens et al., 2007). Intriguingly, synaptic loss is not only a feature of neural development but is also a key pathological feature of neurodegenerative diseases (Schafer and Stevens, 2010, Woodruff et al., 2010). Hence it has been proposed that complement has multiple central roles in the CNS other than its canonical functions associated with host defence (Benard et al., 2008, Rahpeymai et al., 2006, Stevens et al., 2007). Therefore dysregulation or imbalance of the complement system in the CNS can be harmful to the neurons and may lead to, or contribute to, neurodegenerative diseases including ALS.

5. Clinical evidence of complement involvement in ALS

Several studies have been conducted on ALS patients in an attempt to identify whether complement components are up-regulated in disease progression (Table 1). It has been proposed that the classical complement system is involved in the pathophysiology of ALS, as studies have shown that activation fragments of complement components C3 and C4 are increased in the serum, cerebrospinal fluid (CSF), and neurological tissue (including spinal cord and motor cortex) of ALS patients (Annunziata and Volpi, 1985, Apostolski et al., 1991, Goldknopf et al., 2006, Kawamata et al., 1992, Trbojevic-Cepe et al., 1998). The first of these studies examined C3 immunofluorescence in spinal cord and motor cortex of 16 ALS patients and demonstrated significant C3 deposition, which appeared to be on astrocyte-like cells with no apparent neuronal staining (Donnenfeld et al., 1984). Subsequent studies measured C3c, C4, C1 inactivator and C3 activator fractions in the serum and CSF of 13 ALS patients but only detected increased levels of C3c in the CSF of ALS patients compared to normal individuals (Annunziata and Volpi, 1985). Furthermore Apopstolski and colleagues (1991) measured serum C4, C3 and Factor B levels in 33 ALS patients and found an increase in C4 levels when compared to normal individuals. Increased clusters of C3d and C4d coated fibers on oligodendroglia and degenerating neurites in spinal cord and motor cortex was also found in 8 ALS patients compared to 5 normal individuals (Kawamata et al., 1992). Two separate studies also investigated C1q, C4d and C4 levels in the serum and CSF of ALS patients and found C4d levels significantly increased in 15 ALS patients which also correlated with disease severity (Tsuboi and Yamada, 1994); another study also detected upregulation of C4 in ALS patients (Trbojevic-Cepe et al., 1998). Studies by Grewal and colleagues (Grewal et al., 1999) and Jiang and colleagues (Jiang et al., 2005) have identified increased mRNA of upstream complement components (C1q and C2) in the spinal cord of ALS patients. Recently, Sta and colleagues have found increased levels of C1q, C3c, C3d and C5b-9 in the spinal cord and motor cortex of ALS patients compared to normal individuals (Sta et al., 2011). The expression of these complement components was observed in glial cells rather than neurons (Sta et al., 2011). Lastly, complement component C3 was also found to be upregulated in the CSF of 71 ALS patients when compared to 40 normal individuals (Ganesalingam et al., 2011).

These findings of upregulated complement components and activation fragments, predominantly composing the classical pathway, in the serum, CSF, and neurological tissue in ALS patients strongly suggest that the classical complement pathway is involved in the progression of disease in ALS. However it is currently unknown where these complement factors originate, and what initiates their activation. Complement factors can be produced by various cells of the CNS and thus these complement factors could be produced locally in response to disturbance in CNS homeostasis due to immunoglobulin deposits and auto-antibodies in the CNS of ALS patients (Donnenfeld et al., 1984, Niebroj-Dobosz et al., 2006). Also the circulation could be a source of these complement factors as there is BBB breakdown in the end stages of ALS (Apostolski et al., 1991). Overall, evidence from these clinical studies helps us to propose that complement system activation occurs in ALS patients, and may play a role in the disease pathology. This is also supported by evidence of studies showing involvement of complement factors in animal models of ALS.

Complement factors	mRNA/Protein	Sample	Methods
C3	Protein	Spinal Cord, Motor cortex	Immunofluorescence
C3c	Protein	Serum, CSF	Single radial immuno-diffusion
C4	Protein	Serum	Single radial immuno-diffusion
C3d, C4d	Protein	Spinal Cord, Motor cortex	Immunohistochemistry
C4d	Protein	CSF	Sandwich ELISA
C4	Protein	CSF	Laser nephelometry
C1q	mRNA	Spinal Cord, Motor cortex	Northern blot, *In situ* hybridization
C2	mRNA	Spinal Cord	Microarray
C3c, C3dg, Factor H	Protein	Serum	2D gel electrophoresis
C1q, C3c, C3d, C5b-9	mRNA/Protein	Spinal Cord, Motor cortex	qPCR, immunohistochemistry
C3	Protein	CSF	Sandwich ELISA

Table 1. Clinical evidence of complement activation in ALS patients

6. Experimental evidence of complement involvement in ALS

Many studies in animal models of ALS have shown the involvement of the complement system during disease progression, supporting findings in ALS patients (Table 2). Although the SOD1 gene mutation only accounts for 2% of total ALS cases, mouse models carrying over-expression of mutant SOD1 enzyme are widely used, as it leads to progressive symptoms which are very similar to the human condition.

Complement factors	mRNA/Protein	Transgenic model	Reference
C1q	mRNA	Mouse SOD1 [G93A]	(Perrin et al., 2005)
C1q, DAF	mRNA	Mouse SOD1 [G37R] and SOD1 [G85R]	(Lobsiger et al., 2007)
C1q, C4	mRNA/Protein	Mouse SOD1 [G93A]	(Ferraiuolo et al., 2007)
C1q	mRNA	Mouse SOD1 [L126delTT]	(Fukada et al., 2007)
CD88	mRNA/Protein	Rat SOD1 [G93A]	(Woodruff et al., 2008a)
CD88	mRNA/Protein	Mouse NFL -/-	(Humayun et al., 2009)
C1q, C3	mRNA/Protein	Mouse SOD1 [G93A]	(Heurich et al., 2011)

Table 2. Experimental evidence of complement activation in animal models of ALS

The first study to demonstrate experimentally the involvement of complement factors in a SOD1 transgenic mouse model was performed by Perrin and colleagues in 2005. They isolated the ventral motor neurons from the lumbar spinal cord of SOD1[G93A] transgenic mouse using laser-capture micro-dissection and then using microarray analysis they detected increased levels of all subcomponents of C1q in these mice at early symptomatic and end stage when compared to motor neurons from wild-type mice (~5 and ~8 fold respectively) (Perrin et al., 2005).

Subsequent studies in two distinct SOD1 transgenic mouse models also used laser-capture micro-dissection to isolate lumbar motor neurons from SOD1[G37R] and SOD1[G85R] transgenic mice which showed upregulation of genes for all three C1q subcomponents when compared to SOD1[WT] mice 2 months prior to clinical onset (P105) (Lobsiger et al., 2007). In addition, this group demonstrated that the complement regulatory molecule, decay accelerating factor (DAF) also decreased at this time point (Lobsiger et al., 2007). Furthermore they showed that C1q protein was expressed by motor neurons using immunohistochemistry or spinal cord sections of both SOD1[G37R] and SOD1[G85R] transgenic mice but absent in the age-matched control mice (Lobsiger et al., 2007).

A separate group also used laser-capture microdissection to isolate the lumbar motor neurons from SOD1^{G93A} transgenic mice. Using microarray analysis and real time quantitative PCR, they showed there were increased levels of C1q (subcomponent B) and C4 mRNA at disease onset (P90) and late-stage disease (P120) (~7 and ~8 fold respectively) (Ferraiuolo et al., 2007). A similar study also used microarray analysis in a separate SOD1 transgenic mouse model using whole lumbar spinal cord homogenate (Fukada et al., 2007). This study used SOD1^{L126delTT} transgenic mice and showed elevated levels of C1q (subcomponent B) mRNA in post-symptomatic (P154) mice compared to wild-type mice. A very recent study has shown increased levels of C1q in the neuromuscular junction of SOD1^{G93A} transgenic mice compared to wild-type mice (Heurich et al., 2011).

By contrast to the above studies, which indicates a role for the classical complement pathway in the progression of pathology of the SOD1 transgenic mouse, a recent study has demonstrated that when SOD1^{G93A} transgenic mice were bred onto a background deficient in complement C4 (a necessary component of the classical complement pathway, downstream of C1q), there was a difference in the macrophage levels and activation in the peripheral nervous system but no difference in the onset of motor symptoms and survival when compared to wild-type mice (Chiu et al., 2009). This study indicates that other molecular pathways such as the alternative or extrinsic pathway may play compensatory roles in immune activation and macrophage recruitment in the absence of the classical pathway in these mice. To support this, recent studies in SOD1^{G93A} transgenic mouse showed increases in the C3 mRNA and protein levels in the spinal cord when compared to wild-type animals at symptomatic stage (P126) (Heurich et al., 2011). They also observed upregulation of C3 at the motor end plate and nerve terminals in the SOD1^{G93A} transgenic mice at pre-symptomatic stage (P47) when compared to wild-type animal (Heurich et al., 2011).

To further validate the involvement of downstream components of the complement cascade in the disease progression of ALS, upregulation of C5a receptor CD88 mRNA and protein was observed in mice deficient in the low molecular weight neurofilament (NFL) subunit protein, a mouse model of motor neuron degeneration in which neurofilament aggregates in a similar fashion to that in ALS patients (Humayun et al., 2009). This study showed there was a 4 and 3 fold increase in CD88 mRNA expression level at 2 and 3 months respectively, a time which is early in the disease process (Humayun et al., 2009). There was also an increased immunoreactivity of CD88 in motor neurons of NFL deficient mice when compared to wild-type mice at 3, 4 and 5 months. Our own findings also support a pathogenic role for C5a in ALS (Woodruff et al., 2008a). Chronic administration of a specific C5a receptor antagonist, developed in our laboratories (Wong et al., 1998) in SOD1^{G93A} transgenic rats, markedly delayed the onset of motor symptoms and increased survival, compared to untreated animals (Woodruff et al., 2008a). We also showed upregulation of CD88 in the lumbar spinal cord of SOD1^{G93A} transgenic rats, which increased as disease progressed (Woodruff et al., 2008a).

These findings of upregulated complement components in different animal models of ALS suggest that the activation of complement system is critically linked with disease progression in ALS. Whilst inhibition of one component of the classical and lectin complement pathway, C4, failed to ameliorate disease in SOD1^{G93A} transgenic mice, inhibition of the classical receptor for C5a, CD88, reduced disease pathology in SOD1^{G93A} transgenic rats. It should be noted that C5a is expressed following activation of all complement pathways (Figure 1). Hence inhibiting central components of the complement system, at the C3 and C5 level, may have benefits in slowing disease progression in ALS, as opposed to inhibiting an individual activation pathway. Specifically, our studies suggest that inhibiting the pro-inflammatory C5 activation fragment, C5a, which is central to, and generated by, all complement pathways, may be a novel therapeutic strategy to treat ALS.

7. Future directions: Therapeutic applications

To date, riluzole (Rilutek, Aventis Pharmaceuticals Inc) is the only approved therapeutic to treat ALS; it is known to prevent the pre-synaptic release of glutamine (Bellingham, 2011, Miller et al., 2007). In clinical trials, it has been shown to extend survival by around 2 ~ 3 months and delay the onset of ventilator dependence or tracheostomy (Bellingham, 2011, Miller et al., 2007). It is not clear that the drug improves the quality of life, however. Given this modest extension of ~2-3 months in survival there is an urgent need to develop new therapeutics which will significantly extend survival and also decrease morbidity in ALS.

Recent studies have suggested that the innate immune system is important in sensing ALS progression and its subsequent upregulation may drive the progression of this disease (Woodruff et al., 2008b). The complement system would be a logical and viable pathway to target, given the steadily accumulating clinical evidence of complement involvement in this disease. This is also supported by our findings where using specific C5a receptor antagonist improved motor symptoms and extended survival in the SOD1^{G93A} transgenic rat (Woodruff et al., 2008a).

Our laboratories have developed a series of cyclic peptide C5a receptor antagonists which are potent inhibitors of C5a receptors on human inflammatory cells (Woodruff et al., 2011). PMX53 (AcF-[OPdChaWR] and PMX205 (hydrocinnamate-[OPdChaWR]) are orally active cyclic hexapeptides, which were derived from the linear CD88 antagonist, Me-FKPdChaWR (Konteatis et al., 1994) that were cyclised to induce structural and metabolic stability(Finch et al., 1999, March et al., 2004). These drugs have been shown to display therapeutic efficacy in numerous rodent models of inflammatory disease including rheumatoid arthritis (Woodruff et al., 2002), ischemic reperfusion injuries (Arumugam et al., 2004) and inflammatory bowel disease (Woodruff et al., 2003), as well as acute neurodegeneration (Woodruff et al., 2006). PMX205 is more lipophilic than the original CD88 antagonist PMX53, which results in increased potency in certain inflammatory models (Woodruff et al., 2005) and increased CNS penetrance (Woodruff et al., 2006). Hence, it has been used to reduce disease severity and prolong survival in animal models of neural degeneration including Huntington's disease, Alzheimer's disease and ALS (Ager et al., 2010, Fonseca et al., 2009, Woodruff et al., 2006, Woodruff et al., 2008a). As a result of this work, PMX205 would be the particular PMX series compound we would promote for any future clinical trialling in ALS.

In addition to inhibiting C5a receptors, targeting other factors of the complement system may provide viable therapeutic options to treat ALS. Several complement inhibitors have been developed over the years and compounds such as sCR1, C5 antibodies, compstatin or others could be used as potential therapies for ALS. However, due to the need to chronically administer a drug in ALS, a small, orally active and BBB permeable complement inhibitor, such as PMX205, would be required. The selectivity of PMX205 towards the classical C5a receptor leaves other components of the complement system intact, allowing for the production of complement factors including the MAC, thus reducing immune suppression -

a likely side effect of other inhibitors of complement which act more upstream in the system, were they are to be used chronically. Finally, PMX53, an analogue to PMX205 has already been shown to be safe when administered to humans, successfully completing three Phase I/IIa clinical trials, thus promoting the safety of these classes of drugs in humans (Woodruff et al., 2011).

In addition to anti-complement agents, combined therapies targeting multiple and disparate pathways will most likely be needed to effectively treat ALS. Extensive controlled clinical trials will need to be conducted in order to ascertain any potential therapeutic benefit of a complement inhibitor to treat the devastating and intractable nature of ALS.

8. Conclusion

There is increasing evidence that implicates the involvement of the innate immune system in the progression of ALS. In particular, the inappropriate activation or dysregulation of the complement system may play a role in ALS pathology. Evidence for this includes elevated levels of complement activation fragments in the serum, CSF, spinal cord and motor cortex of ALS patients. This has also been supported with elevated levels of complement activation fragments in various animal models of ALS. Moreover, inhibition of the C5a receptor using a specific C5a receptor antagonist ameliorated disease symptoms in a rat model of ALS. Collectively, these studies suggest that complement activation may play a crucial role in the progression of ALS. Hence reducing complement-induced inflammation using inhibitors to target complement factors could be an important therapeutic strategy to treat ALS.

9. Acknowledgments

We acknowledge the funding support of the Motor Neuron Disease Research Institute of Australia (Charles & Shirley Graham MND Research Grant 2010), and the National Health and Medical Research Council of Australia (Project Grants 455856 and APP1004455).

10. References

Ager, R. R., Fonseca, M. I., Chu, S. H., Sanderson, S. D., Taylor, S. M., Woodruff, T. M. & Tenner, A. J. (2010). Microglial C5aR (CD88) expression correlates with amyloid-beta deposition in murine models of Alzheimer's disease. *J Neurochem*, Vol.113, No.2, (April 2010), pp.389-401, ISSN 1471-4159.

Akira, S., Takeda, K. & Kaisho, T. (2001). Toll-like receptors: critical proteins linking innate and acquired immunity. *Nature immunology*, Vol.2, No.8, (August 2001), pp.675-680, ISSN 1529-2908.

Amatruda, T. T., 3RD, Gerard, N. P., Gerard, C. & Simon, M. I. (1993). Specific interactions of chemoattractant factor receptors with G-proteins. *The Journal of biological chemistry*, Vol.268, No.14, (May 1993), pp.10139-10144, ISSN 0021-9258.

Andersson, A., Covacu, R., Sunnemark, D., Danilov, A. I., Dal Bianco, A., Khademi, M., Wallstrom, E., Lobell, A., Brundin, L., Lassmann, H. & Harris, R. A. (2008). Pivotal advance: HMGB1 expression in active lesions of human and experimental multiple sclerosis. *Journal of leukocyte biology*, Vol.84, No.5, (November 2008), pp.1248-1255, ISSN 0741-5400.

Annunziata, P. & Volpi, N. (1985). High levels of C3c in the cerebrospinal fluid from amyotrophic lateral sclerosis patients. *Acta neurologica Scandinavica*, Vol.72, No.1, (July 1985), pp.61-64, ISSN 0001-6314.

Apostolski, S., Nikolic, J., Bugarski-Prokopljevic, C., Miletic, V., Pavlovic, S. & Filipovic, S. (1991). Serum and CSF immunological findings in ALS. *Acta neurologica Scandinavica*, Vol.83, No.2, (February 1991), pp.96-98, ISSN 0001-6314.

Aravalli, R. N., Peterson, P. K. & Lokensgard, J. R. (2007). Toll-like receptors in defense and damage of the central nervous system. *Journal of neuroimmune pharmacology : the official journal of the Society on NeuroImmune Pharmacology*, Vol.2, No.4, (December 2007), pp.297-312, ISSN 1557-1904.

Arumugam, T. V., Shiels, I. A., Woodruff, T. M., Granger, D. N. & Taylor, S. M. (2004). The role of the complement system in ischemia-reperfusion injury. *Shock*, Vol.21, No.5, (May 2004), pp.401-409, ISSN 1073-2322.

Bamberg, C. E., Mackay, C. R., Lee, H., Zahra, D., Jackson, J., Lim, Y. S., Whitfeld, P. L., Craig, S., Corsini, E., Lu, B., Gerard, C. & Gerard, N. P. (2010). The C5a receptor (C5aR) C5L2 is a modulator of C5aR-mediated signal transduction. *Journal of Biological Chemistry*, Vol.285, No.10, (March 2010), pp.7633-7644, ISSN 1083-351X.

Barnum, S. R. (1995). Complement biosynthesis in the central nervous system. *Crit Rev Oral Biol Med*, Vol.6, No.2, (January 1995), pp.132-146, ISSN 1045-4411.

Bellingham, M. C. (2011). A review of the neural mechanisms of action and clinical efficiency of riluzole in treating amyotrophic lateral sclerosis: what have we learned in the last decade? *CNS neuroscience & therapeutics*, Vol.17, No.1, (February 2011), pp.4-31, ISSN 1755-5949.

Benard, M., Raoult, E., Vaudry, D., Leprince, J., Falluel-Morel, A., Gonzalez, B. J., Galas, L., Vaudry, H. & Fontaine, M. (2008). Role of complement anaphylatoxin receptors (C3aR, C5aR) in the development of the rat cerebellum. *Molecular immunology*, Vol.45, No.14, (August 2008), pp.3767-3774, ISSN 0161-5890.

Bianchi, M. E. & Manfredi, A. A. (2007). High-mobility group box 1 (HMGB1) protein at the crossroads between innate and adaptive immunity. *Immunological reviews*, Vol.220, (December 2007), pp.35-46, ISSN 0105-2896.

Bianchi, M. E. & Manfredi, A. A. (2009). Immunology. Dangers in and out. *Science*, Vol.323, No.5922, (March 2009), pp.1683-1684, ISSN 1095-9203.

Boillee, S., Vande Velde, C. & Cleveland, D. W. (2006). ALS: a disease of motor neurons and their nonneuronal neighbors. *Neuron*, Vol.52, No.1, (October 2006), pp.39-59, ISSN 0896-6273.

Bowman, C. C., Rasley, A., Tranguch, S. L. & Marriott, I. (2003). Cultured astrocytes express toll-like receptors for bacterial products. *Glia*, Vol.43, No.3, (September 2003), pp.281-291, ISSN 0894-1491.

Bruijn, L. I. & Cleveland, D. W. (1996). Mechanisms of selective motor neuron death in ALS: insights from transgenic mouse models of motor neuron disease. *Neuropathol Appl Neurobiol*, Vol.22, No.5, (October 1996), pp.373-387, ISSN 0305-1846.

Bruijn, L. I., Miller, T. M. & Cleveland, D. W. (2004). Unraveling the mechanisms involved in motor neuron degeneration in ALS. *Annu Rev Neurosci*, Vol.27, (June 2004), pp.723-749, ISSN 0147-006X.

Buhl, A. M., Avdi, N., Worthen, G. S. & Johnson, G. L. (1994). Mapping of the C5a receptor signal transduction network in human neutrophils. *Proc Natl Acad Sci U S A*, Vol.91, No.19, (September 1994), pp.9190-9194, ISSN 0027-8424.

Cain, S. A. & Monk, P. N. (2002). The orphan receptor C5L2 has high affinity binding sites for complement fragments C5a and C5a des-Arg(74). *Journal of Biological Chemistry*, Vol.277, No.9, (March 2002), pp.7165-7169, ISSN 0021-9258.

Casula, M., Iyer, A. M., Spliet, W. G., Anink, J. J., Steentjes, K., Sta, M., Troost, D. & Aronica, E. (2011). Toll-like receptor signaling in amyotrophic lateral sclerosis spinal cord tissue. *Neuroscience*, Vol.179, (April 2011), pp.233-243, ISSN 1873-7544.

Chiu, I. M., Phatnani, H., Kuligowski, M., Tapia, J. C., Carrasco, M. A., Zhang, M., Maniatis, T. & Carroll, M. C. (2009). Activation of innate and humoral immunity in the peripheral nervous system of ALS transgenic mice. *Proceedings of the National Academy of Sciences of the United States of America*, Vol.106, No.49, (December 2009), pp.20960-20965, ISSN 1091-6490.

Cockcroft, S. (1992). G-protein-regulated phospholipases C, D and A2-mediated signalling in neutrophils. *Biochim Biophys Acta*, Vol.1113, No.2, (August 1992), pp.135-160, ISSN 0006-3002.

Cozzolino, M., Ferri, A. & Carri, M. T. (2008). Amyotrophic lateral sclerosis: from current developments in the laboratory to clinical implications. *Antioxid Redox Signal*, Vol.10, No.3, (March 2008), pp.405-443, ISSN 1523-0864.

Donnenfeld, H., Kascsak, R. J. & Bartfeld, H. (1984). Deposits of IgG and C3 in the spinal cord and motor cortex of ALS patients. *Journal of neuroimmunology*, Vol.6, No.1, (February 1984), pp.51-57, ISSN 0165-5728.

Ferraiuolo, L., Heath, P. R., Holden, H., Kasher, P., Kirby, J. & Shaw, P. J. (2007). Microarray analysis of the cellular pathways involved in the adaptation to and progression of motor neuron injury in the SOD1 G93A mouse model of familial ALS. *The Journal of neuroscience : the official journal of the Society for Neuroscience*, Vol.27, No.34, (August 2007), pp.9201-9219, ISSN 1529-2401.

Finch, A. M., Wong, A. K., Paczkowski, N. J., Wadi, S. K., Craik, D. J., Fairlie, D. P. & Taylor, S. M. (1999). Low-molecular-weight peptidic and cyclic antagonists of the receptor for the complement factor C5a. *Journal of medicinal chemistry*, Vol.42, No.11, (June 1999), pp.1965-1974, ISSN 0022-2623.

Fonseca, M. I., Ager, R. R., Chu, S. H., Yazan, O., Sanderson, S. D., Laferla, F. M., Taylor, S. M., Woodruff, T. M. & Tenner, A. J. (2009). Treatment with a C5aR antagonist decreases pathology and enhances behavioral performance in murine models of Alzheimer's disease. *J Immunol*, Vol.183, No.2, (July 2009), pp.1375-1383, ISSN 1550-6606.

Fukada, Y., Yasui, K., Kitayama, M., Doi, K., Nakano, T., Watanabe, Y. & Nakashima, K. (2007). Gene expression analysis of the murine model of amyotrophic lateral sclerosis: studies of the Leu126delTT mutation in SOD1. *Brain research*, Vol.1160, (July 2007), pp.1-10, ISSN 0006-8993.

Ganesalingam, J., An, J., Shaw, C. E., Shaw, G., Lacomis, D. & Bowser, R. (2011). Combination of neurofilament heavy chain and complement C3 as CSF biomarkers for ALS. *Journal of neurochemistry*, Vol.117, No.3, (May 2011), pp.528-537, ISSN 1471-4159.

Gasque, P., Singhrao, S. K., Neal, J. W., Gotze, O. & Morgan, B. P. (1997). Expression of the receptor for complement C5a (CD88) is up-regulated on reactive astrocytes, microglia, and endothelial cells in the inflamed human central nervous system. *Am J Pathol*, Vol.150, No.1, (January 1997), pp.31-41, ISSN 0002-9440.

Goldknopf, I. L., Sheta, E. A., Bryson, J., Folsom, B., Wilson, C., Duty, J., Yen, A. A. & Appel, S. H. (2006). Complement C3c and related protein biomarkers in amyotrophic lateral sclerosis and Parkinson's disease. *Biochem Biophys Res Commun*, Vol.342, No.4, (April 2006), pp.1034-1039, ISSN 0006-291X.

Gomez-Cambronero, J., Di Fulvio, M. & Knapek, K. (2007). Understanding phospholipase D (PLD) using leukocytes: PLD involvement in cell adhesion and chemotaxis. *J Leukoc Biol*, Vol.82, No.2, (August 2007), pp.272-281, ISSN 0741-5400.

Grewal, R. P., Morgan, T. E. & Finch, C. E. (1999). C1qB and clusterin mRNA increase in association with neurodegeneration in sporadic amyotrophic lateral sclerosis. *Neurosci Lett*, Vol.271, No.1, (August 1999), pp.65-67, ISSN 0304-3940.

Guo, R. F. & Ward, P. A. (2005). Role of C5a in inflammatory responses. *Annu Rev Immunol*, Vol.23, (March 2005), pp.821-852, ISSN 0732-0582.

Hanisch, U. K., Johnson, T. V. & Kipnis, J. (2008). Toll-like receptors: roles in neuroprotection? *Trends in neurosciences*, Vol.31, No.4, (April 2008), pp.176-182, ISSN 0166-2236.

Heurich, B., El Idrissi, N. B., Donev, R. M., Petri, S., Claus, P., Neal, J., Morgan, B. P. & Ramaglia, V. (2011). Complement upregulation and activation on motor neurons and neuromuscular junction in the SOD1 G93A mouse model of familial amyotrophic lateral sclerosis. *Journal of neuroimmunology*, Vol.235, No.1-2, (June 2011), pp.104-109, ISSN 1872-8421.

Hreggvidsdottir, H. S., Ostberg, T., Wahamaa, H., Schierbeck, H., Aveberger, A. C., Klevenvall, L., Palmblad, K., Ottosson, L., Andersson, U. & Harris, H. E. (2009). The alarmin HMGB1 acts in synergy with endogenous and exogenous danger signals to promote inflammation. *Journal of leukocyte biology*, Vol.86, No.3, (September 2009), pp.655-662, ISSN 1938-3673.

Huang, R., Lian, J. P., Robinson, D. & Badwey, J. A. (1998). Neutrophils stimulated with a variety of chemoattractants exhibit rapid activation of p21-activated kinases (Paks): separate signals are required for activation and inactivation of paks. *Mol Cell Biol*, Vol.18, No.12, (December 1998), pp.7130-7138, ISSN 0270-7306.

Huber-Lang, M., Sarma, J. V., Zetoune, F. S., Rittirsch, D., Neff, T. A., Mcguire, S. R., Lambris, J. D., Warner, R. L., Flierl, M. A., Hoesel, L. M., Gebhard, F., Younger, J. G., Drouin, S. M., Wetsel, R. A. & Ward, P. A. (2006). Generation of C5a in the absence of C3: a new complement activation pathway. *Nat Med*, Vol.12, No.6, (June 2006), pp.682-687, ISSN 1078-8956.

Huber-Lang, M., Younkin, E. M., Sarma, J. V., Riedemann, N., Mcguire, S. R., Lu, K. T., Kunkel, R., Younger, J. G., Zetoune, F. S. & Ward, P. A. (2002). Generation of C5a by phagocytic cells. *Am J Pathol*, Vol.161, No.5, (November 2002), pp.1849-1859, ISSN 0002-9440.

Humayun, S., Gohar, M., Volkening, K., Moisse, K., Leystra-Lantz, C., Mepham, J., Mclean, J. & Strong, M. J. (2009). The complement factor C5a receptor is upregulated in

NFL-/- mouse motor neurons. *J Neuroimmunol,* Vol.210, No.1-2, (May 2009), pp.52-62, ISSN 1872-8421.

Ilzecka, J. (2009). Serum-soluble receptor for advanced glycation end product levels in patients with amyotrophic lateral sclerosis. *Acta neurologica Scandinavica,* Vol.120, No.2, (August 2009), pp.119-122, ISSN 1600-0404.

Jiang, H., Burdick, D., Glabe, C. G., Cotman, C. W. & Tenner, A. J. (1994). beta-Amyloid activates complement by binding to a specific region of the collagen-like domain of the C1q A chain. *Journal of immunology,* Vol.152, No.10, (May 1994), pp.5050-5059, ISSN 0022-1767.

Jiang, Y. M., Yamamoto, M., Kobayashi, Y., Yoshihara, T., Liang, Y., Terao, S., Takeuchi, H., Ishigaki, S., Katsuno, M., Adachi, H., Niwa, J., Tanaka, F., Doyu, M., Yoshida, M., Hashizume, Y. & Sobue, G. (2005). Gene expression profile of spinal motor neurons in sporadic amyotrophic lateral sclerosis. *Ann Neurol,* Vol.57, No.2, (February 2005), pp.236-251, ISSN 0364-5134.

Johswich, K. & Klos, A. (2007). C5L2--an anti-inflammatory molecule or a receptor for acylation stimulating protein (C3a-desArg)? *Advances in experimental medicine and biology,* Vol.598, (September 2007), pp.159-180, ISSN 0065-2598.

Kastl, S. P., Speidl, W. S., Kaun, C., Rega, G., Assadian, A., Weiss, T. W., Valent, P., Hagmueller, G. W., Maurer, G., Huber, K. & Wojta, J. (2006). The complement component C5a induces the expression of plasminogen activator inhibitor-1 in human macrophages via NF-kappaB activation. *J Thromb Haemost,* Vol.4, No.8, (August 2006), pp.1790-1797, ISSN 1538-7933.

Kawamata, T., Akiyama, H., Yamada, T. & Mcgeer, P. L. (1992). Immunologic reactions in amyotrophic lateral sclerosis brain and spinal cord tissue. *The American journal of pathology,* Vol.140, No.3, (March 1992), pp.691-707, ISSN 0002-9440.

Konteatis, Z. D., Siciliano, S. J., Van Riper, G., Molineaux, C. J., Pandya, S., Fischer, P., Rosen, H., Mumford, R. A. & Springer, M. S. (1994). Development of C5a receptor antagonists. Differential loss of functional responses. *Journal of immunology,* Vol.153, No.9, (November 1994), pp.4200-4205, ISSN 0022-1767.

Lehnardt, S. (2010). Innate immunity and neuroinflammation in the CNS: the role of microglia in Toll-like receptor-mediated neuronal injury. *Glia,* Vol.58, No.3, (February 2010), pp.253-263, ISSN 1098-1136.

Letiembre, M., Liu, Y., Walter, S., Hao, W., Pfander, T., Wrede, A., Schulz-Schaeffer, W. & Fassbender, K. (2009). Screening of innate immune receptors in neurodegenerative diseases: a similar pattern. *Neurobiology of aging,* Vol.30, No.5, (May 2009), pp.759-768, ISSN 1558-1497.

Liew, F. Y., Xu, D., Brint, E. K. & O'neill, L. A. (2005). Negative regulation of toll-like receptor-mediated immune responses. *Nature reviews. Immunology,* Vol.5, No.6, (June 2005), pp.446-458, ISSN 1474-1733.

Liszewski, M. K., Farries, T. C., Lublin, D. M., Rooney, I. A. & Atkinson, J. P. (1996). Control of the complement system. *Advances in immunology,* Vol.61, (January 1996), pp.201-283, ISSN 0065-2776.

Liu, Y., Hao, W., Dawson, A., Liu, S. & Fassbender, K. (2009). Expression of amyotrophic lateral sclerosis-linked SOD1 mutant increases the neurotoxic potential of microglia via TLR2. *The Journal of biological chemistry*, Vol.284, No.6, (February 2009), pp.3691-3699, ISSN 0021-9258.

Lobsiger, C. S., Boillee, S. & Cleveland, D. W. (2007). Toxicity from different SOD1 mutants dysregulates the complement system and the neuronal regenerative response in ALS motor neurons. *Proc Natl Acad Sci U S A*, Vol.104, No.18, (May 2007), pp.7319-7326, ISSN 0027-8424.

March, D. R., Proctor, L. M., Stoermer, M. J., Sbaglia, R., Abbenante, G., Reid, R. C., Woodruff, T. M., Wadi, K., Paczkowski, N., Tyndall, J. D., Taylor, S. M. & Fairlie, D. P. (2004). Potent cyclic antagonists of the complement C5a receptor on human polymorphonuclear leukocytes. Relationships between structures and activity. *Mol Pharmacol*, Vol.65, No.4, (April 2004), pp.868-879, ISSN 0026-895X.

Marjan, J., Xie, Z. & Devine, D. V. (1994). Liposome-induced activation of the classical complement pathway does not require immunoglobulin. *Biochimica et biophysica acta*, Vol.1192, No.1, (June 1994), pp.35-44, ISSN 0006-3002.

Mastellos, D., Germenis, A. E. & Lambris, J. D. (2005). Complement: an inflammatory pathway fulfilling multiple roles at the interface of innate immunity and development. *Current drug targets. Inflammation and allergy*, Vol.4, No.1, (February 2005), pp.125-127, ISSN 1568-010X.

Melendez, A. J. & Ibrahim, F. B. (2004). Antisense knockdown of sphingosine kinase 1 in human macrophages inhibits C5a receptor-dependent signal transduction, Ca2+ signals, enzyme release, cytokine production, and chemotaxis. *J Immunol*, Vol.173, No.3, (August 2004), pp.1596-1603, ISSN 0022-1767.

Miller, R. G., Mitchell, J. D., Lyon, M. & Moore, D. H. (2007). Riluzole for amyotrophic lateral sclerosis (ALS)/motor neuron disease (MND). *Cochrane Database Syst Rev*, No.1, (January 2007), pp.CD001447, ISSN 1469-493X.

Mouri, F., Tsukada, J., Mizobe, T., Higashi, T., Yoshida, Y., Minami, Y., Izumi, H., Kominato, Y., Kohno, K. & Tanaka, Y. (2008). Intracellular HMGB1 transactivates the human IL1B gene promoter through association with an Ets transcription factor PU.1. *European journal of haematology*, Vol.80, No.1, (January 2008), pp.10-19, ISSN 1600-0609.

Mullmann, T. J., Siegel, M. I., Egan, R. W. & Billah, M. M. (1990). Complement C5a activation of phospholipase D in human neutrophils. A major route to the production of phosphatidates and diglycerides. *J Immunol*, Vol.144, No.5, (March 1990), pp.1901-1908, ISSN 0022-1767.

Nataf, S., Levison, S. W. & Barnum, S. R. (2001). Expression of the anaphylatoxin C5a receptor in the oligodendrocyte lineage. *Brain Res*, Vol.894, No.2, (March 2001), pp.321-326, ISSN 0006-8993.

Nguyen, M. D., D'aigle, T., Gowing, G., Julien, J. P. & Rivest, S. (2004). Exacerbation of motor neuron disease by chronic stimulation of innate immunity in a mouse model of amyotrophic lateral sclerosis. *The Journal of neuroscience : the official journal of the Society for Neuroscience*, Vol.24, No.6, (February 2004), pp.1340-1349, ISSN 1529-2401.

Niebroj-Dobosz, I., Dziewulska, D. & Janik, P. (2006). Auto-antibodies against proteins of spinal cord cells in cerebrospinal fluid of patients with amyotrophic lateral sclerosis (ALS). *Folia neuropathologica / Association of Polish Neuropathologists and Medical*

Research Centre, Polish Academy of Sciences, Vol.44, No.3, (October 2006), pp.191-196, ISSN 1641-4640.

O'barr, S. A., Caguioa, J., Gruol, D., Perkins, G., Ember, J. A., Hugli, T. & Cooper, N. R. (2001). Neuronal expression of a functional receptor for the C5a complement activation fragment. *J Immunol,* Vol.166, No.6, (March 2001), pp.4154-4162, ISSN 0022-1767.

Okinaga, S., Slattery, D., Humbles, A., Zsengeller, Z., Morteau, O., Kinrade, M. B., Brodbeck, R. M., Krause, J. E., Choe, H. R., Gerard, N. P. & Gerard, C. (2003). C5L2, a nonsignaling C5A binding protein. *Biochemistry,* Vol.42, No.31, (August 2003), pp.9406-9415, ISSN 0006-2960.

Olson, J. K. & Miller, S. D. (2004). Microglia initiate central nervous system innate and adaptive immune responses through multiple TLRs. *Journal of immunology,* Vol.173, No.6, (September 2004), pp.3916-3924, ISSN 0022-1767.

Pangburn, M. K., Schreiber, R. D. & Muller-Eberhard, H. J. (1981). Formation of the initial C3 convertase of the alternative complement pathway. Acquisition of C3b-like activities by spontaneous hydrolysis of the putative thioester in native C3. *The Journal of experimental medicine,* Vol.154, No.3, (September 1981), pp.856-867, ISSN 0022-1007.

Parker, L. C., Whyte, M. K., Vogel, S. N., Dower, S. K. & Sabroe, I. (2004). Toll-like receptor (TLR)2 and TLR4 agonists regulate CCR expression in human monocytic cells. *Journal of immunology,* Vol.172, No.8, (April 2004), pp.4977-4986, ISSN 0022-1767.

Perianayagam, M.C., Balakrishnan, V.S., King, A.J., Pereira, B.J., Jaber, B.L., (2002). C5a delays apoptosis of human neutrophils by a phosphatidylinositol 3-kinase signaling pathway. *Kidney Int,* Vol.61, No.2, (February 2002), pp.456-463, ISSN 0085-2538.

Perrin, F. E., Boisset, G., Docquier, M., Schaad, O., Descombes, P. & Kato, A. C. (2005). No widespread induction of cell death genes occurs in pure motoneurons in an amyotrophic lateral sclerosis mouse model. *Human molecular genetics,* Vol.14, No.21, (November 2005), pp.3309-3320, ISSN 0964-6906.

Podack, E. R., Tschoop, J. & Muller-Eberhard, H. J. (1982). Molecular organization of C9 within the membrane attack complex of complement. Induction of circular C9 polymerization by the C5b-8 assembly. *The Journal of experimental medicine,* Vol.156, No.1, (July 1982), pp.268-282, ISSN 0022-1007.

Rabiet, M. J., Huet, E. & Boulay, F. (2007). The N-formyl peptide receptors and the anaphylatoxin C5a receptors: an overview. *Biochimie,* Vol.89, No.9, (Septmeber 2007), pp.1089-1106, ISSN 0300-9084.

Rahpeymai, Y., Hietala, M. A., Wilhelmsson, U., Fotheringham, A., Davies, I., Nilsson, A. K., Zwirner, J., Wetsel, R. A., Gerard, C., Pekny, M. & Pekna, M. (2006). Complement: a novel factor in basal and ischemia-induced neurogenesis. *The EMBO journal,* Vol.25, No.6, (March 2006), pp.1364-1374, ISSN 0261-4189.

Ricklin, D., Hajishengallis, G., Yang, K. & Lambris, J. D. (2010). Complement: a key system for immune surveillance and homeostasis. *Nature immunology,* Vol.11, No.9, (September 2010), pp.785-797, ISSN 1529-2916.

Rollins, T. E., Siciliano, S., Kobayashi, S., Cianciarulo, D. N., Bonilla-Argudo, V., Collier, K. & Springer, M. S. (1991). Purification of the active C5a receptor from human polymorphonuclear leukocytes as a receptor-Gi complex. *Proceedings of the National Academy of Sciences of the United States of America,* Vol.88, No.3, (February 1991), pp.971-975, ISSN 0027-8424.

Rosen, D. R., Siddique, T., Patterson, D., Figlewicz, D. A., Sapp, P., Hentati, A., Donaldson, D., Goto, J., O'regan, J. P., Deng, H. X. & Et Al. (1993). Mutations in Cu/Zn superoxide dismutase gene are associated with familial amyotrophic lateral sclerosis. *Nature,* Vol.362, No.6415, (March 1993), pp.59-62, ISSN 0028-0836.

Scaffidi, P., Misteli, T. & Bianchi, M. E. (2002). Release of chromatin protein HMGB1 by necrotic cells triggers inflammation. *Nature,* Vol.418, No.6894, (July 2002), pp.191-195, ISSN 0028-0836.

Schafer, D. P. & Stevens, B. (2010). Synapse elimination during development and disease: immune molecules take centre stage. *Biochem Soc Trans,* Vol.38, No.2, (April 2010), pp.476-481, ISSN 1470-8752.

Sta, M., Sylva-Steenland, R. M., Casula, M., De Jong, J. M., Troost, D., Aronica, E. & Baas, F. (2011). Innate and adaptive immunity in amyotrophic lateral sclerosis: evidence of complement activation. *Neurobiology of disease,* Vol.42, No.3, (June 2011), pp.211-220, ISSN 1095-953X.

Stevens, B., Allen, N. J., Vazquez, L. E., Howell, G. R., Christopherson, K. S., Nouri, N., Micheva, K. D., Mehalow, A. K., Huberman, A. D., Stafford, B., Sher, A., Litke, A. M., Lambris, J. D., Smith, S. J., John, S. W. & Barres, B. A. (2007). The classical complement cascade mediates CNS synapse elimination. *Cell,* Vol.131, No.6, (December 2007), pp.1164-1178, ISSN 0092-8674.

Strong, M. J. (2003). The basic aspects of therapeutics in amyotrophic lateral sclerosis. *Pharmacology & Therapeutics,* Vol.98, No.3, (n.d.), pp.379-414, ISSN 01637258.

Tang, S. C., Arumugam, T. V., Xu, X., Cheng, A., Mughal, M. R., Jo, D. G., Lathia, J. D., Siler, D. A., Chigurupati, S., Ouyang, X., Magnus, T., Camandola, S. & Mattson, M. P. (2007). Pivotal role for neuronal Toll-like receptors in ischemic brain injury and functional deficits. *Proceedings of the National Academy of Sciences of the United States of America,* Vol.104, No.34, (August 2007), pp.13798-13803, ISSN 0027-8424.

Thoman, M. L., Meuth, J. L., Morgan, E. L., Weigle, W. O. & Hugli, T. E. (1984). C3d-K, a kallikrein cleavage fragment of iC3b is a potent inhibitor of cellular proliferation. *Journal of immunology,* Vol.133, No.5, (November 1984), pp.2629-2633, ISSN 0022-1767.

Torres, M. & Forman, H. J. (1999). Activation of several MAP kinases upon stimulation of rat alveolar macrophages: role of the NADPH oxidase. *Arch Biochem Biophys,* Vol.366, No.2, (June 1999), pp.231-239, ISSN 0003-9861.

Trbojevic-Cepe, M., Brinar, V., Pauro, M., Vogrinc, Z. & Stambuk, N. (1998). Cerebrospinal fluid complement activation in neurological diseases. *Journal of the neurological sciences,* Vol.154, No.2, (February 1998), pp.173-181, ISSN 0022-510X.

Tsai, H. R., Yang, L. M., Tsai, W. J. & Chiou, W. F. (2004). Andrographolide acts through inhibition of ERK1/2 and Akt phosphorylation to suppress chemotactic migration. *Eur J Pharmacol,* Vol.498, No.1-3, (September 2004), pp.45-52, ISSN 0014-2999.

Tsuboi, Y. & Yamada, T. (1994). Increased concentration of C4d complement protein in CSF in amyotrophic lateral sclerosis. *Journal of neurology, neurosurgery, and psychiatry,* Vol.57, No.7, (July 1994), pp.859-861, ISSN 0022-3050.

Van Beek, J., Elward, K. & Gasque, P. (2003). Activation of complement in the central nervous system: roles in neurodegeneration and neuroprotection. *Ann N Y Acad Sci,* Vol.992, (May 2003), pp.56-71, ISSN 0077-8923.

Van Lith, L. H., Oosterom, J., Van Elsas, A. & Zaman, G. J. (2009). C5a-stimulated recruitment of beta-arrestin2 to the nonsignaling 7-transmembrane decoy receptor C5L2. *J Biomol Screen,* Vol.14, No.9, (October 2009), pp.1067-1075, ISSN 1552-454X.

Wong, A. K., Finch, A. M., Pierens, G. K., Craik, D. J., Taylor, S. M. & Fairlie, D. P. (1998). Small molecular probes for G-protein-coupled C5a receptors: conformationally constrained antagonists derived from the C terminus of the human plasma protein C5a. *Journal of medicinal chemistry,* Vol.41, No.18, (August 1998), pp.3417-3425, ISSN 0022-2623.

Woodruff, T. M., Ager, R. R., Tenner, A. J., Noakes, P. G. & Taylor, S. M. (2010). The role of the complement system and the activation fragment C5a in the central nervous system. *Neuromolecular Med,* Vol.12, No.2, (June 2010), pp.179-192, ISSN 1559-1174.

Woodruff, T. M., Arumugam, T. V., Shiels, I. A., Reid, R. C., Fairlie, D. P. & Taylor, S. M. (2003). A potent human C5a receptor antagonist protects against disease pathology in a rat model of inflammatory bowel disease. *J Immunol,* Vol.171, No.10, (November 2003), pp.5514-5520, ISSN 0022-1767.

Woodruff, T. M., Costantini, K. J., Crane, J. W., Atkin, J. D., Monk, P. N., Taylor, S. M. & Noakes, P. G. (2008a). The complement factor C5a contributes to pathology in a rat model of amyotrophic lateral sclerosis. *J Immunol,* Vol.181, No.12, (Dec ember 2008), pp.8727-8734, ISSN 1550-6606.

Woodruff, T. M., Costantini, K. J., Taylor, S. M. & Noakes, P. G. (2008b). Role of complement in motor neuron disease: animal models and therapeutic potential of complement inhibitors. *Adv Exp Med Biol,* Vol.632, (November 2008), pp.143-158, ISSN 0065-2598.

Woodruff, T. M., Crane, J. W., Proctor, L. M., Buller, K. M., Shek, A. B., De Vos, K., Pollitt, S., Williams, H. M., Shiels, I. A., Monk, P. N. & Taylor, S. M. (2006). Therapeutic activity of C5a receptor antagonists in a rat model of neurodegeneration. *FASEB J,* Vol.20, No.9, (July 2006), pp.1407-1417, ISSN 1530-6860.

Woodruff, T. M., Nandakumar, K. S. & Tedesco, F. (2011). Inhibiting the C5-C5a receptor axis. *Molecular immunology,* Vol.48, No.14, (August 2011), pp.1631-1642, ISSN 1872-9142.

Woodruff, T. M., Pollitt, S., Proctor, L. M., Stocks, S. Z., Manthey, H. D., Williams, H. M., Mahadevan, I. B., Shiels, I. A. & Taylor, S. M. (2005). Increased potency of a novel complement factor 5a receptor antagonist in a rat model of inflammatory bowel disease. *J Pharmacol Exp Ther,* Vol.314, No.2, (August 2005), pp.811-817, ISSN 0022-3565.

Woodruff, T. M., Strachan, A. J., Dryburgh, N., Shiels, I. A., Reid, R. C., Fairlie, D. P. & Taylor, S. M. (2002). Antiarthritic activity of an orally active C5a receptor antagonist against antigen-induced monarticular arthritis in the rat. *Arthritis Rheum,* Vol.46, No.9, (September 2002), pp.2476-2485, ISSN 0004-3591.

Worms, P. M. (2001). The epidemiology of motor neuron diseases: a review of recent studies. *Journal of the neurological sciences*, Vol.191, No.1-2, (October 2001), pp.3-9, ISSN 0022-510X.

Zhao, W., Beers, D. R., Henkel, J. S., Zhang, W., Urushitani, M., Julien, J. P. & Appel, S. H. (2010). Extracellular mutant SOD1 induces microglial-mediated motoneuron injury. *Glia*, Vol.58, No.2, (January 2010), pp.231-243, ISSN 1098-1136.

The Astrocytic Contribution in ALS: Inflammation and Excitotoxicity

Kim Staats[1,2] and Ludo Van Den Bosch[1,2]
[1]University of Leuven,
[2]VIB Vesalius Research Center,
Belgium

1. Introduction

Amyotrophic Lateral Sclerosis (ALS) is a devastating progressive neurodegenerative disease, due to the loss of motor neurons and denervation of muscle fibres, resulting in increasing muscle weakness and paralysis. The disease has an incidence of 2.7 cases per 100,000 people in Europe (Longroscino et al., 2010). It is diagnosed from teen years onward, but is more prevalent in the later years of life. In lack of a medical cure, average life expectancy post diagnosis is between 2 and 5 years, though 10% of all patients live longer than 10 years. Patients mainly succumb to the disease by respiratory insufficiency or may opt for euthanasia where legislature permits (Maessen et al., 2010). Although ALS is characterised by degeneration of central nervous system tissue, mental functions remain largely unaffected resulting in a locked-in state (Kotchoubey et al., 2003). At current, there is but one medicine to treat the disease, riluzole, slowing disease progression moderately (Miller et al., 2007).

1.1 Basic genetics of ALS

Mutations in the ubiquitously expressed Cu/Zn superoxide dismutase 1 (SOD1) gene can cause ALS. SOD1 detoxifies cell damaging free radicals and its mutations account for 20% of the ALS patients suffering from the disease by familial origin (fALS) worldwide. The remaining 90% of ALS patients suffer from the disease by unknown sporadic causes (sALS), though a common mechanism is predicted as fALS and sALS patients display indistinguishable clinical phenotypes. Overexpression of mutant forms of human SOD1 causes the ALS phenotype of transgenic SOD1 mice, accounting for an invaluable contribution to ALS research (Gurney et al., 1994). Many hallmarks of the disease are shared between patients and this rodent model, including specific motor neuron loss, aggregate formation, astrogliosis, microgliosis and progressive paralysis. As the genetic ablation of SOD1 does not produce an ALS-like phenotype in mice (Reaume et al., 1996; Shefner et al., 1999) the pathogenic mechanism of mutant SOD1 is a toxic gain of function. This gain of function may be exerted by protein misfolding, aggregation, impaired proteasome functioning, impaired retrograde transport, excitotoxic cell death or other mechanisms (reviewed in Bruijn et al., 2004). Mutations in other genes also cause familial ALS, including mutations in vesicle-associated membrane protein-associated protein B (VAPB), TAR DNA binding protein (TDP-43), fused in sarcoma/translocated in liposarcoma (FUS/TLS), optineurin and valsolin containing protein (VCP) (Johnson et al.; Maruyama et al.; Rutherford et al., 2008; Van Deerlin et al., 2008; Del Bo et al., 2009; Kwiatkowski et al., 2009; Vance et al., 2009). Unfortunately, the discovery of these mutant genes has not yet progressed into useful ALS model organisms, so most of the work described below was conducted with mutant SOD1-based ALS models.

1.2 Non-cell autonomous ALS

Multiple cell types contribute to the pathology making ALS a non-cell autonomous disease (Boillee et al., 2006a). By addition or deletion of mutant SOD1 in specific cell types, it is known that mutant SOD1 influences the disease depending on the cell type, including astrocytes (Yamanaka et al., 2008; Wang et al., 2011a), microglia (Boillee et al., 2006b), Schwann cells (Lobsiger et al., 2009) and motor neurons (Jaarsma et al., 2008). Additionally, ablation of T-cells (Beers et al., 2008; Chiu et al., 2008), B-cells (Naor et al., 2009), CD4+ and CD8+ cells (Beers et al., 2008) decrease survival of ALS mice, demonstrating the role of immune cells in disease progression. Although ALS is a non-cell autonomous disease, mutant SOD1 expressed solely in motor neurons is sufficient to initiate the disease, albeit with a slower disease progression (Jaarsma et al., 2008). Motor neurons in the motor cortex, brainstem and spinal cord undergo cell death selectively in patients. A number of hypotheses attempt to explain this cell type selectivity, including the long axons of the motor neurons (Fischer and Glass, 2007), their poor intracellular calcium buffering capacity (Grosskreutz et al., 2010) and motor neuron specific cell death pathways (Raoul et al., 2002; Raoul et al., 2006; Genestine et al., 2011).

The contribution of mutant SOD1 expressing astrocytes in the non-cell autonomous character of ALS has been studied by excising mutant SOD1 from astrocytes which increases survival in two different mutant SOD1 mouse models (Yamanaka et al., 2008; Wang et al., 2011a). These results denote the toxic character of mutant SOD1 in astrocytes that accelerate disease progression significantly by mechanisms such as, but not exclusively, the below described mechanisms of neuroinflammation and excitotoxicity. This is schematically presented in figure 1.

1.3 Neuroinflammation observed in ALS

Neuroinflammation occurs in a number of neurodegenative diseases, including ALS (reviewed in Papadimitriou et al., 2010 and Philips and Robberecht, 2011), and entails the reactive state of astrocytes (astrogliosis) and microglia (microgliosis) and the infiltration of lymphocytes. Initially perceived as a bystander effect, neuroinflammation is currently seen as beneficial at first, removing damaged cells and secreting supportive factors, and potentially detrimental thereafter by excessive release of cytokines (Beers et al., 2011a). Evidence of inflammation is detected in post mortem tissue (Schiffer et al., 1996; Anneser et al., 2004; Casula et al., 2011; Sta et al., 2011; Wang et al., 2011b), in cerebrospinal fluid (CSF) (Baron et al., 2005; Tateishi et al., 2010) and in blood samples of ALS patients (Poloni et al., 2000). In accordance, similar parameters of neuroinflammation are detected in ALS rodent models (among many others in Kiaei et al., 2006; Keller et al., 2009; Beers et al., 2011b). Inflammation is generally perceived as hazardous in ALS, as increasing inflammation in ALS models exacerbates disease progression and diminishes survival (Nguyen et al., 2004; Gowing et al., 2009). Fittingly, therapeutic strategies targeting inflammation are often advantageous in ALS rodent models (see below).

1.4 Excitotoxicity in ALS

An additional detrimental mechanism in ALS is excitotoxicity; an overstimulation of neurons causing neurodegeneration. Glutamate binds to the N-methyl D-aspartate (NMDA) or α-amino-3-hydroxy-5-methyl-4-isoxazole proprionic acid (AMPA) receptors, allowing extracellular sodium and calcium to enter motor neurons. Increased levels of intracellular calcium consequently cause neuronal cell death. The importance of excitotoxicity in ALS is demonstrated by the beneficial effects obtained by treating patients with riluzole. Although the precise mechanism of this drug is not yet known, it blocks NMDA receptors, enhances re-uptake of glutamate from the synaptic cleft and inhibits glutamate release by blocking voltage-gated sodium channels (Siniscalhi et al., 1999), thus preventing motor neuron cell death. Riluzole treatment increases predicted lifespan with a significant 12% in ALS mice (Bensimon et al., 1994; Lacomblez et al., 1996) and increases the probability of one year survival in patients by 9% (Miller et al., 2007). Unfortunately, it does not halt disease progression.

An overview of the current knowledge of the astrocytic contribution in ALS will be addressed in this chapter separately for the mechanisms inflammation and excitotoxicity.

2. Astrocytes in inflammation

Despite that microglia are the main immune cells of the central nervous system (reviewed in Ransohoff, 2010), astrocytes can also become reactive and contribute to neuroinflammation and are the focus of this chapter, with microglial inflammatory effects residing beyond the scope of this chapter. During neuroinjury or neurodegeneration the production of cytokines induce astrogliosis in which astrocytes increase glial fibrillary acidic protein (GFAP) and vimentin expression as well as an array of other genes. This response increases neuronal survival and includes both supportive factors (e.g. growth factors and glutamate transporters) and cytokines to sustain/promote neuroinflammation. Interestingly, during neuroinflammation the number of astrocytes increases by the differentiation of chondroitin sulfate proteoglycan, NG2, positive cells to astrocytes and not by astrocytic proliferation (Gowing et al., 2008).

2.1 Increasing inflammation in ALS

To assess the effect of inflammation in ALS and thus to discover whether boosting the inherent inflammation would be beneficial, lipopolysaccharide (LPS) was daily administered to ALS mice (Nguyen et al., 2004). The effect of this treatment was a clear decrease in lifespan, implying that an increase of inflammation is detrimental in ALS (Nguyen et al., 2004). Another study, initially intended to decrease inflammation, administered macrophage colony stimulating factor (M-CSF) to ALS mice and observed an unexpected increase of microgliosis also leading to a decreased survival (Gowing et al., 2009). Although not directed specifically at astrocytes, this work has led to the understanding of the hazardous character of neuroinflammation in ALS.

2.2 Astrogliosis in ALS

Reactive astrocytes alter gene expression including an upregulation of the intermediate filaments GFAP and vimentin that allow for visualisation of astrogliosis by increased immunoreactivity of these filaments in patient and ALS model tissue. Post mortem spinal cord tissue from fALS and sALS patients display astrogliosis (Schiffer et al., 1996), implying that reactivity of astrocytes is not limited to the familial form of ALS. Interestingly, astrogliosis levels are similar between long surviving and short surviving ALS patients, although this is not the case for microglial activation and the amount of dendritic cells (Sta et al., 2011). An extra facet of astrogliosis in ALS is an increased immunoreactivity of toll-like receptor 4 in astrocytes of sALS patients (Casula et al., 2011). Astrogliosis in ALS mice is present at symptomatic stages preceeding microgliosis (Kiaei et al., 2006; Keller et al., 2009; Yang et al., 2011). Interestingly, GFAP is not necessary for astrogliosis as GFAP deficient astrocytes can still become reactive and do not affect survival of ALS mice (Yoshii et al., 2011).

2.3 Mutant SOD1 affects astrocytic inflammatory behaviour

The expression of mutant SOD1 in astrocytes alters their function in vivo and in vitro. To begin, deletion of mutant SOD1 in astrocytes in two distinct ALS models demonstrates the detrimental effect of mutant SOD1 in astrocytes mainly post onset, as deletion increased lifespan of ALS mice (Yamanaka et al., 2008; Wang et al., 2011a). Intriguingly, astrogliosis was unaltered, implying that the negative effect of mutant SOD1 in astrocytes is not due to altered levels of astrogliosis (Yamanaka et al., 2008), but potentially by astrocytes inducing microgliosis (Yamanaka et al., 2008; Wang et al., 2011a). An alternative approach arrives from the field of transplantation in which non-transgenic mesenchymal stem cells are transplanted into the spinal cord of ALS rats and differentiate into astrocytes, thus diluting the mutant SOD1 positive astrocytes in the spinal cord (Boucherie et al., 2009). This approach also shows unaltered astrogliosis, but also decreased microgliosis and cyclooxygenase 2 (COX2) expression, and extends murine ALS life span (Boucherie et al., 2009). The processes explaining this hazardous effect of mutant SOD1 in astrocytes has been investigated in vitro. To begin, an interesting approach of transducing human astrocytes with wild-type SOD1 or mutant SOD1 increases inflammation in mutant SOD1 cultures (Marchetto et al., 2008). In addition, the mutant SOD1 transduced astrocytes provide a less viable environment for human embryonic stem cell derived motor neurons (Marchetto et al., 2008). The latter was rescued by using a NADPH oxidase 2 (NOX2) inhibitor, apocynin (Marchetto et al., 2008). Other studies concur that mutant SOD1 primary astrocytes exhibit a higher gene expression of cytokines on baseline and when stimulated by interferon γ (IFNγ) or tumor necrosis factor α (TNFα) (Hensley et al., 2006), implying once again that mutant SOD1 expression may affect the threshold of astrocytes to produce proinflammatory cytokines. Accordingly, the expression of interferon simulated genes is detected in astrocytes of presymptomatic ALS mice (Wang et al., 2011b) and genetic ablation and knockdown of the interferon alpha receptor type 1 (IFNAR1) increase ALS mouse survival by 5% and 10%, respectively (Wang et al., 2011b). Intriguingly, Aebischer et al. stress the importance of interferon signalling in mutant SOD1 astrocytes by demonstrating that mutant SOD1 astrocytes trigger the selective death of motor neurons mediated by IFNγ (Aebischer et al., 2011). This mechanism is dependent on the activation of the lymphotoxin-β receptor by LIGHT (TNFSF14) and genetic ablation of LIGHT extends survival of ALS mice by 13%, but does not postpone disease onset (Aebischer et al., 2011). Although this is a large increase in disease survival, clearly other mechanisms remain to play a role.

The above described altered functioning of mutant SOD1 expressing astrocytes is induced by an overexpression of multiple copies of mutant SOD1. It is unclear whether these effects also play a role in fALS patients with only 1 allele of mutant SOD1 or in fALS/sALS patients without disease causing SOD1 mutations. Remarkable work by Haidet-Phillips et al., (2011) shows that astrocytes collected post mortem from fALS and sALS are both able to induced motor neuron selective death which is not observed with astrocytes obtained from controls (Haidet-Phillips et al., 2011). Gene expression analysis of the the fALS and sALS astrocytes demonstrated increased expression chemokines, proinflammatory cytokines and components of the complement pathway (Haidet-Phillips et al., 2011). This study confirms that the astrocytic inflammatory effects found in vitro and in vivo in ALS mice may also contribute to disease pathology in humans.

2.4 Genetic tools to minimise astrogliosis
Attempts to minimise the inflammatory effect of astrocytes in ALS include genetic strategies targeting astrocytic knockdown of certain cytokines. Targeting of nuclear factor κB (NF-κB) activation specifically in astrocytes does not alter disease onset nor life span in ALS mice (Crosio et al., 2011). Which may be in part due to the mere decreased astrogliosis at presymtomatic stage (Crosio et al., 2011). Additionally, complete ablation of TNFα does not affect disease parameters (Gowing et al., 2006), also implying deletion of a single cytokine may not be sufficient to affect disease progression, as a general decrease in inflammation can be beneficial (see below). Instead of targeting cytokine production, ablating proliferating astrocytes was attempted in ALS, showing no effect on survival (Lepore et al., 2008a). This may be explained by the inability of astrocytes to proliferate in ALS (Gowing et al., 2008).

2.5 Therapeutic strategies targeting inflammation in ALS
A number of strategies have been utilized to diminish inflammation in ALS mice, though often not specifically targeting astrocytes. It is worthwhile to note that it is commonly unclear whether anti-inflammatory strategies truly exert an anti-inflammatory function due to the age-matched analysis of astrogliosis instead of disease stage-matched analysis with drugs that successfully extend lifespan. Among these therapeutic strategies are those intended to pharmacologically block the cyclooxygenase (COX) pathway by administration of celecoxib, a selective COX-2 inhibitor, and deletion of the prostaglandin E2 receptor. Both strategies diminish inflammation, postpone disease onset and prolong survival in ALS mice (Drachman et al., 2002; Liang et al., 2008). Similarly, celastrol administration also postponed disease onset extended lifespan, while decreasing TNFα, nitric oxide synthases (iNOS), cluster of differentiation 40 (CD40) immunoreactivity and astrogliosis when assessing age-matched spinal cord tissue (Kiaei et al., 2005). Similar effects are obtained when providing ALS mice with folic acid (Zhang et al., 2008) or bee venom (Yang et al., 2010). Thalidomide extends survival in ALS mice by destabilising cytokine mRNA including TNFα (Kiaei et al., 2006). Additionally, its analog lenalidomide also prolongs survival (Kiaei et al., 2006), even when administered after symptom onset (Neymotin et al., 2009). To conclude, minocycline has shown a dramatic increase in survival of ALS mice and postpones symptom onset (Kriz et al., 2002; Van Den Bosch et al., 2002; Zhu et al., 2002). Interestingly, this effect is moment of administration dependent, as administration of minocycline post disease onset increases the astrocytic and microglial response in ALS mice, decreasing survival (Keller et al., 2011).

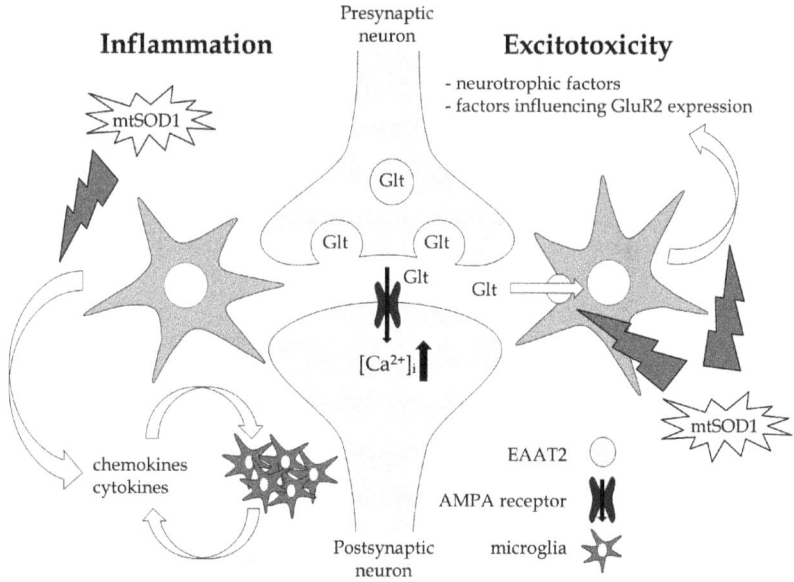

Fig. 1. Mutant SOD1 in astrocytes affecting (motor) neuron survival.

3. Astrocytes in excitotoxicity

In addition to the clear inflammatory role that astrocytes play in ALS, they also contribute to the mechanism of excitotoxicity. Their effect in the latter mechanism is two-fold: firstly, astrocytes facilitate the removal of excessive glutamate at the synaptic cleft and secondly, they affect the calcium permeability of AMPA receptors of motor neurons.

3.1 Excitotoxicity in ALS explained

Glutamate is the initiator of excitotoxicity in ALS. This neurotransmitter is the most abundant excitatory neurotransmitter in the brain and binds to NMDA, AMPA, and kainate (ionotropic) and metabotropic glutamate receptors (mGluR). Packaged into vesicles by the pre-synaptic neuron, glutamate is released into the synaptic cleft by the fusion of vesicles to the membrane of the neuron to excite the post synaptic neuron. This process is inhibited by riluzole (Siniscalhi et al., 1999). Increased levels of glutamate are detected in fALS, sALS (Fiszman et al., 2010; Spreux-Varoquaux et al., 2002) and is confirmed in spinal cords of ALS mice and rats. The detrimental role of glumate in the disease is demonstrated by the pronounced cell death that occurs to neurons in vitro when exposed to low levels of glutamate, even as low as physiologically detected in CSF (Cid et al., 2003). To further illustrate the detrimental role of glutamate in ALS, administration of compounds that block the formation of glutamate increase cell survival, both in vivo and in vitro (Cid et al., 2003).

3.2 Astrocytes in excitotoxicity in ALS: EAAT2/GLT-1

After glutamate release from the pre-synaptic neuron and binding of glutamate to ionotropic or metabotropic receptors on the post-synapse (increasing the concentration of intracellular calcium), glutamate is recycled for further use by the glial and endothelial cells, including astrocytes. Astrocytic glutamate re-uptake occurs by the glutamate transporters excitatory amino acid transporter 1 (EAAT1) and excitatory amino acid transporter 2 (EAAT2; also known as glutamate aspartate transporter (GLAST1) and glutamate transporter 1 (GLT-1), respectively). These transporters internalise glutamate, eg. into the astrocyte, for conversion to glutamine that is returned to the pre-synaptic neuron to be release again as glutamate (Laake et al., 1995).

Decreased glutamate uptake and EAAT2 protein levels are a common feature in both fALS and sALS and both in vitro and in vivo model systems (Staats and Van Den Bosch, 2009). In vitro transfection of primary cultured astrocytes with either mutant SOD1 or wild type human SOD1 down-regulates EAAT2 post transcriptionally (Tortarolo et al., 2004) and decreases EAAT2 transcription (Yang et al., 2009). Accordingly, glutamate transport is decreased in a neuronal cell line by mutant SOD1 transfection (Sala et al., 2005). Interestingly, this down-regulation also occurs in ALS model rats at pre-symptomatic stages through to end stage (Howland et al., 2002), at end stage only (Warita et al., 2002), in ALS model mice at end stage (Bendotti et al., 2001; Guo et al., 2010) and in post mortem patient spinal cords (Sasaki et al., 2001). In addition, in patient material the loss of EAAT2 and decreased tissue glutamate transport does not coincide with decreased levels of gene expression (Bristol and Rothstein, 1996), indicating that the loss is induced post transcriptionally, also in humans. Interestingly, a decrease of EAAT2 protein levels is not only in mutant SOD1 ALS models, but also a model of ALS/PDC (Wilson et al., 2003). In this model wild-type mice are fed with washed cycad flour containing β-methylamino-alanine (BMAA), which causes an ALS-like phenotype (Wilson et al., 2002). Although the loss of EAAT2 in ALS is apparent, it remains unclear whether this post transcriptional loss of EAAT2 proceeds or follows the loss of motor neurons.

3.3 Targeting (astrocytic) EAAT2

To assess whether the loss of glutamate transport or the loss of EAAT2 specifically results in motor neuron loss, pharmacological and genetic tools have been used. To begin, research conducted by pharmacologically inhibiting glutamate transport in the rat spinal cord, failed to show any motor neuron loss despite the increased levels of glutamate (Tovar et al., 2009). In contrast, a similar experiment has been performed to address whether EAAT2 loss specifically induces motor neuron loss. EAAT2 null mice live for approximately 6 weeks before they succumb to epileptic seizures and are vulnerability to acute brain injury (Tanaka et al., 1997). To this end, heterozygous mice demonstrated the effect of approximately 40% knockdown of EAAT2 in the spinal cord in ALS mice (Pardo et al., 2006). This knockdown resulted in a non-significant decrease of symptom onset and significant, but moderate, decrease of lifespan in ALS mice (Pardo et al., 2006).

To assess the expected beneficial role of EAAT2 in ALS, transgenic mice overexpressing human EAAT2 in specifically astrocytes were crossbred with mutant SOD1 mice. Although glutamate uptake is increased in vivo and an overexpression of human EAAT2 is protective on cortical neurons in vitro, an effect on symptom onset or lifespan was absent (Guo et al., 2003). Possibly, the expression levels were insufficient to induce an effect or human EAAT2 is not as efficient as murine EAAT2 in mouse, as administration of ceftriaxone (a β-lactam antibiotic) and GPI-1046 (a synthetic, non-immunosuppressive derivative of FK506) increase EAAT2 protein levels and extend lifespan of ALS mice (Rothstein et al., 2005; Ganel et al.,

2006) by enhancing EAAT2 transcription (Lee et al., 2008). In addition, EAAT2 is also expressed by other cells types than astrocytes alone (Anderson and Swanson, 2000), which are not targeted in this genetic experimental design. Interestingly, removal of mutant SOD1 from astrocytes leads to prolonged survival without affecting astrogliosis, but does preserve EAAT2 levels potentially explaining the extended lifespan (Wang et al., 2011a).

3.4 Astrocytic replacement therapy in ALS mice

The beneficial effect of EAAT2 is often used as an explanation of positive effects found by cell transfers in ALS model rodents. For instance, the systemic transplantation of c-kit positive cell from bone marrow in mutant SOD1 mice significantly increased the lifespan, which is, at least in part, attributed to increased EAAT2 expression induced by the transferred cells (Corti et al., 2010). The same holds true for the prolonged survival of ALS rats when treated with focal transplantation-based astrocyte replacement with wild type glial-restricted precursors (GRPs) (Lepore et al., 2008b). This study also focussed on EAAT2 by also transplanting EAAT2 overexpressing GRPs and EAAT2 null GRPs. The ALS mice treated with the EAAT2 overexpressing GRPs showed no additional increase of lifespan compared to wild type GRP treated ALS mice (already increased compared to controls). Intriguingly, this positive effect of transplantation of the wild type GRPs is diminished in mice transplanted with EAAT2 null GRPs (Lepore et al., 2008b). In addition, co-cultures of human adipose-derived stem cells with astrocytes induce higher levels of EAAT2 in astrocytes (Gu et al., 2010), though this treatment has not (yet) been shown to affect motor neuron survival in vitro or in vivo.

3.5 Astrocytes in excitotoxicity in ALS: AMPA receptor permeability

After the release of glutamate from the pre-synaptic neuron into the synaptic cleft, glutamate binds to NMDA, AMPA receptors or the metabotropic receptors. High levels of calcium entering through AMPA receptors into the post-synaptic neuron can cause neuronal death. The AMPA receptor is formed as a tetramer combining, usually pairwise, a combination of its four different subunits (glutamate receptor unit 1-4 (GluR1-4)) (Shi et al., 1999). Each subunit can bind glutamate and the channel opens after occupation of at least 2 binding locations (Mayer, 2005). The importance of this receptor in ALS is demonstrated by the ablation of glutamate induced apoptosis in cortical neurons in vitro (Cid et al., 2003) and in vivo when administering an AMPA receptor antagonist (Van Damme et al., 2003; Tortarolo et al., 2006).

The AMPA receptor plays an imperative role in excitotoxicity by its calcium permeability that is determined by the incorporation of the GluR2 subunit in the receptor complex. In most conditions, the AMPA receptor complex contains at least one GluR2 subunit and it prevents the influx of extracellular calcium into the neuron (Seeburg et al., 2001). In contrast, receptors lacking the GluR2 subunit are highly calcium permeable (Seeburg et al., 2001). A general decrease of GluR2 is found in ALS model mice, portraying an increased vulnerability of these mice to excitotoxic insults (Tortarolo et al., 2006; Zhao et al., 2008). The role of GluR2 in ALS is investigated by genetically ablating GluR2 in ALS mice, which decreases survival in vivo and decreases cell survival in vitro (Van Damme et al., 2005). The opposite has been shown by up-regulating GluR2 expression in motor neurons of ALS mice, as hereby survival is increased (Tateno et al., 2002). In addition, pharmacological inhibition of the AMPA receptor prolonged survival in ALS model mice (Van Damme et al., 2003; Tortarolo et al., 2006).

Interestingly, the surrounding astrocytes influence the expression level of the GluR2 subunit in motor neurons, as soluble factor(s) released from astrocytes effect GluR2 gene expression and neuronal vulnerability to excitotoxic insults, both in vitro and in vivo (Van Damme et al., 2007). Moreover, the presence of mutant SOD1 interferes with the production and/or secretion of this factor(s) to increase GluR2 expression and thus decreases motor neuronal resistance to excitotoxicity (Van Damme et al., 2007).

4. Conclusions and future directions

Astrocytes clearly contribute to ALS decrease progression in both neuroinflammation and excitotoxicity. An intriguing aspect of astrocytes in ALS disease pathology is whether the mutant SOD1 astrocytic properties, of LIGHT dependent cell death and diminished GluR2 editing for example, are also important in other ALS causing mutations and in sporadic cases of ALS. Initial work performed implies that these characteristics are not solely dependent on mutant SOD1 in patients. In addition, both mechanisms in which astrocytes function seem successfully targetable in mice. Future research may benefit from further assessing the role of also non-SOD1 ALS causing mutations in astrocytes on ALS and optimizing therapeutic strategies against neuroinflammation and excitotoxicity.

5. References

Aebischer, J., Cassina, P., Otsmane, B., Moumen, A., Seilhean, D., Meininger, V., Barbeito, L., Pettmann, B., and Raoul, C. (2011). IFNgamma triggers a LIGHT-dependent selective death of motoneurons contributing to the non-cell-autonomous effects of mutant SOD1. *Cell Death Differ* 18, 754-768.

Anderson, C.M., and Swanson, R.A. (2000). Astrocyte glutamate transport: review of properties, regulation, and physiological functions. *Glia* 32, 1-14.

Anneser, J.M., Chahli, C., Ince, P.G., Borasio, G.D., and Shaw, P.J. (2004). Glial proliferation and metabotropic glutamate receptor expression in amyotrophic lateral sclerosis. *J Neuropathol Exp Neurol* 63, 831-840.

Baron, P., Bussini, S., Cardin, V., Corbo, M., Conti, G., Galimberti, D., Scarpini, E., Bresolin, N., Wharton, S.B., Shaw, P.J., *et al.* (2005). Production of monocyte chemoattractant protein-1 in amyotrophic lateral sclerosis. *Muscle Nerve* 32, 541-544.

Beers, D.R., Henkel, J.S., Zhao, W., Wang, J., and Appel, S.H. (2008). CD4+ T cells support glial neuroprotection, slow disease progression, and modify glial morphology in an animal model of inherited ALS. *Proc Natl Acad Sci U S A* 105, 15558-15563.

Beers, D.R., Henkel, J.S., Zhao, W., Wang, J., Huang, A., Wen, S., Liao, B., and Appel, S.H. (2011a). Endogenous regulatory T lymphocytes ameliorate amyotrophic lateral sclerosis in mice and correlate with disease progression in patients with amyotrophic lateral sclerosis. *Brain* 134, 1293-1314.

Beers, D.R., Zhao, W., Liao, B., Kano, O., Wang, J., Huang, A., Appel, S.H., and Henkel, J.S. (2011b). Neuroinflammation modulates distinct regional and temporal clinical responses in ALS mice. *Brain Behav Immun* 25, 1025-1035.

Bendotti, C., Tortarolo, M., Suchak, S.K., Calvaresi, N., Carvelli, L., Bastone, A., Rizzi, M., Rattray, M., and Mennini, T. (2001). Transgenic SOD1 G93A mice develop reduced

GLT-1 in spinal cord without alterations in cerebrospinal fluid glutamate levels. *J Neurochem* 79, 737-746.

Bensimon, G., Lacomblez, L., and Meininger, V. (1994). A controlled trial of riluzole in amyotrophic lateral sclerosis. ALS/Riluzole Study Group. *N Engl J Med* 330, 585-591.

Boillee, S., Vande Velde, C., and Cleveland, D.W. (2006a). ALS: a disease of motor neurons and their nonneuronal neighbors. *Neuron* 52, 39-59.

Boillee, S., Yamanaka, K., Lobsiger, C.S., Copeland, N.G., Jenkins, N.A., Kassiotis, G., Kollias, G., and Cleveland, D.W. (2006b). Onset and progression in inherited ALS determined by motor neurons and microglia. *Science* 312, 1389-1392.

Boucherie, C., Schafer, S., Lavand'homme, P., Maloteaux, J.M., and Hermans, E. (2009). Chimerization of astroglial population in the lumbar spinal cord after mesenchymal stem cell transplantation prolongs survival in a rat model of amyotrophic lateral sclerosis. *J Neurosci Res* 87, 2034-2046.

Bristol, L.A., and Rothstein, J.D. (1996). Glutamate transporter gene expression in amyotrophic lateral sclerosis motor cortex. *Ann Neurol* 39, 676-679.

Bruijn, L.I., Miller, T.M., and Cleveland, D.W. (2004). Unraveling the mechanisms involved in motor neuron degeneration in ALS. *Annu Rev Neurosci* 27, 723-749.

Casula, M., Iyer, A.M., Spliet, W.G., Anink, J.J., Steentjes, K., Sta, M., Troost, D., and Aronica, E. (2011). Toll-like receptor signaling in amyotrophic lateral sclerosis spinal cord tissue. *Neuroscience* 179, 233-243.

Chiu, I.M., Chen, A., Zheng, Y., Kosaras, B., Tsiftsoglou, S.A., Vartanian, T.K., Brown, R.H., Jr., and Carroll, M.C. (2008). T lymphocytes potentiate endogenous neuroprotective inflammation in a mouse model of ALS. *Proc Natl Acad Sci U S A* 105, 17913-17918.

Cid, C., Alvarez-Cermeno, J.C., Regidor, I., Salinas, M., and Alcazar, A. (2003). Low concentrations of glutamate induce apoptosis in cultured neurons: implications for amyotrophic lateral sclerosis. *J Neurol Sci* 206, 91-95.

Corti, S., Nizzardo, M., Nardini, M., Donadoni, C., Salani, S., Simone, C., Falcone, M., Riboldi, G., Govoni, A., Bresolin, N., *et al.* (2010). Systemic transplantation of c-kit+ cells exerts a therapeutic effect in a model of amyotrophic lateral sclerosis. *Hum Mol Genet* 19, 3782-3796.

Crosio, C., Valle, C., Casciati, A., Iaccarino, C., and Carri, M.T. (2011). Astroglial inhibition of NF-kappaB does not ameliorate disease onset and progression in a mouse model for amyotrophic lateral sclerosis (ALS). *PLoS One* 6(3): e17187. doi:10.1371/journal.pone.0017187.

Del Bo, R., Ghezzi, S., Corti, S., Pandolfo, M., Ranieri, M., Santoro, D., Ghione, I., Prelle, A., Orsetti, V., Mancuso, M., *et al.* (2009). TARDBP (TDP-43) sequence analysis in patients with familial and sporadic ALS: identification of two novel mutations. *Eur J Neurol* 16, 727-732.

Drachman, D.B., Frank, K., Dykes-Hoberg, M., Teismann, P., Almer, G., Przedborski, S., and Rothstein, J.D. (2002). Cyclooxygenase 2 inhibition protects motor neurons and prolongs survival in a transgenic mouse model of ALS. *Ann Neurol* 52, 771-778.

Fischer, L.R., and Glass, J.D. (2007). Axonal degeneration in motor neuron disease. *Neurodegener Dis* 4, 431-442.

Fiszman, M.L., Ricart, K.C., Latini, A., Rodriguez, G., and Sica, R.E. (2010). In vitro neurotoxic properties and excitatory aminoacids concentration in the cerebrospinal fluid of amyotrophic lateral sclerosis patients. Relationship with the degree of certainty of disease diagnoses. *Acta Neurol Scand* 121, 120-126.

Ganel, R., Ho, T., Maragakis, N.J., Jackson, M., Steiner, J.P., and Rothstein, J.D. (2006). Selective up-regulation of the glial Na+-dependent glutamate transporter GLT1 by a neuroimmunophilin ligand results in neuroprotection. *Neurobiol Dis* 21, 556-567.

Genestine, M., Caricati, E., Fico, A., Richelme, S., Hassani, H., Sunyach, C., Lamballe, F., Panzica, G.C., Pettmann, B., Helmbacher, F., *et al.* (2011). Enhanced neuronal Met signalling levels in ALS mice delay disease onset. *Cell Death Dis* 2, e130; doi:10.1038/cddis.2011.11.

Gowing, G., Dequen, F., Soucy, G., and Julien, J.P. (2006). Absence of tumor necrosis factor-alpha does not affect motor neuron disease caused by superoxide dismutase 1 mutations. *J Neurosci* 26, 11397-11402.

Gowing, G., Lalancette-Hebert, M., Audet, J.N., Dequen, F., and Julien, J.P. (2009). Macrophage colony stimulating factor (M-CSF) exacerbates ALS disease in a mouse model through altered responses of microglia expressing mutant superoxide dismutase. *Exp Neurol* 220, 267-275.

Gowing, G., Philips, T., Van Wijmeersch, B., Audet, J.N., Dewil, M., Van Den Bosch, L., Billiau, A.D., Robberecht, W., and Julien, J.P. (2008). Ablation of proliferating microglia does not affect motor neuron degeneration in amyotrophic lateral sclerosis caused by mutant superoxide dismutase. *J Neurosci* 28, 10234-10244.

Grosskreutz, J., Van Den Bosch, L., and Keller, B.U. (2010). Calcium dysregulation in amyotrophic lateral sclerosis. *Cell Calcium* 47, 165-174.

Gu, R., Hou, X., Pang, R., Li, L., Chen, F., Geng, J., Xu, Y., and Zhang, C. (2010). Human adipose-derived stem cells enhance the glutamate uptake function of GLT1 in SOD1(G93A)-bearing astrocytes. *Biochem Biophys Res Commun* 393, 481-486.

Guo, H., Lai, L., Butchbach, M.E., Stockinger, M.P., Shan, X., Bishop, G.A., and Lin, C.L. (2003). Increased expression of the glial glutamate transporter EAAT2 modulates excitotoxicity and delays the onset but not the outcome of ALS in mice. *Hum Mol Genet* 12, 2519-2532.

Guo, Y., Duan, W., Li, Z., Huang, J., Yin, Y., Zhang, K., Wang, Q., Zhang, Z., and Li, C. (2010). Decreased GLT-1 and increased SOD1 and HO-1 expression in astrocytes contribute to lumbar spinal cord vulnerability of SOD1-G93A transgenic mice. *FEBS Lett* 584, 1615-1622.

Gurney, M.E., Pu, H., Chiu, A.Y., Dal Canto, M.C., Polchow, C.Y., Alexander, D.D., Caliendo, J., Hentati, A., Kwon, Y.W., Deng, H.X., *et al.* (1994). Motor neuron degeneration in mice that express a human Cu,Zn superoxide dismutase mutation. *Science* 264, 1772-1775.

Haidet-Phillips, A.M., Hester, M.E., Miranda, C.J., Meyer, K., Braun, L., Frakes, A., Song, S., Likhite, S., Murtha, M.J., Foust, K.D., *et al.* (2011). Astrocytes from familial and sporadic ALS patients are toxic to motor neurons. *Nat Biotechnol* doi: 10.1038/nbt.1957

Hensley, K., Abdel-Moaty, H., Hunter, J., Mhatre, M., Mou, S., Nguyen, K., Potapova, T., Pye, Q.N., Qi, M., Rice, H., *et al.* (2006). Primary glia expressing the G93A-SOD1 mutation present a neuroinflammatory phenotype and provide a cellular system for studies of glial inflammation. *J Neuroinflammation* 3, 2.

Howland, D.S., Liu, J., She, Y., Goad, B., Maragakis, N.J., Kim, B., Erickson, J., Kulik, J., DeVito, L., Psaltis, G., et al. (2002). Focal loss of the glutamate transporter EAAT2 in a transgenic rat model of SOD1 mutant-mediated amyotrophic lateral sclerosis (ALS). Proc Natl Acad Sci U S A 99, 1604-1609.

Jaarsma, D., Teuling, E., Haasdijk, E.D., De Zeeuw, C.I., and Hoogenraad, C.C. (2008). Neuron-specific expression of mutant superoxide dismutase is sufficient to induce amyotrophic lateral sclerosis in transgenic mice. J Neurosci 28, 2075-2088.

Johnson, J.O., Mandrioli, J., Benatar, M., Abramzon, Y., Van Deerlin, V.M., Trojanowski, J.Q., Gibbs, J.R., Brunetti, M., Gronka, S., Wuu, J., et al. Exome sequencing reveals VCP mutations as a cause of familial ALS. Neuron 68, 857-864.

Keller, A.F., Gravel, M., and Kriz, J. (2009). Live imaging of amyotrophic lateral sclerosis pathogenesis: disease onset is characterized by marked induction of GFAP in Schwann cells. Glia 57, 1130-1142.

Keller, A.F., Gravel, M., and Kriz, J. (2011). Treatment with minocycline after disease onset alters astrocyte reactivity and increases microgliosis in SOD1 mutant mice. Exp Neurol 228, 69-79.

Kiaei, M., Kipiani, K., Petri, S., Chen, J., Calingasan, N.Y., and Beal, M.F. (2005). Celastrol blocks neuronal cell death and extends life in transgenic mouse model of amyotrophic lateral sclerosis. Neurodegener Dis 2, 246-254.

Kiaei, M., Petri, S., Kipiani, K., Gardian, G., Choi, D.K., Chen, J., Calingasan, N.Y., Schafer, P., Muller, G.W., Stewart, C., et al. (2006). Thalidomide and lenalidomide extend survival in a transgenic mouse model of amyotrophic lateral sclerosis. J Neurosci 26, 2467-2473.

Kriz, J., Nguyen, M.D., and Julien, J.P. (2002). Minocycline slows disease progression in a mouse model of amyotrophic lateral sclerosis. Neurobiol Dis 10, 268-278.

Kotchoubey, B., Lang, S., Winter, S., and Birbaumer, N. (2003). Cognitive processing in completely paralyzed patients with amyotrophic lateral sclerosis. Eur J Neurol 10, 551-558.

Kwiatkowski, T.J., Jr., Bosco, D.A., Leclerc, A.L., Tamrazian, E., Vanderburg, C.R., Russ, C., Davis, A., Gilchrist, J., Kasarskis, E.J., Munsat, T., et al. (2009). Mutations in the FUS/TLS gene on chromosome 16 cause familial amyotrophic lateral sclerosis. Science 323, 1205-1208.

Laake, J.H., Slyngstad, T.A., Haug, F.M., and Ottersen, O.P. (1995). Glutamine from glial cells is essential for the maintenance of the nerve terminal pool of glutamate: immunogold evidence from hippocampal slice cultures. J Neurochem 65, 871-881.

Lacomblez, L., Bensimon, G., Leigh, P.N., Guillet, P., and Meininger, V. (1996). Dose-ranging study of riluzole in amyotrophic lateral sclerosis. Amyotrophic Lateral Sclerosis/Riluzole Study Group II. Lancet 347, 1425-1431.

Lee, S.G., Su, Z.Z., Emdad, L., Gupta, P., Sarkar, D., Borjabad, A., Volsky, D.J., and Fisher, P.B. (2008). Mechanism of ceftriaxone induction of excitatory amino acid transporter-2 expression and glutamate uptake in primary human astrocytes. J Biol Chem 283, 13116-13123.

Lepore, A.C., Dejea, C., Carmen, J., Rauck, B., Kerr, D.A., Sofroniew, M.V., and Maragakis, N.J. (2008a). Selective ablation of proliferating astrocytes does not affect disease outcome in either acute or chronic models of motor neuron degeneration. Exp Neurol 211, 423-432.

Lepore, A.C., Rauck, B., Dejea, C., Pardo, A.C., Rao, M.S., Rothstein, J.D., and Maragakis, N.J. (2008b). Focal transplantation-based astrocyte replacement is neuroprotective in a model of motor neuron disease. *Nat Neurosci* 11, 1294-1301.

Liang, X., Wang, Q., Shi, J., Lokteva, L., Breyer, R.M., Montine, T.J., and Andreasson, K. (2008). The prostaglandin E2 EP2 receptor accelerates disease progression and inflammation in a model of amyotrophic lateral sclerosis. *Ann Neurol* 64, 304-314.

Lobsiger, C.S., Boillee, S., McAlonis-Downes, M., Khan, A.M., Feltri, M.L., Yamanaka, K., and Cleveland, D.W. (2009). Schwann cells expressing dismutase active mutant SOD1 unexpectedly slow disease progression in ALS mice. *Proc Natl Acad Sci U S A* 106, 4465-4470.

Logroscino, G., Traynor, B.J., Hardiman, O., Chio, A., Mitchell, D., Swingler, R.J., Millul, A., Benn, E., and Beghi, E. (2010). Incidence of amyotrophic lateral sclerosis in Europe. *J Neurol Neurosurg Psychiatry* 81(4):385-90

Maessen, M., Veldink, J.H., van den Berg, L.H., Schouten, H.J., van der Wal, G., and Onwuteaka-Philipsen, B.D. (2010). Requests for euthanasia: origin of suffering in ALS, heart failure, and cancer patients. *J Neurol* 257, 1192-1198.

Marchetto, M.C., Muotri, A.R., Mu, Y., Smith, A.M., Cezar, G.G., and Gage, F.H. (2008). Non-cell-autonomous effect of human SOD1 G37R astrocytes on motor neurons derived from human embryonic stem cells. *Cell Stem Cell* 3, 649-657.

Maruyama, H., Morino, H., Ito, H., Izumi, Y., Kato, H., Watanabe, Y., Kinoshita, Y., Kamada, M., Nodera, H., Suzuki, H., *et al.* Mutations of optineurin in amyotrophic lateral sclerosis. *Nature* 465, 223-226.

Mayer, M.L. (2005). Glutamate receptor ion channels. *Curr Opin Neurobiol* 15, 282-288.

Miller, R.G., Mitchell, J.D., Lyon, M., and Moore, D.H. (2007). Riluzole for amyotrophic lateral sclerosis (ALS)/motor neuron disease (MND). *Cochrane Database Syst Rev*, CD001447.

Naor, S., Keren, Z., Bronshtein, T., Goren, E., Machluf, M., and Melamed, D. (2009). Development of ALS-like disease in SOD-1 mice deficient of B lymphocytes. *J Neurol* 256, 1228-1235.

Neymotin, A., Petri, S., Calingasan, N.Y., Wille, E., Schafer, P., Stewart, C., Hensley, K., Beal, M.F., and Kiaei, M. (2009). Lenalidomide (Revlimid) administration at symptom onset is neuroprotective in a mouse model of amyotrophic lateral sclerosis. *Exp Neurol* 220, 191-197.

Nguyen, M.D., D'Aigle, T., Gowing, G., Julien, J.P., and Rivest, S. (2004). Exacerbation of motor neuron disease by chronic stimulation of innate immunity in a mouse model of amyotrophic lateral sclerosis. *J Neurosci* 24, 1340-1349.

Papadimitriou, D., Le Verche, V., Jacquier, A., Ikiz, B., Przedborski, S., and Re, D.B. (2010). Inflammation in ALS and SMA: sorting out the good from the evil. *Neurobiol Dis* 37, 493-502.

Pardo, A.C., Wong, V., Benson, L.M., Dykes, M., Tanaka, K., Rothstein, J.D., and Maragakis, N.J. (2006). Loss of the astrocyte glutamate transporter GLT1 modifies disease in SOD1(G93A) mice. *Exp Neurol* 201, 120-130.

Philips, T., and Robberecht, W. (2011). Neuroinflammation in amyotrophic lateral sclerosis: role of glial activation in motor neuron disease. *Lancet Neurol* 10, 253-263.

Poloni, M., Facchetti, D., Mai, R., Micheli, A., Agnoletti, L., Francolini, G., Mora, G., Camana, C., Mazzini, L., and Bachetti, T. (2000). Circulating levels of tumour necrosis factor-alpha and its soluble receptors are increased in the blood of patients with amyotrophic lateral sclerosis. *Neurosci Lett* 287, 211-214.

Ransohoff, R.M., and Cardona, A.E. (2010). The myeloid cells of the central nervous system parenchyma. *Nature* 468, 253-262.

Raoul, C., Buhler, E., Sadeghi, C., Jacquier, A., Aebischer, P., Pettmann, B., Henderson, C.E., and Haase, G. (2006). Chronic activation in presymptomatic amyotrophic lateral sclerosis (ALS) mice of a feedback loop involving Fas, Daxx, and FasL. *Proc Natl Acad Sci U S A* 103, 6007-6012.

Raoul, C., Estevez, A.G., Nishimune, H., Cleveland, D.W., deLapeyriere, O., Henderson, C.E., Haase, G., and Pettmann, B. (2002). Motoneuron death triggered by a specific pathway downstream of Fas. potentiation by ALS-linked SOD1 mutations. *Neuron* 35, 1067-1083.

Reaume, A.G., Elliott, J.L., Hoffman, E.K., Kowall, N.W., Ferrante, R.J., Siwek, D.F., Wilcox, H.M., Flood, D.G., Beal, M.F., Brown, R.H., Jr., *et al.* (1996). Motor neurons in Cu/Zn superoxide dismutase-deficient mice develop normally but exhibit enhanced cell death after axonal injury. *Nat Genet* 13, 43-47.

Rothstein, J.D., Patel, S., Regan, M.R., Haenggeli, C., Huang, Y.H., Bergles, D.E., Jin, L., Dykes Hoberg, M., Vidensky, S., Chung, D.S., *et al.* (2005). Beta-lactam antibiotics offer neuroprotection by increasing glutamate transporter expression. *Nature* 433, 73-77.

Rutherford, N.J., Zhang, Y.J., Baker, M., Gass, J.M., Finch, N.A., Xu, Y.F., Stewart, H., Kelley, B.J., Kuntz, K., Crook, R.J., *et al.* (2008). Novel mutations in TARDBP (TDP-43) in patients with familial amyotrophic lateral sclerosis. *PLoS Genet* 4, e1000193.

Sala, G., Beretta, S., Ceresa, C., Mattavelli, L., Zoia, C., Tremolizzo, L., Ferri, A., Carri, M.T., and Ferrarese, C. (2005). Impairment of glutamate transport and increased vulnerability to oxidative stress in neuroblastoma SH-SY5Y cells expressing a Cu,Zn superoxide dismutase typical of familial amyotrophic lateral sclerosis. *Neurochem Int* 46, 227-234.

Sasaki, S., Warita, H., Abe, K., Komori, T., and Iwata, M. (2001). EAAT1 and EAAT2 immunoreactivity in transgenic mice with a G93A mutant SOD1 gene. *Neuroreport* 12, 1359-1362.

Schiffer, D., Cordera, S., Cavalla, P., and Migheli, A. (1996). Reactive astrogliosis of the spinal cord in amyotrophic lateral sclerosis. *J Neurol Sci* 139 Suppl, 27-33.

Seeburg, P.H., Single, F., Kuner, T., Higuchi, M., and Sprengel, R. (2001). Genetic manipulation of key determinants of ion flow in glutamate receptor channels in the mouse. *Brain Res* 907, 233-243.

Shefner, J.M., Reaume, A.G., Flood, D.G., Scott, R.W., Kowall, N.W., Ferrante, R.J., Siwek, D.F., Upton-Rice, M., and Brown, R.H., Jr. (1999). Mice lacking cytosolic copper/zinc superoxide dismutase display a distinctive motor axonopathy. *Neurology* 53, 1239-1246.

Shi, S.H., Hayashi, Y., Petralia, R.S., Zaman, S.H., Wenthold, R.J., Svoboda, K., and Malinow, R. (1999). Rapid spine delivery and redistribution of AMPA receptors after synaptic NMDA receptor activation. *Science* 284, 1811-1816.

Siniscalchi, A., Zona, C., Sancesario, G., D'Angelo, E., Zeng, Y.C., Mercuri, N.B., and Bernardi, G. (1999). Neuroprotective effects of riluzole: an electrophysiological and histological analysis in an in vitro model of ischemia. *Synapse* 32, 147-152.

Spreux-Varoquaux, O., Bensimon, G., Lacomblez, L., Salachas, F., Pradat, P.F., Le Forestier, N., Marouan, A., Dib, M., and Meininger, V. (2002). Glutamate levels in cerebrospinal fluid in amyotrophic lateral sclerosis: a reappraisal using a new HPLC method with coulometric detection in a large cohort of patients. *J Neurol Sci* 193, 73-78.

Sta, M., Sylva-Steenland, R.M., Casula, M., de Jong, J.M., Troost, D., Aronica, E., and Baas, F. (2011). Innate and adaptive immunity in amyotrophic lateral sclerosis: evidence of complement activation. *Neurobiol Dis* 42, 211-220.

Staats, K.A., and Van Den Bosch, L. (2009). Astrocytes in amyotrophic lateral sclerosis: direct effects on motor neuron survival. *J Biol Phys* 35(4): p. 337-46.

Tanaka, K., Watase, K., Manabe, T., Yamada, K., Watanabe, M., Takahashi, K., Iwama, H., Nishikawa, T., Ichihara, N., Kikuchi, T., *et al.* (1997). Epilepsy and exacerbation of brain injury in mice lacking the glutamate transporter GLT-1. *Science* 276, 1699-1702.

Tateishi, T., Yamasaki, R., Tanaka, M., Matsushita, T., Kikuchi, H., Isobe, N., Ohyagi, Y., and Kira, J. (2010). CSF chemokine alterations related to the clinical course of amyotrophic lateral sclerosis. *J Neuroimmunol* 222, 76-81.

Tateno, M., Sugimoto, H., Tanaka, S., Itohara, H., Hama, A., Miyawaki, R.M., Shin, M.M., Masumada, T., Aosaki, H., Misawa, R., *et al.* (2002). GluR2 overexpression in motor neurons renders AMPA receptors impermeable to calcium and delays disease onset in an ALS transgenic mouse model. *Soc for Neurosci Abstr* 789.21

Tortarolo, M., Crosshwaite, A.J., Conforti, L., Spencer, J.P., Williams, R.J., Bendotti, C., and Rattray, M. (2004). Expression of SOD1 G93A or wild-type SOD1 in primary cultures of astrocytes down-regulates the glutamate transporter GLT-1: lack of involvement of oxidative stress. *J Neurochem* 88, 481-493.

Tortarolo, M., Grignaschi, G., Calvaresi, N., Zennaro, E., Spaltro, G., Colovic, M., Fracasso, C., Guiso, G., Elger, B., Schneider, H., *et al.* (2006). Glutamate AMPA receptors change in motor neurons of SOD1(G93A) transgenic mice and their inhibition by a noncompetitive antagonist ameliorates the progression of amytrophic lateral sclerosis-like disease. *J Neurosci Res* 83, 134-146.

Tovar, Y.R.L.B., Santa-Cruz, L.D., Zepeda, A., and Tapia, R. (2009). Chronic elevation of extracellular glutamate due to transport blockade is innocuous for spinal motoneurons in vivo. *Neurochem Int* 54, 186-191.

Van Damme, P., Bogaert, E., Dewil, M., Hersmus, N., Kiraly, D., Scheveneels, W., Bockx, I., Braeken, D., Verpoorten, N., Verhoeven, K., *et al.* (2007). Astrocytes regulate GluR2 expression in motor neurons and their vulnerability to excitotoxicity. *Proc Natl Acad Sci U S A* 104, 14825-14830.

Van Damme, P., Braeken, D., Callewaert, G., Robberecht, W., and Van Den Bosch, L. (2005). GluR2 deficiency accelerates motor neuron degeneration in a mouse model of amyotrophic lateral sclerosis. *J Neuropathol Exp Neurol* 64, 605-612.

Van Damme, P., Leyssen, M., Callewaert, G., Robberecht, W., and Van Den Bosch, L. (2003). The AMPA receptor antagonist NBQX prolongs survival in a transgenic mouse model of amyotrophic lateral sclerosis. *Neurosci Lett* 343, 81-84.

Van Deerlin, V.M., Leverenz, J.B., Bekris, L.M., Bird, T.D., Yuan, W., Elman, L.B., Clay, D., Wood, E.M., Chen-Plotkin, A.S., Martinez-Lage, M., *et al.* (2008). TARDBP mutations in amyotrophic lateral sclerosis with TDP-43 neuropathology: a genetic and histopathological analysis. *Lancet Neurol* 7, 409-416.

Van Den Bosch, L., Tilkin, P., Lemmens, G., and Robberecht, W. (2002). Minocycline delays disease onset and mortality in a transgenic model of ALS. *Neuroreport* 13, 1067-1070.

Vance, C., Rogelj, B., Hortobagyi, T., De Vos, K.J., Nishimura, A.L., Sreedharan, J., Hu, X., Smith, B., Ruddy, D., Wright, P., *et al.* (2009). Mutations in FUS, an RNA processing protein, cause familial amyotrophic lateral sclerosis type 6. *Science* 323, 1208-1211.

Wang, L., Gutmann, D.H., and Roos, R.P. (2011a). Astrocyte loss of mutant SOD1 delays ALS disease onset and progression in G85R transgenic mice. *Hum Mol Genet* 20, 286-293.

Wang, R., Yang, B., and Zhang, D. (2011b). Activation of interferon signaling pathways in spinal cord astrocytes from an ALS mouse model. *Glia* 59, 946-958.

Warita, H., Manabe, Y., Murakami, T., Shiote, M., Shiro, Y., Hayashi, T., Nagano, I., Shoji, M., and Abe, K. (2002). Tardive decrease of astrocytic glutamate transporter protein in transgenic mice with ALS-linked mutant SOD1. *Neurol Res* 24, 577-581.

Wilson, J.M., Khabazian, I., Pow, D.V., Craig, U.K., and Shaw, C.A. (2003). Decrease in glial glutamate transporter variants and excitatory amino acid receptor down-regulation in a murine model of ALS-PDC. *Neuromolecular Med* 3, 105-118.

Wilson, J.M., Khabazian, I., Wong, M.C., Seyedalikhani, A., Bains, J.S., Pasqualotto, B.A., Williams, D.E., Andersen, R.J., Simpson, R.J., Smith, R., *et al.* (2002). Behavioral and neurological correlates of ALS-parkinsonism dementia complex in adult mice fed washed cycad flour. *Neuromolecular Med* 1, 207-221.

Yamanaka, K., Chun, S.J., Boillee, S., Fujimori-Tonou, N., Yamashita, H., Gutmann, D.H., Takahashi, R., Misawa, H., and Cleveland, D.W. (2008). Astrocytes as determinants of disease progression in inherited amyotrophic lateral sclerosis. *Nat Neurosci* 11, 251-253.

Yang, E.J., Jiang, J.H., Lee, S.M., Yang, S.C., Hwang, H.S., Lee, M.S., and Choi, S.M. (2010). Bee venom attenuates neuroinflammatory events and extends survival in amyotrophic lateral sclerosis models. *J Neuroinflammation* 7, 69.

Yang, W.W., Sidman, R.L., Taksir, T.V., Treleaven, C.M., Fidler, J.A., Cheng, S.H., Dodge, J.C., and Shihabuddin, L.S. (2011). Relationship between neuropathology and disease progression in the SOD1(G93A) ALS mouse. *Exp Neurol* 227, 287-295.

Yang, Y., Gozen, O., Watkins, A., Lorenzini, I., Lepore, A., Gao, Y., Vidensky, S., Brennan, J., Poulsen, D., Won Park, J., *et al.* (2009). Presynaptic regulation of astroglial excitatory neurotransmitter transporter GLT1. *Neuron* 61, 880-894.

Yoshii, Y., Otomo, A., Pan, L., Ohtsuka, M., and Hadano, S. (2011). Loss of glial fibrillary acidic protein marginally accelerates disease progression in a SOD1(H46R) transgenic mouse model of ALS. *Neurosci Res* 70, 321-329.

Zhang, X., Chen, S., Li, L., Wang, Q., and Le, W. (2008). Folic acid protects motor neurons against the increased homocysteine, inflammation and apoptosis in SOD1 G93A transgenic mice. *Neuropharmacology* 54, 1112-1119.

Zhao, P., Ignacio, S., Beattie, E.C., and Abood, M.E. (2008). Altered presymptomatic AMPA and cannabinoid receptor trafficking in motor neurons of ALS model mice: implications for excitotoxicity. *Eur J Neurosci* 27, 572-579.

Zhu, S., Stavrovskaya, I.G., Drozda, M., Kim, B.Y., Ona, V., Li, M., Sarang, S., Liu, A.S., Hartley, D.M., Wu du, C., *et al.* (2002). Minocycline inhibits cytochrome c release and delays progression of amyotrophic lateral sclerosis in mice. *Nature* 417, 74-78.

The Role of TNF-Alpha in ALS: New Hypotheses for Future Therapeutic Approaches

Cristina Cereda[1]*, Stella Gagliardi[1]*,
Emanuela Cova[1], Luca Diamanti[2,3] and Mauro Ceroni[2,3]
[1]*Laboratory of Experimental Neurobiology, IRCCS,
National Neurological Institute "C. Mondino", Pavia,*
[2]*General Neurology Department, IRCCS,
National Neurological Institute "C. Mondino", Pavia,*
[3]*Department of Neurological Sciences, University of Pavia, Pavia,
Italy*

1. Introduction

The pathophysiological origins of neurodegenerative disorders are a complex combination of both environmental and genetic factors. However, in many of these disorders, processes such as inflammation and oxidative stress activate common and final pathways leading to toxicity and cellular death. High levels of oxidative damage within the brain and the activation of neuroinflammation factors are a prominent feature in patients with Alzheimer's disease (AD), Parkinson's disease (PD), Huntington's disease (HD), Amyotrophic Lateral Sclerosis (ALS) and inherited ataxias (Halliwell, 2006; Lin & Beal, 2006). Regarding the immunological point of view, the brain was considered an immune privileged organ because it was isolated from the systemic circulation by protective blood-brain barrier that controls the infiltration of pathogens, the transition of pro or anti inflammatory factors and peripheral blood cells (Itzhaki et al., 2004). Despite that, in recent years, the relationship between neuroinflammation and neurodegeneration has been described with particular attention to the lymphocytes activation and cytokines production (Appel, 2009; Tansey et al., 2007). Moreover, it is well known the implication of glial cells in the progression of neurodegeneration: they are involved in many types of damage, they migrate to the damaged cells and also they have a role in clearing the debris of the dead cells. Through such processes, microglia releases reactive oxygen species, proinflammatory cytokines, complement factors, and neurotoxic molecules, leading to further neuronal dysfunction and death (Heneka et al., 2011; Lasiene et al., 2011). In addition, the implication of the peripheral system and its participation in the cellular mechanisms that direct to neurodegeneration, as white blood cells, is well documented (Calvo et al., 2010; Ghezzi et al., 1998; Gowing et al., 2006). Many data from autoptic spinal cord and blood examinations of the ALS patients, animal and cellular models support an immune system involvement in ALS pathogenesis. Since

---

These authors contributed equally to this work.

1984 the presence of an autoimmunity component in ALS was proven when immunoglobulin depositories have been described in spinal cord (Donnenfeld et al., 1984). At present the implication of the neuronal and non-neuronal immunological cells and activation of the inflammatory processes have been extensively described in ALS (Engelhardt et al., 1995; Henkel et al., 2004; Troost et al., 1990).

Starting from literature data about implication of the innate and adaptive immunity in ALS, we would like to point out the role of the TNF alpha (TNF-α) system and its interactions in ALS pathway with particular attention to SOD1 protein, the most important player in the ALS pathogenesis. We will focus this book section on TNF-α cytokine because its involvement both in immunological pathways and in oxidative stress is known in ALS disease. Moreover we will try to define the immunological actors that exert a protective function and how they could be used in a possible therapy.

2. ALS and immunity

In the last decades, increasing numbers of experimental and clinical observations have reported inflammatory reactions in ALS tissues which indicate the involvement of both the innate and adaptive immune responses (Fig. 1) (McGeer & McGeer, 2006; Moisse & Strong, 2006; Sta et al., 2011; Weydt et al., 2002).

So far it is not clear how immune system is involved in ALS disease, whether the adaptive or innate immunity has a major role and whether immunity is part of damaging or neuroprotective response to the pathological process.

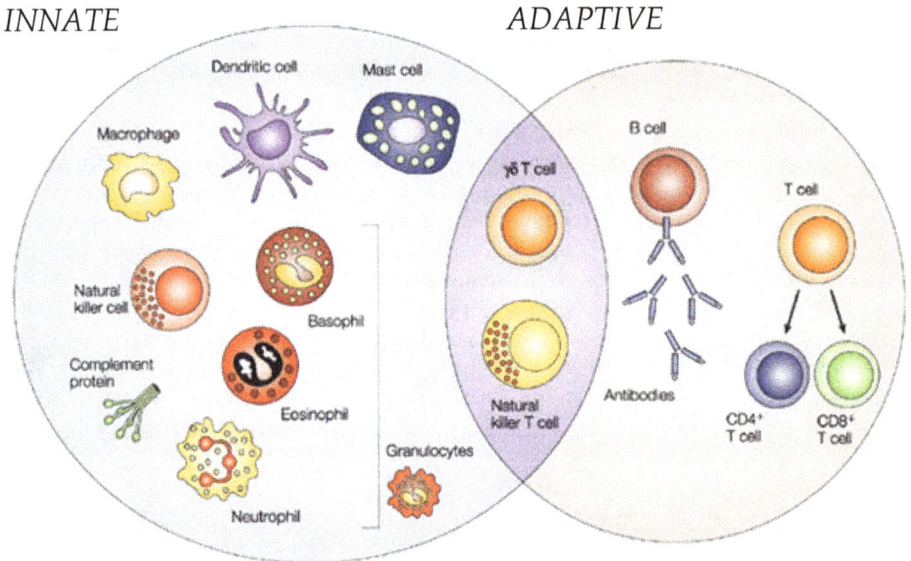

Fig. 1. Innate and adaptive immunity.

2.1 Innate immune system

Innate immunity is naturally present and is not stimulated by antigens or mediated by antibodies. It is therefore non-specific and is executed by a variety of cells: granulocytes, as eosinophils and basophils, white blood cells as natural killer and mast cells. Instead, microglia belongs to the central nervous system and is involved in the local innate immunity. Inflammation is one of the aspects of the innate immune response.

Interactions between innate immune system, brain and neurodegenerative diseases are known (Ghezzi et al., 1998; Gowing et al., 2006) and it has been reported that mast cells, macrophages, dendritic cells, microglia, complement and cytokines participate in limiting the damage (Calvo et al., 2010).

Innate system was found activated in central and in peripheral system of ALS patients (Chandels et al., 2001; Elliott et al., 2001; Sta et al., 2011).

Several studies regarding peripheral innate immune system changes in sporadic ALS reveal that there are increased levels of circulating monocytes and macrophages (Harman et al., 1991; Hemnani et al, 1998). The presence of T cells, IgG, activated microglia, macrophages, and reactive astrocytes, as well as other indications of inflammation are found in ALS spinal cord tissue (Henkel et al., 2004; Engelhardt et al., 1995; Troost et al., 1990).

In ALS there is morphological and neurochemical evidence for the proliferation and activation of microglia in areas of significant motor neuron loss, as spinal cord (Henkel et al., 2004; Kawamata et al., 1992; Moisse et al., 2006). This activation may be a consequence of stressed neurons that induced proliferation and activation of microglial cells activating complement system and pro-cytokine response involved in neuronal death (Fig. 2). Motor neuron loss and immune system activation may increase neuron stress leading to increase of neuroinflammation.

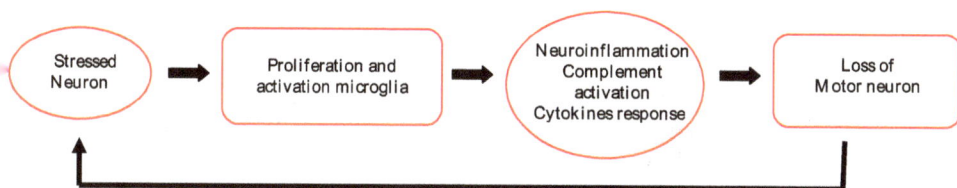

Fig. 2. Hypothesis of activation of innate immunity in ALS.

2.2 Adaptive immune system

As innate immunity, adaptive immunity has a role in ALS (Sta et al., 2011). Unlike innate immune responses, the adaptive responses are highly specific and they consist of antibodies, lymphocytes activation and cell mediated response. The cells of the adaptive immune system are B and T lymphocytes: B cells, which are derived from the bone marrow, become the cells that produce antibodies. T cells can cross-talk with neurons and microglia, and either damage or protect neurons from stressful stimuli (Alexaniu et al., 2001), also in spinal cord and brain (Chiu et al., 2008).

T-helper cells have been observed in proximity of degenerating corticospinal tracts; T-helper and T-suppressor cells, with a variable number of macrophages, have been found in ventral horns of the spinal cord (Troost et al., 1990).

Infiltration of T cells compatible with adaptive response have been found in the areas of motor neuron destruction in the CNS but no correlation was found between clinical parameters and infiltrating T cells (Holmoy et al., 2008). The majority of T cells characterized in the infiltration were CD8+ cytotoxic T cells, but a substantial number of T CD4+ cells were also present (Beers et al., 2008).

Alterations of total lymphocyte count (Provinciali et al., 1988; Tavolato et al., 1975) and T subset distribution in peripheral system of ALS patients (Westall et al., 1983) have been reported. Low T cells numbers and decreased proliferative capacity in T cells are found in the blood of ALS patients (Holmoy et al., 2008).

As concerned CD8+ and natural killer T cells, they were found increased in ALS patients compared to control cohort (Rentzos et al., 2011).

Interestingly, ALS patients showed a reduction of CD4+/CD25+ regulatory T cells that are known to interact with the local microglia, reinforcing the hypothesis of the involvement of the adaptive immune system associated with neuroinflammatory process in ALS (Mantovani et al., 2009). Beers and colleagues (Beers et al., 2011) observed that regulatory T cells as CD4+/CD25+/FoxP3 correlated with disease progression; in fact, the number of T cells were found inversely correlated with disease progression rate.

Animal studies showed that in ALS model T cells deficiency decreases microglia reactivity and accelerates ALS disease progression; specific and progressive accumulation of monocytes/macrophages was observed along the length of degenerating nerve fibers and activated microglia was detected in spinal cord of ALS model mice (Chiu et al., 2009).

No infiltrating B-cells have been found even if a role of B lymphocytes in the pathogenesis of ALS has been hypothesized, as secreted autoantibodies by B cells identified in CSF and serum from ALS patients (Naor et al., 2009).

As concern antibodies, since the eighties the presence of IgG in serum or tissues of ALS patients has been documented (anti-ganglioside GM1, anti-sulfoglucuronyl paragloboside, anti-neurofilaments and anti-Fas) (Sengun & Appel, 2003; Yi et al., 2000). Indeed, IgG deposits have been demonstrated in motor cortex, spinal cord and in motor neurons from ALS patients (Donnenfeld et al., 1984; Engelhardt & Appel, 1990; Fishman & Drachman, 1995). Serum immunoglobulins from ALS patients showed enhanced binding to rat spinal cord cells *in vitro* (Digby et al., 1985), demonstrating cytotoxic effects when they were added to a motor neuron cell cultures (Alexianu et al., 1994; Demestre et al., 2005) and that the presence of an immune response to spinal cord cell membrane components in patients with motor neuron disease was a damaging event.

IgG from ALS patients reacts with the skeletal muscle DHP (bisognerebbe spiegare cosa è)-sensitive Ca^{2+} channels reducing the peak of the Ca^{2+} current and the charge movement in single cut fibres from the rat extensor muscle (Delbono et al., 1991). About 60% of ALS sera contained different monoclonal immunoglobulins: in particular IgG (72.7%) and IgM (27.3%) have been found (Duarte et al., 1991).

2.3 Cytokines

Different interactions have been found between innate and adaptive immunity in ALS, as concern cytokines involvement. Cytokines have an effect on the expression of other inflammatory factors and on each other, and these functional relationships are non-linear: the causal relationships of cytokines and disease are complex and difficult to prove (Marklund et al., 1992).

Several studies regarding immune system changes in sporadic ALS reveal that there are increased levels of circulating monocytes and macrophages, producing cytokines as IL-1 and IFN-γ, (Harman et al., 1991; Hemnani et al., 1998). Furthermore, high cytokine levels have been described in plasma, serum and cerebral fluid (CSF) from ALS patients and sometimes correlate with the clinical status (Kelly et al., 1994; Lee et al., 2005; Khule et al., 2009; Tateishi et al., 2010).

As concern inflammatory cytokines (IL-7, 9, 12, 17 and IL-1β) levels were found higher in CSF of sporadic ALS patients (Tateishi et al., 2010). IL-15 and IL-12 serum levels, they also have been found higher in patients with ALS (Rentzos et al., 2010). The same authors measured IL-17 and IL-23 levels in serum and CSF from ALS patients that were found increased compared to controls (Rentzos et al., 2010). TGF-β1 concentrations in the serum and CSF of ALS patients did not differ from controls, but TGF-β1 serum concentration was significantly higher in ALS patients at the terminal clinical status (Ilzecka et al., 2002). Higher amount of IL-6 has been found in sera and CSF from sporadic ALS patients and it has been related to hypoxemia severity rather than pathological condition (Moreau et al., 2005).

Plasma concentration of TNF-α, TNF-R1 and TNF-R2 and their time course during disease progression were studied in ALS patients in order to assess the TNF-α system implication in ALS pathogenesis. In all plasma patients soluble forms of the TNF-α and its receptors are found increased already at disease onset and remain over the normal range during the disease progression time (Cereda et al., 2008). In addition TNF-α amounts have been found higher in sera from sporadic ALS patients but no correlation was found with the clinical criteria (Poloni et al., 2000; Cereda et al., 2008). TNF-α role in neurodegeneration will be further highlight in the next paragraph.

3. Tumor necrosis factor-alpha (TNF-α)

The Tumour Necrosis Factor Alpha (TNF-α) is a pro-inflammatory cytokine produced by monocytes/macrophages and activated by mast cells, endothelial cells, fibroblasts, neurons and glial cells during acute inflammation and it is responsible for a wide range of cell signals about cell viability, gene expression, homeostasis control and synaptic integrity.

TNF-α was described for the first time by Carswell et al. in 1975 as a protein component of serum of mice stimulated with bacterial antigens, and was brought to light the ability to induce death in cancer cell lines in vitro and in vivo to destroy transplanted sarcomas. Characteristically, this cytokine was able to cause tumor cells death without compromising the viability of healthy cells. The subsequent isolation and molecular characterization of the gene have provided information on the structure and functioning of this molecule.

3.1 TNF-α gene

The gene coding for TNF-α is located on chromosome 6 within the region encoding the Major Histocompatibility Complex (MCH), HLA in human, between the HLA-DR class II and HLA-B class I genes (Fig. 3). Its location and strict linkage disequilibrium present between some alleles of class I and class II genes has permitted to hypothesize associations between TNF-α alleles and some diseases. The gene for TNF-α include about 3 Kb and contains four exons (almost 80% of the protein is codified by the exon four) and three introns.

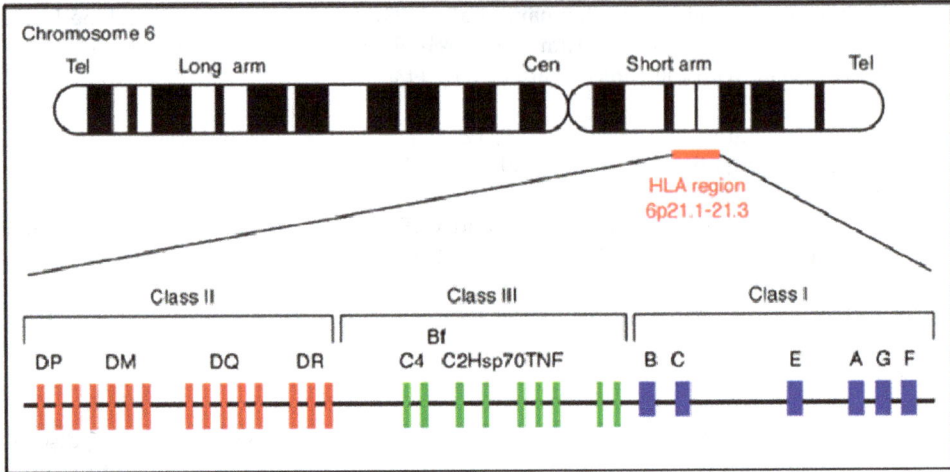

Fig. 3. Localization of TNF-α gene on chromosome 6 (6p21.3)

TNF-α gene codifies for a protein of 233 amino acids with a molecular weight of 25.6 kDa. TNF-α is, at the beginning, a transmembrane protein of 212 amino acids associated to homotrimers; the N-terminal portion loses 76 amino acid by cleavage of TNF-α converting enzyme (TACE or ADAM-17), producing a soluble monomeric TNF-α form (17 kD) and next, the trimetric form of 51 kD (Bazzoni & Beutler, 1996; Reddy et al., 2000).

The trimer is the biological active soluble form because of its ability to bind its receptors. However, the trimeric soluble form spontaneously tends to dissociate into a monomeric inactive form, that is a physiological process that allows to limit the deleterious effects of excessive concentration of TNF-α (Smith et al., 1987).

TNF-α response to a variety of extracellular signals is very rapid and transient and includes a transcriptional component as well as posttranscriptional events. Its transcriptional control occurs predominantly at the level of transcriptional initiation.

The approximately 1000 base pairs of the TNF-α gene's 5' flanking region contains a number of important regulatory elements that affect TNF-α transcription in response to various stimuli. The basic promoter region is defined by TATA box sequence, located about 20 bp upstream from the transcription site and about 200 bp form the translation start codon. Multiple potential regulatory sites, including consensus sequences for the AP-1 (Activator Protein-1) and AP-2 (Activator Protein-2) sites, the cAMP-responsive element, and sequences similar to the NF-kB, (Nuclear Factor kappa-light-chain-enhancer of activated B cells) sequences found in immunoglobulin and cytokine regulatory elements are present in 5' flanking region. This sequence has been demonstrated to be responsive to LPS (lipolysaccharide) and TNF-α stimulation. The 3' untranslated region contains a sequence element affecting posttranslational control of TNF-α through mRNA stability and translation efficiency.

Many polymorphisms have been described in TNF-α promoter region (-308, -857, -863, -238, -1031) defining its correlation with TNF-α mRNA amounts: wild-308G allele is responsible for a higher transcription gene (Helmig et al., 2011), as the A mutated allele at position -857 results in a high production of TNF-α (McCusker et al., 2001).

As concerned -238 polymorphism, has been described a direct effect on gene expression, although studies suggest that this region contains a strong repressor site (-280 to -172). -238 TNFG/A allele genotype may be in linkage disequilibrium with a functional polymorphism that impacts TNF production (Liu et al., 2008).
Several of these polymorphisms have been studied extensively in some diseases, mainly -308 and -857 SNPs.
The mutated allele -308A is a marker of susceptibility to several autoimmune and inflammatory diseases such as lupus erythematosus, celiac disease and Alzheimer's disease (Candor et al., 2002 and 2004), but so far it has been published in a very large number of works in order to reach the correct conclusions on the role of these polymorphisms.
Most SNPs (-863, -238, -1031) do not affect the levels of expression but their pathologic involvement is related to the variation of allelic or genotypic frequencies.
As concerned SNPs in coding region, some polymorphisms are described (http://www.ncbi.nlm.nih.gov/SNP) but they are not correlated with any diseases or functions.

3.2 TNF-α protein function

The functions of TNF-α are biologically dependent on the amount of cytokine produced. If it is present in small amounts, TNF-α acts locally as autocrine and paracrine mediator of inflammation in leukocytes and endothelial cells, determines the expression of surface receptors for leukocyte migration, acting as an angiogenic factor, such as fibroblast growth factor and induces apoptosis in certain cell types. If it is present in high amounts, however, is distributed in the systemic circulation where it stimulates the production of IL-1 and IL-6 by leukocytes and the synthesis of acute phase proteins in the liver (such as fibrinogen) and activates the intravascular thrombus formation.
TNF-α exerts many of its effects by binding, as a trimer, the cell membrane receptor TNF-R1 of 55 kDa (p55) or TNF-R2 of 75 kDa (p75) belonging to the superfamily of TNF receptors, which also includes FAS, CD40, CD27 and RANK.
TNF-R1 is expressed in almost all tissues and may be activated by trimeric soluble form and also by membrane-associated form of TNF-α; TNF-R2 is expressed only by cells of the immune system and it is activated only by trimeric soluble form of the TNF-α. Differently from TNF-R1, TNF-R2 do not own a death domain (DD), and its activation may only induce the survival pathway (Fig. 4).
Instead, the binding of TNF-α to the TNF-R1 may cause both cell death or survival depending on which pathway is activated and it also depends on the second signal involved (Hsu et al., 1996; Darnay et al.,1997). Following the binding of TNF-α, TNF-R1 produces a conformational change that determines the separation of the intracellular death domain (DD). This dissociation allows the adapter protein TRADD to bind the domain of death (DD) to induce apoptosis or form a platform for the subsequent binding proteins to make cell survival. If TRADD directly binds FADD, which in turn recruits caspase-8, the apoptosis way is activated. High concentrations of caspase-8 induce its proteolytic activation and subsequent cleavage of downstream caspases, leading to cell apoptosis. Cell death induced by TNF-α plays a minor role compared to the role of this cytokine in inflammation. Its ability to induce apoptosis is in fact modest when compared to that of other members of the family as Fas and often masked by the anti-apoptotic effects.

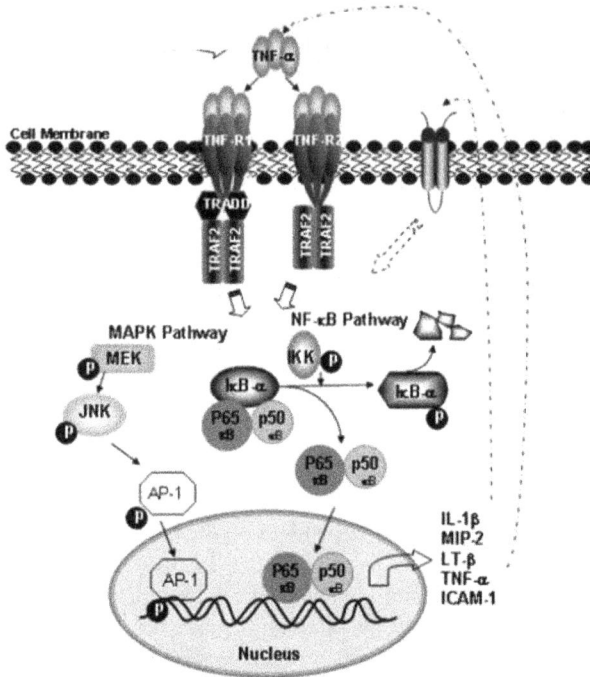

Fig. 4. TNF-α and TNFR pathway (Rosenquist M., 2003)

Both TNF-α receptors activate different survival intracellular signalling pathways, especially because of the IkB kinase (IKK) and the cascade of MAP kinases (MAPKs) that control the gene expression through NF-kB, and AP-1 respectively. In detail the term NF-kB refers to a family of five structurally-related transcription factors (p50, p52, RelA/ p65, c-Rel and RelB), all containing the Rel homology domain (RHD) within the N-terminus and acting as homo- and heterodimeric DNA binding complexes (O'Dea et al., 2010). Several studies showed that NF-kB activity is induced in most cell types in response to a broad variety of stimuli, ranging from cytokines, radiation and reactive oxygen species (ROS) (such as exposure to H_2O_2), with major roles in coordinating innate and adaptative immunity, cell activation and proliferation, survival, development and apoptosis (Ghosh et al., 2008; Vallabhapurapu et al., 2009).

TRADD recruits TRAF2 (TNF receptor-associated factor 2) and RIP (receptor interacting protein). TRAF2 in turn recruits the protein kinase IKK (inhibitor of nuclear factor kappa-B kinase), which is activated by RIP. The IKBα inhibitory protein that normally binds the NF-kB and inhibits its translocation, is phosphorylated by IKK and then is degraded, releasing NF-kB. The latter NF-kB is a transcription factor that translocates into the nucleus and mediates the transcription of a wide variety of genes and theirs products involved in survival and cell proliferation, in the inflammatory response and anti-apoptotic factors.

As concerns the activation of MAP kinase (MAPK), TNF-α induces a strong activation of JNK (c-Jun N-terminal Kinase), one of three major cascades of MAPK, evokes a moderate response of the p38-MAPK, and is responsible of a minimal activation of ERK. TRAF2 actives MEKK1 and ASK1 directly or indirectly, which phosphorylate MKK7, which in turn activates JNK. The latter AP-1 translocates into the nucleus and activates transcription factors such as c-Jun and AFT2. The way of JNK is involved in differentiation, cell proliferation and apoptosis.

3.3 TNF-α and nervous system

In the central nervous system TNF-α is produced by astrocytes, microglia and neurons in response to several stimuli both intra and extracellular, and seems to play a central role in the genesis and perpetuation of neuroinflammatory signal. An alteration in the regulatory mechanisms of TNF-α was found in a wide variety of disorders such as depression, carcinogenesis, and Alzheimer's disease. In the nervous system different TNF-α activities were defined, as inducer or inhibitor of neuronal apoptosis underlining how complex TNF-α pathway may be.

Moreover, electrophysiological experiments have shown a negative effect determined by TNF-α on neuronal function. Studies of hippocampal sections showed that the addition of pro-inflammatory cytokines decreased the long-term potentiation (Long-term potentiation, LTP), a correlate of learning and memory processes (Tancredi et al., 1992). The mechanism by which this occurs is still under investigation, but it has been suggested that activation of p38 plays a major role in reducing the early phase of LTP in response to TNF-α, while the protein expression changes would play a role in the late phase (Butler et al., 2004).

However, other studies have shown that TNF-α alone is not able to initiate apoptosis in the absence of a second signal and may actually prevent apoptosis in response to certain types of cell damage (Badiola et al., 2009). In fact, although apoptosis is primarily triggered by the TRADD, TNF-α may also be associated with cell survival signals, because it is also able to facilitate the binding of other molecules such as JNK and NF-kB, which were instead important in cells endurance, indicating how complex are the signalling pathways of TNF-α. In fact, TNF-α facilitates axonal regeneration, induces neuronal survival through the anti-apoptotic pathway mediated by NF-kB, limits the demyelination in experimental autoimmune encephalomyelitis, but these effects appear to be highly dose-dependent and related to the exposure time and interaction with other factors (Schwartz et al., 1991).

The protective effect of the cascade triggered by TNF-α has been documented experimentally: mice lacking the receptor for TNF-α were subjected to cerebral ischemia. This result was attributed to an increase of reactive oxygen species, suggesting that TNF-α could induce an antioxidant protection due to ischemic events (Bruce et al., 1996). Similarly, in a model of glutamatergic excitotoxicity, stimulation of TNF-R2 with TNF-α led to protection against this toxicity (Marchetti et al., 2004). In conclusion, these data suggest that TNF-α could affect neuronal viability in different ways depending on the receptor subtype involved and the presence/absence of secondary signals from endogenous or exogenous stimuli.

In neurodegenerative disease, as Parkinson's (PD) and Alzheimer's (AD), neuroinflammatory processes appear to play key roles in neuronal dysfunction and death (Hakansson et al., 2005). TNF-α was found increased in striatum and CSF from PD patients compared to controls (Nagatsu et al., 2000), and a large number of TNF-α immunoreactive glial cells were detected in CSN from PD patients (Imamura et al., 2003).

As concern AD, TNF-α was found upregulated in both CSF and serum, and its levels correlate with disease severity (Dickson, 1997; Fillit et al., 1991; Paganelli et al., 2002); examination of post-mortem AD brains reveals that TNF-α increased and co-localizes with Aβ plaques (Montgomery et al., 2011). AD patients showed elevated levels of TNF-α in the brain (Tarkowski et al., 2000) and in vitro studies have shown that TNF-α induces the production of Aβ peptides through the regulation of the gamma secretase complex (Blasko et al., 1999).

4. TNF-α system and ALS

Starting from TNF-α literature in ALS disease, the data often come from ALS animal model: TNF-α mRNA was found in the spinal cord of G93A mice in the early stages of the disease (4 months of age) in correlation with the astroglia activation (Hensley et al., 2003) . Moreover gene expression in mice increases with age up to a peak at the final stages of the disease (7-8 months). Although transcripts of both receptors, TNF-R1 and TNF-R2, have been identified in the spinal cord of the G93A rat (Elliot et al., 2001; Hensley et al., 2003). Yoshihara et al. (2002) have shown that the expression of TNF-α in the marrow of G93A mice overlaps with the activation of microglia already in a pre-symptomatic stage. Then, using immunohistochemistry approach authors found that TNF-α was located mainly at the level of motor neurons and microglia. Some genes involved in apoptosis showed the same pattern of TNF-α gene expression, suggesting a correlation between the inflammatory reaction and the apoptotic pathway (Yoshihara et al., 2002). To this regard, Hensley et al. (2003) have characterized the relationship between the inflammatory genes, oxidative stress and apoptotic events in the G93A mice. In the spinal cord of mice at the presymptomatic stadium expression of FADD and TNF-R1 and many members of the caspase apoptotic cascade were found increased; however, they were expressed at the highest level only in the early stage of the disease, during which an increased protein oxidation was also observed.

Kiaei et al. (2006) have seen an increase in immunoreactivity for TNF-α in sections of the spinal cord of G93A mice and familial or sporadic ALS patients; in G93A mice treatment with thalidomide and lenalidomide, drugs capable of inhibiting the expression of TNF-α, attenuates disease progression was. This result is a further confirmation of the hypothesis that TNF-α plays an important role in the pathogenesis of ALS, probably giving rise to an apoptotic pathway (Kiaei et al., 2006).

Veglianese et al. (2006), showed p38MAPK activation in the G93A mice in the presymptomatic stage at the level of motor neurons, and in later phase also in astrocytes and microglia. It has also been demonstrated to be involved in the activation of kinases upstream of MAPK pathway. An increased expression of both receptors of TNF-α is also observed in the presymptomatic stage, confirming the activation, mediated by TNF-α, of the signalling cascade that leads to MAPK. The MAPK seems to be implicated in the development and disease progression in G93A mice, as already said. Once activated it is able to phosphorylate neurofilaments, causing their accumulation within motor neurons, which is considered one of the pathogenetic features of ALS. In addition, p38MAPK is able to stimulate nitric oxide synthase in neurons and in glia, leading to the formation of peroxynitrite (Wengenack et al., 2004). The generation of SOD1 knock-out mice for TNF-α, however, has shown that the absence of TNF-α has no effect on axonal degeneration but influences onset, severity and progression of the disease in G93A mice; these data suggest that TNF-α, despite its high expression during disease, is not the only factor involved in the degeneration caused by mutations in SOD1 motor neurons in animal models (Gowing et al., 2006).

4.1 TNF-α level in peripheral blood of ALS patients

TNF-α and its soluble receptors, sTNFRs, were already found significantly higher in plasma of ALS patients than in those of healthy controls (Poloni et al., 2000). They found a significant correlation between levels of TNF-α and sTNF-R1 and sTNF-R2, confirming that a general activation of the TNF-α system occurred in ALS patients. Activation of the TNF-α system however did not correlate neither with the disease duration nor with the disease severity. Even after dividing the patients in two subgroups, with high and low TNF-α levels, they did not find any difference in terms of clinical parameters of the disease (Poloni et al., 2000).

Our research group analyzed the possible implication of TNF-α pathway in ALS pathogenesis (Cereda et al., 2008). We assayed both the levels of TNF-α and its soluble receptors in plasma from ALS patients overtime during disease progression. We assayed the concentrations of TNF-α and its soluble receptors in plasma of 88 patients with sporadic ALS and 40 healthy controls; blood sample from each patient was taken since two months after diagnosis up to death, or along 80 months. We found that circulating levels of TNF-α and its two soluble receptors were significantly increased in the plasma of patients with sporadic ALS. Our data show that TNF-α high plasma concentration is present already at disease onset in the majority of ALS patients and remains over the normal range during the whole disease progression time, even though it slightly decreases during disease progression.

We hypothesised that in the majority of ALS patients TNF-α plasma concentration has already reached its peak at disease onset, remains high during all disease duration and starts to decrease at the end of the disease. This finding suggests that TNF-α pathway could be activated in the first stage of the disease and it decreases its effect with the progression of the disease (Cereda et al., 2008).

4.2 Polymorphisms and TNF-α transcription gene

Preliminary genetic analysis are documented in ALS only about (-308, -857) TNF-α promoter polymorphisms and they do not show statistically significant differences in allelic and genotypic frequencies (Cereda et al., 2008). In 2008 over 100 sporadic ALS patients' DNA samples collected at the Neurological Institute "C. Mondino" (Pavia, Italy) and DNA sample from 228 healthy controls were used to study polymorphisms of TNF-α, TNF-R1 and TNF-R2 genes by RFLP.

In our work we studied -308 G/A and -857 A/G. Moreover, we investigated MspaI polymorphism in exon 1 TNF-R1 gene, a SNP at +36 A/G positions, and Nla III polymorphism in exon 6 TNF-R2 that identified a SNP (T/G) at 196 codon, which leads to an amino acid substitution (Met/Arg). We found no statistically significant differences in allele and genotype frequencies between patients and controls for polymorphisms considered. In our recent work, we performed a molecular study of polymorphisms of many cytokines (IL-1α, IL-1β, IL-1R, IL-1R, IL-4Rα, IL-12, IFN-γ, TGF-β1, IL-2, IL-4, IL-6, IL-10) including -238 TNF-α on 70 ALS patients (unpublished data). Although no difference was found in allele frequencies of this polymorphism, we observed a statistical significance in AA genotype of the TNF-α -238 SNPs comparing ALS patients respect to healthy control. The most common G allele of -238 polymorphism of TNF-α gene is associated with high production of TNF-α (Huizinga et al., 1991; Wilson et al., 1997) but no data is available on the relationship between the minor allele and transcriptional level. Indeed the results obtained from studies on multiple sclerosis, a chronic inflammatory disease, suggest a possible protective effect of A allele in -238 position.

Our study shows that mRNAs of TNF-α were expressed at higher level in lymphocytes of sporadic ALS patients than in controls but there was not relationship with site of disease onset (spinal or bulbar), disease duration at the time of blood sample withdrawal or disease severity. We suppose that mRNA level increase may be due to an ALS disease's point common, as oxidative stress involvement, in all patients analyzed (Carrì et al., 1997; Ciriolo et al., 2002). Interaction between TNF-α, oxidative stress and SOD1 will be better described in the next paragraph.

4.3 TNF-α and SOD1 pathways

Several data support the hypothesis that TNF-α and SOD1 may not only take part to a common cellular pathway but they may also regulate directly and indirectly their self. In fact, an inverse correlation between the expression of SOD1 and TNF-α has been described: cytotoxic effects of TNF-α can be reduced by increasing levels of SOD1 as inhibition of SOD1 mRNA and protein may result in a decrease in the protective effect of SOD1 against inflammation (Meier et al.,1989; Wong & Goeddel ,1988).

In 2006 Afonso and collaborators demonstrated that, in U937 cells, TNF-α down-regulated SOD1 protein expression in a time-dependent manner (Alfonso et al., 2006). Afonso and colleagues performed different experiments treating U937 cells with TNF-α (10 ng/ml) for 1, 4 , 24 hours and their data showed a decline of SOD1 mRNA at 1 hour (22%), maximal suppressor at 4 h (54%) and lesser at 24h (38%).

Although SOD1 activity is modified in some specific situations, the direct effect of the proinflammatory cytokine TNF-α on SOD1 promoter has not been reported. Variable results were reported regarding SOD1 regulation by TNF-α (Chovolou et al.,2003), confirmed by gene expression studies that show the same tendency of SOD1 and TNF-α and suggest that these two genes may have a common system, or, at least, they may take part to the same one.

As concern SOD1 and TNF-α, it is well documented that both TNF-α and SOD1 pathways are regulated by reactive oxygen species (ROS) concentration and we suppose that oxidative stress is a common regulation point thought NF-kB activation.

The important role of ROS is reported in TNF-α signalling although it is unclear whether the TNF-α action may be producer or reducer of ROS concentration. In fact, TNF-α has been reported to increase ROS production from electron transport in mitochondria, plasma membrane NADPH oxidase and cytosolic phospholipase A2-linked cascade through signal transduction pathways triggered by TNFR-related proteins (Chandel et al., 2001; Micheau et al., 2003; Woo et al., 2000). Multimerization of TNFRs may lead to recruitment of TRAFs (TNFR-associated factors) by the receptors resulting in activation of kinases and transcription factors, such as c-Jun and NF-kB (Chandel et al., 2001).

About the reducer role, in a mice model it was demonstrated that TNF-α stimulation in mice deficient in TNF receptor-associated factor 2 (TRAF2) or p65 NF-kB subunit did not induce ROS accumulation, indicating that TRAF-mediated NF-kB activation normally suppresses the TNF-induced ROS accumulation (Sakon et al., 2003). ROS in lower concentrations may function as second messengers in mediating TNF-α activated signal transduction pathways that regulate the NF-kB system (Grisham et al.,1998; Janssen-Heininger et al.,2000).

As concern ROS role, Scott and collaborators demonstrated that ROS may up-regulate TACE activity and consequently, this increased activity may change TNF-α cleavage by TACE (Scott et al., 2011).

In fact, hydrogen peroxide serves as a messenger mediating directly or indirectly the activation of transcription factors such as NF-kB that mediates the induction of various proinflammatory genes (Schreck et al.,1991).

Regarding NF-kB, its pathway is also involved in SOD1, NF-κB was one of the first transcription factor shown to be redox-regulated. Rojo and colleagues (Rojo et al., 2004) showed that cell treatment with H_2O_2 initiates the PI3K/Akt cascades, which participates in NF-κB activation and in subsequent SOD1 transcriptional induction. Indeed, NF-κB binding site was identified in the human SOD1 promoter (GGTAAGTCCC) demonstrating that Akt-activated NF-κB presents increased binding to this sequence, mediating the up-regulation of SOD1 expression.

About ALS disease, we have already underlined the importance of NF-kB role in SOD1 activity, which altered expression and mutations are implicated in ALS disease. Our laboratory studied SOD1 mRNA expression (Gagliardi et al., 2010), we demonstrated that SOD1 mRNA level were altered in ALS patients. In fact we found that the SOD1 gene expression was increased in ALS patients than in controls population. Our unpubblished data show that TNF-α mRNA level is higher in patients' lymphocytes than controls as mRNA SOD1 gene. Unfortunately only few data are available about NF-kB and ALS, that may help to understand the relationship between SOD1 and ALS, so far NF-kB have been studied in ALS mouse model but the inhibition of NF-kB pathway has not effect on the progression of the disease (Crosio et al., 2011).

5. Therapeutic strategies

5.1 Classic immunotherapy in ALS

Several trials both controlled and uncontrolled using immunomodulating agents have been conduced in patients with ALS. These have included plasma exchange, steroids, azathioprine, cyclophosphamide, recombinant human IFN, cyclosporine, immunoglobulin, glatiramer acetate, minocycline.

High-dose therapy with intravenous immunoglobulins was used in ALS, the rationale was strengthened by observations that Ig was effective in improving the muscle strength of patients with a paraproteinemic or conduction block polyneuropathy and also in other autoimmune neuromuscular disease. The authors (Meucci et al. 1996, Dalakas et al. 1994) concluded that IVIg had no apparent therapeutic role in improving the symptoms or arresting the progression in ALS patients (Meucci et al. 1996). Meucci et al included in the study seven patients with a diagnosis of definite or probable ALS according to El Escorial criteria. All patients were treated with intravenous infusions of IVIg 0,4 g/kg/die for 5 consecutive days, followed by monthly, two day infusions at the same daily dosage for 4 to 13 months. All patients were concomitantly treated with oral cyclophosphamide, 1-2 mg/kg/die, as this therapy is effective delaying the frequency of IVIg maintenance infusions in other diseases. The response to treatment was assessed by the Medical Research Council rating scale for muscle strength on ten muscles per limb, a clinical bulbar function scale, a modified Rankin disability scale. The effect of treatment on the progression of the disease was evaluated by comparing the monthly rate of progression of upper and lower limb muscle weakness before and during treatment. All patients continued to deteriorate during treatment, reflected by the worsening of scores after treatment compared with the scores before therapy. The monthly rate of progression of limb weakness during therapy was not better and possibly worse than that estimated in the period before therapy. No major side effect was reported by the patients.

Dalakas and collaborators (Dalakas et al. 1994) used intravenous infusions of high-dose immunoglobulin administered once a month for 3 months (total dose 2g/kg, divided into two daily doses) in nine ALS patients (El Escorial criteria) with a rapidly progressive course of disease. The efficacy of treatment was assessed by objective measurement of maximum voluntary isometric contraction in all muscle groups of two limbs or with Medical Research Council sores, before and after therapy. All patients worsened during the study and, by the end of the third month, their mean total muscle scores had declined. The pace of progression did not change during the observation period. All patients tolerated the intravenous immunoglobulin infusions well and adverse effects were noted.

Another approach was designed by Drachman lab's group (Drachman et al., 1994), who assessed a more powerful and prolonged immunosuppression obtained by total lymphoid irradiation (TLI) in ALS patients. The discovery that TLI produces powerful immunosuppression in humans led to its use in the treatment of autoimmune diseases. The basic principles of TLI therapy involve the lymphoid organs while shielding non-lymphoid tissues and delivering the radiation in multiple small fractions. The study included thirty patients with ALS. The radiation field consisted of an extended mantle, a para-aortic field and an inverted-Y including the spleen. Patients received anterior and posterior irradiation 5 days/week at a rate of 1,8 Gy/day. Blood counts were obtained 1 to 3 times/week as needed to detect haematological toxicity. Four types of parameters of motor function were evaluated: quantitative dynamometry (4 pairs of muscles in the upper extremities and 5 pairs of muscles in the lower extremities), manual muscle testing, functional tests (swallowing, breathing), activity indexes. Tests of immune function were: leukocytes (absolute lymphocyte counts, decrease in CD4 cells, CD4/CD8 ratio), cell-mediated immunity (negative conversion of skin tests), humoral immunity (tetanus antibody response). To assess whether the effectiveness of immunosuppression had an influence on the course of ALS, they analysed the relationships between parameters of immunosuppression and the measures of progression of ALS. This analysis showed that evidence of more effective immunosuppression did not correlate with a more favourable disease course.

Another immunotherapy tried in ALS was liquorpheresis (Andrich et al. 1996; Finsterer et al., 1999) with no results both in sporadic and familial ALS.

IFNs alpha and beta cytokines can regulate the major histocompatibility complex and the presentation of antigens to T-cell receptors. They have been used in variable doses for up to 6 months in small trials in ALS patients with negative results, however the small sample size, the possibility inadequate dose and the short period of follow-up prevented definite conclusions about the efficacy of IFNs. For these reasons a study was undertaken in which recombinant IFNbeta-1a was used in a large patient population at a dose twice as large as that found to be effective in patient with MS. Beghi et al. (2000) recruited patients with 6 to 24 months history of confirmed ALS, that received 12 mIU of IFN subcutaneously three times a week for 6 months and were followed up for an additional 6 months. Medical Research Council scale, Norris scale, bulbar scores were used to assess disability; selected electrophysiologic measures were also used. There were no significant differences of disease progression and disability in patients treated with IFN. Common adverse events were flu-like syndrome, local erythema, gastrointestinal symptomps.

Glatiramer acetate (GA) is a synthetic copolymer composed of four amino acids, used in MS for reduction of the frequency of relapses. GA induces a wide variety of actions on T-cells and leads to generalized, antigen-non-specific alterations of various types of antigen presenting cells in such a way that they stimulate Th2-like responses. It blocks the release of TNF-α and interleukin in monocytes and dendritic cells. So GA has neuroprotective as well as immunomodulatory actions. Meininger and collaborators (Meininger et al., 2009) recruited patients with El Escorial definite, probable or laboratory probable ALS of less than three years duration. Patients were given 40 mg GA daily for a period of 52 weeks. The prospectively defined primary efficacy outcome was the slope of ALSFRS score, the secondary efficacy outcome was time to death, tracheostomy or positive pressure ventilation more than 23 h per day. Additional functional endpoints included mean change from baseline and across visits in ALSFRS score, manuasl muscle testing score and slow vital capacity. GA was shown to be safe and well tolerated, the most significant adverse event was the injection site reaction. This study suggested that glatiramer acetate didn't show any beneficial effect in ALS patients either for course or survival.

Minocycline has anti-apoptotic and anti-inflammatory effects in vitro in CNS, so several trials are planned or are in progress to assess whether minocycline slows human neurodegeneration. Gordon (Gordon et al., 2007) did a multicentre trial in which patients with diagnosis of ALS (according to El Escorial criteria) received minocycline escalating doses of up to 400 mg/day for 9 months (started at 100 mg twice per day and increased every week by 50 mg twice per day to the highest dose of 400 mg). The primary outcome measures was the changes in ALSFRS-r, the secondary outcome measures were forced vital capacity, manual muscle testing, quality of life, time of tracheostomy, chronic assisted ventilation, survival and safety. ALSFRS-r score deterioration was faster in the minocycline group of patients and greater mortality during the 9-months treatment phase was registered in the same group.

Adverse events were most commonly reported in the respiratory system, gastrointestinal system (nausea, diarrhoea, costipation), neurological system (dizziness, fatigue).

5.2 TNF-α and new approaches in immunotherapy

The discovery, in 1988, of a naturally occurring TNF-α inhibitor in human urine (Seckinger et al., 1990), which was identified as a soluble form of the TNF-receptor that acted by neutralizing the cytokine, opened the way to immunotherapy. Subsequently two TNF-binding proteins were purified that were capable of inhibiting the binding of TNF-α to cells (Engelmann et al., 1990). The identification of soluble TNF-α receptors paved the way for the development of soluble TNF-α receptors antibodies currently used for the treatment of several systemic inflammatory diseases, including rheumatoid arthritis, juvenile polyarticular rheumatoid arthritis, inflammatory bowel diseases, psoriatic arthritis and ankylosing spondylitis (Sfikakis et al., 2010).

There are three anti-TNF-α agents approved for clinical use: Etancercept, Infliximab, Adalimumab. The latter two are full-length bivalent IgG monoclonal antibodies specific for sTNF and tmTNF, whereas Etanercept is a genetically engineered Fc fusion protein generated from the extracellular domain of human TNF-R2 and functions as a decoy receptor to block sTNF, tmTNF and distinct ligands of lymphotoxin, a TNF-related protein (Tracey et al., 2005).

The important side effects that have been most extensively related to TNF-α inhibitors include: lymphoma (hepatosplenic T-cell lymphoma in young patients being treated for

Chron disease and ulcerative colitis), infections (fungal infections such as histoplasmosis, coccidioidomycosis, blastomycosis and tuberculosis), congestive heart failure, demyelinating disease, a lupus-like syndrome, induction of auto-antibodies, injection site reactions and systemic side effects (Scheinfeld et al., 2006).

Clinical trials examining the effects of TNF-α inhibition have been conducted on patients with Multiple Sclerosis (MS) and Alzheimer disease (AD).

Strategies to inhibit TNF-α in MS seemed promising in preclinical applications but have widely failed in human clinical trials due to the lack of therapeutic selectivity. During an open-label phase I trial, a monoclonal TNF-α antibody was infused into two human patients exhibiting rapidly progressing disease. Subsequently, in a double-blinded, placebo controlled, multicentered phase II study, 168 relapsing-remitting MS patients were administered Lenercept, a sTNF-R1 fusion protein that neutralizes TNF-α. Lenercept-treated individuals experienced higher occurrence of relapse and increased neurological deficits (Van oosten et al., 1996). The ineffectiveness of anti-TNF-α therapy in MS may be a consequence of divergent roles for the TNF receptors, considering that blocking TNF-R1 in mouse models dampens disease severity, while suppressing TNF-R2, the receptor that induces remyelination and harbors immunosuppressive properties, results in exacerbated disease (Arnett et al., 2001; Kassiotis et al., 2011). Recently, pharmacological agents selectively targeting TNF-R1 have been investigated. Using phage display technology, a TNF-R1 antagonist was developed and upon evaluation in mice it was found that administration of this selective antagonist improved clinical scores, reduced cerebral demyelination and suppressed the number of infiltrating inflammatory cells (Nomura et al., 2011).

TNF-α intervention in AD has been evaluated in open-labeled phase I clinical trials where perispinal extrathecal administration of Etanercept was administered weekly to a small number of patients ranging from mild to severe AD for a short duration of 6 months that claimed substantial cognitive and behavioural improvements, including verbal fluency and aphasia (Tobinick et al., 2006; Tobinick et al., 2008). Currently a phase II study is recruiting to evaluate the safety and tolerability of Etanercept in AD. These results seem promising but conclusions regarding the promise of such a therapeutic strategy should be reserved until after extensive chronic suppression of TNF-α activity is performed in preclinical models and double-blind human clinical trials have been conducted and results critically reviewed by the research community.

Trails on the immunological hypothesis in ALS are not yet established although TNF-α system implications have been described for a long time. This therapeutic approach was not considered using neither synthetic TNF-α-receptor inhibitors nor monoclonal anti-TNF-α antibody.

6. Conclusions

There is no doubt that TNF-α play key roles in degenerative conditions afflicting CNS, also in ALS. The precise role TNF-α plays remain highly controversial due to the complexity and pleiotropic nature of this cytokine and its activities during critical developmental and homeostatic cellular processes. Multiple factors determine whether TNF-α will exert deleterious or beneficial effects for neuronal survival and some of these differential actions relate to its duration of expression, concentration, receptor conformation. Despite the elaborate and promising data collected thus far to assign function to TNF-α in neurodegeneration, surprisingly little is still known about the cellular and stage-specific roles of this cytokine.

The data reported in this chapter also underline the importance of TNF-α pathways in ALS pathology due to the interaction with SOD1 gene.

In fact, the data that demonstrated the down-regulation of SOD1 after treatment with TNF-α (Afonso et al., 2006), related to the up-regulation of SOD1 mRNA expression in ALS patients suggest to carry on the studies about TNF-α in ALS disease to better define the TNF-α function in neurodegeneration. A better understanding of SOD1 regulation related to TNF-α function may permit to develop novel immunotherapy application in ALS disease.

7. Acknowledgement

We are grateful to "our" ALS patients and their families that trust our work. Moreover we would like to thank National and International Research Agencies and Italian Health Minister that found our research projects.

8. References

Aisen P.S., J. Schmeidler, G.M. Pasinetti. (2002). Randomized pilot study of nimesulide treatment in Alzheimer disease. Neurology, 58, 1050-1054.

Aisen P.S., K.A. Schafer, M Grundman, E. Pfeiffer, M. Sano, K.L. Davis, M.R. Farlow, S. Jin, R.G. Thomas, L.J. Thal. (2003). Effects of rofecoxib or naproxen vs placebo on Alzheimer disease progression: a randomized controlled trial. JAMA, 289, 2819-2826.

Aisen P.S., K.L. Davis, J.D. Berg, K. Schafer, K. Campbell, R.G. Thomas, M.F. Weiner, M.R. Farlow, M. Sano, M. Grundman, L.J. Thal. (2000). A randomized controlled trial of prednisone in Alzheimer disease. Neurology, 54, 588-593. Alexianu ME, Kozovska M, Appel SH. (2001) Immune reactivity in a mouse model of familial ALS correlates with disease progression. Neurology.57:1282-1289.

Arnett H.A., J. Mason, M. Marino, K. Suzuki, G.K. Matsushima, J.P. Ting. (2001). TNF-alpha promotes proligeration of oligdendrocyte progenitors and remyelination. Nat Neurosci, 4, 1116-1122.

Badiola N, Malagelada C, Llecha N, Hidalgo J, Comella JX, Sabriá J, Rodríguez-Alvarez J. (Sep 2009). Activation of caspase-8 by tumour necrosis factor receptor 1 is necessary for caspase-3 activation and apoptosis in oxygen-glucose deprived cultured cortical cells. Neurobiol Dis.;35(3):438-47. Epub 2009 Jun 23.

Baker SJ, Reddy EP.Modulation of life and death by the TNF receptor superfamily. Oncogene. (Dec 1998). 24;17(25):3261-70.

Bazzoni F, Beutler B. The tumor necrosis factor ligand and receptor families. N Engl J Med. (Jun 1996) 27;334(26):1717-25.

Beers DR, Henkel JS, Zhao W, Wang J, Appel. (Oct 2008). SH.CD4+ T cells support glial neuroprotection, slow disease progression, and modify glial morphology in an animal model of inherited ALS.Proc Natl Acad Sci U S A. 7;105(40):15558-63. Epub 2008 Sep 22.

Beghi E, A. Chiò, M. Inghilleri, L. Mazzini, A. Micheli, G. Mora, M. Poloni, R. Riva, L. Serlenga, D. Testa, P. Tonali; A randomized controlled trial of recombinant interferon beta-1a in ALS. Neurology,. (2000). 54, 469-474.

Blasko I, Marx F, Steiner. E, Hartmann T, Grubeck-Loebenstein B. (Jan 1999). TNFalpha plus IFNgamma induce the production of Alzheimer beta-amyloid peptides and decrease the secretion of APPs.FASEB J.13(1):63-8.

Bruce AJ, Boling W, Kindy MS, Peschon J, Kraemer PJ, Carpenter MK, Holtsberg FW, Mattson MP. (Jul 1996). Altered neuronal and microglial responses to excitotoxic and ischemic brain injury in mice lacking TNF receptors.Nat Med.2(7):788-94.

Bruijn LI, Houseweart MK, Kato S, Anderson KL, Anderson SD, Ohama E, Reaume AG, Scott RW, Cleveland DW. (Sep 1998). Aggregation and motor neuron toxicity of an ALS-linked SOD1 mutant independent from wild-type SOD1. Science. 281(5384):1851-4.

Butler MP, O'Connor JJ, Moynagh PN. (2004). Dissection of tumor-necrosis factor-alpha inhibition of long-term potentiation (LTP) reveals a p38 mitogen-activated protein kinase-dependent mechanism which maps to early-but not late-phase LTP. Neuroscience.124(2):319-26.

Calvo A., C. Moglia, M. Balma, A. Chiò. (2010). Involvement of immune response in the pathogenesis of Amyotrofic Lateral Sclerosis: a therapeutic opportunity? CNS & neurological disorders – Drugs Targets, , 9, 325-330.

Carlo-Stella N, Badulli C, De Silvestri A, Bazzichi L, Martinetti M, Lorusso L, Bombardieri S, Salvaneschi L, Cuccia M. (2006). A first study of cytokine genomic polymorphisms in CFS: Positive association of TNF-857 and IFNgamma 874 rare alleles. Clin Exp Rheumatol.24:179 182.

Carswell EA, Old LJ, Kassel RL, Green S, Fiore N, Williamson B. (Sep 1975). An endotoxin-induced serum factor that causes necrosis of tumors. Proc Natl Acad Sci U S A.72(9):3666-70.

Cereda C, Boiocchi C, Bongioanni P, Cova E, Guareschi S, Metelli MR, Rossi B, Sbalsi I, Cuccia MC, Ceroni M. (2008). TNF and sTNFR1/2 plasma levels in ALS patients. J Neuroimmunol. 194:123-131,.

Chandel NS, Schumacker PT, Arch RH. (2001). Reactive oxygen species are downstream products of TRAF-mediated signal transduction. J. Biol. Chem. 276: 42728-42736,.

Chiu IM, (2008). T lymphocytes potentiate endogenous neuroprotective inflammation in a mouse model of ALS. Proc Natl Acad Sci USA.;105:17913–17918

Chovolou Y, Watjen W, Kampkotter A, Kahl R. (Aug 2003). Resistance to tumor necrosis factor-alpha (TNF-alpha)-induced apoptosis in rat hepatoma cells expressing TNF-alpha is linked to low antioxidant enzyme expression. J Biol Chem. 8;278(32):29626-32. Epub 2003 May 29.

Crosio C, Valle C, Casciati A, Iaccarino C, Carrì MT. (Mar 2011). Astroglial inhibition of NF-κB does not ameliorate disease onset and progression in a mouse model for amyotrophic lateral sclerosis (ALS). PLoS One. 6(3):e17187.

Cudkowicz ME, Katz J, Moore DH, O'Neill G, Glass JD, Mitsumoto H, Appel S, Ravina B, Kieburtz K, Shoulson I, Kaufmann P, Khan J, Simpson E, Shefner J, Levin B, Cwik V, Schoenfeld D, Aggarwal S, McDermott MP, Miller RG. (May 2010). Toward more efficient clinical trials for amyotrophic lateral sclerosis. Amyotroph Lateral Scler. 11(3):259-65. Review.

Dal Canto MC, Gurney ME. (1994). Development of central nervous system pathology in a murine transgenic model of human amyotrophic lateral sclerosis. Am J Clin Pathol.;145:1271–9.

Dalakas M.C., D.P. Stein, C. Otero, E. Sekul, E.J. Cupler, S. McCrosky. (1994). Effect of high-dose intravenous immunoglobulin on ALS and multifocal motor neuropathy. Arch. Neurol., , 51, 861-864

Darnay BG. and Aggarwal B.B., (1997). Early events in TNF signaling : a story of associations and dissociations. Journal of Leukocyte Biology 61:559-566

Dickson DW (1997) The pathogenesis of senile plaques. J Neuropathol Exp Neurol 56:321–339

Drachman D.B, V. Chaudhry, D. Cornblath, R.W. Kuncl, A. Pestronk, L. Clawson, E.D Mellits, S. Quaskey, T. Quinn, A. Calkins, S. Order. (1994). Trial of immunosuppression in ALS using total lymphoid irradiation. Ann. Neurol., 35, 142-150

Elliott J.L., (2001). Cytokine upregulation in a murine model of familial amyotrophic lateral sclerosis. Brain Res. Mol. Brain Res. 95:172-178

Engelhardt JI, Tajti J, Appel SH. Lymphocytic infiltrates in the spinal cord in amyotrophic lateral sclerosis. Arch Neurol 1993;50:30 –36.

Engelmann H., D. Novick, D. Wallach. (1990). Two TNF-binding proteins purified from human urine, evidence for immunological cross-reactivity with cell surface TNF-receptors. J. Biol. Chem., , 265, 1531-1536.-Estevez AY, O'Regan MH, Song D, Phillis JW. (1999). Hyposmotically induced amino acid release from the rat cerebral cortex: role of phospholipases and protein kinases. Brain Res. Oct 9;844(1-2):1-9.

Fillit H, Ding WH, Buee L, Kalman J, Altstiel L, Lawlor B, Wolf- Klein G (1991) Elevated circulating tumor necrosis factor levels

Finsterer, B. Mamoli. (1999). Liquorpheresis in familial ALS. Spinal Cord., , 37, 592-593

Ghosh S, Hayden MS. (2008). New regulators of NF-κB in inflammation. Nat Rev Immunol 8: 837–848.

Glezer I, Simard AR, Rivest S. (Jul 2007). Neuroprotective role of the innate immune system by microglia. Neuroscience. 147(4):867-83. Apr 24. Review.

Gordon P.H., D.H. Moore, R.G. Miller, J.M. Florence, J.L. Verheijde, C. Doorish, J.F. Hilton, G.M. Spitalny, R.B. MacArthur, H. Mitsumoto, H.E. Neville, K. Boylan, T. Mozaffar, J.M. Belsh, J. Ravits, R.S. Bedlack, M.C. Graves, L.F. Mccluskey, R.J. Barohn, R. Tundan. (2007), Efficacy of minocycline in patients with ALS: a phase III randomized trial. Lancet Neurol., 6, 1045-1053

Gowing G, Dequen F, Soucy G, Julien JP. (2006). Absence of tumor necrosis factor-alpha does not affect motor neuron disease caused by superoxide dismutase 1 mutations. J Neurosci. 26(44):11397-402

Grisham MB, Granger DN, Lefer DJ. (1998). Modulation of leukocyte-endothelial interactions by reactive metabolites of oxygen and nitrogen: relevance to ischemicheart disease. Free Radic. Biol. Med. 25: 404-433.

Halliwell B. (Jun 2006). Oxidative stress and neurodegeneration: where are we now? J Neurochem.97(6):1634-58. Review.

Hemnani T and Parihar MS. (1998). Reactive oxygen species and oxidative DNA damage. Ind. J. Physiol. Pharmacol. 42: 440-452.

Heneka M. T., J. J. Rodr´ıguez, and A. Verkhratsky. (2010). Neuroglia in neurodegeneration, Brain Research Reviews, vol. 63, no. 1- 2, pp. 189–211.

Hensley K., Fedynyshyn J., Ferrell S., Floyd R.A., Gordon B., Grammas P., Hamdheydari L., Mhatre M., Mou S., Pye Q.N., Stewart C., West M., West S., Williamson K.S. (2003). Message and protein-level elevation of tumor necrosis factor alpha (TNF alpha) and TNF alphamodulating cytokines in spinal cords of the G93A-SOD1 mouse model for amyotrophiclateral sclerosis. Neurobiol. Dis. 14:74-80

Holmøy T. (Apr 2008). T cells in amyotrophic lateral sclerosis. Eur J Neurol.15(4):360-6. Epub 2008 Feb 11. Review.

Hsu H., Shu H.B., Pan M.G., Goeddel D.V., (1996). TRADD-TRAF2 and TRADD-FADD interactions define two distinct TNF receptor 1 signal transduction pathways. Cell 84:299-308

Huizinga TW, Westendorp RG, Bollen EL, Keijsers V, Brinkman BM, Langermans JA, et al. (1997). TNF-alpha promoter polymorphisms, production and susceptibility to multiple sclerosis in different groups of patients. J Neuroimmunol.;72:149 153.

Håkansson A, Westberg L, Nilsson S, Buervenich S, Carmine A, Holmberg B, Sydow O, Olson L, Johnels B, Eriksson E, Nissbrandt H. (2005). Investigation of genes coding for inflammatory components in Parkinson's disease. Mov Disord. May;20(5):569-73.

Iłzecka J, Stelmasiak Z, Dobosz B. (Dec 2002). Transforming growth factor-Beta 1 (tgf-Beta 1) in patients with amyotrophic lateral sclerosis. Cytokine. 7;20(5):239-43.

Ilzecka J, Stelmasiak, Z, Dobosz B. (2002). Transforming growth factor-Beta 1 (tgf-Beta 1) in patients with amyotrophic lateral sclerosis. Cytokine;20:239 243.

Imamura K, Hishikawa N, Sawada M, Nagatsu T, Yoshida M, Hashizume Y. (1988). Distribution of major histocompatibility complex class II-positive microglia and cytokine profile of Parkinson's disease brains.Immunity assessment in the early stages of amyotrophic lateral sclerosis: a study of virus antibodies and lymphocyte subsets. Acta Neurol Scand. Dec;78(6):449-54.

Itzhaki RF, Wozniak MA, Appelt DM, Balin BJ. (2004). Infiltration of the brain by pathogens causes Alzheimer's disease.Neurobiol Aging. May-Jun;25(5):619-27. Review.

Janssen-Heininger YMW, Poynter ME, Baeuerle PA. (2000). Recent advances towards understanding redox mechanisms in the activation of nuclear factor kappaB. Radic. Biol. Med. 28: 1317-1327,

Kassiotis G., G. Kollias. (2001). Uncoupling the proinflammatory from the immunosuppressive properties of TNF at the p55 TNF receptor level: implications for pathogenesis and therapy of autoimmune demyelination. J Exp Med, , 193, 427-434.

Kawamata T, Akiyama H, Yamada T, McGeer PL. (Mar 1992). Immunologic reactions in amyotrophic lateral sclerosis brain and spinal cord tissue.Am J Pathol.140(3):691-707.

Kelly KA, Hill MR, Youkhana K, Wanker F, Gimble JM. (1994). Dimethyl sulfoxide modulates NF-kappa B and cytokine activation in lipopolysaccharide-treated murine macrophages. Infect. Immun. 62: 3122-3128,.

Kiaiei M. et al., (2006). Thalidomide and Lenalidomide extend survival in a transgenic mouse model of amyotrophic lateral sclerosis. The Journal of Neuroscience, 26(9):2467-2473

Kuhle, R. L. P. Lindberg, A. Regeniter, M. Mehling, A. J. Steck, L. Kappos and A. Czaplinski (2009). Increased levels of inflammatory chemokines in amyotrophic lateral sclerosis. European Journal of Neurology, 16: 771-774

Lasiene J, Yamanaka K. Glial cells in amyotrophic lateral sclerosis (2011). Neurol Res Int. 2011;2011:718987. Epub Jun 7.

Lee ,Choi EM. Biochanin A. (2005) stimulates osteoblastic differentiation and inhibits hydrogen peroxide-induced production of inflammatory mediators in MC3T3-E1 cells. Biol. Pharm. Bull. 28:1948-1953

Li N, Karin M. (1999). Is NF-kappaB the sensor of oxidative stress? FASEB J. 13(10):1137-43.

Lin MT, Beal MF. Mitochondrial dysfunction and oxidative stress in neurodegenerative diseases. Nature. 2006 Oct 19;443(7113):787-95. Review.

Liu C, Wang J, Zhou S, Wang B, Ma X. (Sep 2010). Association between -238 but not -308 polymorphism of Tumor necrosis factor alpha (TNF-alpha)v and unexplained recurrent spontaneous abortion (URSA) in Chinese population. Reprod Biol Endocrinol.8:114.

Manna SK, Mukhopadhyay A, Aggarwal BB. (2000). Resveratrol suppresses TNF-induced activation of nuclear transcription factors NF-kappa B, activator protein-1, and apoptosis: potential role of reactive oxygen intermediates and lipid peroxidation. J. Immunol. 164: 6509-6519,.

Mantovani S, Garbelli S, Pasini A, Alimonti D, Perotti C, Melazzini M, Bendotti C, Mora G. (May 2009). Immune system alterations in sporadic amyotrophic lateral sclerosis patients suggest an ongoing neuroinflammatory process. J Neuroimmunol. 210(1-2):73-9.

Marchetti L, Klein M, Schlett K, Pfizenmaier K, Eisel UL. (2004). Tumor necrosis factor (TNF)-mediated neuroprotection against glutamate-induced excitotoxicity is enhanced by N-methyl-D-aspartate receptor activation. Essential role of a TNF receptor 2-mediated phosphatidylinositol 3-kinase-dependent NF-kappa B pathway. J Biol Chem. Jul 30;279(31):32869-81.

McGeer, P.L., McGeer, E.G., (2006). Inflammatory processes in amyotrophic lateral sclerosis. Muscle Nerve 26, 459-470.

Meier B, Radeke HH, Selle S, Younes M, Sies H, Resch K, Habermehl GG. (1989). Human fibroblasts release reactive oxygen species in response to interleukin-1 or tumour necrosis factor-alpha. Biochem. J. 269:539-545,.

Meininger V, V.E. Drory, P.N. Leigh, A. Ludolph, W. Robberecht, V. Silani (2009). Glatiramer acetate has no impact on disease progression in ALS at 40 mg/day: a double-blind, randomized, multicentre, placebo-controlled trial. Amyotrofic Lat. Scler., 10, 378-383

Meucci N, E. Nobile-Orazio, G. Scarlato. (1996). Intravenous immunoglobulin therapy in ALS. J. Neurol., 243, 117-120

Micheau O., J. Tschopp. (2003). Induction of TNF receptor I-mediated apoptosis via two sequential signaling complexes, Cell 114 181-190.

Moisse, K., Strong, M.J. (2006). Innate immunity in amytrophic lateral sclerosis. Biochim. Biophys. Acta 1762, 1083-1093.

Montgomery S.L., W.J. Bowers. (2011). Tumor necrosis factor-alpha and the roles it plays in homeostatic and degenerative processes within the central nervous system. J Neuroimmune Pharmacol,.

Moodie FM, Marwick JA, Anderson CS, Szulakowski P, Biswas SK, Bauter MR, Kilty I, Rahman I. (2004). Oxidative stress and cigarette smoke alter chromatin remodeling but differentially regulate NF-kappaB activation and proinflammatory cytokine release in alveolar epithelial cells. FASEB J. 18: 1897-1899,.

Moon DO, Kim MO, Lee JD, Choi YH, Kim GY. (2009). Rosmarinic acid sensitizes cell death through suppression of TNF-alpha-induced NF-kappaB activation and ROS generation in human leukemia U937 cells. Cancer Lett. 2010 Feb 28;288(2):183-91. Jul 19.

Moreau C, Devos D, Brunaud-Danel V, Defebvre L, Perez T, Destée A, Tonnel AB, Lassalle P, Just N. (Dec 2005). Elevated IL-6 and TNF-alpha levels in patients with ALS: inflammation or hypoxia? Neurology. 27;65(12):1958-60.

Nagatsu T, Mogi M, Ichinose H, Togari A. (Dec 2003). Changes in cytokines and neurotrophins in Parkinson's disease. J Neural Transm Suppl. 2000;(60):277-90. Review. Acta Neuropathol.;106(6):518-26.

Naor S, Keren Z, Bronshtein T, Goren E, Machluf M, Melamed D. (Aug 2009). Development of ALS-like disease in SOD-1 mice deficient of B lymphocytes.J Neurol.256(8):1228-35. Epub 2009 Mar 12.

Nomura et al. T. (2011). Therapeutic effect of PEGylated TNF-R1 selective antagonistic mutant TNF in experimental autoimmune encephalomyelitis mice. J Control Release, 149, 8-14.

O'Dea E, Hoffmann A. (2010) The regulatory logic of the NF-kappaB signaling system. Cold Spring Harb Perspect Biol. Jan;2(1):a000216.

Oppenheim RW. (1996). Neurotrophic survival molecules for motoneurons: an embarrassment of riches. Neuron 17:195–197,

Paganelli R, Di Iorio A, Patricelli L, Ripani F, Sparvieri E, Faricelli R, Iarlori C, Porreca E, Di Gioacchino M, Abate G (2002) Proinflammatory cytokines in sera of elderly patients with dementia: levels in vascular injury are higher than those of mild-moderate Alzheimers disease patients. Exp Gerontol 37:257–263

Pettmann B, Henderson CE (Feb 1998) Neuronal cell death. Neuron 20:633–647. Presence of dendritic cells, MCP-1, and activated microglia/macrophages in amyotrophic lateral sclerosis spinal cord tissue. Ann Neurol. 2004;55(2):221-35.

Provinciali L, Laurenzi MA, Vesprini L, Giovagnoli AR, Bartocci C, Montroni M, Bagnarelli P, Clementi M, Varaldo PE. Reaume AG, Elliott JL, Hoffman EK, Kowall NW, Ferrante RJ, Siwek DF, Wilcox HM, Flood DG, Beal MF, Brown RH Jr, Scott RW, Snider WD. (May 1996) Motor neurons in Cu/Zn superoxide dismutase-deficient mice develop normally but exhibit enhanced cell death after axonal injury.Nat Genet.13(1):43-7.

Reddy P, Slack JL, Davis R, Cerretti DP, Kozlosky CJ, Blanton RA, Shows D, Peschon JJ, Black RA. (2000) Functional analysis of the domain structure of tumor necrosis factor-alpha converting enzyme. J Biol Chem. May 12;275(19):14608-14.

Rentzos M, Evangelopoulos E, Sereti E, Zouvelou V, Marmara S, Alexakis T, Evdokimidis I. (2011). Alterations of T cell subsets in ALS: a systemic immune activation? Acta Neurol Scand. Jun 9. doi: 10.1111/j.1600-0404.2011.01528.x. [Epub ahead of print]

Rentzos M, Rombos A, Nikolaou C, Zoga M, Zouvelou V, Dimitrakopoulos A, Alexakis T, Tsoutsou A, Samakovli A, Michalopoulou M, Evdokimidis I. (2010). Interleukin-15 and interleukin-12 are elevated in serum and cerebrospinal fluid of patients with amyotrophic lateral sclerosis. Eur Neurol.;63(5):285-90. Epub 2010 Apr 14.

Rentzos M, Rombos A, Nikolaou C, Zoga M, Zouvelou V, Dimitrakopoulos A, Alexakis T, Tsoutsou A, Samakovli A, Michalopoulou M, Evdokimidis J. (2010). Interleukin-17 and interleukin-23 are elevated in serum and cerebrospinal fluid of patients with ALS: a reflection of Th17 cells activation? Acta Neurol Scand. Dec;122(6):425-9.

Rojo AI, Salinas M, Martín D, Perona R, Cuadrado A. (2004). Regulation of Cu/Zn-superoxide dismutase expression via the phosphatidylinositol 3 kinase/Akt pathway and nuclear factor-kappaB. J Neurosci. Aug 18;24(33):7324-34.

Rosenquist M. 14-3-3 proteins in apoptosis. Braz J Med Biol Res. (Apr 2003).;36(4):403-8. Epub 2003 Apr 8. Review.

Sakon S, Xue X, Takekawa M, Sasazuki T, Okazaki T, Kojima Y, Piao JH, Yagita H, Okumura K, Doi T, Nakano H. (2003). NF-kappaB inhibits TNF-induced accumulation of ROS that mediate prolonged MAPK activation and necrotic cell death. EMBO J. 22: 3898-3909.

Scharf S., A. Mander, A. Ugoni, F. Vajda, N. Christophidis. (2003) A double-blind, placebo-controlled trial of diclofenac/misoprostol in Alzheimer disease. Neurology, 53, 197-201.

Scheinfeld N. (2004) A comprehensive review and evaluation of the side effects of the TNF blockers etanercept, infliximab and adalimumab. J Dermatolog Treat, 15, 280-294.

Schreck R, Rieber P, Baeuerle PA. (Aug 1991). Reactive oxygen intermediates as apparently widely used messengers in the activation of the NF-kappa B transcription factor and HIV-1. EMBO J.10(8):2247-58.

Schwartz M, Solomon A, Lavie V, Ben-Bassat S, Belkin M, Cohen A. (1991). Tumor necrosis factor facilitates regeneration of injured central nervous system axons. Brain Res. Apr 5;545(1-2):334-8.

Scott AJ, O'Dea KP, O'Callaghan D, Williams L, Dokpesi JO, Tatton L, Handy JM, Hogg PJ, Takata M. (2011). Reactive oxygen species and p38 MAPK mediate TNF-alpha converting enzyme (TACE/ADAM17) activation in primary human monocytes. J Biol Chem. Aug 24. [Epub ahead of print]

Seckinger P., J.H. Zhang, B. Hauptmann, J.M. Dayer. (1990). Characterization of a TNF-alpha inhibitor: evidence of immunological cross-reactivity with the TNF receptor. Proc. Natl. Acad. Sci., 87, 5188-5192.

Sfikakis P.P. (2010). The first decade of biologic TNF antagonists in clinical practice: lessons learned, unresolved issues and future directions. Curr. Dir. Autoimmun, , 11, 180-210.

Smith RA, Baglioni C.The active form of tumor necrosis factor is a trimer.J Biol Chem. (1987) May 25;262(15):6951-4.

Sta M, Sylva-Steenland RM, Casula M, de Jong JM, Troost D, Aronica E, Baas F. (2011). Innate and adaptive immunity in amyotrophic lateral sclerosis: Evidence of complement activation. Neurobiol Dis. [Epub ahead of print]

Stewart W.F., C. Kawas, M. Corrada, E.J. Metter. (1997) Risk of Alzheimer disease and duration of NSAID use. Neurology, 48, 626-632.

Tancredi V, D'Arcangelo G, Grassi F, Tarroni P, Palmieri G, Santoni A, Eusebi F. (1992). Tumor necrosis factor alters synaptic transmission in rat hippocampal slices. Neurosci Lett. Nov 9;146(2):176-8.

Tansey MG, Frank-Cannon TC, McCoy MK, Lee JK, Martinez TN, McAlpine FE, Ruhn KA, Tran TA. (2008). Neuroinflammation in Parkinson's disease: is there sufficient evidence for mechanism-based interventional therapy? Front Biosci. Jan 1;13:709-17. Review.

Tarkowski E, Ringqvist A, Blennow K, Wallin A, Wennmalm A. (2000). Intrathecal release of nitric oxide in Alzheimer's disease and vascular dementia.Dement Geriatr Cogn Disord. Nov-Dec;11(6):322-6.

Tateishi T, Yamasaki R, Tanaka M, Matsushita T, Kikuchi H, Isobe N, Ohyagi Y, Kira JI. (2010). CSF chemokine alterations related to the clinical course of amyotrophic lateral sclerosis. J Neuroimmunol. Apr 8. [Epub ahead of print]

Tavolato BF. (1975). Immunoglobulin G distribution in multiple sclerosis brain. An immunofluorescence study. J Neurol Sci. Jan;24(1):1-11.

Tobinick E., H. Gross, A. Weinberger, H. Cohen. (2006). TNF-alpha modulation for treatment of Alzheimer disease: a 6-month pilot study. MedGenMed, 8, 25.

Tobinick E., H. Gross. (2008). Rapid improvement in verbal fluency and aplasia following perispinal etanercept in Alzheimer disease. BMC Neurol, 8, 27.

Tracey D., L. Klareskog, E.H. Sasso, J.G. Salfeld, P.P. Tak. (2008). TNF antagonist mechanisms of action : a comprehensive review. Pharmacol Ther, 117, 244-279.

Troost D, Van den Oord JJ, Vianney de Jong JM. (1990). Immunohistochemical characterization of the inflammatory infiltrate in amyotrophic lateral sclerosis. Neuropathol Appl Neurobiol. Oct;16(5):401-10.

Van oosten B.W., F. Barkhof, L. Truyen, J.B. Boringa, F.W. Bertelsmann, B.M. Von Blomberg, J.N. Woody, H.P. Hartung, C.H. Polman (1996). Increased MRI activity and immune activation in two multiple sclerosis patients treated with the monoclonal anti-TNF antibody cA2. Neurology, 47, 1531-1534.

Veglianese P, Lo Coco D, Bao Cutrona M, Magnoni R, Pennacchini D, Pozzi B, Gowing G, Julien JP, Tortarolo M, Bendotti C. (2006). Activation of the p38MAPK cascade is associated with upregulation of TNF alpha receptors in the spinal motor neurons of mouse models of familial ALS. Mol Cell Neurosci. 31(2):218-31

Wengenack TM. (2004). Activation of programmed cell death markers in ventral horn motor neurons during early presyntomatic stages of amyotrophic lateral sclerosis in a transgenic mouse model. Brain Res. 1027:73-86

Westall FC, Rubin R, Gospodarowicz D. (1983). Brain-derived fibroblast growth factor: a study of its inactivation. Life Sci. Dec 12;33(24):2425-9.

Weydt, P., Weiss, M.D., Möller, T., Carter, G.T. (2002). Neuro-inflammation as a therapeutic target amyotrophic lateral sclerosis. Curr. Opin. Investig. Drugs 12, 1720–1724.

Wilson AG, Symons JA, McDowell TL, McDevitt HO, Duff GW. (1997). Effects of a polymorphism in the human tumor necrosis factor alpha pronoter on transcriptional activation. Proc Natl Acad Sci USA; 94:3195-3199.

Vlahopoulos S, Boldogh I, Casola A, Brasier AR. (1999). Nuclear factor-kappaB-dependent induction of interleukin-8 gene expression by tumor necrosis factor alpha: evidence for an antioxidant sensitive activating pathway distinct from nuclear translocation. Blood 94: 1878-1889.

Wong GHW and Goeddel DV. (1988). Induction of manganous superoxide dismutase by tumor necrosis factor: possible protective mechanism. Science 242: 941-944.

Woo CH, Eom YW, Yoo MH, You HJ, Han HJ, Song WK, Yoo YJ, Chun JS, Kim JH. (2000). Tumor necrosis factor-alpha generates reactive oxygen species via acytosolic phospholipase A2-linked cascade. J. Biol. Chem. 275: 32357-32362.

Yoshihara T., Ishigaki S., Yamamoto M., Liang Y., Niwa J., Takeuchi H., Doyu M., Sobue G. (2002). Differential expression of inflammation- and apoptosis-related genes in spinal cords of a mutant SOD1 transgenic mouse model of familial amyotrophic lateral sclerosis. J.Neurochem. 80:158-167

Zhao X, Bausano B, Pike BR, Newcomb-Fernandez JK, Wang KK, Shohami E, Ringger NC, DeFord SM, Anderson DK, Hayes RL. (2001). TNF-alpha stimulates caspase-3 activation and apoptotic cell death in primary septo-hippocampal cultures. J Neurosci Res 64:121–131

4

Glial Cells as Therapeutic Targets for ALS

Amanda M. Haidet-Phillips and Nicholas J. Maragakis

*Department of Neurology, Johns Hopkins University, Baltimore, Maryland,
USA*

1. Introduction

Although Amyotrophic Lateral Sclerosis (ALS) is a neurodegenerative disease characterized by motor neuron death, recent studies now implicate the non-neuronal environment as a major contributor to motor neuron loss. This body of evidence has been amassed over the past 10-15 years and highlights glial cells as new therapeutic targets for ALS. Glial cells, once thought to be simply the "glue" of the central nervous system (CNS), are now realized to actively participate in neural transmission and serve complex roles in regulation of the CNS environment.

Several glial cell types including astrocytes, microglia, and oligodendrocytes exist in the CNS; each serves a distinct function. Astrocytes comprise the majority of the CNS cellular space and act to regulate neurotransmitter concentrations at synapses, provide trophic support for neurons, and maintain metabolic and ionic homeostasis. Astrocytes can participate in the immune response, however, microglia serve as the resident immune cell of the CNS. Microglia are mobile, phagocytic, and constantly screening the CNS for possible infection or injury. Upon activation, microglia can secrete pro-inflammatory cytokines and chemokines to promote the clearance of any infectious agents and recruit other immune cells to the site of injury. Depending on the stimuli, microglia also are known to release neurotrophic growth factors and anti-inflammatory molecules to aid in repair and resolution of neural damage. Oligodendrocytes are the myelinating glia of the CNS which intimately interact with, and provide metabolic support to neurons. Oligodendrocytes are capable of producing myelin sheaths which insulate axons and aid in the conduction of action potentials.

Ongoing research strives to define exactly how glial cells affect motor neuron survival in ALS. Furthermore, translation of these studies to the clinical setting begs for novel approaches to treat this new target for ALS.

2. Non-neuronal cells contribute to motor neuron death in ALS

The bulk of work on glial cells in ALS is derived from studies in rodent ALS models. The most widely used ALS models are rodents that ubiquitously express the human mutant superoxide dismutase 1 (SOD1) protein associated with dominantly-inherited familial ALS (fALS) (Gurney et al., 1994). Currently, 12 different SOD1 mutations have been expressed in lines of transgenic mice leading to development of motor neuron disease. By far, the most commonly used model is the SOD1 G93A mutant mouse which contains 25 copies of the human SOD1 G93A transgene corresponding to a 10-15 fold increase in SOD1 protein (Chiu et al., 1995; Gurney et al., 1994). These mice develop a severe motor neuron disease which resembles many of the clinical and pathological features of human ALS. One of the first indications that non-neuronal cells were involved in disease came from studies where the mutant SOD1 gene was expressed only in neurons instead of ubiquitously. Lines of transgenic mice were generated where mutant SOD1 expression was driven by either the Thy1 promoter or neurofilament light chain promoter (Jaarsma et al., 2008; Lino et al., 2002; Pramatarova et al., 2001). In two of these three studies (Lino et al., 2002; Pramatarova et al., 2001), the mice did not develop any neurological disease phenotype leading to the hypothesis that mutant SOD1 must be expressed in multiple cell types to trigger ALS. A subsequent study did report motor neuron disease with neuronal mutant SOD1 expression, however, the disease onset was very late (~500 days of age) and highly variable, suggesting a possible contribution of mutant non-neuronal cells in disease (Jaarsma et al., 2008).

Further studies combining various approaches continue to support this hypothesis (Clement et al., 2003; Miller et al., 2005). To evaluate the contribution of mutant SOD1 expression in different cell populations, chimeric mice were generated from a mixture of wild-type cells and cells that expressed mutant SOD1 (Clement et al., 2003). It was observed that mice with a greater proportion of wild-type cells to mutant SOD1 cells had extended survival. In addition, motor neurons expressing mutant SOD1 that were surrounded by wild-type non-neuronal cells had less severe pathology. Likewise, wild-type motor neurons surrounded by non-neuronal cells expressing mutant SOD1 appeared to be degenerating, suggesting that neighboring non-neuronal cells may play a direct role in the death of MNs. To more directly discern the contribution of mutant SOD1 in motor neurons, transgenic mice were created where mutant SOD1 was removed by Hb9-driven cre recombinase solely in motor neurons. Although these mice have greatly reduced mutant SOD1 expression in motor neurons, they still develop motor neuron disease albeit a significant delay in disease onset (Boillee et al., 2006a). Furthermore, targeting only the motor neurons with an siRNA to reduce mutant SOD1 levels showed only a transient effect of motor neuron protection, suggesting that other cell types were contributing to the ultimate demise of motor neurons (Miller et al., 2005). Collectively, these studies suggest that ALS is a non-cell autonomous disease; non-neuronal mutant SOD1-expressing cells can directly cause wild-type motor neurons to exhibit a disease phenotype.

2.1 Astrocytes influence the course of disease in ALS

Specific populations of glial cells have been analyzed to determine their precise role in motor neuron death in ALS. Astrocytes are glial cells with diverse roles including regulation of the extracellular CNS environment, maintenance of cell-cell communication, CNS vascular control, growth factor production, and neurotransmitter metabolism (Maragakis & Rothstein, 2006). Astrocytes can also become reactive and proliferative in response to neuronal death or CNS injury. Indeed, reactive astrocytosis and inflammation are prominent features in both the human ALS spinal cord as well as in rodent ALS models. Moreover, astrocytes have long been suspected to exacerbate motor neuron death due to their reported loss of glial glutamate transporter 1 (GLT1) [excitatory amino acid transporter 2 (EAAT2) in humans](Bendotti et al., 2001; Bristol & Rothstein, 1996; Bruijn et al., 1997; Rothstein et al., 1995). GLT1 is a glutamate transporter responsible for removing 90% of the extrasynaptic glutamate to prevent continued neuronal firing. Increased levels of glutamate have been found in the cerebrospinal fluid of ALS patients (Rothstein et al., 1990; Shaw et al., 1995). Chronic reduction in glutamate uptake results in a buildup of extracellular glutamate, leading to increased neuronal synaptic transmission and excitotoxic neuronal death. The ALS-linked GLT1 loss is found in both human ALS and in several rodent models and signifies astrocyte pathology as consistent theme in ALS pathobiology. However, it is difficult to discern whether astrocytes become dysfunctional due to motor neuron degeneration or whether dysfunction is a secondary event in the disease course.

Recent studies aim to answer these questions by evaluating how mutant SOD1 expression in astrocytes affects disease course in the mutant SOD1 mouse model. In these sets of experiments, cre recombinase was driven using the GFAP promoter to excise the floxed mutant SOD1 gene solely in astrocytes. Depending on which SOD1 mutation was present, the reduction of mutant SOD1 in astrocytes either slows disease progression (SOD1 G37R)(Yamanaka et al., 2008b) or slows disease onset and progression (SOD1 G85R)(Wang et al., 2011). Microgliosis was reduced and astrocytic GLT1 expression was maintained in one study (Wang et al., 2011), however, the exact mechanism for prolonged survival in these mice is still undefined. Nevertheless, it seems that the mutant SOD1 protein directly causes astrocytes to become aberrant in the SOD1 mouse model and rescue of diseased astrocytes can significantly influence disease course. It is also interesting to note that complete ablation of proliferating mutant SOD1 astrocytes in the SOD1 mouse model does not affect any measure of motor neuron disease in these mice. Therefore, astrocyte proliferation itself or the presence of mutant SOD1 in the proliferating astrocyte population does not seem to contribute to motor neuron degeneration (Lepore et al., 2008a).

2.2 Microglia direct disease progression in ALS mouse models

In addition to astrocytes, microglia are another important glial cell type in ALS pathogenesis due to their phagocytic properties and capacity to produce a wide array of cytokines and chemokines, attracting other cells to the site of injury. Indeed, extensive microglial activation and proliferation characterizes sites of motor neuron injury in human ALS and rodent models and this microgliosis increases as disease worsens (Henkel et al., 2009). Interestingly, investigations are ongoing as to whether microglia are neuroprotective, neurotoxic, or situationally both in ALS.

To directly assess the role of mutant SOD1 in microglia of the SOD1 mouse model, two parallel studies sought to remove the mutant SOD1 G37R specifically from microglia in these transgenic mice. In one study, the floxed mutant SOD1 gene was excised from microglia using cre recombinase driven by the Cd11b promoter, removing the gene from microglia and peripheral macrophages only (Boillee et al., 2006b). In the other parallel study, microglia were genetically ablated in the mutant SOD1 mouse followed by reconstitution with wild-type microglia through a bone-marrow transplant (Beers et al., 2006). The result from both studies was a slowed disease progression resulting in a dramatic extension in life in these mice. More recently, an additional study also showed slowed disease progression when a different SOD1 mutant, SOD1 G85R, was excised by cre recombinase solely in microglia (Wang et al., 2009). Collectively, these studies suggest the presence of mutant SOD1 in microglia causes these cells to adopt a more neurotoxic phenotype and directly affects motor neuron survival in the mutant SOD1 mouse model.

Other studies suggest that microglia may actually play a neuroprotective role in motor neuron disease. Evidence from other disease and injury models indicates that as microglia become activated, they can adopt either an "M1" proinflammatory phenotype or an "M2" alternatively activated phenotype leading to secretion of anti-inflammatory cytokines and neurotrophic factors (Henkel et al., 2009). Although mutant SOD1 expression seems to cause microglia to lean toward proinflammatory M1 activation, microglia have also been shown to produce anti-inflammatory cytokines and neuroprotective growth factors during the early phase of disease in the ALS mice (Chiu et al., 2008). Interestingly, several studies have indicated that T cells directly influence microglial activation and their differentiation toward a neuroprotective or proinflammatory phenotype. When SOD1 G93A mice were bred with a strain of mice lacking T cells, disease course was accelerated and this worsening of disease was accompanied by a decrease in alternative M2 microglial activation, although astrocytosis remained unchanged (Chiu et al., 2008). In addition, increased numbers of regulatory T cells are associated with the stable phase of disease in both mice and ALS patients and these regulatory T cells can promote microglia to adopt an anti-inflammatory M2 phenotype (Beers et al., 2011). Over the course of disease, these regulatory T cells decrease in number accompanied by a shift in microglia from protective M2 to the proinflammatory M1 phenotype. Therefore, this evidence suggests microglia adopt an activated neuroprotective M2 phenotype during early disease, but then develop into proinflammatory M1 microglia as disease progresses. Therapeutic approaches that promote M2 microglial differentiation or maintenance may prove to be an alternative to the limitation of microglial activation.

2.3 The undefined role of oligodendrocytes and their progenitors in ALS

While focus has been on the involvement of neurons, astrocytes and microglia in ALS pathogenesis, a few studies have investigated other glial cell lineages as well. In particular, myelinating oligodendrocytes of the central nervous system and Schwann cells of the peripheral nervous system form intimate connections with motor neurons and their axons, promote neuronal health through production of neurotrophic factors, and aid in regeneration after neuronal injury. Surprisingly little is known about the role of Schwann cells and oligodendrocytes in ALS, although pathological aberrations in myelin have been reported along peripheral nerves in human patients (Perrie et al., 1993). As with glial inflammation, these myelin abnormalities may be primary or secondary to motor neuron degeneration. To specifically investigate whether mutant SOD1 alters Schwann cells, transgenic mice were created with SOD1 G93A expression restricted to myelinating Schwann cells using the myelin protein zero (P0) promoter (Turner et al., 2010). No evidence of motor neuron disease was observed in these mice, suggesting the mutant SOD1 protein is not detrimental to this Schwann cell population. In contrast, the specific removal of floxed mutant SOD1 in Schwann cells by P0-driven cre recombinase seems to modestly accelerate disease progression in the SOD1 G37R mice (Lobsiger et al., 2009). This curious disease acceleration is hypothesized to be a result of reducing SOD1's normal dismutase activity in Schwann cells, which may serve an unrealized neuroprotective function during the nerve regeneration process. Thus, a clear role of mutant SOD1-expressing Schwann cells has not been determined in rodent ALS models.

Another open question in the field is whether oligodendrocytes and their NG2+ progenitor cells directly affect motor neuron loss in ALS. To date, only one study has investigated how mutant SOD1 in oligodendrocytes influences motor neuron loss and the experimental design causes the results to be difficult to interpret. In this study, chimeric mice were created by mixing embryonic cells expressing SOD1 G37R with wild-type cells lacking the Olig1 transcription factor (Yamanaka et al., 2008a). The Olig1 -/- mice are unable to form motor neurons or oligodendrocytes. Therefore, the motor neurons and oligodendrocytes in the chimeric mice were generated from the mutant SOD1 G37R cells which have normal Olig1 levels. The result is a chimeric mouse with mutant motor neurons and oligodendrocytes, but with all other cells being a mixture of mutant and wild-type cells. These mice did not develop the motor neuron disease typical in the SOD1 G37R mouse model and the authors suggest that mutant SOD1 expression in oligodendrocytes is not a significant contributor to motor neuron degeneration. However, technical limitations prohibited verifying that all oligodendrocytes expressed the mutant SOD1 so it is difficult to draw a strong conclusion from these studies.

Interest in the oligodendrocyte progenitor cells, also called NG2+ cells, has risen in the ALS field due to recent reports of their aberrant proliferation in rodent models. These NG2+ cells are found widely throughout the CNS and are mitotically active, especially in areas of injury or neuronal degeneration. Although the specific functions of these cells is still under investigation, these NG2+ cells can divide and differentiate into myelinating oligodendrocytes, but not into astrocytes or neurons *in vivo* (Kang et al., 2010). Several studies have reported a dramatic (20-fold) increase in proliferation of NG2+ cells over the course of disease in ALS mouse models, with NG2+ cells contributing to over half of the total dividing cell population in the spinal cord of symptomatic mice (Kang et al., 2010; Lepore et al., 2008a; Magnus et al., 2008). Differentiation of these NG2+ cells into oligodendrocytes is also enhanced in mutant SOD1 mice compared to wild-type mice for reasons still unknown (Kang et al., 2010). It has been proposed that oligodendrocytes undergo degeneration in response to motor neuron loss and the NG2+ cell proliferation and differentiation is an attempt to restore these lost oligodendrocytes. However, it will be crucial to dissect what effects are primary and secondary to motor neuron loss and what role, if any, NG2+ cells play in disease course. Studies investigating how mutant SOD1 influences normal NG2+ cell behavior are warranted, including analysis of whether mutant SOD1 NG2+ cells share a similar non-cell autonomous toxicity as astrocytes and microglia.

2.4 Glial cell involvement in TDP43/FUS ALS?

A defining pathological feature in post-mortem ALS tissue is ubiquitin-positive inclusions within neurons and glia in the spinal cord, brainstem, and motor cortex. In patients with SOD1 mutations, these inclusions contain misfolded SOD1 protein (Bruijn et al., 1998). However, in ALS patients lacking SOD1 mutations, these inclusions contain one of two RNA/DNA binding proteins: TAR DNA-binding protein 43 (TDP43) or fused in sarcoma protein (FUS) (Kwiatkowski et al., 2009; Mackenzie et al., 2007; Neumann et al., 2006; Vance et al., 2009). Genetic analyses have also revealed disease-linked mutations in both TDP43 and FUS in subsets of familial and few sporadic ALS patients, adding to evidence that these proteins are involved in ALS pathogenesis (Kabashi et al., 2008; Kwiatkowski et al., 2009; Sreedharan et al., 2008; Vance et al., 2009). However, a major question that remains is whether glial cells play an active role in ALS disease caused by TDP43 or FUS mutations.

Animal models are in development to better understand pathological disease mechanisms in TDP43 and FUS ALS. Thus far, a number of rodent models have been described for TDP43 ALS and these models vary in the TDP43 mutations expressed and the promoter used to drive expression (Cohen et al., 2011). The phenotypes observed in these models have been somewhat perplexing due to the difficulties in dissecting the effects of human TDP43 protein overexpression from mutant-specific effects. Nonetheless, a common theme in these animals is neurodegeneration accompanied by neuronal cytoplasmic aggregates in affected regions. None of the models to this point have reported glial pathology other than an increase in gliosis at sites of neuronal injury which may be secondary to neuronal death. Likewise, in the first reported rodent model for FUS ALS, astrogliosis and microgliosis were the only noted glial-specific pathologies (Huang et al., 2011). In contrast, TDP43- and FUS-positive inclusions are found in glial cells in post-mortem ALS spinal cord and it is difficult to know whether these inclusions were overlooked in the early animal models or whether they represent a discrepancy between human ALS and rodent models (Mackenzie et al., 2010). Careful dissection of the effects of mutant TDP43 and FUS in astrocytes, microglia, and oligodendrocytes (as well as NG2+ progenitors) will be essential to determine whether the non-cell autonomous disease nature extensively noted in SOD1 ALS is also recapitulated in TDP43- and FUS-mediated ALS.

3. ALS disease modeling using glial cells

Transgenic mouse models have played a key role in elucidating how glial cells affect the disease course of ALS. There are obvious advantages to *in vivo* models; however, it is often difficult to dissect the specific contributions of various cell populations from other influences in the CNS milieu. In parallel with these *in vivo* studies, several groups have established novel *in vitro* ALS models that recapitulate the glial-mediated motor neuron toxicity observed in transgenic ALS mouse models. Most of these *in vitro* models involve a co-culture where wildtype motor neurons are co-cultured with mutant SOD1 glia or wild-type glia. The goal is to determine the direct effects of diseased glia on motor neurons. Furthermore, *in vitro* models allow for the study of human cells derived from ALS patients. Most studies striving to correlate work from the ALS rodent model with human ALS rely on post-mortem tissue analysis, which makes it difficult to sort out primary contributors to motor neuron loss from secondary effects caused by neurodegeneration and the inflammatory response in the endstage spinal cord. These *in vitro* models provide a unique avenue to study human ALS in real-time and evaluate therapeutics and disease mechanisms.

3.1 Motor neuron-glial cell co-cultures recapitulate glial-derived motor neuron damage

Transgenic models have shown that removing the mutant SOD1 gene in microglia reduces motor neuron loss in the mutant SOD1 mouse model (Beers et al., 2006; Boillee et al., 2006b). Similar work has recapitulated this motor neuron loss using primary microglia isolated from mutant SOD1 mice in a co-culture with motor neurons. These studies have demonstrated that mutant SOD1-expressing microglia are more neurotoxic compared to wild-type microglia (Beers et al., 2006; Weydt et al., 2004; Xiao et al., 2007) which is not surprising given that mutant SOD1 microglia release an array of toxic inflammatory factors including nitric oxide, reactive oxygen species, TNF-α, and IL-1 (Almer et al., 1999; Henkel et al., 2009; Hensley et al., 2003; Nguyen et al., 2001; Sasaki et al., 2000; Weydt et al., 2004; Xiao et al., 2007). Motor neurons co-cultured with mutant SOD1-expressing microglia show a reduction in the number and length of neurites and reduced survival in the co-culture paradigm (Xiao et al., 2007). In addition, microglia treated with extracellular mutant SOD1 protein become inflamed and damaging to motor neurons in co-culture (Urushitani et al., 2006; Zhao et al., 2010). The extracellular mutant SOD1 only caused motor neuron death when microglia were added into the culture, indicating the motor neuron damage was directly initiated by microglia (Zhao et al., 2010). These *in vitro* systems could provide a platform for testing therapeutics that could potentially block neurotoxic microglia. For example, *in vitro* treatment with IL-4 caused mutant SOD1-expressing microglia to differentiate from an "M1" proinflammatory phenotype to an "M2" neuroprotective phenotype and improved motor neuron survival in co-culture (Zhao et al., 2006). It remains to be determined whether IL-4 will have the same effect when delivered to microglia *in vivo*. More efforts have focused on studying aberrant astrocyte function in mutant SOD1-based *in vitro* ALS models. Several studies have demonstrated that astrocytes isolated from mutant SOD1 mice (Di Giorgio et al., 2007; Nagai et al., 2007) as well as astrocytes derived from neural stem cells from these mice (Dodge et al., 2008) are toxic to wild-type motor neurons in co-culture. In these studies, primary motor neurons as well as motor neurons derived from mouse embryonic stem cells were shown to die more quickly *in vitro* when cultured on top of SOD1 G93A astrocytes compared to wild-type astrocytes. It has also been recently shown that human motor neurons differentiated from embryonic stem cells are susceptible to the same astrocytes isolated from the SOD1 G93A mouse model (Di Giorgio et al., 2008). Furthermore, human motor neurons derived from embryonic stem cells die in the presence of human fetal primary astrocytes overexpressing mutant SOD1 by lentivirus (Marchetto et al., 2008). These *in vitro* models support that mutant SOD1-expressing astrocytes are toxic to motor neurons regardless of the species and provide a way to study familial ALS utilizing human cells. While these results have been exciting, no consistent pathway has been implicated in these *in vitro* studies for causing motor neuron death; however, one common finding is that the toxicity is transferred through the media, suggesting a secreted factor may be responsible. Future studies will hopefully identify the specific factor(s) involved in this toxicity.

3.2 ALS disease modeling using human-derived cells

Development of *in vitro* ALS models provides another tool to investigate disease mechanisms and test therapeutics for ALS. Unfortunately, there has been a disconnect in the translation of drugs from rodent models of ALS to human clinical trials. While various drugs have shown promise in rodent models, there continues to be disappointment in clinical trials which may be a result of various factors including poor preclinical testing regimen, ineffective clinical design and delivery, or use of an animal model that does not accurately reflect human disease (Benatar, 2007). Indeed, most ALS models currently used for therapeutic testing are based on fALS caused by SOD1 mutations. Since fALS only accounts for 5-10% of ALS cases and SOD1 mutations are only present in 20% of these fALS patients, rodent ALS models may only represent 2% of all ALS cases. Thus, efforts have been focused on developing *in vitro* cell based models for sALS, representing the majority of the patient population. Human ALS-based *in vitro* models could be a helpful tool to identify drugs which modulate glial activity and be utilized as a complement to the mutant SOD1 mouse model to select more effective drugs for further clinical development.

Several methods can be employed to derive patient-specific glia for *in vitro* study. While it is difficult to isolate primary astrocytes or microglia from post-mortem tissue in large enough quantities, neural progenitor cells can be harvested from post-mortem brain and spinal cord tissue (Palmer et al., 2001). These human neural progenitor cells can be continuously expanded *in vitro* and differentiated into neurons, astrocytes, or oligodendrocytes for study. Recently, it has been shown that isolation of neural progenitor cells from post-mortem ALS spinal cord is feasible and astrocytes can be generated from these progenitors (Haidet-Phillips et al., 2011). Astrocytes derived from a fALS patient harboring a SOD1 mutation were co-cultured with wild-type motor neurons and a 50% increase in neuronal cell death was observed compared to co-culture with astrocytes from non-ALS controls, recapitulating evidence from the mutant SOD1 mouse model. However, it was also shown for the first time that astrocytes derived from sALS patients, which represent the majority of ALS patients, were similarly toxic to motor neurons in co-culture. The motor neuron death was shown to be triggered by conditioned astrocyte media, suggesting toxic secreted factors are responsible for motor neuron damage as seen in the mouse astrocyte co-culture studies. These results indicate a shared mechanism leading to motor neuron death between fALS and sALS through astrocyte-mediated toxicity and suggest therapies directed at astrocytes may be beneficial for both ALS populations.

In addition to neural progenitor cells, there are other stem cell sources which can be potentially used to derive patient-specific glial cells or motor neurons *in vitro*. With the development of induced pluripotent stem cell (iPSC) technology, many groups are also striving to create populations of neurons and astrocytes from iPSCs for disease modeling. iPSCs are pluripotent stem cells generated by reprogramming somatic cells through forced expression of specific pluripotency transcription factors. Like embryonic stem cells, iPSCs are characterized by an immense proliferative capacity and the ability to differentiate into all three germ lineages (endoderm, ectoderm, and mesoderm) which can eventually give rise to all tissues of the body (Yamanaka & Blau, 2010). A variety of different cell types have now been reprogrammed into iPSCs including both mouse and human somatic cells (Okita et al., 2007; Park et al., 2008; Takahashi et al., 2007; Takahashi & Yamanaka, 2006; Wernig et al., 2007; Yu et al., 2007). Importantly, protocols have also been developed for the differentiation of motor neurons, astrocytes, and oligodendrocytes from human iPSCs, which allow for *in vitro* ALS disease modeling (Czepiel et al., 2011; Dimos et al., 2008; Krencik et al., 2011; Liu et al., 2011).

Several groups have reprogrammed human fibroblasts from ALS patients into iPSCs and successfully differentiated motor neurons from these iPSCs (Boulting et al., 2011; Dimos et al., 2008). However, the major hurdle thus far has been demonstration of a disease-related phenotype in the iPSC-derived motor neurons. It may be necessary to either stress the iPSC-derived motor neurons or co-culture with astrocytes also generated from ALS patient iPSCs in order to observe motor neuron damage. Still, it may be difficult to reproduce a relevant *in vitro* phenotype when working with diseases that are complex and likely multifactorial such as sALS. Another question posed by these experiments is whether or not reprogramming a cell and concordant epigenetic remodeling causes the loss of the ALS "signature". If sporadic ALS is triggered in part by epigenetic modifications, reprogramming may eliminate this epigenetic profile leaving essentially a "wild-type" cell. Therefore, comparisons between cells derived from ALS post-mortem tissues (not reprogrammed) and ALS-derived iPSCs may be crucial for dissecting these issues.

Although still in development, these *in vitro*-based ALS models provide a valuable platform for further mechanistic and therapeutic studies. Many of these models employ the use of Hb9-GFP reporter cell lines to generate motor neurons allowing for easy visualization of motor neuron survival over time in co-culture. With the reported ability to track motor neuron survival in real-time in a 96 well plate format (Haidet-Phillips et al., 2011), the development of high-throughput screens is foreseeable. Therapeutic compounds could be quickly screened for motor neuron protection against glial-cell mediated toxicity in this format. Additionally, one could envision genetic screens for modifiers of glial-cell derived motor neuron damage, leading to new therapeutic approaches or insights into disease mechanisms. Since there are currently no models for sALS, these *in vitro*-based systems utilizing either post-mortem neural progenitor or iPS-derived cells could provide a much needed novel platform for drug discovery. Although promising, some limitations do exist for *in vitro* modeling systems. For example, the time course for modeling motor neuron disease *in vitro* is short (days to weeks) whereas ALS is a late onset disorder which usually does not develop until 40-60 years of age. Additionally, the heterogeneity of ALS cases may pose another challenge, requiring a large number of both disease and control samples in order to identify relevant disease-related changes *in vitro*. Lastly, although *in vitro* modeling allows for dissection of cell-specific phenotypes, it will be important to evaluate any noticed changes in an *in vivo* context where many cell types interact and can influence disease.

4. Therapeutic advances to target glial cells in ALS

In recent years, much emphasis has been placed on the role of glial cells in mutant SOD1 mouse models and some of these findings have been recapitulated *in vitro* using human ALS patient-derived cells. Thus, many groups are devoting significant efforts to development of therapies directed at modulating glial cell activity. Indeed, glial cells have been suggested to affect both disease onset and progression in ALS mouse models. Since the majority of ALS patients are only diagnosed well after the onset of disease, therapies targeting disease progression by modification of glial cells may be beneficial in slowing symptomatic disease processes.

4.1 Therapeutic agents to target astrocytes and microglia

Currently, there is only one US Food and Drug Administration (FDA)-approved drug for the treatment of ALS and its therapeutic effects are hypothesized to derive from counteracting aberrant glutamate metabolism. Riluzole is an inhibitor of presynaptic glutamate release which may offset excitotoxicity seen in ALS. Riluzole has been confirmed to alter ALS disease survival in four independent clinical trials providing strong support for its therapeutic benefits (Miller et al., 2007). Unfortunately, riluzole only extends lifespan in ALS patients by an average of 3 months so efforts have focused on identifying other compounds which can counteract glutamate excitotoxicity. A variety of other drugs targeting glutamatergic pathways (talampanel, memantine, topiramate, lamotrigine, gabapentin, ONO-2506) have been evaluated in ALS patients, but the results have not suggested a benefit on disease course (Cudkowicz et al., 2003; de Carvalho et al., 2010; Miller et al., 2001; Ryberg et al., 2003; Zinman & Cudkowicz, 2011).

To identify new medications which may modulate glutamatergic pathways, an *in vitro* screening of over 1000 compounds already approved by the US Food and Drug Administration was completed (Rothstein et al., 2005). From this screen, β-lactam antibiotics were found to upregulate expression of the glutamate transporter, GLT1, and one of these antibiotics, ceftriaxone, was shown to significantly delay disease progression in the SOD1 G93A mouse model. Clinical trials testing intravenous ceftriaxone administration in ALS patients have already passed safety and tolerability stages and are currently in the final phase III of evaluation (Zinman & Cudkowicz, 2011).

In contrast to specific targeting of glutamatergic pathways, a variety of anti-inflammatory agents have been tested with hopes to combat the extensive glial reaction observed in ALS patient brain and spinal cord. Prostaglandins are mediators of the inflammatory response that can be released in response to immune stimuli and production of prostaglandins is increased in the spinal cord of ALS patients (Kondo et al., 2002). Prostaglandin stimulation can be reduced by inhibiting cyclooxygenase 2 (COX2), an inducible enzyme involved in the synthesis of prostaglandins. Treatment of SOD1 G93A mice with COX2 inhibitors lowers prostaglandin levels and prolongs survival in these mice (Drachman et al., 2002; Klivenyi et al., 2004; Pompl et al., 2003). Unfortunately, the COX2 inhibitor, celecoxib, was ineffective at increasing survival in a clinical trial of ALS patients (Cudkowicz et al., 2006). However, prostaglandin E2 levels in the CSF of these patients was unaltered by celecoxib therapy indicating the dose may have been too low to reach therapeutic levels in the CNS (Aggarwal & Cudkowicz, 2008).

Additional efforts to modulate the immune response in ALS have also been unsuccessful. The anti-microbial drug, minocycline, was shown to inhibit microglial activation and lengthen survival in mouse models of ALS (Kriz et al., 2002; Van Den Bosch et al., 2002; Zhu et al., 2002). Nonetheless, in a multicenter, randomized, phase III clinical trial of over 400 ALS patients, minocycline did not increase survival and in fact, was shown to worsen disease course in these patients (Gordon et al., 2007). The apparent divergence in results between preclinical animal studies and the clinical trial may have been due to the timing of minocycline treatment. When tested in animal models, minocycline was administered prior to symptomatic disease onset, whereas patients received the drug only after clinical onset of ALS. Indeed, a recent study showed that treatment of SOD1 G93A mice with minocycline administered after disease onset conferred no survival benefit and highlights the importance of a clinically-relevant testing regimen in ALS mouse studies (Keller et al., 2011). Compounds which modify neuroinflammation already present in the spinal cord, in contrast to preventing inflammation, may be more successful in the clinical setting.

4.2 Stem cell therapies for ALS

Because mounting data indicate that pathogenic glial cells actively contribute to motor neuron loss in ALS, one developing strategy is to replace the diseased glia with healthy cells which may alter the endogenous spinal cord environment and promote motor neuron survival. Transplantation of terminally differentiated glia to the CNS may pose technical difficulties since these cells are typically mature with limited proliferative and migratory capacity. Therefore, exploration of stem cells as a source for glial replacement has been sought after by many groups.

Mutant SOD1-expressing microglia are key drivers of disease progression in mouse models of fALS. Since microglia are derived from the hematopoietic lineage, hematopoietic stem cells are one possible source for microglial cell replacement. When SOD1 mice lacking microglia are given bone marrow transplants from wild-type mice, the microglial cell population is reconstituted with healthy microglia and survival is prolonged (Beers et al., 2006). In translating this line of investigation to ALS patients, allogeneic peripheral blood hematopoietic stem cells were transplanted into ALS patients following full body irradiation (Appel et al., 2008). Although transplanted cells remarkably migrated to sites of motor neuron injury, no clinical change in disease was observed. It is possible that either the transplanted cells did not differentiate into microglia or that a large proportion of endogenous microglia survived post-irradiation which outnumbered healthy, transplanted stem cells. Trials are ongoing to similarly test intraparenchymal transplantation of hematopoietic stem cells to ALS patients (Deda et al., 2009), but results may be difficult to interpret based on the use of autologous (and potentially diseased) stem cells as a source instead of allogeneic (from a matched donor) derived stem cells. Further studies are needed in ALS rodent models to determine the optimal cell type, number, and delivery method for transplantation to establish a critical proof-of-principle for these paradigms.

Further efforts have focused on replacement of diseased astrocytes using various cell sources and delivery approaches. In contrast to microglia, astrocytes are derived from the neural lineage and can be differentiated from several stem cell sources including both glial-restricted precursors as well as neural stem and progenitor cells. Thus far, transplantation of neural progenitor cells to rodent ALS models has resulted in either a lack of differentiation *in vivo* (Klein et al., 2005; Suzuki et al., 2007) or differentiation to mostly neurons after neural stem cell transplantation, but not to astrocytes (Xu et al., 2009; Xu et al., 2011).

In contrast, glial-restricted precursors are lineage-restricted and can only become astrocytes or oligodendrocytes. Transplantation of glial-restricted precursors to the cervical spinal cord of SOD1 G93A rats led to extensive differentiation of grafted cells into astrocytes (>85% of transplanted cells) which reduced significant motor neuron loss (Lepore et al., 2008b). The graft-derived astrocytes expressed increased levels of GLT1 in comparison to endogenous diseased astrocytes, which likely played a major role in protecting motor neurons. Importantly, rats receiving transplants also survived longer and showed preserved forelimb grip strength and respiratory function, attributable to the focal delivery of glial-restricted precursor cells to the cervical region of the spinal cord. This work provides a proof-of-principle for astrocyte replacement in ALS and sets the stage for future clinical trials testing transplantation of human glial-restricted precursors in ALS patients. Questions still remain as to whether human glial-restricted precursors will survive and differentiate after transplantation into humans and which spinal cord regions are most practical for targeting in ALS patients.

With the advancement of stem cell technology, astrocytes as well as neural progenitors (and possibly glial-restricted precursors) can now be derived from human iPS cells. This novel stem cell source provides another option for glial-cell replacement therapies since iPS cells have immense expansive abilities *in vitro*. A major potential advantage to iPS cells is that these cells can be derived directly from a living patient. In theory, use of autologous iPS cells for transplantation therapies may lessen worries of graft rejection and obviate the need for continued immunosuppressive therapy. However, one study testing this paradigm documented rejection of mouse iPS cells after transplantation to an autologous recipient, cautioning that transplantation of these cells may be more complex than originally thought (Zhao et al., 2011). Another issue is whether stem cells derived from ALS patients carry the disease phenotype. If so, any cells differentiated from the patient iPS cells may not provide the desired therapeutic benefit. In cases where there exists a disease-associated mutation such as SOD1, ex-vivo genetic correction of the mutation through homologous recombination, viral vectors, or zinc finger technology may be possible (Amabile & Meissner, 2009). However, most ALS patients have no identified genetic mutation responsible for the disease. Additionally, there remain many unresolved challenges with iPS cell therapy such as obtaining efficient differentiation of the iPS cells to the desired cell population, purifying a safe and non-tumorgenic population for transplantation, and optimizing delivery methods for transplantation of the iPS-derived cells back to the patient. In addition to benefits derived from replacing diseased glia, transplanted populations of stem cells may also be used to deliver therapeutics to the brain and spinal cord. Stem cells can be genetically modified *in vitro* by transduction with viral vectors which can integrate into the genome and stably express therapeutic genes long-term. Since many therapeutic proteins have short half-lives after direct injection, genetically modified stem cells transplanted to the brain or spinal cord would allow for continuous production of the desired protein at the site of neurodegeneration, serving as "therapeutic pumps" *in vivo*. For example, human neural progenitor cells transduced with a lentivirus expressing glial-derived neurotrophic factor (GDNF) and transplanted to the ALS rat spinal cord can produce GDNF *in vivo* and protect motor neurons (Klein et al., 2005; Suzuki et al., 2007). One could envision using stem cells to deliver not only neuroprotective factors, but also therapies to modulate the glial environment such as anti-inflammatory proteins or anti-glutamatergic agents.

4.3 Gene-targeted therapies for ALS

The mechanisms leading to motor neuron death in ALS are still unclear; however, it is generally agreed in the field that in cases of SOD1 fALS, the mutant SOD1 protein harbors a toxic gain-of-function and reduction of mutant SOD1 is likely to be beneficial in these patients. Additionally, several studies have implicated a pathogenic role for wild-type SOD1 in cases of sALS (Bosco et al., 2010; Gruzman et al., 2007), including a potential role in glial cells (Haidet-Phillips et al., 2011). Therefore, therapies aimed at reducing SOD1 levels may potentially be applicable for not only SOD1 fALS patients, but for other ALS patient populations as well.

A variety of approaches have been attempted to reduce SOD1 levels in rodent models of ALS. RNA interference (RNAi) is a post-transcriptional gene-silencing mechanism initiated by small interfering RNAs (siRNA) which are double-stranded pieces of RNA 21-23 nucleotides in length (Sah & Aronin, 2011). Within the cytoplasm, the siRNA gets recognized and directed to the RNA-induced silencing complex. The silencing complex then uses the sequence-specific information on the siRNA to initiate degradation of endogenous complementary mRNA sequences, leading to subsequent gene silencing. Targeted siRNA can be exogenously delivered to a cell although naked siRNA is instable with a relatively short half life (Sah & Aronin, 2011). Alternatively, viral vectors can be used to continuously transcribe RNA containing short complementary sequences (Miller et al., 2008). These complementary sequences can bind, leading to duplex hairpin formation (short hairpin RNA or shRNA). Once transcribed, the shRNA gets recognized by the cellular machinery and cleaved by the Dicer enzyme to produce short, double-stranded siRNA sequences.

Sequences of siRNA targeted against SOD1 mRNA have been designed to reduce levels of the mutant SOD1 protein. Similar to many small molecule therapies, siRNA does not cross the blood-brain-barrier, creating challenges for delivery to the CNS (Sah & Aronin, 2011). Viral-mediated delivery of SOD1 shRNA has been attempted in rodent models of ALS with successful knockdown of SOD1 levels by both lentivirus and adeno-associated virus (AAV) (Miller et al., 2005; Ralph et al., 2005; Towne et al., 2011). However, these studies have targeted only motor neurons, transduced after retrograde transport from muscles injected with the virus. These strategies were unsuccessful in slowing disease progression, most likely due to the fact that motor neurons were solely targeted, although glial cells play a significant role in the disease process.

Other approaches have strived to target both motor neurons and glial cells with SOD1 shRNA. Intraparenchymal injection to the lumbar spinal cord of a lentivirus encoding SOD1 shRNA was shown to reduce SOD1 levels and retard disease onset and progression in the SOD1 G93A mouse (Raoul et al., 2005). Yet, the vast anatomical distribution of diseased cells throughout the motor cortex, brain stem and spinal cord pose a hurdle for direct injection of viral therapy with limited diffusive capacity. A novel version of AAV, AAV serotype 9, has recently shown potential for extensive targeting of CNS tissues (Foust et al., 2009). In this study, AAV9 was able to cross the blood-brain-barrier after vascular delivery and transduce over 60% of astrocytes in the brain and spinal cord. Additional evaluation in non-human primates verified that AAV9 is capable of efficiently targeting both motor neurons and glia in the brain and spinal cord after vascular delivery to a large species (Bevan et al., 2011). Use of this virus to deliver SOD1 shRNA is conceivable, although steps may be needed to target viral expression away from peripheral organs and only to CNS tissues.

Instead of using a viral vector to deliver shRNA sequences, others have sought to create more stable siRNA for direct delivery through chemically modifying the siRNA (Wang et al., 2008). Intrathecal infusion of chemically-modified SOD1 siRNA using an osmotic pump generated a 15% knockdown in SOD1 protein levels and a modest therapeutic effect in the SOD1 G93A mice. One potential advantage to infusion of naked, stabilized siRNA over viral delivery is the ability to halt the treatment at any time following adverse effects. Therefore, this type of RNAi therapy seems promising at least for treatment of ALS patients with SOD1 mutations.

A similar approach to RNAi therapy involves the use of antisense oligonucleotides to enact post-transcriptional gene silencing (Sah & Aronin, 2011). Antisense oligonucleotides are short (15-25 nucleotides) single stranded pieces of synthetic DNA which can bind to complementary mRNA sequences in the cytoplasm. Once bound, these DNA-mRNA complexes are targeted for degradation by the enzyme RNase H. Additionally, translation of mRNA bound by antisense oligonucleotides can be physically blocked, leading to further gene silencing for targeted mRNA sequences. Antisense oligonucleotides are generally more stable than naked siRNA with a half life of 2-6 weeks after delivery to the mouse and monkey CNS (Sah & Aronin, 2011). Like siRNA, antisense oligonucleotides can be absorbed by both neurons and glia to execute gene silencing. Sequence specific targeting of antisense oligonucleotides to SOD1 mRNA has been attainable, with a 50% reduction in SOD1 protein levels in the brain and spinal cord of SOD1 G93A rats infused for 28 days with antisense oligonucleotides into the right ventricle (Smith et al., 2006). The rats treated with SOD1 antisense oligonucleotides showed a slowed disease progression and this same SOD1 antisense oligonucleotide was demonstrated to lower SOD1 levels in fibroblasts isolated from an ALS patient. A phase I clinical trial has been initiated in fALS patients with SOD1 mutations testing intrathecal infusion of this same antisense oligonucleotide against SOD1. This dose-escalation trial will evaluate safety, tolerability, and pharmacokinetics in patients treated with antisense oligonucleotide infusion for 12 hours. If proven safe, this strategy holds considerable promise to treat SOD1 fALS patients.

While a great deal of progress has been made in the development of anti-SOD1 therapies, additional work needs to be focused on advancing novel treatments for non-SOD1 ALS patient populations. As additional genetic mutations are linked to ALS, these genes might present new targets for gene-based therapeutic approaches. However, in the case of TDP43 and FUS mutations, a great deal of basic research is still required to evaluate whether a loss-of-function or gain-of-function mechanism is responsible for disease caused by these mutations and whether glial cells are also a target in these cases. Until these crucial questions are answered, it will be difficult to develop RNAi or gene therapy treatments for these patients. Efforts to reach a broad ALS patient population may benefit most from the design of therapies which interfere with downstream mechanisms prevalent in most patients, such as glial-mediated glutamate excitotoxicity or neuroinflammation. Many of the siRNA and antisense oligonucleotide approaches can be amenable to inhibit potentially damaging genes involved in these glial responses. Additionally, viral vectors have been developed that can deliver gene therapies to glial cells in the CNS, allowing for potential immune modulation. With increasingly innovative developments in RNAi and gene therapy, the door is open for novel gene-based therapies to alter the ALS disease process.

5. Conclusion

The field of ALS research has progressed significantly in recent years with the identification of glial cells as an active contributor to the disease process. Specifically, astrocytes and microglia have been recognized as glial cell types which undeniably influence survival in rodent models of ALS. Efforts are underway to test therapies aimed at modifying the glial cell population in hopes of slowing ALS disease progression and extending patient survival. While rodent models of ALS have been key in revealing glial cells as a disease contributor in SOD1 fALS, it still remains to be determined to what extent glial cells are involved in disease processes in other patient populations. New genes have been recently linked ALS including TDP43 and FUS, suggesting a possible role for RNA metabolism in disease pathogenesis. Creation of both rodent and *in vitro* models mimicking these forms of ALS is underway and will hopefully reveal whether glial cells are also a target in patients harboring these mutations.

Although glial cell targets have been identified, much work remains to elucidate the mechanisms behind their neural toxicity. Several groups have been able to model the glial-motor neuron interface *in vitro* using unique stem-cell based models to study the effects of diseased glia on motor neurons. While these studies have yet to identify relevant mechanisms involved in glial-mediated toxicity, *in vitro* models present the opportunity to study human patient-derived glial cells from both fALS and sALS patients. With the development of iPSC technology, there exists potential to study patient-specific glial cells and evaluate therapies in a high-throughput fashion.

Discovery of mechanisms involved in glial pathogenicity will likely lead to the development of promising therapeutic interventions. Detection of additional pathways of importance will hopefully shed light on new compounds which may be capable of targeting glial-mediated motor neuron damage. Furthermore, stem cell and gene-based therapies have reached evaluation in clinical trials, creating excitement and optimism in the field. As new knowledge of disease mechanisms arises, there is great hope for novel interventions to target glial cells and significantly change the ALS disease course.

6. References

Aggarwal, S. & Cudkowicz, M., (2008). ALS drug development: reflections from the past and a way forward. *Neurotherapeutics*. Vol. 5, No. 4, pp. 516-27.

Almer, G., Vukosavic, S., Romero, N. & Przedborski, S., (1999). Inducible nitric oxide synthase up-regulation in a transgenic mouse model of familial amyotrophic lateral sclerosis. *J Neurochem*. Vol. 72, No. 6, pp. 2415-25.

Amabile, G. & Meissner, A., (2009). Induced pluripotent stem cells: current progress and potential for regenerative medicine. *Trends Mol Med*. Vol. 15, No. 2, pp. 59-68.

Appel, S.H., Engelhardt, J.I., Henkel, J.S., Siklos, L., Beers, D.R., Yen, A.A., Simpson, E.P., Luo, Y., Carrum, G., Heslop, H.E., Brenner, M.K. & Popat, U., (2008). Hematopoietic stem cell transplantation in patients with sporadic amyotrophic lateral sclerosis. *Neurology*. Vol. 71, No. 17, pp. 1326-34.

Beers, D.R., Henkel, J.S., Xiao, Q., Zhao, W., Wang, J., Yen, A.A., Siklos, L., McKercher, S.R. & Appel, S.H., (2006). Wild-type microglia extend survival in PU.1 knockout mice with familial amyotrophic lateral sclerosis. *Proc Natl Acad Sci U S A*. Vol. 103, No. 43, pp. 16021-6.

Beers, D.R., Henkel, J.S., Zhao, W., Wang, J., Huang, A., Wen, S., Liao, B. & Appel, S.H., (2011). Endogenous regulatory T lymphocytes ameliorate amyotrophic lateral sclerosis in mice and correlate with disease progression in patients with amyotrophic lateral sclerosis. *Brain*. Vol. 134, No. Pt 5, pp. 1293-314.

Benatar, M., (2007). Lost in translation: treatment trials in the SOD1 mouse and in human ALS. *Neurobiol Dis*. Vol. 26, No. 1, pp. 1-13.

Bendotti, C., Tortarolo, M., Suchak, S.K., Calvaresi, N., Carvelli, L., Bastone, A., Rizzi, M., Rattray, M. & Mennini, T., (2001). Transgenic SOD1 G93A mice develop reduced GLT-1 in spinal cord without alterations in cerebrospinal fluid glutamate levels. *J Neurochem*. Vol. 79, No. 4, pp. 737-46.

Bevan, A.K., Duque, S., Foust, K.D., Morales, P.R., Braun, L., Schmelzer, L., Chan, C.M., McCrate, M., Chicoine, L.G., Coley, B.D., Porensky, P.N., Kolb, S.J., Mendell, J.R., Burghes, A.H. & Kaspar, B.K., (2011). Systemic Gene Delivery in Large Species for Targeting Spinal Cord, Brain, and Peripheral Tissues for Pediatric Disorders. *Mol Ther*. Vol., No., pp.

Boillee, S., Vande Velde, C. & Cleveland, D.W., (2006a). ALS: a disease of motor neurons and their nonneuronal neighbors. *Neuron*. Vol. 52, No. 1, pp. 39-59.

Boillee, S., Yamanaka, K., Lobsiger, C.S., Copeland, N.G., Jenkins, N.A., Kassiotis, G., Kollias, G. & Cleveland, D.W., (2006b). Onset and Progression in Inherited ALS Determined by Motor Neurons and Microglia. *Science*. Vol. 312, No. 5778, pp. 1389-92.

Bosco, D.A., Morfini, G., Karabacak, N.M., Song, Y., Gros-Louis, F., Pasinelli, P., Goolsby, H., Fontaine, B.A., Lemay, N., McKenna-Yasek, D., Frosch, M.P., Agar, J.N., Julien, J.P., Brady, S.T. & Brown, R.H., Jr., (2010). Wild-type and mutant SOD1 share an aberrant conformation and a common pathogenic pathway in ALS. *Nat Neurosci*. Vol. 13, No. 11, pp. 1396-403.

Boulting, G.L., Kiskinis, E., Croft, G.F., Amoroso, M.W., Oakley, D.H., Wainger, B.J., Williams, D.J., Kahler, D.J., Yamaki, M., Davidow, L., Rodolfa, C.T., Dimos, J.T., Mikkilineni, S., MacDermott, A.B., Woolf, C.J., Henderson, C.E., Wichterle, H. & Eggan, K., (2011). A functionally characterized test set of human induced pluripotent stem cells. *Nat Biotechnol.* Vol. 29, No. 3, pp. 279-86.

Bristol, L.A. & Rothstein, J.D., (1996). Glutamate transporter gene expression in amyotrophic lateral sclerosis motor cortex. *Ann Neurol.* Vol. 39, No. 5, pp. 676-9.

Bruijn, L.I., Becher, M.W., Lee, M.K., Anderson, K.L., Jenkins, N.A., Copeland, N.G., Sisodia, S.S., Rothstein, J.D., Borchelt, D.R., Price, D.L. & Cleveland, D.W., (1997). ALS-linked SOD1 mutant G85R mediates damage to astrocytes and promotes rapidly progressive disease with SOD1-containing inclusions. *Neuron.* Vol. 18, No. 2, pp. 327-38.

Bruijn, L.I., Houseweart, M.K., Kato, S., Anderson, K.L., Anderson, S.D., Ohama, E., Reaume, A.G., Scott, R.W. & Cleveland, D.W., (1998). Aggregation and motor neuron toxicity of an ALS-linked SOD1 mutant independent from wild-type SOD1. *Science.* Vol. 281, No. 5384, pp. 1851-4.

Chiu, A.Y., Zhai, P., Dal Canto, M.C., Peters, T.M., Kwon, Y.W., Prattis, S.M. & Gurney, M.E., (1995). Age-dependent penetrance of disease in a transgenic mouse model of familial amyotrophic lateral sclerosis. *Mol Cell Neurosci.* Vol. 6, No. 4, pp. 349-62.

Chiu, I.M., Chen, A., Zheng, Y., Kosaras, B., Tsiftsoglou, S.A., Vartanian, T.K., Brown, R.H., Jr. & Carroll, M.C., (2008). T lymphocytes potentiate endogenous neuroprotective inflammation in a mouse model of ALS. *Proc Natl Acad Sci U S A.* Vol. 105, No. 46, pp. 17913-8.

Clement, A.M., Nguyen, M.D., Roberts, E.A., Garcia, M.L., Boillee, S., Rule, M., McMahon, A.P., Doucette, W., Siwek, D., Ferrante, R.J., Brown, R.H., Jr., Julien, J.P., Goldstein, L.S. & Cleveland, D.W., (2003). Wild-type nonneuronal cells extend survival of SOD1 mutant motor neurons in ALS mice. *Science.* Vol. 302, No. 5642, pp. 113-7.

Cohen, T.J., Lee, V.M. & Trojanowski, J.Q., (2011). TDP-43 functions and pathogenic mechanisms implicated in TDP-43 proteinopathies. *Trends Mol Med.* Vol., No., pp.

Cudkowicz, M.E., Shefner, J.M., Schoenfeld, D.A., Brown, R.H., Jr., Johnson, H., Qureshi, M., Jacobs, M., Rothstein, J.D., Appel, S.H., Pascuzzi, R.M., Heiman-Patterson, T.D., Donofrio, P.D., David, W.S., Russell, J.A., Tandan, R., Pioro, E.P., Felice, K.J., Rosenfeld, J., Mandler, R.N., Sachs, G.M., Bradley, W.G., Raynor, E.M., Baquis, G.D., Belsh, J.M., Novella, S., Goldstein, J. & Hulihan, J., (2003). A randomized, placebo-controlled trial of topiramate in amyotrophic lateral sclerosis. *Neurology.* Vol. 61, No. 4, pp. 456-64.

Cudkowicz, M.E., Shefner, J.M., Schoenfeld, D.A., Zhang, H., Andreasson, K.I., Rothstein, J.D. & Drachman, D.B., (2006). Trial of celecoxib in amyotrophic lateral sclerosis. *Ann Neurol.* Vol. 60, No. 1, pp. 22-31.

Czepiel, M., Balasubramaniyan, V., Schaafsma, W., Stancic, M., Mikkers, H., Huisman, C., Boddeke, E. & Copray, S., (2011). Differentiation of induced pluripotent stem cells into functional oligodendrocytes. *Glia.* Vol. 59, No. 6, pp. 882-92.

de Carvalho, M., Pinto, S., Costa, J., Evangelista, T., Ohana, B. & Pinto, A., (2010). A randomized, placebo-controlled trial of memantine for functional disability in amyotrophic lateral sclerosis. *Amyotroph Lateral Scler.* Vol. 11, No. 5, pp. 456-60.

Deda, H., Inci, M.C., Kurekci, A.E., Sav, A., Kayihan, K., Ozgun, E., Ustunsoy, G.E. & Kocabay, S., (2009). Treatment of amyotrophic lateral sclerosis patients by autologous bone marrow-derived hematopoietic stem cell transplantation: a 1-year follow-up. *Cytotherapy.* Vol. 11, No. 1, pp. 18-25.

Di Giorgio, F.P., Carrasco, M.A., Siao, M.C., Maniatis, T. & Eggan, K., (2007). Non-cell autonomous effect of glia on motor neurons in an embryonic stem cell-based ALS model. *Nat Neurosci.* Vol. 10, No. 5, pp. 608-614.

Di Giorgio, F.P., Boulting, G.L., Bobrowicz, S. & Eggan, K.C., (2008). Human embryonic stem cell-derived motor neurons are sensitive to the toxic effect of glial cells carrying an ALS-causing mutation. *Cell Stem Cell.* Vol. 3, No. 6, pp. 637-48.

Dimos, J.T., Rodolfa, K.T., Niakan, K.K., Weisenthal, L.M., Mitsumoto, H., Chung, W., Croft, G.F., Saphier, G., Leibel, R., Goland, R., Wichterle, H., Henderson, C.E. & Eggan, K., (2008). Induced pluripotent stem cells generated from patients with ALS can be differentiated into motor neurons. *Science.* Vol. 321, No. 5893, pp. 1218-21.

Dodge, J.C., Haidet, A.M., Yang, W., Passini, M.A., Hester, M., Clarke, J., Roskelley, E.M., Treleaven, C.M., Rizo, L., Martin, H., Kim, S.H., Kaspar, R., Taksir, T.V., Griffiths, D.A., Cheng, S.H., Shihabuddin, L.S. & Kaspar, B.K., (2008). Delivery of AAV-IGF-1 to the CNS extends survival in ALS mice through modification of aberrant glial cell activity. *Mol Ther.* Vol. 16, No. 6, pp. 1056-64.

Drachman, D.B., Frank, K., Dykes-Hoberg, M., Teismann, P., Almer, G., Przedborski, S. & Rothstein, J.D., (2002). Cyclooxygenase 2 inhibition protects motor neurons and prolongs survival in a transgenic mouse model of ALS. *Ann Neurol.* Vol. 52, No. 6, pp. 771-8.

Foust, K.D., Nurre, E., Montgomery, C.L., Hernandez, A., Chan, C.M. & Kaspar, B.K., (2009). Intravascular AAV9 preferentially targets neonatal neurons and adult astrocytes. *Nat Biotechnol.* Vol. 27, No. 1, pp. 59-65.

Gordon, P.H., Moore, D.H., Miller, R.G., Florence, J.M., Verheijde, J.L., Doorish, C., Hilton, J.F., Spitalny, G.M., MacArthur, R.B., Mitsumoto, H., Neville, H.E., Boylan, K., Mozaffar, T., Belsh, J.M., Ravits, J., Bedlack, R.S., Graves, M.C., McCluskey, L.F., Barohn, R.J. & Tandan, R., (2007). Efficacy of minocycline in patients with amyotrophic lateral sclerosis: a phase III randomised trial. *Lancet Neurol.* Vol. 6, No. 12, pp. 1045-53.

Gruzman, A., Wood, W.L., Alpert, E., Prasad, M.D., Miller, R.G., Rothstein, J.D., Bowser, R., Hamilton, R., Wood, T.D., Cleveland, D.W., Lingappa, V.R. & Liu, J., (2007). Common molecular signature in SOD1 for both sporadic and familial amyotrophic lateral sclerosis. *Proc Natl Acad Sci U S A.* Vol. 104, No. 30, pp. 12524-9.

Gurney, M.E., Pu, H., Chiu, A.Y., Dal Canto, M.C., Polchow, C.Y., Alexander, D.D., Caliendo, J., Hentati, A., Kwon, Y.W., Deng, H.X. & et al., (1994). Motor neuron degeneration in mice that express a human Cu,Zn superoxide dismutase mutation. *Science.* Vol. 264, No. 5166, pp. 1772-5.

Haidet-Phillips, A.M., Hester, M.E., Miranda, C.J., Meyer, K., Braun, L., Frakes, A., Song, S., Likhite, S., Murtha, M.J., Foust, K.D., Rao, M., Eagle, A., Kammesheidt, A., Christensen, A., Mendell, J.R., Burghes, A.H. & Kaspar, B.K., (2011). Astrocytes from familial and sporadic ALS patients are toxic to motor neurons. *Nat Biotechnol.* Vol., No., pp.

Henkel, J.S., Beers, D.R., Zhao, W. & Appel, S.H., (2009). Microglia in ALS: The Good, The Bad, and The Resting. *J Neuroimmune Pharmacol.* Vol., No., pp.

Hensley, K., Fedynyshyn, J., Ferrell, S., Floyd, R.A., Gordon, B., Grammas, P., Hamdheydari, L., Mhatre, M., Mou, S., Pye, Q.N., Stewart, C., West, M., West, S. & Williamson, K.S., (2003). Message and protein-level elevation of tumor necrosis factor alpha

(TNF alpha) and TNF alpha-modulating cytokines in spinal cords of the G93A-SOD1 mouse model for amyotrophic lateral sclerosis. *Neurobiol Dis.* Vol. 14, No. 1, pp. 74-80.

Huang, C., Zhou, H., Tong, J., Chen, H., Liu, Y.J., Wang, D., Wei, X. & Xia, X.G., (2011). FUS transgenic rats develop the phenotypes of amyotrophic lateral sclerosis and frontotemporal lobar degeneration. *PLoS Genet.* Vol. 7, No. 3, pp. e1002011.

Jaarsma, D., Teuling, E., Haasdijk, E.D., De Zeeuw, C.I. & Hoogenraad, C.C., (2008). Neuron-specific expression of mutant superoxide dismutase is sufficient to induce amyotrophic lateral sclerosis in transgenic mice. *J Neurosci.* Vol. 28, No. 9, pp. 2075-88.

Kabashi, E., Valdmanis, P.N., Dion, P., Spiegelman, D., McConkey, B.J., Vande Velde, C., Bouchard, J.P., Lacomblez, L., Pochigaeva, K., Salachas, F., Pradat, P.F., Camu, W., Meininger, V., Dupre, N. & Rouleau, G.A., (2008). TARDBP mutations in individuals with sporadic and familial amyotrophic lateral sclerosis. *Nat Genet.* Vol. 40, No. 5, pp. 572-4.

Kang, S.H., Fukaya, M., Yang, J.K., Rothstein, J.D. & Bergles, D.E., (2010). NG2+ CNS glial progenitors remain committed to the oligodendrocyte lineage in postnatal life and following neurodegeneration. *Neuron.* Vol. 68, No. 4, pp. 668-81.

Keller, A.F., Gravel, M. & Kriz, J., (2011). Treatment with minocycline after disease onset alters astrocyte reactivity and increases microgliosis in SOD1 mutant mice. *Exp Neurol.* Vol. 228, No. 1, pp. 69-79.

Klein, S.M., Behrstock, S., McHugh, J., Hoffmann, K., Wallace, K., Suzuki, M., Aebischer, P. & Svendsen, C.N., (2005). GDNF delivery using human neural progenitor cells in a rat model of ALS. *Hum Gene Ther.* Vol. 16, No. 4, pp. 509-21.

Klivenyi, P., Kiaei, M., Gardian, G., Calingasan, N.Y. & Beal, M.F., (2004). Additive neuroprotective effects of creatine and cyclooxygenase 2 inhibitors in a transgenic mouse model of amyotrophic lateral sclerosis. *J Neurochem.* Vol. 88, No. 3, pp. 576-82.

Kondo, M., Shibata, T., Kumagai, T., Osawa, T., Shibata, N., Kobayashi, M., Sasaki, S., Iwata, M., Noguchi, N. & Uchida, K., (2002). 15-Deoxy-Delta(12,14)-prostaglandin J(2): the endogenous electrophile that induces neuronal apoptosis. *Proc Natl Acad Sci U S A.* Vol. 99, No. 11, pp. 7367-72.

Krencik, R., Weick, J.P., Liu, Y., Zhang, Z.J. & Zhang, S.C., (2011). Specification of transplantable astroglial subtypes from human pluripotent stem cells. *Nat Biotechnol.* Vol. 29, No. 6, pp. 528-34.

Kriz, J., Nguyen, M.D. & Julien, J.P., (2002). Minocycline slows disease progression in a mouse model of amyotrophic lateral sclerosis. *Neurobiol Dis.* Vol. 10, No. 3, pp. 268-78.

Kwiatkowski, T.J., Jr., Bosco, D.A., Leclerc, A.L., Tamrazian, E., Vanderburg, C.R., Russ, C., Davis, A., Gilchrist, J., Kasarskis, E.J., Munsat, T., Valdmanis, P., Rouleau, G.A., Hosler, B.A., Cortelli, P., de Jong, P.J., Yoshinaga, Y., Haines, J.L., Pericak-Vance, M.A., Yan, J., Ticozzi, N., Siddique, T., McKenna-Yasek, D., Sapp, P.C., Horvitz, H.R., Landers, J.E. & Brown, R.H., Jr., (2009). Mutations in the FUS/TLS gene on chromosome 16 cause familial amyotrophic lateral sclerosis. *Science.* Vol. 323, No. 5918, pp. 1205-8.

Lepore, A.C., Dejea, C., Carmen, J., Rauck, B., Kerr, D.A., Sofroniew, M.V. & Maragakis, N.J., (2008a). Selective ablation of proliferating astrocytes does not affect disease outcome in either acute or chronic models of motor neuron degeneration. *Exp Neurol.* Vol. 211, No. 2, pp. 423-32.

Lepore, A.C., Rauck, B., Dejea, C., Pardo, A.C., Rao, M.S., Rothstein, J.D. & Maragakis, N.J., (2008b). Focal transplantation-based astrocyte replacement is neuroprotective in a model of motor neuron disease. *Nat Neurosci*. Vol. 11, No. 11, pp. 1294-301.

Lino, M.M., Schneider, C. & Caroni, P., (2002). Accumulation of SOD1 mutants in postnatal motoneurons does not cause motoneuron pathology or motoneuron disease. *J Neurosci*. Vol. 22, No. 12, pp. 4825-32.

Liu, Y., Jiang, P. & Deng, W., (2011). OLIG gene targeting in human pluripotent stem cells for motor neuron and oligodendrocyte differentiation. *Nat Protoc*. Vol. 6, No. 5, pp. 640-55.

Lobsiger, C.S., Boillee, S., McAlonis-Downes, M., Khan, A.M., Feltri, M.L., Yamanaka, K. & Cleveland, D.W., (2009). Schwann cells expressing dismutase active mutant SOD1 unexpectedly slow disease progression in ALS mice. *Proc Natl Acad Sci U S A*. Vol. 106, No. 11, pp. 4465-70.

Mackenzie, I.R., Bigio, E.H., Ince, P.G., Geser, F., Neumann, M., Cairns, N.J., Kwong, L.K., Forman, M.S., Ravits, J., Stewart, H., Eisen, A., McClusky, L., Kretzschmar, H.A., Monoranu, C.M., Highley, J.R., Kirby, J., Siddique, T., Shaw, P.J., Lee, V.M. & Trojanowski, J.Q., (2007). Pathological TDP-43 distinguishes sporadic amyotrophic lateral sclerosis from amyotrophic lateral sclerosis with SOD1 mutations. *Ann Neurol*. Vol. 61, No. 5, pp. 427-34.

Mackenzie, I.R., Rademakers, R. & Neumann, M., (2010). TDP-43 and FUS in amyotrophic lateral sclerosis and frontotemporal dementia. *Lancet Neurol*. Vol. 9, No. 10, pp. 995-1007.

Magnus, T., Carmen, J., Deleon, J., Xue, H., Pardo, A.C., Lepore, A.C., Mattson, M.P., Rao, M.S. & Maragakis, N.J., (2008). Adult glial precursor proliferation in mutant SOD1G93A mice. *Glia*. Vol. 56, No. 2, pp. 200-8.

Maragakis, N.J. & Rothstein, J.D., (2006). Mechanisms of Disease: astrocytes in neurodegenerative disease. *Nat Clin Pract Neurol*. Vol. 2, No. 12, pp. 679-89.

Marchetto, M.C., Muotri, A.R., Mu, Y., Smith, A.M., Cezar, G.G. & Gage, F.H., (2008). Non-cell-autonomous effect of human SOD1 G37R astrocytes on motor neurons derived from human embryonic stem cells. *Cell Stem Cell*. Vol. 3, No. 6, pp. 649-57.

Miller, R.G., Moore, D.H., 2nd, Gelinas, D.F., Dronsky, V., Mendoza, M., Barohn, R.J., Bryan, W., Ravits, J., Yuen, E., Neville, H., Ringel, S., Bromberg, M., Petajan, J., Amato, A.A., Jackson, C., Johnson, W., Mandler, R., Bosch, P., Smith, B., Graves, M., Ross, M., Sorenson, E.J., Kelkar, P., Parry, G. & Olney, R., (2001). Phase III randomized trial of gabapentin in patients with amyotrophic lateral sclerosis. *Neurology*. Vol. 56, No. 7, pp. 843-8.

Miller, R.G., Mitchell, J.D., Lyon, M. & Moore, D.H., (2007). Riluzole for amyotrophic lateral sclerosis (ALS)/motor neuron disease (MND). *Cochrane Database Syst Rev*. Vol., No. 1, pp. CD001447.

Miller, T.M., Kaspar, B.K., Kops, G.J., Yamanaka, K., Christian, L.J., Gage, F.H. & Cleveland, D.W., (2005). Virus-delivered small RNA silencing sustains strength in amyotrophic lateral sclerosis. *Ann Neurol*. Vol. 57, No. 5, pp. 773-6.

Miller, T.M., Smith, R.A., Kordasiewicz, H. & Kaspar, B.K., (2008). Gene-targeted therapies for the central nervous system. *Arch Neurol*. Vol. 65, No. 4, pp. 447-51.

Nagai, M., Re, D.B., Nagata, T., Chalazonitis, A., Jessell, T.M., Wichterle, H. & Przedborski, S., (2007). Astrocytes expressing ALS-linked mutated SOD1 release factors selectively toxic to motor neurons. *Nat Neurosci*. Vol. 10, No. 5, pp. 615-622.

Neumann, M., Sampathu, D.M., Kwong, L.K., Truax, A.C., Micsenyi, M.C., Chou, T.T., Bruce, J., Schuck, T., Grossman, M., Clark, C.M., McCluskey, L.F., Miller, B.L., Masliah, E., Mackenzie, I.R., Feldman, H., Feiden, W., Kretzschmar, H.A., Trojanowski, J.Q. & Lee,

V.M., (2006). Ubiquitinated TDP-43 in frontotemporal lobar degeneration and amyotrophic lateral sclerosis. *Science*. Vol. 314, No. 5796, pp. 130-3.

Nguyen, M.D., Julien, J.P. & Rivest, S., (2001). Induction of proinflammatory molecules in mice with amyotrophic lateral sclerosis: no requirement for proapoptotic interleukin-1beta in neurodegeneration. *Ann Neurol*. Vol. 50, No. 5, pp. 630-9.

Okita, K., Ichisaka, T. & Yamanaka, S., (2007). Generation of germline-competent induced pluripotent stem cells. *Nature*. Vol. 448, No. 7151, pp. 313-7.

Palmer, T.D., Schwartz, P.H., Taupin, P., Kaspar, B., Stein, S.A. & Gage, F.H., (2001). Cell culture. Progenitor cells from human brain after death. *Nature*. Vol. 411, No. 6833, pp. 42-3.

Park, I.H., Zhao, R., West, J.A., Yabuuchi, A., Huo, H., Ince, T.A., Lerou, P.H., Lensch, M.W. & Daley, G.Q., (2008). Reprogramming of human somatic cells to pluripotency with defined factors. *Nature*. Vol. 451, No. 7175, pp. 141-6.

Perrie, W.T., Lee, G.T., Curtis, E.M., Sparke, J., Buller, J.R. & Rossi, M.L., (1993). Changes in the myelinated axons of femoral nerve in amyotrophic lateral sclerosis. *J Neural Transm Suppl*. Vol. 39, No., pp. 223-33.

Pompl, P.N., Ho, L., Bianchi, M., McManus, T., Qin, W. & Pasinetti, G.M., (2003). A therapeutic role for cyclooxygenase-2 inhibitors in a transgenic mouse model of amyotrophic lateral sclerosis. *FASEB J*. Vol. 17, No. 6, pp. 725-7.

Pramatarova, A., Laganiere, J., Roussel, J., Brisebois, K. & Rouleau, G.A., (2001). Neuron-specific expression of mutant superoxide dismutase 1 in transgenic mice does not lead to motor impairment. *J Neurosci*. Vol. 21, No. 10, pp. 3369-74.

Ralph, G.S., Radcliffe, P.A., Day, D.M., Carthy, J.M., Leroux, M.A., Lee, D.C., Wong, L.F., Bilsland, L.G., Greensmith, L., Kingsman, S.M., Mitrophanous, K.A., Mazarakis, N.D. & Azzouz, M., (2005). Silencing mutant SOD1 using RNAi protects against neurodegeneration and extends survival in an ALS model. *Nat Med*. Vol. 11, No. 4, pp. 429-33.

Raoul, C., Abbas-Terki, T., Bensadoun, J.C., Guillot, S., Haase, G., Szulc, J., Henderson, C.E. & Aebischer, P., (2005). Lentiviral-mediated silencing of SOD1 through RNA interference retards disease onset and progression in a mouse model of ALS. *Nat Med*. Vol. 11, No. 4, pp. 423-8.

Rothstein, J.D., Tsai, G., Kuncl, R.W., Clawson, L., Cornblath, D.R., Drachman, D.B., Pestronk, A., Stauch, B.L. & Coyle, J.T., (1990). Abnormal excitatory amino acid metabolism in amyotrophic lateral sclerosis. *Ann Neurol*. Vol. 28, No. 1, pp. 18-25.

Rothstein, J.D., Van Kammen, M., Levey, A.I., Martin, L.J. & Kuncl, R.W., (1995). Selective loss of glial glutamate transporter GLT-1 in amyotrophic lateral sclerosis. *Ann Neurol*. Vol. 38, No. 1, pp. 73-84.

Rothstein, J.D., Patel, S., Regan, M.R., Haenggeli, C., Huang, Y.H., Bergles, D.E., Jin, L., Dykes Hoberg, M., Vidensky, S., Chung, D.S., Toan, S.V., Bruijn, L.I., Su, Z.Z., Gupta, P. & Fisher, P.B., (2005). Beta-lactam antibiotics offer neuroprotection by increasing glutamate transporter expression. *Nature*. Vol. 433, No. 7021, pp. 73-7.

Ryberg, H., Askmark, H. & Persson, L.I., (2003). A double-blind randomized clinical trial in amyotrophic lateral sclerosis using lamotrigine: effects on CSF glutamate, aspartate, branched-chain amino acid levels and clinical parameters. *Acta Neurol Scand*. Vol. 108, No. 1, pp. 1-8.

Sah, D.W. & Aronin, N., (2011). Oligonucleotide therapeutic approaches for Huntington disease. *J Clin Invest*. Vol. 121, No. 2, pp. 500-7.

Sasaki, S., Shibata, N., Komori, T. & Iwata, M., (2000). iNOS and nitrotyrosine immunoreactivity in amyotrophic lateral sclerosis. *Neurosci Lett*. Vol. 291, No. 1, pp. 44-8.

Shaw, P.J., Forrest, V., Ince, P.G., Richardson, J.P. & Wastell, H.J., (1995). CSF and plasma amino acid levels in motor neuron disease: elevation of CSF glutamate in a subset of patients. *Neurodegeneration*. Vol. 4, No. 2, pp. 209-16.

Smith, R.A., Miller, T.M., Yamanaka, K., Monia, B.P., Condon, T.P., Hung, G., Lobsiger, C.S., Ward, C.M., McAlonis-Downes, M., Wei, H., Wancewicz, E.V., Bennett, C.F. & Cleveland, D.W., (2006). Antisense oligonucleotide therapy for neurodegenerative disease. *J Clin Invest*. Vol. 116, No. 8, pp. 2290-6.

Sreedharan, J., Blair, I.P., Tripathi, V.B., Hu, X., Vance, C., Rogelj, B., Ackerley, S., Durnall, J.C., Williams, K.L., Buratti, E., Baralle, F., de Belleroche, J., Mitchell, J.D., Leigh, P.N., Al-Chalabi, A., Miller, C.C., Nicholson, G. & Shaw, C.E., (2008). TDP-43 mutations in familial and sporadic amyotrophic lateral sclerosis. *Science*. Vol. 319, No. 5870, pp. 1668-72.

Suzuki, M., McHugh, J., Tork, C., Shelley, B., Klein, S.M., Aebischer, P. & Svendsen, C.N., (2007). GDNF secreting human neural progenitor cells protect dying motor neurons, but not their projection to muscle, in a rat model of familial ALS. *PLoS One*. Vol. 2, No. 8, pp. e689.

Takahashi, K. & Yamanaka, S., (2006). Induction of pluripotent stem cells from mouse embryonic and adult fibroblast cultures by defined factors. *Cell*. Vol. 126, No. 4, pp. 663-76.

Takahashi, K., Tanabe, K., Ohnuki, M., Narita, M., Ichisaka, T., Tomoda, K. & Yamanaka, S., (2007). Induction of pluripotent stem cells from adult human fibroblasts by defined factors. *Cell*. Vol. 131, No. 5, pp. 861-72.

Towne, C., Setola, V., Schneider, B.L. & Aebischer, P., (2011). Neuroprotection by gene therapy targeting mutant SOD1 in individual pools of motor neurons does not translate into therapeutic benefit in fALS mice. *Mol Ther*. Vol. 19, No. 2, pp. 274-83.

Turner, B.J., Ackerley, S., Davies, K.E. & Talbot, K., (2010). Dismutase-competent SOD1 mutant accumulation in myelinating Schwann cells is not detrimental to normal or transgenic ALS model mice. *Hum Mol Genet*. Vol. 19, No. 5, pp. 815-24.

Urushitani, M., Sik, A., Sakurai, T., Nukina, N., Takahashi, R. & Julien, J.P., (2006). Chromogranin-mediated secretion of mutant superoxide dismutase proteins linked to amyotrophic lateral sclerosis. *Nat Neurosci*. Vol. 9, No. 1, pp. 108-18.

Van Den Bosch, L., Tilkin, P., Lemmens, G. & Robberecht, W., (2002). Minocycline delays disease onset and mortality in a transgenic model of ALS. *Neuroreport*. Vol. 13, No. 8, pp. 1067-70.

Vance, C., Rogelj, B., Hortobagyi, T., De Vos, K.J., Nishimura, A.L., Sreedharan, J., Hu, X., Smith, B., Ruddy, D., Wright, P., Ganesalingam, J., Williams, K.L., Tripathi, V., Al-Saraj, S., Al-Chalabi, A., Leigh, P.N., Blair, I.P., Nicholson, G., de Belleroche, J., Gallo, J.M., Miller, C.C. & Shaw, C.E., (2009). Mutations in FUS, an RNA processing protein, cause familial amyotrophic lateral sclerosis type 6. *Science*. Vol. 323, No. 5918, pp. 1208-11.

Wang, H., Ghosh, A., Baigude, H., Yang, C.S., Qiu, L., Xia, X., Zhou, H., Rana, T.M. & Xu, Z., (2008). Therapeutic gene silencing delivered by a chemically modified small interfering RNA against mutant SOD1 slows amyotrophic lateral sclerosis progression. *J Biol Chem*. Vol. 283, No. 23, pp. 15845-52.

Wang, L., Sharma, K., Grisotti, G. & Roos, R.P., (2009). The effect of mutant SOD1 dismutase activity on non-cell autonomous degeneration in familial amyotrophic lateral sclerosis. *Neurobiol Dis*. Vol. 35, No. 2, pp. 234-40.

Wang, L., Gutmann, D.H. & Roos, R.P., (2011). Astrocyte loss of mutant SOD1 delays ALS disease onset and progression in G85R transgenic mice. *Hum Mol Genet*. Vol. 20, No. 2, pp. 286-93.

Wernig, M., Meissner, A., Foreman, R., Brambrink, T., Ku, M., Hochedlinger, K., Bernstein, B.E. & Jaenisch, R., (2007). In vitro reprogramming of fibroblasts into a pluripotent ES-cell-like state. *Nature*. Vol. 448, No. 7151, pp. 318-24.

Weydt, P., Yuen, E.C., Ransom, B.R. & Moller, T., (2004). Increased cytotoxic potential of microglia from ALS-transgenic mice. *Glia*. Vol. 48, No. 2, pp. 179-82.

Xiao, Q., Zhao, W., Beers, D.R., Yen, A.A., Xie, W., Henkel, J.S. & Appel, S.H., (2007). Mutant SOD1(G93A) microglia are more neurotoxic relative to wild-type microglia. *J Neurochem*. Vol. 102, No. 6, pp. 2008-19.

Xu, L., Ryugo, D.K., Pongstaporn, T., Johe, K. & Koliatsos, V.E., (2009). Human neural stem cell grafts in the spinal cord of SOD1 transgenic rats: differentiation and structural integration into the segmental motor circuitry. *J Comp Neurol*. Vol. 514, No. 4, pp. 297-309.

Xu, L., Shen, P., Hazel, T., Johe, K. & Koliatsos, V.E., (2011). Dual transplantation of human neural stem cells into cervical and lumbar cord ameliorates motor neuron disease in SOD1 transgenic rats. *Neurosci Lett*. Vol. 494, No. 3, pp. 222-6.

Yamanaka, K., Boillee, S., Roberts, E.A., Garcia, M.L., McAlonis-Downes, M., Mikse, O.R., Cleveland, D.W. & Goldstein, L.S., (2008a). Mutant SOD1 in cell types other than motor neurons and oligodendrocytes accelerates onset of disease in ALS mice. *Proc Natl Acad Sci U S A*. Vol. 105, No. 21, pp. 7594-9.

Yamanaka, K., Chun, S.J., Boillee, S., Fujimori-Tonou, N., Yamashita, H., Gutmann, D.H., Takahashi, R., Misawa, H. & Cleveland, D.W., (2008b). Astrocytes as determinants of disease progression in inherited amyotrophic lateral sclerosis. *Nat Neurosci*. Vol., No., pp.

Yamanaka, S. & Blau, H.M., (2010). Nuclear reprogramming to a pluripotent state by three approaches. *Nature*. Vol. 465, No. 7299, pp. 704-12.

Yu, J., Vodyanik, M.A., Smuga-Otto, K., Antosiewicz-Bourget, J., Frane, J.L., Tian, S., Nie, J., Jonsdottir, G.A., Ruotti, V., Stewart, R., Slukvin, II & Thomson, J.A., (2007). Induced pluripotent stem cell lines derived from human somatic cells. *Science*. Vol. 318, No. 5858, pp. 1917-20.

Zhao, T., Zhang, Z.N., Rong, Z. & Xu, Y., (2011). Immunogenicity of induced pluripotent stem cells. *Nature*. Vol. 474, No. 7350, pp. 212-5.

Zhao, W., Xie, W., Xiao, Q., Beers, D.R. & Appel, S.H., (2006). Protective effects of an anti-inflammatory cytokine, interleukin-4, on motoneuron toxicity induced by activated microglia. *J Neurochem*. Vol. 99, No. 4, pp. 1176-87.

Zhao, W., Beers, D.R., Henkel, J.S., Zhang, W., Urushitani, M., Julien, J.P. & Appel, S.H., (2010). Extracellular mutant SOD1 induces microglial-mediated motoneuron injury. *Glia*. Vol. 58, No. 2, pp. 231-43.

Zhu, S., Stavrovskaya, I.G., Drozda, M., Kim, B.Y., Ona, V., Li, M., Sarang, S., Liu, A.S., Hartley, D.M., Wu, D.C., Gullans, S., Ferrante, R.J., Przedborski, S., Kristal, B.S. & Friedlander, R.M., (2002). Minocycline inhibits cytochrome c release and delays progression of amyotrophic lateral sclerosis in mice. *Nature*. Vol. 417, No. 6884, pp. 74-8.

Zinman, L. & Cudkowicz, M., (2011). Emerging targets and treatments in amyotrophic lateral sclerosis. *Lancet Neurol*. Vol. 10, No. 5, pp. 481-90.

5

Stem Cell Application for Amyotrophic Lateral Sclerosis: Growth Factor Delivery and Cell Therapy

Masatoshi Suzuki, Chak Foon Tso and Michael G. Meyer
University of Wisconsin-Madison
U. S. A.

1. Introduction

1.1 ALS and the SOD1 rodent models

Amyotrophic lateral sclerosis (ALS) is a progressive disorder that leads to degeneration of upper and lower motor neurons, muscular atrophy, and (ultimately) death. A clinical diagnosis of ALS requires signs of progressive degeneration in both upper and lower motor neurons, with no evidence that suggest that the signs can be explained by other disease processes (Brooks et al., 1994, 2000). The incidence rate of the disease is around 2 in 100,000 people (Hirtz et al., 2007). The onset age of sporadic and most familial form of ALS is between 50-60 years, and is generally fatal within 1-5 years of onset (Cleveland & Rothstein, 2001). Riluzile is the only drug that demonstrates a beneficial effect on ALS patients, but only increases survival by a matter of months (Zoccolella et al., 2009).

Motor neuron cell death in ALS probably involves multiple pathways. Most ALS cases are sporadic in nature, while ~10% arise from a dominantly inherited trait (familial ALS or FALS) (Brown, 1995). The cause for sporadic ALS remains unclear, while 20% of FALS patients have a point mutation in the cytosolic Cu^{2+}/Zn^{2+} superoxide dismutase 1 (SOD1) gene (Rosen et al., 1993). Recent reports suggested that other causes of FALS also include mutations in TDP-43 (the 43-KDa TAR DNA binding protein) and FUS (Fused in sarcoma/translocated in liposarcoma) genes (Ticozzi et al, 2011). From various lines of transgenic mice, we can observe that motor neuron disease is developed in mutants with elevated SOD1 levels (ex. hSOD1-G93A line), while no symptoms are observed in SOD1 knockout mice. The combined effect shows that SOD1 acts through a toxic gain of function rather than loss of dismutase activity (Julien et al., 2001). Both mouse and rat models over-expressing SOD1 genes show similar disease phenotypes and disease progression to those observed in human ALS patients (Gurney, 1994; Nagai et al., 2001; Howland et al., 2002).

The mechanism underlying motor neuron death in ALS is still unknown. However, SOD1 mutant induces non-cell-autonomous motor neuron killing by an unknown gain of toxicity, which means the gain of toxicity arises from damage to cells other than motor neurons (Boillée et al., 2006a). Multiple mechanisms account for the selective vulnerability of motor neurons including protein misfolding, mitochondrial dysfunction, oxidative damage, defective axonal transport, excitotoxicity, insufficient growth factor signaling, and inflammation (Boillée et al., 2006a). Of course there are a lot of shortcomings for using

G93A and other SOD1 transgenic rodent models as SOD1 mutation is only found in a small proportion of human ALS patients. However, it is still an excellent tool for ALS researchers as transgenic mice have proven to be one of the most useful tools to understand the complexity of neurodegenerative diseases because of their usefulness to unveil underlying mechanisms of the disease and evaluating potential treatments (Rothstein, 2004). In this review we will overview the extensive use of SOD1 transgenic rodent models in ALS research and how those findings can be transferred to treat human ALS patients.

1.2 Chapter overview

Topics covered in this chapter include growth factor therapy and stem cell therapy for ALS. For growth factor therapy, we will introduce different delivery methods and injection sites. As for stem cell transplantation therapy, we will look into strategies that aim to replace or protect motor neurons. After that, we will summarize studies that utilize stem cells as a tool to deliver growth factors. We will conclude the chapter by looking forward to future development in the field.

2. Growth factors and gene therapy in ALS

2.1 Growth factors and the nervous system

Growth factors are a class of naturally occurring proteins that are capable of stimulating cell growth, proliferation, and differentiation. In development of the nervous system, they are crucial because they are essential for neuronal survival and differentiation. For adults, they are also required in some cases to maintain normal function of the nervous system, but only at very low levels. However, the presence of low levels of growth factors in adult tissues is critical because motor neurons rely on them for survival and repair upon stress and injury. Experiments have been performed to investigate the effect of growth factors on alleviating the symptoms of ALS. Those growth factors includes glial cell line-derived neurotrophic factor (GDNF), insulin growth factor 1 (IGF-1), vascular endothelial growth factor (VEGF), and brain derived neurotrophic factor (BDNF). For each of the growth factors listed above, there are studies on hSOD1-G93A transgenic rodent models that show some degree of improvement, which includes some or all of the following: delay onset, slow disease progression, decrease motor neuron loss, preserve neuromuscular junction and prolong survival.

2.2 Strategies of growth factor delivery
2.2.1 Methods of delivery

Currently, three different methods of have been used to deliver the growth factor into the motor nervous system to ALS patients or rodent models. The first is subcutaneous injection of the growth factor protein. The obvious advantage of this method is the ease and simplicity to administrate. Some growth factors are pharmaceutically available to treat other neurodevelopmental diseases, such as IGF-1 to treat IGF deficiency in children. This is the reason why it is the only method of delivery that has been tested on human ALS patients. However, a statistically significant result has not been observed in this method of delivery. The only successful case is the North American study on IGF-1 in 1997 (Lai et al., 1997), but was immediately challenged by an almost identical study in Europe in 1998 (Borasio et al., 1998) and other later studies. The failure of this classical method of delivery to alleviate ALS symptoms includes (i) inability of some of the chemical of interest to pass the blood-brain barrier; (ii) unwanted side effects in non-targeted sites, and (iii) a relative short half-life of the protein. The significance of these issues is amplified in the human nervous system because of greater cross-sectional area when compared to rodents. Further penetration is needed for the injected growth factor to reach the deep structure in the brain or spinal cord to give its desired effect. Similar issues are found in clinical trials for patients with Parkinson's disease using the same strategy to deliver growth factors.

The second method is to deliver the chemical of interest by implanting a catheter directly into the site of the brain that needs the growth factor, as seen in a couple Parkinson's disease studies (Gill et al., 2003; Slevin et al., 2005). It is better than the previous method as it overcomes the distance problem seen in large animals. However, there are a couple of drawbacks if this is applied to ALS patients to deliver the growth factor into the spinal cord instead of the brain for Parkinson's disease. The implanted catheter might interrupt the ascending and/or descending white matter track, and the natural movement of the spinal cord in patients increase the shearing forces may cause further damage. Therefore catheter delivery would not be a desirable method of ALS growth factor delivery.

The last approach uses viral vectors to circumvent all those issues. Those viruses include lentivirus (Cisterni et al., 2000; Hottinger et al., 2000; Azzouz et al., 2004), adenovirus (Acsadi et al., 2002; Hasse et al., 2007), and adeno-associated virus (AAV) (Kasper et al., 2003; Wang et al., 2002). They are used because of the ability to deliver genes to non-dividing cells, which includes mature neurons. Thus they are ready to be engineered to encode the therapeutic protein. Extensive studies of AAV delivery of potential drugs to specific brain regions have been published, suggesting viral vector delivery is a practical method.

2.2.2 Sites of delivery

Studies have been done to inject vectors encoding the growth factor of interest into two distinctive types of tissues: (i) limb/respiratory muscles and (ii) the connecting motor neurons. In most ALS studies the vectors are injected in the muscle. Although positive results are shown in studies with GDNF and IGF-1, researchers believes that motor neurons may detach from the muscle at early stages of the disease (Fischer et al., 2004), or the cellular transport mechanism is heavily impaired (Williamson & Cleveland, 1999; De Vos et al., 2007). Again due to their large cross-sectional area, retrograde transport is more severely affected in larger mammals when compared to mice, and thus requires a longer distance of transport. This factor may slow the translation of this successful strategy to clinical trials. To overcome the potential problems of retrograde transport that may be encountered in muscle injections in humans, studies that inject vectors directly to motor neurons within spinal cord has been performed. Surprisingly, only a few studies have been published on this approach and the effect is less significant than the muscle injection studies. In a GDNF study on ALS mice, neuroprotection is only seen on facial but not lumbar motor neurons (Guillot, 2004). Another study supports the above idea by showing that GDNF is neuroprotective when it is overexpressed in skeletal muscles, but has no effect when the growth factor is overexpressed in motor neurons (Li et al., 2007). Disease progression is only slowed when GDNF is expressed in skeletal muscles, but not when it is expressed in the motor neurons.

2.3 Insights from growth factor studies to understand ALS disease progression

Although the ultimate goal of growth factor therapy for ALS is to alleviate symptoms, prolong survival, delay onset, and slow disease progression, during the course of investigation several interesting findings have been observed and may provide insights to better understand the underlying mechanism of the disease. For example, finding growth factors' targets may help us find how the disease is initiated. Currently, the growth factors' targets are not fully known. It could be the degenerating motor neuron itself, the neighboring neuron, or surrounding glial cells. But a recent report about wild type non-neuronal cells extending survival of SOD1 mutant motor neurons in chimeric ALS mice (Clement et al., 2003) may provide adequate evidence showing that the growth factor's target is the supporting glia instead of neurons.

Another point of interest is the similarity of the growth factors that have been used. All GDNF, IGF-1, VEGF, and BDNF interact with receptor tyrosine kinases to produce downstream effects. Experiments have shown that those growth factors indeed work in a similar pathway and mechanism as there is no additional improvement observed when they work in combination (IGF-1 and VEGF) as compared to working individually (Dodge et al. 2010). Another article reports that VEGF promotes motor neuron survival by blocking Caspase through Phosphoinositide 3-kinase/ protein kinase B (PI3K/Akt) pathway (Lunn et al., 2009). Further investigation on the PI3K/Akt pathway may provide clues on how motor neuron death is triggered in ALS.

3. Stem cell therapy for ALS

3.1 The motor neuron replacement strategy

As motor neuron loss is the key diagnostic feature of ALS, the most straightforward strategy is to derive motor neurons from various types of stem cells and try to use them to replace the dead motor neurons in patients. For adult stem cells, cells expressing neuron and glial lineage markers were successfully derived from trans-differentiation of human umbilical cord blood cells (McGuckin et al., 2004) and mouse bone marrow stem cells (Croft et al. 2006). However, those cells' electrophysiological properties, survival, differentiation, and efficacy of integration to functional neurons and glial cells either *in vitro* or *in vivo* were not tested. Neural stem cells are the only type of adult stem cells which have successfully derived motor neurons that are functional *in vivo* (Gao et al., 2005). Human neural stem cells, which are scarce in the human body, are usually derived from embryonic stem cells or fetal brain tissues (Tai & Svendsen, 2004).

More promising results were shown in experiments using pluripotent stem cells. From mouse embryonic stem (ES) cells, motor neurons were successfully generated by induction of developmentally relevant signaling factors. The derived cells survive when transplanted into chick embryonic spinal cord, extend axons, and exhibit signs of presynaptic specialization when reaching targeted muscles (Wichterle et al., 2002). Another study shows that those cells possess immunohistochemical and electrophysiological features of normal motor neurons (Miles et al., 2004). Similar to mouse ES cells, human ES cells have been reported to form functional neurons (Li et al., 2005; Lee et al., 2007).

Functional motor neurons can also be derived from human induced pluripotent stem (iPS) cells, a possible alternative that may avoid the ethical concerns for the use of human ES cells (Karumbayaram et al., 2009). iPS cells are somatic cells that are reprogrammed into pluripotent stem cells (Yu et al., 2007; Takahashi, 2007), with great similarity to embryonic stem cells. They are capable of deriving patient-specific differentiated cells like neurons and glia, which allows them to potentially be used for autologous cell replacement in ALS patients. iPS cells have been generated from ALS patients and the cells are capable of differentiating into motor neurons

(Dimos, 2008).   However, introduction of new genes during the production of iPS cells may give rise to additional technical concerns when translating to clinical studies.

Mouse ES-derived motor neurons reportedly grow around the ventral horn when transplanted into the spinal cord of rats with impaired motor neurons (Harper et al., 2004). In combination with chemicals that overcome myelin-mediated repulsion and GDNF that stimulates axon guidance towards skeletal muscles, further improvement in survival and engraftment of the transplanted cells was observed.   Improvement in motor function of the paralyzed rats was also observed (Despande et al., 2006).

Despite the excitement that these transplantation studies brings to the field, the fact that these studies were performed on static models of motor neuron loss does not guarantee success in progressive motor neuron diseases like ALS. In addition, in order for the motor neuron replacement strategy to be successful, the transplanted motor neuron will first need to receive synaptic input from the presynaptic neurons and extend it's axon all the way to the targeted muscle at a rate of 1-3 mm/day, which takes months to years in humans, before innervation to the targeted muscle can be possible (Papadeas & Maragakis, 2009). Therefore motor neuron replacement may not be a legitimate treatment at this moment.

3.2 The neuroprotection strategy
3.2.1 Non-cell autonomous nature of motor neuron death in ALS

Previously, little attention has been paid to the function of glial cells in the nervous system. However, we now know that glial cells modulate neuronal functions such as glutamate uptake, synaptic plasticity, trophic factor support, and even neuronal transmission (Kirchhoff et al., 2001). Studies also show that motor neuron death in ALS is non-cell autonomous, or mediated by astrocytes and microglia (Hall et al., 1998; Barbeito et al., 2004). Researchers also hypothesize that astrocytes and/or microglia form a positive feedback loop with motor neurons that leads to further propagation of the disease (Rao & Weiss, 2004). Moreover, chimeric mice with increased proportion of healthy, wild type glial cells increase survival of nearby human SOD1 mutant neurons *in vivo* (Clement et al., 2003). Using a CRE-lox system, selective reduction of the mutant gene in microglia and astrocytes in SOD1 transgenic mice slows disease progression, but has no effect on disease onset (Boillée et al., 2006b; Yamanaka et al., 2008).

Additional evidence is provided by stem cell–derived motor neurons/astrocytes co-culture. A study in 2007 shows that primary and ES cell-derived motor neurons are complementary in an *in vitro* motor neuron/astrocytes study for ALS (Nagai et al., 2007). From then on, studies using the following combinations have been performed: hES cell derived motor neurons with primary hSOD1-G93A or wild type mouse primary astrocytes (Di Giorgio et al. 2008); hSOD1-G93A mouse ES derived motor neuron with hSOD1-G93A derived mouse primary astrocytes (Di Giorgio 2007); and hES cells derived motor neuron with primary human astrocytes transfected with hSOD1-G47R genes (Marchetto, 2008). The Marchetto paper also uses that approach to verify a potential drug that has been beneficial in ALS rodent models. The success in this approach provides an easily accessible *in vitro* testing platform for cell-cell interactions in ALS and underlying disease mechanisms.   Drug discovery will also accelerate as high throughput drug screening can be performed on the cultures.

3.2.2 Astrocyte replacement

Based on non-cell autonomous nature of motor neuron death in ALS, astrocyte replacement is another feasible strategy for ALS stem cell therapy.   Researchers transplant glial restricted precursor (GRP) cells (lineage-restricted as derived from developing spinal cord) focally to cervical spinal cord that controls respiratory function in SOD1 rats (Lepore et al., 2008). The effect of the GRP transplant is significant: GRP cells survive and differentiated into mature astrocytes *in vivo*. The treatment also reduces microgliosis, prolongs survival, ameliorates motor neuron loss, and slows motor function decline. The group also found that the ALS rats with grafted GRP cells maintain normal level of glutamate transporter (GLT-1), an astrocyte-specific protein that has reduced expression in both ALS model rats and human patients (Howland et al., 2002; Rothstein et al., 1995). This may provide further evidence that astrocyte replacement is a sound strategy for ALS cell therapy.

3.2.3 Immunomodulation

Other than replacement strategies, some stem cell therapies modulate the immunological environment around the degenerating motor neurons to prevent them from dying. Bone marrow cells provide a rich source of mesenchymal stem cells (MSCs) and hematopoietic stem cells (HSCs). HSCs can give rise to a great variety of blood cells and cells in the immune system, but will particularly differentiate into microglia when introduced to the nervous system (Vitry et al., 2003). MSCs do not have the ability to differentiate into cells in the nervous system, but contribute to improved locomotion by differentiating into cells in the skeletal muscle lineage (Corti et al., 2004). Bone marrow transplanted into irradiated SOD1^{G93A}/PU1$^{-/-}$ double mutants (born without microglia and peripheral immune cells) prolonged survival and slowed disease progression (Beers et al., 2006). Another similar experiment confirms the result (Corti et al., 2004). This led to clinical trials of MSC and HSC transplants to sporadic ALS patients (Appel et al., 2008; Mazzini et al., 2008). Some of these studies show promising results **(Table 1)**.

3.3 Protective effect of neural stem cell and other cells in the neural lineage

Although most transplantations involving cells in the neural lineage were aimed at replacement of motor neurons, researchers now find that neuro-protection was instead the main effect. Various cell transplantations have been performed on hSOD1-G93A rodent models. They include: i) human embryonic germ cell delivered to cerebral spinal fluid (Kerr et al., 2003); ii) human neural stem cells grafted into the spinal cord (Yan et al., 2006); iii) hNT neurons derived from a human teratocarcinoma cell line grafted into spinal cord (Garbuzova-Davis et al., 2002); mouse Sertoli cells into parenchyma (Hemendinger et al., 2005); and human umbilical cord blood cells transfused into the systemic circulation (Habisch et al., 2007). In each of the cases, there was some degree of positive effect on motor neuron survival and life span of the animals. In addition, in most cases the positive effect is related to growth factor release (Suzuki & Svendsen, 2008). However, these studies do not specify which cell types are eventually exerting the protective effect or releasing the growth factors, though they are expected to be astrocytes (See Section 3.2 of this chapter). However, one human neural stem cell (NSC) transplant study suggests that the neuroprotective effect of host motor neurons stems from the ability of NSCs to differentiate into neuronal subtypes other than motor neurons such as GABAergic neurons that forms synaptic connection between grafted and host motor neurons (Xu et al., 2009). These neurons may provide additional benefits other than that from glial cells.

Cell type	Subject	Injection Site	Effect	Paper
Mouse GRP	hSOD1-G93A rats	bilateral cervival spinal cord injection	cells survive and differentiated into mature astrocytes; reduces microgliosis; prolongs survival, ameliorates motor neuron loss and slows down motor function decline; normal GLT-1 level	Lepore et al. 2008
Mouse bone marrow cell	hSOD1-G93A /PU1-/- double mutant mice	i.p. injection	cells effectively differentiated into microglia cells; prolongs survival; suppressed cytotoxicity; restore glial activation	Beers et al. 2006
Mouse Bone marrow transplant	hSOD1-G93A mice	i.p. injection	delayed onset, increase life span	Corti et al. 2004
Human embryonic germ cell	rats with diffused motor neuron injury	i.c.v injection (CSF)	cells distributed extensively over the rostrocaudal length of the spinal cord and migrated into the spinal cord parenchymal partially recovered motor function 12 and 24 weeks after transplantation	Kerr et al. 2003
hNT cell	hSOD1-G93A mice	L4-L5 segments of the ventral horn spinal cord	delay onset, prolong survival,	Garbuzova-Davis et al. 2002
Mouse Sertoli cell	hSOD1-G93A	unilateral spinal injection into the L4-L5 ventral horn	significant increase in motor neuron survival; no effect on disease onset and progression	Hemendiner et al. 2005
Neuroectodermal derivatives of hUBS (hUBS-NSCs)	hSOD1-G93A	direct injection into the CSF (the cisterna magna).	No effect	Habisch et al. 2007

Cell type	Subject	Injection Site	Effect	Paper
hUBC	hSOD1-G93A mice	i.v. injection	reduce microgliosis; increased lifespan; delayed disease progrssion	Garbuzova-Davis et al. 2008
hNPC-GDNF	hSOD1-G93A rats	Unilateral lumbar spinal cord injection	Robust migration of the transplanted cells into the degenerating region; efficient delivery of GDNF as well as preservation of a large proportion of motor neurons; no continued innervations of motor neuron to the skeletal muscle end plates, no effect on ipsilateral hind limb function.	Suzuki et al. 2007
hMSC-GDNF	hSOD1-G93A rats	Skeletal muscles	Transplanted cells survive within host skeletal muscles and release GDNF; significant increase in neuromuscular junctions; improves motor neuron survival	Suzuki et al. 2008
CD34+ HSCs, HLA-matched sibling donors	ALS patients	i.v. injection	No clinical benefits	Appel et al. 2008
Autologous bone marrow derived MSCs	ALS patients	multiple thoracic spinal cord injection	Decelerated linear decline of the forced vital capacity and of the ALS-FRS score in some patients	Mazzini et al. 2010
Autologous CD133+ cells	ALS patients	bilateral injection into frontal motor cortex	lives 47 months more than the control group	Martinez et al. 2009

Table 1. Stem Cell Trials for ALS GRP. Glial restricted precursor; hUBC: human umbilical cord blood cells; NSCs: neural stem cells; hNPC: human neural progenitor cell; hMSC: human mesenchymal stem cell; HSCs: hematopoietic stem cells.

4. Working in combination: Genetically engineered stem cells as a tool of growth factor delivery for ALS

We have introduced two successful strategies for slowing ALS disease progression in the previous sections of this chapter. Although both of them in some degree involve the release of neuroprotective growth factors, both strategies have their shortcomings. In viral delivery of growth factors, the cells still carry the mutant SOD1 gene or has the disease phenotype. Therefore the cells that are delivering the treatment are indeed still doing harm on the surrounding cells at the same time. On the other hand, neuroprotective strategy of stem cell transplants, though increases the proportion of wild type (normal) cells around the injection site(s), the transplanted cells may not naturally produce the desired neuroprotective growth factors in a pharmaceutically adequate amount (Gonzalez, 2009). Therefore, it is reasonable for us to combine the two strategies and see if they can complement each other and produce a great synergic effect.

4.1 hNPC-GDNF injection to spinal cord

Based on the logic above, our group genetically engineered human neural progenitor cells (hNPC) that express and secrete GDNF through lentiviral infection (Klein et al., 2005; Suzuki et al., 2007). hNPC are comprised of multiple classes of neural stem cells and lineage-restricted precursors. They are isolated from fetal brain cortical tissue (Svendsen et al., 1996; Keyoung et al., 2001; Tamaki et al., 2006; Suslov, 2002) and can be maintained for over 50 weeks in the presence of mitogen while retaining the ability to differentiate into astrocytes (Wright et al, 2003). With their special properties, hNPC can thus serve as "mini-pumps" to provide glial replacement and deliver trophic factors through transplantation into specific sites in the brain and spinal cord of diseased animals and patients. hNPC-GDNF were transplanted to the lumbar region of the spinal cord of hSOD1-G93A rats. We observed robust migration of the transplanted cells into the degenerating region, efficient delivery of GDNF, as well as preservation of a large proportion of motor neurons at both early and late stages of the disease within chimeric regions (Suzuki et al. 2007). However, the preservation of motor neurons does not accompany with continued innervations of motor neuron to the skeletal muscle end plates, thus had no effect on ipsilateral hind limb function.

4.2 hMSC-GDNF injection to skeletal muscles

Skeletal muscles clearly play an important role in guiding and attracting the developing neurons; and provide trophic support to maintain motor neuron function (Dobrowolny et al., 2005). A previous study showed that transplants of genetically engineered myoblasts (a kind of skeletal muscle precursor which has the ability to fuse with mature myofibers) secreting GDNF ameliorates motor neuron loss in ALS mice (Mohajeri et al., 1999). Thus we genetically engineered human MSCs (hMSCs) that express and secrete GDNF and transplanted them to three muscle groups in hSOD1-G93A rats (Suzuki et al., 2008). MSCs can be easily obtained from bone marrow from donations and have the ability to differentiate into the skeletal muscle lineage (Caplan & Arnold, 2009). The transplanted cells survives in the host skeletal muscle and releases GDNF. Moreover, it significantly increases the number of functional neuromuscular junctions and improves motor neuron survival in spinal cord at the mid-stage of disease. Furthermore, intramuscular hMSC-GDNF transplantation remarkably prolongs disease progression, increasing overall life span up to 28 days, which is one of the greatest improvements ever observed in familial ALS model rats.

4.3 Future research directions

From the two sets of experiments described in this section, we can conclude that stem cell delivery of growth factors is an effective strategy for ALS treatment. We also know that different sets of delivery tools are needed for the motor neuron cell bodies in the spinal cord and their synaptic connections to the skeletal muscles. Our current knowledge leads us to an initial thought for future development of the field of ALS growth factor/stem cell therapy. Motor neuron cell body protection will be provided by stem cell derived wild type astrocytes and microglia (from hNPC for example); while synaptic/axonal protection will be provided by stem cell derived myoblasts (from hMSC for example). Those cells will be genetically modified to enhance delivery of neurotrophic factors. Lastly, GDNF is only one of the many neurotrophic factors that showed to have beneficial effect on ALS rodent models as mentioned in Section 2 of this chapter. We expect there will soon be tests on the other neurotrophic factors.

5. Clinical translation

Despite the exciting breakthroughs in stem cell research aiming to treat ALS, there is still a long way to go to translate those successes to the clinic and help patients. Since we are still uncertain about the fate of stem cells after transplantation, thorough safety tests are needed. Then, optimal cell dose, source of cells, stage of cells, route of delivery, injection sites, and immunosuppressive regimen (to ensure grafted cell survival in host) will need to be determined as well (Papadeas and Margaskis, 2009).

Clinical trials that involve stem cells on ALS patients are in the initial stage. In 2010 the phrase I clinical trial of hMSC transplantation performed in Italy was reported. (Mazzini et. al., 2010) Autologous MSC isolated from bone marrow derived cells were transplanted to the thoracic region of 9 ALS patients. Neither adverse effect nor significant improvement was found. However, it provides initial evidence that MSC injection is safe. Large volume (1 mL) of cells can be infused to the spinal cord without causing observable defects.

Neuralstem and Emory ALS center have begun the phase I trial of spinal cord derived stem cells for patients with ALS. The advantages of using neural stem cells derived from human fetal spinal cord are no tumor formation and minimal HLA (human leukocyte antigen) expression, thus, resulting in a low overall antigenicity of the cells. The first surgery of the trial took place a year ago, and the 9th surgery was performed earlier in 2011, without the need for patients to be on ventilators or to be taken to intensive care post-operation. The trial was staged, first enrolling non-ambulatory patients, and the first ambulatory patient was enrolled early 2011.

6. Conclusion

In this chapter, we introduced the current application of stem cells in ALS (summarized in Figure 1). There are three points we should keep in mind about this topic. First, stem cell therapy design should be aimed at neuroprotection rather than motor neuron replacement. Motor neuron replacement is technically difficult to achieve. Also, in theory it will not bring much improvement to the patients because the evidence shows that glial cells are the actual determinant of ALS disease progression. Secondly, combining stem cell transplantation and growth factor delivery provides the best result in slowing disease progression and prolonging survival, as the two greatly complement each other. Finally, we are now convinced that injections of stem cells in multiple sites are needed in order to alleviate symptoms of ALS. There should be at least one injection that focuses on protecting cell bodies of motor neurons and another that aims to maintain neuromuscular connections. To sum up, stem cell applications have made a lot of contributions to ALS research and have great potential to bring breakthroughs to the field in the near future.

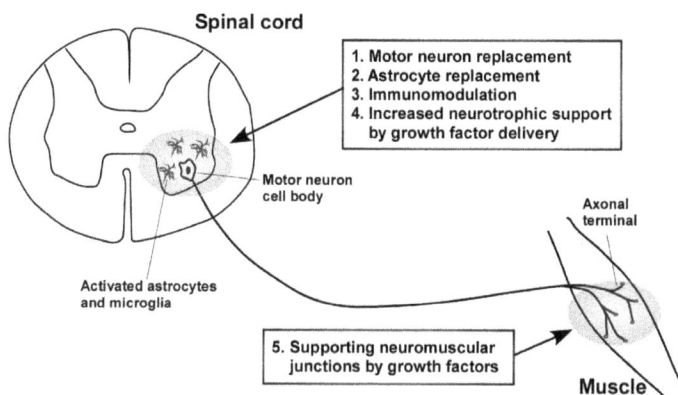

Fig. 1. Schematic illustration of possible stem cell interventions for ALS therapies. These could include: (1) Motor neuron replacement, differentiation of neural progenitor cells to motor neurons and projection to the periphery; (2) Differentiation and replacement of dysfunctional astrocytes; (3) Modulation of immunological environment around the degenerating motor neuron; (4) Trophic/growth factor delivery via stem cells to provide neuroprotective support for the endogenous populations; (5) Local delivery of growth factors to support neuromuscular junctions and axon integrity.

7. Acknowledgment

This work was support by grants from the ALS association, NIH/NINDS (R21NS06104), the University of Wisconsin Foundation, and the Les Turner ALS Foundation.

8. References

Acsadi G, Anguelov RA, Yang H, Toth G, Thomas R, Jani A, Wang Y, Ianakova E, Mohammad S, Lewis RA & Shy ME. (2002) Increased survival and function of SOD1 mice after glial cell-derived neurotrophic factor gene therapy. *Hum Gene Ther*. 2002 Jun 10; Volume 13(9); Pages 1047-59.

Appel SH, Engelhardt JI, Henkel JS, Siklos L, Beers DR, Yen AA, Simpson EP, Luo Y, Carrum G, Heslop HE, Brenner MK & Popat U. (2008) Hematopoietic stem cell transplantation in patients with sporadic amyotrophic lateral sclerosis. *Neurology*. 2008 Oct 21; Volume 71(17); Pages 1326-34.

Azzouz M, Ralph GS, Storkebaum E, Walmsley LE, Mitrophanous KA, Kingsman SM, Carmeliet P & Mazarakis ND. (2004) VEGF delivery with retrogradely transported lentivector prolongs survival in a mouse ALS model. *Nature.* 2004 May 27; Volume 429(6990); Pages 413-7.

Barbeito LH, Pehar M, Cassina P, Vargas MR, Peluffo H, Viera L, Estévez AG & Beckman JS. (2004) A role for astrocytes in motor neuron loss in amyotrophic lateral sclerosis. *Brain Res Brain Res Rev.* 2004 Dec; Volume 47(1-3): Pages 263-74.

Beers DR, Henkel JS, Xiao Q, Zhao W, Wang J, Yen AA, Siklos L, McKercher SR & Appel SH. (2006) Wild-type microglia extend survival in PU.1 knockout mice with familial amyotrophic lateral sclerosis. *Proc Natl Acad Sci U S A.* 2006 Oct 24; Volume 103(43); Pages 16021-6.

Boillée S, Vande Velde C & Cleveland DW. (2006a) ALS: a disease of motor neurons and their nonneuronal neighbors. *Neuron.* 2006 Oct 5; Volume 52(1): Pages 39-59.

Boillée S, Yamanaka K, Lobsiger CS, Copeland NG, Jenkins NA, Kassiotis G, Kollias G & Cleveland DW. (2006b) Onset and progression in inherited ALS determined by motor neurons and microglia. *Science.* 2006 Jun 2; Volume 312(5778); Pages 1389-92.

Borasio GD, Robberecht W, Leigh PN, Emile J, Guiloff RJ, Jerusalem F, Silani V, Vos PE, Wokke JH & Dobbins T. (1998) A placebo-controlled trial of insulin-like growth factor-I in amyotrophic lateral sclerosis. European ALS/IGF-I Study Group. *Neurology.* 1998 Aug; Volume 51(2); Pages 583-6.

Brooks BR (1994) El escorial World Federation of Neurology criteria for the diagnosis of amyotrophic lateral sclerosis. *Journal of the Neurological Sciences.* Volume 124 (Supplement 1), 1994 July, Pages 96-107, ISSN 0022-510X

Brooks BR, Miller RG, Swash M & Munsat TL. (2000) World Federation of Neurology Research Group on Motor Neuron Diseases. El Escorial revisited: revised criteria for the diagnosis of amyotrophic lateral sclerosis. *Amyotroph Lateral Scler Other Motor Neuron Disord.* 2000 Dec; Volume 1(5); Pages 293-9.

Brown RH Jr. (1995) Superoxide dismutase in familial amyotrophic lateral sclerosis: models for gain of function. *Curr Opin Neurobiol.* 1995 Dec; Volume 5(6); Pages 841-6.

Caplan, Arnold I. (2009) Mesenchymal Stem Cell, In: *Essentials of Stem Cell Biology*, Robert Lanza, pp 485-496, Academic Press, ISBN 9780123747297, U. S. A.

Cisterni C, Henderson CE, Aebischer P, Pettmann B & Déglon N. (2000) Efficient gene transfer and expression of biologically active glial cell line-derived neurotrophic factor in rat motoneurons transduced wit lentiviral vectors. *J Neurochem.* 2000 May; Volume 74(5); Pages 1820-8.

Clement AM, Nguyen MD, Roberts EA, Garcia ML, Boillée S, Rule M, McMahon AP, Doucette W, Siwek D, Ferrante RJ, Brown RH Jr, Julien JP, Goldstein LS & Cleveland DW. (2003) Wild-type nonneuronal cells extend survival of SOD1 mutant motor neurons in ALS mice. *Science.* 2003 Oct 3; Volume 302(5642); Pages 113-7. Erratum in: *Science.* 2003 Oct 24; Volume 302(5645): Page 568.

Cleveland DW & Rothstein JD. (2001) From Charcot to Lou Gehrig: deciphering selective motor neuron death in ALS. *Nat Rev Neurosci.* 2001 Nov; Volume 2(11); Pages 806-19.

Croft AP & Przyborski SA. (2006) Formation of neurons by non-neural adult stem cells: potential mechanism implicates an artifact of growth in culture. *Stem Cells.* 2006 Aug; Volume 24(8); Pages 1841-51.

Corti S, Locatelli F, Donadoni C, Guglieri M, Papadimitriou D, Strazzer S, Del Bo R & Comi GP. (2004) Wild-type bone marrow cells ameliorate the phenotype of SOD1-G93A

ALS mice and contribute to CNS, heart and skeletal muscle tissues. *Brain*. 2004 Nov; Volume 127(Pt 11); Pages 2518-32..

Deshpande DM, Kim YS, Martinez T, Carmen J, Dike S, Shats I, Rubin LL, Drummond J, Krishnan C, Hoke A, Maragakis N, Shefner J, Rothstein JD & Kerr DA. (2006) Recovery from paralysis in adult rats using embryonic stem cells. *Ann Neurol*. 2006 Jul; Volume 60(1); Pages 32-44.

De Vos KJ, Chapman AL, Tennant ME, Manser C, Tudor EL, Lau KF, Brownlees J, Ackerley S, Shaw PJ, McLoughlin DM, Shaw CE, Leigh PN, Miller CC & Grierson AJ. (2007) Familial amyotrophic lateral sclerosis-linked SOD1 mutants perturb fast axonal transport to reduce axonal mitochondria content. *Hum Mol Genet*. 2007 Nov 15; Volume 16(22); Pages 2720-8.

Dimos JT, Rodolfa KT, Niakan KK, Weisenthal LM, Mitsumoto H, Chung W, Croft GF, Saphier G, Leibel R, Goland R, Wichterle H, Henderson CE & Eggan K. (2008) Induced pluripotent stem cells generated from patients with ALS can be differentiated into motor neurons. *Science*. 2008 Aug 29; Volume 321(5893); Pages 1218-21..

Di Giorgio FP, Carrasco MA, Siao MC, Maniatis T & Eggan K. (2007) Non-cell autonomous effect of glia on motor neurons in an embryonic stem cell-based ALS model. *Nat Neurosci*. 2007 May; Volume 10(5); Pages 608-14.

Di Giorgio FP, Boulting GL, Bobrowicz S & Eggan KC. (2008) Human embryonic stem cell-derived motor neurons are sensitive to the toxic effect of glial cells carrying an ALS-causing mutation. *Cell Stem Cell*. 2008 Dec 4; Volume 3(6); Pages 637-48.

Dobrowolny G, Giacinti C, Pelosi L, Nicoletti C, Winn N, Barberi L, Molinaro M, Rosenthal N & Musarò A. (2005) Muscle expression of a local Igf-1 isoform protects motor neurons in an ALS mouse model. *J Cell Biol*. 2005 Jan 17; Volume 168(2): Pages 193-9.

Dodge JC, Treleaven CM, Fidler JA, Hester M, Haidet A, Handy C, Rao M, Eagle A, Matthews JC, Taksir TV, Cheng SH, Shihabuddin LS & Kaspar BK. (2010) AAV4-mediated expression of IGF-1 and VEGF within cellular components of the ventricular system improves survival outcome in familial ALS mice. *Mol Ther*. 2010 Dec; Volume 18(12): Pages 2075-84.

Fischer LR, Culver DG, Tennant P, Davis AA, Wang M, Castellano-Sanchez A, Khan J, Polak MA & Glass JD. (2004) Amyotrophic lateral sclerosis is a distal axonopathy: evidence in mice and man. *Exp Neurol*. 2004 Feb; Volume 185(2) Pages 232-40.

Gao J, Coggeshall RE, Tarasenko YI, Wu P. (2005) Human neural stem cell-derived cholinergic neurons innervate muscle in motoneuron deficient adult rats. *Neuroscience*. 2005; Volume 131(2); Pages 257-62.

Garbuzova-Davis S, Willing AE, Milliken M, Saporta S, Zigova T, Cahill DW & Sanberg PR. (2002) Positive effect of transplantation of hNT neurons (NTera 2/D1 cell-line) in a model of familial amyotrophic lateral sclerosis. *Exp Neurol*. 2002 Apr; Volume 174(2): Pages 169-80. Erratum in: *Exp Neurol* 2002 Jun; Volume 175(2); Pages 451.

Garbuzova-Davis S, Sanberg CD, Kuzmin-Nichols N, Willing AE, Gemma C, Bickford PC, Rossi R, & Sanberg PR. (2008) Human umbilical cord blood treatment in a mouse model of ALS: optimization of cell dose. *PLoS One*. 2008 Jun; Volume 3(6); Page e2494.

Gill SS, Patel NK, Hotton GR, O'Sullivan K, McCarter R, Bunnage M, Brooks DJ, Svendsen CN & Heywood P. (2003) Direct brain infusion of glial cell line-derived neurotrophic factor in Parkinson disease. *Nat Med.* 2003 May; Volume 9(5); Pages 589-95.

Gonzalez, Rodolfo. (2009) Neural Stem Cells for Central Nervous System Repair, In: *Essentials of Stem Cell Biology*, Robert Lanza, pp 485-496, Academic Press, ISBN 9780123747297, U. S. A.

Guillot S, Azzouz M, Déglon N, Zurn A & Aebischer P. (2004) Local GDNF expression mediated by lentiviral vector protects facial nerve motoneurons but not spinal motoneurons in SOD1(G93A) transgenic mice. *Neurobiol Dis.* 2004 Jun; Volume 16(1); Pages 139-49.

Gurney ME. (1994) Transgenic-mouse model of amyotrophic lateral sclerosis. *N Engl J Med.* 1994 Dec 22; Volume 331(25); Pages 1721-2.

Haase G, Kennel P, Pettmann B, Vigne E, Akli S, Revah F, Schmalbruch H & Kahn A. (1997) Gene therapy of murine motor neuron disease using adenoviral vectors for neurotrophic factors. *Nat Med.* 1997 Apr; Volume 3(4); Pages 429-36.

Habisch HJ, Janowski M, Binder D, Kuzma-Kozakiewicz M, Widmann A, Habich A, Schwalenstöcker B, Hermann A, Brenner R, Lukomska B, Domanska-Janik K, Ludolph AC & Storch A. (2007) Intrathecal application of neuroectodermally converted stem cells into a mouse model of ALS: limited intraparenchymal migration and survival narrows therapeutic effects. *J Neural Transm.* 2007; Volume 114(11); Pages 1395-406.

Hall ED, Oostveen JA & Gurney ME. (1998) Relationship of microglial and astrocytic activation to disease onset and progression in a transgenic model of familial ALS. *Glia.* 1998 Jul; Volume 23(3); Pages 249-56.

Harper JM, Krishnan C, Darman JS, Deshpande DM, Peck S, Shats I, Backovic S, Rothstein JD & Kerr DA. (2004) Axonal growth of embryonic stem cell-derived motoneurons in vitro and in motoneuron-injured adult rats. *Proc Natl Acad Sci U S A.* 2004 May 4; Volume 101(18):Pages 7123-8.

Hemendinger R, Wang J, Malik S, Persinski R, Copeland J, Emerich D, Gores P, Halberstadt C & Rosenfeld J. (2005) Sertoli cells improve survival of motor neurons in SOD1 transgenic mice, a model of amyotrophic lateral sclerosis. *Exp Neurol.* 2005 Dec; Volume 196(2); Pages 235-43.

Hirtz D, Thurman DJ, Gwinn-Hardy K, Mohamed M, Chaudhuri AR & Zalutsky R. (2007) How common are the "common" neurologic disorders? *Neurology.* 2007 Jan 30; Volume 68(5); Pages 326-37.

Hottinger AF, Azzouz M, Déglon N, Aebischer P & Zurn AD. (2000) Complete and long-term rescue of lesioned adult motoneurons by lentiviral-mediated expression of glial cell line-derived neurotrophic factor in the facial nucleus. *J Neurosci.* 2000 Aug 1; Volume 20(15); Pages 5587-93.

Howland DS, Liu J, She Y, Goad B, Maragakis NJ, Kim B, Erickson J, Kulik J, DeVito L, Psaltis G, DeGennaro LJ, Cleveland DW & Rothstein JD. (2002) Focal loss of the glutamate transporter EAAT2 in a transgenic rat model of SOD1 mutant-mediated amyotrophic lateral sclerosis (ALS). *Proc Natl Acad Sci U S A.* 2002 Feb 5; Volume 99(3): Pages 1604-9.

Julien JP. (2001) Amyotrophic lateral sclerosis. unfolding the toxicity of the misfolded. *Cell.* 2001 Feb 23; Volume 104(4) Pages 581-91..

Karumbayaram S, Novitch BG, Patterson M, Umbach JA, Richter L, Lindgren A, Conway AE, Clark AT, Goldman SA, Plath K, Wiedau-Pazos M, Kornblum HL & Lowry WE. (2009) Directed differentiation of human-induced pluripotent stem cells generates active motor neurons. *Stem Cells.* 2009 Apr; Volume 27(4); Pages 806-11.

Kaspar BK, Lladó J, Sherkat N, Rothstein JD & Gage FH. (2003) Retrograde viral delivery of IGF-1 prolongs survival in a mouse ALS model. *Science.* 2003 Aug 8; Volume 301(5634); Pages 839-42.

Kerr DA, Lladó J, Shamblott MJ, Maragakis NJ, Irani DN, Crawford TO, Krishnan C, Dike S, Gearhart JD & Rothstein JD. (2003) Human embryonic germ cell derivatives facilitate motor recovery of rats with diffuse motor neuron injury. *J Neurosci.* 2003 Jun 15; Voluem 23(12); Pages 5131-40.

Keyoung HM, Roy NS, Benraiss A, Louissaint A Jr, Suzuki A, Hashimoto M, Rashbaum WK, Okano H & Goldman SA. (2001) High-yield selection and extraction of two promoter-defined phenotypes of neural stem cells from the fetal human brain. *Nat Biotechnol.* 2001 Sep; Volume 19(9); Pages 843-50.

Kirchhoff F, Dringen R & Giaume C. (2001) Pathways of neuron-astrocyte interactions and their possible role in neuroprotection. *Eur Arch Psychiatry Clin Neurosci.* 2001 Aug; Volume 251(4); Pages 159-69..

Klein SM, Behrstock S, McHugh J, Hoffmann K, Wallace K, Suzuki M, Aebischer P & Svendsen CN. (2005) GDNF delivery using human neural progenitor cells in a rat model of ALS. *Hum Gene Ther.* 2005 Apr; Volume 16(4); Pages 509-21.

Lai EC, Felice KJ, Festoff BW, Gawel MJ, Gelinas DF, Kratz R, Murphy MF, Natter HM, Norris FH & Rudnicki SA. (1997) Effect of recombinant human insulin-like growth factor-I on progression of ALS. A placebo-controlled study. The North America ALS/IGF-I Study Group. *Neurology.* 1997 Dec;Volume 49(6); Pages 1621-30.

Lee H, Shamy GA, Elkabetz Y, Schofield CM, Harrsion NL, Panagiotakos G, Socci ND, Tabar V & Studer L. (2007) Directed differentiation and transplantation of human embryonic stem cell-derived motoneurons. *Stem Cells.* 2007 Aug; Voluem 25(8); Pages 1931-9.

Lepore AC, Rauck B, Dejea C, Pardo AC, Rao MS, Rothstein JD & Maragakis NJ. (2008) Focal transplantation-based astrocyte replacement is neuroprotective in a model of motor neuron disease. *Nat Neurosci.* 2008 Nov; Volume 11(11): Pages 1294-301.

Li W, Brakefield D, Pan Y, Hunter D, Myckatyn TM & Parsadanian A. (2007) Muscle-derived but not centrally derived transgene GDNF is neuroprotective in G93A-SOD1 mouse model of ALS. *Exp Neurol.* 2007 Feb; Volume 203(2); Pages 457-71.

Li XJ, Du ZW, Zarnowska ED, Pankratz M, Hansen LO, Pearce RA & Zhang SC. (2005) Specification of motoneurons from human embryonic stem cells. *Nat Biotechnol.* 2005 Feb; Volume 23(2); Pages 215-21..

Lunn JS, Sakowski SA, Kim B, Rosenberg AA & Feldman EL. (2009) Vascular endothelial growth factor prevents G93A-SOD1-induced motor neuron degeneration. *Dev Neurobiol.* 2009 Nov; Volume 69(13); Pages 871-84.

Marchetto MC, Muotri AR, Mu Y, Smith AM, Cezar GG & Gage FH. (2008) Non-cell-autonomous effect of human SOD1 G37R astrocytes on motor neurons derived from human embryonic stem cells. *Cell Stem Cell*. 2008 Dec 4; Volume 3(6); Pages 649-57.

Martinez HR, Gonzalez-Garza MT, Moreno-Cuevas JE, Caro E, Gutierrez-Jimenez E & Segura JJ. (2009) Stem-cell transplantation into the frontal motor cortex in amyotrophic lateral sclerosis patients. *Cytotherapy*. 2009; Volume 11(1); Pages 26-34.

Mazzini L, Mareschi K, Ferrero I, Vassallo E, Oliveri G, Nasuelli N, Oggioni GD, Testa L & Fagioli F. (2008) Stem cell treatment in Amyotrophic Lateral Sclerosis. *J Neurol Sci*. 2008 Feb 15; Volume 265(1-2); Pages 78-83.

Mazzini L, Ferrero I, Luparello V, Rustichelli D, Gunetti M, Mareschi K, Testa L, Stecco A, Tarletti R, Miglioretti M, Fava E, Nasuelli N, Cisari C, Massara M, Vercelli R, Oggioni GD, Carriero A, Cantello R, Monaco F & Fagioli F. (2010) Mesenchymal stem cell transplantation in amyotrophic lateral sclerosis: A Phase I clinical trial. *Exp Neurol*. 2010 May; Volume 223(1); Pages 229-37.

McGuckin CP, Forraz N, Allouard Q & Pettengell R. (2004) Umbilical cord blood stem cells can expand hematopoietic and neuroglial progenitors in vitro. *Exp Cell Res*. 2004 May 1; Volume 295(2); Pages 350-9.

Miles GB, Yohn DC, Wichterle H, Jessell TM, Rafuse VF & Brownstone RM. (2004) Functional properties of motoneurons derived from mouse embryonic stem cells. *J Neurosci*. 2004 Sep 8; Volume 24(36); Pages 7848-58.

Mohajeri MH, Figlewicz DA & Bohn MC. (1999) Intramuscular grafts of myoblasts genetically modified to secrete glial cell line-derived neurotrophic factor prevent motoneuron loss and disease progression in a mouse model of familial amyotrophic lateral sclerosis. *Hum Gene Ther*. 1999 Jul 20; Volume 10(11): Pages1853-66.

Nagai M, Aoki M, Miyoshi I, Kato M, Pasinelli P, Kasai N, Brown RH Jr & Itoyama Y. (2001) Rats expressing human cytosolic copper-zinc superoxide dismutase transgenes with amyotrophic lateral sclerosis: associated mutations develop motor neuron disease. *J Neurosci*. 2001 Dec 1; Volume 21(23); Pages 9246-54.

Nagai M, Re DB, Nagata T, Chalazonitis A, Jessell TM, Wichterle H & Przedborski S. (2007) Astrocytes expressing ALS-linked mutated SOD1 release factors selectively toxic to motor neurons. *Nat Neurosci*. 2007 May; Volume 10(5); Pages 615-22.

Papadeas ST & Maragakis NJ. (2009) Advances in stem cell research for Amyotrophic Lateral Sclerosis. *Curr Opin Biotechnol*. 2009 Oct; Volume 20(5); Pages 545-51.

Rao SD & Weiss JH. (2004) Excitotoxic and oxidative cross-talk between motor neurons and glia in ALS pathogenesis. *Trends Neurosci*. 2004 Jan; Volume 27(1); Pages 17-23.

Rosen DR, Siddique T, Patterson D, Figlewicz DA, Sapp P, Hentati A, Donaldson D, Goto J, O'Regan JP, Deng HX, et al. (1993) Mutations in Cu/Zn superoxide dismutase gene are associated with familial amyotrophic lateral sclerosis. *Nature*. 1993 Mar 4; Volume 362(6415); Pages 59-62. Erratum in: *Nature*. 1993 Jul 22; Volume 364(6435); Page 362.

Rothstein JD, Van Kammen M, Levey AI, Martin LJ & Kuncl RW. (1995) Selective loss of glial glutamate transporter GLT-1 in amyotrophic lateral sclerosis. *Ann Neurol*. 1995 Jul; Volume 38(1): Pages 73-84.

Rothstein J. (2004) Preclinical studies: how much can we rely on?. *Amyotrophic Lateral Sclerosis & Other Motor Neuron Disorders* . September 2, 2004; Volume 5; Pages 22-25.

Slevin JT, Gerhardt GA, Smith CD, Gash DM, Kryscio R & Young B. (2005) Improvement of bilateral motor functions in patients with Parkinson disease through the unilateral intraputaminal infusion of glial cell line-derived neurotrophic factor. *J Neurosurg.* 2005 Feb; Volume 102(2); Pagees 216-22.

Suslov ON, Kukekov VG, Ignatova TN & Steindler DA. (2002) Neural stem cell heterogeneity demonstrated by molecular phenotyping of clonal neurospheres. *Proc Natl Acad Sci U S A.* 2002 Oct 29; Volume 99(22); Pages 14506-11.

Suzuki M, McHugh J, Tork C, Shelley B, Klein SM, Aebischer P, Svendsen CN. (2007) GDNF secreting human neural progenitor cells protect dying motor neurons, but not their projection to muscle, in a rat model of familial ALS. *PLoS One.* 2007 Aug 1; Volume 2(8).

Suzuki M & Svendsen CN. (2008) Combining growth factor and stem cell therapy for amyotrophic lateral sclerosis. *Trends Neurosci.* 2008 Apr; Volume 31(4): Pages 192-8.

Suzuki M, McHugh J, Tork C, Shelley B, Hayes A, Bellantuono I, Aebischer P & Svendsen CN. (2008) Direct muscle delivery of GDNF with human mesenchymal stem cells improves motor neuron survival and function in a rat model of familial ALS. *Mol Ther.* 2008 Dec; Volume 16(12); Pages 2002-10.

Svendsen CN, Clarke DJ, Rosser AE, Dunnett SB. (1996) Survival and differentiation of rat and human epidermal growth factor-responsive precursor cells following grafting into the lesioned adult central nervous system. *Exp Neurol.* 1996 Feb; Volume 137(2); Pages 376-88.

Tai YT & Svendsen CN. (2004) Stem cells as a potential treatment of neurological disorders. *Curr Opin Pharmacol.* 2004 Feb; Volume 4(1); Pages 98-104.

Tamaki S, Eckert K, He D, Sutton R, Doshe M, Jain G, Tushinski R, Reitsma M, Harris B, Tsukamoto A, Gage F, Weissman I & Uchida N. (2002) Engraftment of sorted/expanded human central nervous system stem cells from fetal brain. *J Neurosci Res.* 2002 Sep 15; Volume 69(6); Pages 976-86.

Takahashi K, Tanabe K, Ohnuki M, Narita M, Ichisaka T, Tomoda K & Yamanaka S. (2007) Induction of pluripotent stem cells from adult human fibroblasts by defined factors. *Cell.* 2007 Nov 30; Volume 131(5); Pages 861-72.

Ticozzi N, Tiloca C, Morelli C, Colombrita C, Poletti B, Doretti A, Maderna L, Messina S, Ratti A & Silani V. (2011) Genetics of familial Amyotrophic lateral sclerosis. *Arch Ital Biol.* 2011 Mar; Volume 149(1); Pages 65-82.

Vitry S, Bertrand JY, Cumano A & Dubois-Dalcq M. (2003) Primordial hematopoietic stem cells generate microglia but not myelin-forming cells in a neural environment. *J Neurosci.* 2003 Nov 19; Volume 23(33); Pages 10724-31.

Wang LJ, Lu YY, Muramatsu S, Ikeguchi K, Fujimoto K, Okada T, Mizukami H, Matsushita T, Hanazono Y, Kume A, Nagatsu T, Ozawa K & Nakano I. (2002) Neuroprotective effects of glial cell line-derived neurotrophic factor mediated by an adeno-associated virus vector in a transgenic animal model of amyotrophic lateral sclerosis. *J Neurosci.* 2002 Aug 15; Volume 22(16); Pages 6920-8.

Wichterle H, Lieberam I, Porter JA, Jessell TM. (2002) Directed differentiation of embryonic stem cells into motor neurons. *Cell.* 2002 Aug 9; Volume 110(3); Pages 385-97.

Williamson TL & Cleveland DW. (1999) Slowing of axonal transport is a very early event in the toxicity of ALS-linked SOD1 mutants to motor neurons. *Nat Neurosci.* 1999 Jan; Volume 2(1); Pages 50-6.

Wright LS, Li J, Caldwell MA, Wallace K, Johnson JA & Svendsen CN. (2003) Gene expression in human neural stem cells: effects of leukemia inhibitory factor. *J Neurochem.* 2003 Jul; Volume 86(1): Pages 179-95.

Xu L, Ryugo DK, Pongstaporn T, Johe K & Koliatsos VE. (2009) Human neural stem cell grafts in the spinal cord of SOD1 transgenic rats: differentiation and structural integration into the segmental motor circuitry. *J Comp Neurol.* 2009 Jun 1; Volume 514(4); Pages 297-309.

Yamanaka K, Chun SJ, Boillee S, Fujimori-Tonou N, Yamashita H, Gutmann DH, Takahashi R, Misawa H & Cleveland DW. (2008) Astrocytes as determinants of disease progression in inherited amyotrophic lateral sclerosis. *Nat Neurosci.* 2008 Mar; Volume 11(3); Pages 251-3.

Yan J, Xu L, Welsh AM, Chen D, Hazel T, Johe K & Koliatsos VE. (2006) Combined immunosuppressive agents or CD4 antibodies prolong survival of human neural stem cell grafts and improve disease outcomes in amyotrophic lateral sclerosis transgenic mice. *Stem Cells.* 2006 Aug; Volume 24(8); Pages 1976-85.

Yu J, Vodyanik MA, Smuga-Otto K, Antosiewicz-Bourget J, Frane JL, Tian S, Nie J, Jonsdottir GA, Ruotti V, Stewart R, Slukvin II & Thomson JA. (2007) Induced pluripotent stem cell lines derived from human somatic cells. *Science.* 2007 Dec 21; Volume 318(5858); Pages 1917-20.

Zoccolella S, Santamato A & Lamberti P. (2009) Current and emerging treatments for amyotrophic lateral sclerosis. *Neuropsychiatr Dis Treat.* 2009 May Pages 577-95. Epub 2009 Nov 16.

Part 2

Human Genetics in ALS

6

Genetics of Familial Amyotrophic Lateral Sclerosis

Emily F. Goodall, Joanna J. Bury,
Johnathan Cooper-Knock, Pamela J. Shaw and Janine Kirby
*Sheffield Institute for Translational Neuroscience, University of Sheffield, Sheffield,
United Kingdom*

1. Introduction

Amyotrophic lateral sclerosis (ALS) is a devastating neurodegenerative disorder caused by the selective loss of motor neurones from the cortex, brainstem and spinal cord. For the patient, this results in a progressive loss of muscle function characterised by muscle weakness, atrophy and spasticity that develops into paralysis. Onset is typically in mid-life around ages 50-60 years, however there are juvenile forms with much earlier symptom onset (below 25 years). Disease duration is heterogeneous; however the majority of patients will only survive 2-3 years following initial symptom onset, with death generally resulting from respiratory muscle failure (Worms 2001).

A recent meta-analysis of population based studies revealed that 5% of ALS cases are familial (FALS) and the remaining 95% are sporadic (SALS) with no reported family history (Byrne et al 2011). There is a broad spectrum of inheritance for FALS ranging from fully penetrant, dominantly inherited Mendelian forms to recessive disease with weak penetrance affecting only a few family members (Simpson & Al-Chalabi 2006). The majority of familial cases are clinically and pathologically indistinguishable from sporadic cases, leading to the hypothesis that they share common pathogenic mechanisms. In addition, mutations in several of the FALS genes have also been identified in apparently sporadic disease, suggesting some degree of genetic overlap (Alexander et al 2002; Chio et al 2010; Kabashi et al 2008).

In ALS, cognitive impairment has been reported in up to 51% of cases, with frontotemporal dementia (FTD) present in up to 15% (Gordon et al 2011; Lillo et al 2011; Ringholz et al 2005). In approximately a third of cases, there is a family history of ALS or FTD or both in the family, and genes initially associated with either ALS or FTD are now being found to be associated with both disease phenotypes. This genetic link, in addition to extensive neuropathological evidence (Mackenzie et al 2010) has led to the widely accepted view that ALS and FTD form part of a spectrum of the same neurodegenerative disease process (Geser et al 2010).

2. Overview of genetics of ALS

The inheritance of FALS in many families is atypical with one proband and one or two first/second degree relatives who also have the disease (Valdmanis & Rouleau 2008). The first big breakthrough in the genetics of FALS came in 1993 with the discovery of pathological mutations in the Cu-Zn superoxide dismutase (*SOD1*) gene in ALS patients (Rosen et al 1993). Since then there has been an explosion of research into the mechanism(s) by which *SOD1* mutations cause ALS, however the answer remains elusive. There are now 16 genes associated with Mendelian forms of ALS (Table 1) which have mostly been identified using linkage analysis of rare families with large pedigrees affected by the disease (Lill et al 2011). More recently, studies to identify the proteins found in the ubiquitinated inclusions that are a common neuropathological feature of both ALS and FTD, have identified trans-activation response element (TAR) DNA binding protein of 43kDa (TDP-43) as the major component (Arai et al 2006; Neumann et al 2006). Mutations in the gene encoding TDP-43, *TARDBP*, were subsequently found as a genetic cause of ALS (Sreedharan et al 2008). The genetics of FALS has moved forward rapidly in recent years, providing invaluable insight into disease pathogenesis and allowing the development of animal models to further study the disease and efficacy of therapeutic compounds.

	Type	Locus	Reference
Autosomal Dominant Adult Onset			
Most common genetic causes			
SOD1	ALS1	21q22	(Rosen et al 1993)
TARDBP	ALS10	1p36.22	(Sreedharan et al 2008)
FUS	ALS6	16q12.1-2	(Abalkhail et al 2003)
Less frequent genetic causes			
VAPB	ALS8	20q13.3	(Nishimura et al 2004)
ANG	ALS9	14q11.2	(Greenway et al 2004)
FIG4	ALS11	6q21	(Chow et al 2009)
OPTN	ALS12	10p15-14	(Maruyama et al 2010)
DAO		12q22-23	(Mitchell et al 2010)
VCP		9p13.3	(Johnson et al 2010b)
Autosomal Dominant Juvenile Onset			
SETX	ALS4	9q34	(Chen et al 2004)
Autosomal Recessive			
ALS2	ALS2	2q33-35	(Hentati et al 1994)
ALS+FTD			
SIGMAR1		9p13.3	(Luty et al 2010)
MAPT		17q21	(Sundar et al 2007)
Genetic Loci Linked to Familial ALS			
SPG11	ALS5	15q15-22	(Orlacchio et al 2010)
Unknown	ALS7	20ptel-p13	(Sapp et al 2003)
Unknown	ALS3	18q21	(Hand et al 2002)
UBQLN2	ALSX	Xp11-q12	(Deng et al 2011)
C9ORF72	ALS-FTD1	9p21-q22	(Hosler et al 2000)
Unknown	ALS-FTD2	9p13.2-p21.3	(Vance et al 2006)

Table 1. Summary of the Genetic Causes of Familial ALS

3. Genetic causes of FALS

3.1 Most common genetic causes of autosomal dominant, adult onset ALS

The three most common genetic causes of FALS, together accounting for approximately 30% of cases are mutation of the *SOD1*, *TARDBP* and fused in sarcoma (*FUS*) genes.

3.1.1 ALS1: Cu-Zn superoxide dismutase 1 (*SOD1*)

The first genetic cause of familial ALS was identified by Rosen and colleagues (Rosen et al 1993) when, following analysis of FALS pedigrees demonstrating linkage to chromosome 21, mutations were identified in the *SOD1* gene. Since then, over 150 mutations have been described throughout the 5 exons encoding the gene consisting predominantly of missense mutations, although nonsense mutations, insertions and deletions have also been described (Lill et al 2011). The frequency of *SOD1* mutations is widely reported to be 20% of FALS cases, though this varies across European and North American populations, from 12% in Germany to 23.5% in USA (Andersen 2006). Whilst the majority of mutations are inherited in an autosomal dominant manner, in Scandinavia the p.D90A mutation is polymorphic, (0.5-5% of Scandinavian populations), with the disease manifesting only in individuals who are homozygous (Andersen et al 1995). However, this inheritance pattern is not attributable to the specific amino acid substitution, as p.D90A has been shown to be inherited as an autosomal dominant mutation in other populations. Mutations in *SOD1* have also been identified in sporadic ALS, albeit at lower frequencies, suggesting that some mutations have reduced penetrance. This has been shown in a family where the p.I113T mutation shows age-related penetrance (Lopate et al 2010).

Clinically, *SOD1* mutations are not associated with a distinctive phenotype. Individuals with *SOD1*-related ALS predominantly manifest with limb onset ALS, with symptoms more likely to start in the lower limbs (rather than upper limbs). However, bulbar onset is seen in approximately 7% of *SOD1*-related cases (ALSoD database: http:alsod.iop.kcl.ac.uk). Whilst duration of disease varies widely among *SOD1* mutations, even within members of the same family with the same mutation, the p.A4V mutation has been shown to be associated with a rapid disease progression and only 1-2 years survival (Andersen 2006). In contrast to the indistinguishable clinical phenotype, *SOD1*-related ALS cases appear to have a characteristic pathology distinguished by SOD1 positive, but TDP-43 negative, protein inclusions (Mackenzie et al 2007).

The mature SOD1 protein is a homodimer of 153 amino acid subunits. This free radical scavenging protein converts the superoxide anion to hydrogen peroxide; this in turn is converted to water and oxygen by glutathione peroxidise or catalase. Mutations in *SOD1* cause a toxic gain of function in the resulting mutant protein, though the mechanism(s) by which this brings about selective neurodegeneration of the motor neurones appears to be a complex interplay between multiple interacting pathomechanisms. The main hypotheses involve either an altered redox function or misfolding of the protein leading to aggregation (Rakhit & Chakrabartty 2006). Interestingly, not only have SOD1 positive aggregations been seen in SALS spinal cord, recent work has also shown that a conformation specific antibody raised against mutant SOD1 binds oxidised, but not normal, wild-type SOD1 in a subset of SALS cases thereby linking both *SOD1*-ALS and SALS (Bosco et al 2010).

Identification of *SOD1* led to the generation of many cellular and animal models which mirror aspects of the disease process and enable mechanistic insights and therapeutic approaches to be investigated. Current pathogenic mechanisms associated with mutant

SOD1 include oxidative stress, excitotoxicity, protein aggregation, mitochondrial dysfunction, endoplasmic reticulum stress, inflammatory cascades, involvement of non-neuronal cells and dysregulation of axonal transport. Each of these mechanisms has also been shown to play a role in SALS, demonstrating the relevance of the *SOD1* models to the disease as a whole (Ferraiuolo et al 2011). Therefore, although to date therapeutic agents which have shown promising results in the SOD1 transgenic mouse models have yet to show a beneficial effect in human trials (Benatar 2007), the generation and continued use of these models has greatly extended our knowledge of ALS.

3.1.2 ALS10: Transactive response (TAR) DNA binding protein (*TARDBP*)

The identification of TAR-DNA binding protein (TDP-43) as the major component of ubiquitinated cytoplasmic inclusions in ALS (and FTD) (Neumann et al 2006) led to the gene encoding this protein, *TARDBP*, to be screened in cohorts of FALS. Following the initial report of mutations being identified in exon 6 of the gene (Sreedharan et al 2008), a further 39 nucleotide substitutions have been published; the vast majority of which are in exon 6 and encode non-synonymous changes. The frequency is reported to be 4-5% of FALS cases (Kirby et al 2010; Mackenzie et al 2010), with mutations inherited in an autosomal dominant manner.

Clinically, *TARDBP*-related ALS presents as a classical adult-onset form of ALS; 73% of cases manifest with limb onset and there is a wide range in the age of onset (30-77 years) and disease duration, even in cases carrying the same mutation (e.g. p.M337V), (ALSoD database: http:alsod.iop.kcl.ac.uk). Perhaps the most distinctive feature commented upon, is the absence of dementia in these patients, despite several reports of *TARDBP* mutations in cases of FTD (Borroni et al 2009; Kovacs et al 2009). Neuropathologically, there is no distinction between *TARDBP*-related ALS and SALS cases, with both showing skein and compact ubiquitinated inclusions.

TARDBP encodes several isoforms of a predominantly nuclear protein, of which TDP-43 is the most prevalent. TDP-43 contains 2 RNA recognition motifs (RRM), a nuclear localisation and nuclear export signal, as well as a glycine-rich region in the C-terminus, which is encoded by exon 6. TDP-43 is involved in a variety of roles in the nucleus, including regulation of transcription, RNA splicing, microRNA (miRNA) processing and stabilisation of mRNA. Reports have recently identified RNA molecules which bind to TDP-43 in whole cell extracts using cross linking and immunoprecipitation (CLIP) methodologies (Polymenidou et al 2011; Sephton et al 2011; Tollervey et al 2011; Xiao et al 2011). This has established over 4000 TDP-43 binding targets, including ALS-related genes *FUS* and vasolin containing protein (*VCP*), as well as other RNA processing genes. One target which has been confirmed is the *TARDBP* mRNA. TDP-43 regulates its own transcription by binding to the 3'UTR region of the *TARDBP* mRNA and promoting mRNA instability (Budini & Buratti 2011). In addition, TDP-43 has been shown to interact with mutant, but not wild-type SOD1 mRNA, thereby linking the two distinct genetic pathogenic mechanisms (Higashi et al 2010). In ALS, both in *TARDBP*-related ALS and SALS, TDP-43 is seen to mislocalise to the cytoplasm and form either compact or skein like protein inclusions. It is currently unclear whether a loss of nuclear function or a gain of toxic function (or both) causes motor neuronal cell death. Numerous cellular and animal models for *TARDBP*-related ALS have been generated in multiple species, in order to investigate the mechanisms of TDP-43 associated neurodegeneration (Joyce et al 2011). What is evident from this body of work is that over-expression of not only mutant, but also wild-type *TARDBP* is toxic and that TDP-43 is essential for development, as knockout models show embryonic lethality.

3.1.3 ALS6: Fused in sarcoma (*FUS*)

Mutations in *FUS*, also referred to as translocated in sarcoma (*TLS*), were initially identified both through linkage analysis in a large Cape Verde pedigree manifesting with autosomal recessive ALS and in several autosomal dominant ALS families linked to chr16 (Kwiatkowski et al 2009; Vance et al 2009). Similarly to *TARDBP*, mutations in this second RNA binding protein gene are clustered, rather than spread across the 15 exons encoding FUS; a third occur in exons 5-6 encoding the glycine-rich region and two thirds in exon 13-14 encoding the arginine-glycine-glycine (RGG)-rich domain and the nuclear localisation signal. *FUS* mutations have been shown to account for a further 4-5% of FALS cases (Hewitt et al 2010; Mackenzie et al 2010).

Clinically, *FUS* mutations are associated with limb onset ALS; no bulbar onset cases with *FUS* mutations have been reported to date (ALSoD database: http:alsod.iop.kcl.ac.uk). There is a large range in the age of onset, from 26-80 years and as with *TARDBP* mutations, to date no correlations are evident between specific mutations and clinical characteristics. Pathologically, however, *FUS*-related cases have shown distinctive FUS-positive, TDP-43 negative inclusions. Specifically, those cases with basophilic inclusions and compact neuronal cytoplasmic FUS-positive inclusions had an earlier onset than those ALS cases with skein-like neuronal cytoplasmic inclusions, in whom glial cytoplasmic inclusions were also seen (Baumer et al 2010; Mackenzie et al 2011).

FUS is an RNA/DNA binding protein, which shuttles between the nucleus and cytoplasm. The 526 amino acid protein contains multiple protein domains, including a glutamine-glycine-serine-tyrosine rich domain at the N-terminus, involved in transcriptional activation of oncogenic fusion genes involving *FUS*, a glycine-rich region, a nuclear export signal, an RNA recognition motif and two arginine-glycine-glycine motifs flanking a zinc finger motif. At the C-terminus resides the nuclear localisation signal. Mutations within this region have been shown to disrupt transportin mediated transport of FUS into the nucleus, and cause the formation of FUS containing stress granules in the cytoplasm (Dormann et al 2010; Ito et al 2011a). In contrast, mutations in the glycine-rich region of FUS have yet to demonstrate pathogenicity. The normal function of FUS is poorly understood, though there is evidence for its involvement in alternative splicing, miRNA processing and transportation of mRNA to the dendrites for localised translation. Of the animal and cellular models generated to investigate the mechanisms of mutant FUS, a rat model over-expressing human p.R521C shows progressive paralysis, axonal degeneration and loss of neurones in 1-2 months old rats, whilst rats over-expressing wild-type FUS are pre-symptomatic at 1 year, though they do show learning and memory deficits and loss of cortical neurons (Huang et al 2011). Furthermore, drosophila and yeast models demonstrate FUS toxicity is due to accumulation of mutant protein in the cytoplasm (Kryndushkin et al 2011; Lanson et al 2011).

3.2 Rarer genetic causes of autosomal dominant, adult onset ALS
3.2.1 ALS8: Vesicle associated membrane protein (VAMP) associated protein B (*VAPB*)

ALS8 was first described in a large Brazilian kindred comprised of 28 Caucasian affected male and female family members distributed across four generations. Patients in this family had a characteristic clinical phenotype of a postural tremor, fasciculations and a slowly progressive upper and lower limb weakness with an unusually long duration. Linkage analysis revealed a unique locus at Chr20q13.33 and mutation screening revealed a heterozygous C>T nucleotide substitution, resulting in a p.P56S non-synonymous change within the highly conserved major sperm protein (MSP) domain of VAPB (Nishimura et al 2004).

This exon 2 variant has since been detected in 22 additional individuals from six Brazilian pedigrees in which there is evidence of a founder effect, although it has also been seen in a Japanese and European case (Funke et al 2010; Landers et al 2008; Millecamps et al 2010). The neurodegenerative phenotype associated with this mutation is variable; 3 of the families also had several confirmed cases of autosomal dominant adult onset spinal muscular atrophy (SMA). A second heterozygous point mutation (p.T46I) within the same domain of the VAPB peptide has recently been reported in a single Caucasian from the UK with classical ALS (Chen et al 2010).

VAPB is a type II integral endoplasmic reticulum (ER) membrane protein. It is involved in multiple cellular processes including intracellular trafficking, lipid transport, and the unfolded protein response (Lev et al 2008). Both mutations residing in the MSP domain result in conformational changes which lead to VAPB aggregation and an increase in ER stress (Chen et al 2010; Kim et al 2010; Suzuki et al 2009). Whilst mutations in *VAPB* are only found rarely in FALS patients, *VAPB* shows significantly decreased gene expression in SALS cases compared to age and gender matched neurologically normal controls (Anagnostou et al 2010; Mitne-Neto et al 2011).

3.2.2 ALS9: Angiogenin (*ANG*)

Chr14q11.2 was first proposed as a susceptibility locus for ALS following the strong allelic association in the Irish population with a single nucleotide polymorphism (SNP) (rs11701) residing in the single exon angiogenin (*ANG*) gene (Greenway et al 2004). Mutation screening analysis of a large cohort of Irish, Scottish, English, Swedish and North American ALS cases detected 7 missense mutations in 15 patients, 4 of whom were FALS (Greenway et al 2006). Additional screening of ALS cohorts report *ANG* mutations occurring in both FALS and SALS cases, though at low frequencies (Fernandez-Santiago et al 2009; Gellera et al 2008).

ANG is a member of the pancreatic ribonuclease A (RNaseA) superfamily whose activities are known to be important in protein translation, ribosome biogenesis and cell proliferation (Crabtree et al 2007). The ribonuclease A activity has been shown to be reduced or lost in ANG mutant proteins. ANG is a potent inducer of neovascularization *in vivo* and has been shown to play a key role in neurite outgrowth and pathfinding during early embryonic development (Subramanian et al 2008). Its structure and function are partially homologous to that of vascular endothelial cell growth factor (VEGF); a previously reported genetic susceptibility and disease modifying factor in the development of neurodegeneration (Lambrechts et al 2009), and both VEGF and ANG have been shown to be neuroprotective. A proposed mechanism by which ANG prevents cell death is through inhibiting the translocation of apoptosis inducing factor into the nucleus (Li et al 2011).

3.2.3 ALS11: Factor-induced gene 4 *S.cerevisiae* homolog (*FIG4*)

The Sac1 domain containing protein 3 (SAC3) *FIG4*, located on Chr6q21, was originally identified as the causative gene of Charcot Marie-Tooth disease type 4J (CMT4J); a severe autosomal recessive childhood disorder that is characterised by both sensory and motor deficits (Chow et al 2007). However, in one CMT4J pedigree there was a later onset of disease, with predominantly motor symptoms, similar to ALS (Zhang et al 2008). Screening of a North European cohort of FALS patients revealed 5 heterozygous mutations, resulting in either complete or significant loss of protein (Chow et al 2009). In general, cases of ALS11 are associated with a rapidly progressive disease course of approximately 1-2 years, early bulbar involvement and minimal cognitive dysfunction.

FIG4 encodes the phosphatidylinositol 3,5-bisphosphate 5-phosphatase which controls the cellular abundance of $PI(3,5)P_2$, a signalling lipid that mediates retrograde trafficking of endosomal vesicles to the Golgi apparatus (Michell & Dove 2009). It remains unclear as to whether the deleterious variants of FIG4 exert an effect by a dominant negative mechanism or through a partial loss of function, as seen in CMT4J patients (Chow et al 2007). Human motor neurones are considered to be particularly susceptible to disruptions in this transport network because of their high membrane component turnover demands from long axonal processes over many decades (Ferguson et al 2010).

3.2.4 ALS12: Optineurin (OPTN)

Homozygosity mapping using 4 FALS cases demonstrated linkage to chr10p13 and subsequently mutations in OPTN, a gene previously linked to primary open-angle glaucoma (POAG), were identified in these cases (Maruyama et al 2010; Rezaie et al 2002). Mutations were initially found in both homozygous and heterozygous states. However, mutation screening of subsequent cohorts have identified only heterozygous mutations in ALS cases, occurring at a frequency of 3.4% in Japanese populations whilst this was at much lower frequencies in European and North American populations (Belzil et al 2011; Del Bo et al 2011). Interestingly, OPTN-related ALS is characterised by a lower limb onset with upper motor neurone involvement and a slow clinical progression.

The gene encodes the ubiquitously expressed optic neuropathy inducing protein which localises to the perinuclear region of the cytoplasm, where it is known to associate with the Golgi apparatus, and plays a key role in a number of biological processes, including vesicular trafficking, signal transduction and gene expression (Chalasani et al 2008). It is anticipated where mutations are inherited in an autosomal recessive manner, that reduced protein levels result in neurotoxicity through a loss of function mechanism. Conversely, the heterozygous missense substitution is predicted to exert a dominant negative effect. Examination of autopsy derived spinal cord tissue revealed extensive OPTN staining of TDP-43 positive intracytoplasmic hyaline inclusion bodies, although this was not replicated in a subsequent study (Hortobagyi et al 2011; Ito et al 2011b).

3.2.5 D-amino acid oxidase (DAO)

Following linkage analysis, a rare heterozygous missense mutation in the DAO gene, located on chr12q22-23, has been reported to segregate with disease in a single three generational Caucasian pedigree, though there was evidence of incomplete penetrance (Mitchell et al 2010). Those affected showed a rapidly progressive form of classical ALS with a mean disease duration of 21 months. Early bulbar involvement was apparent with limited signs of cognitive impairment. Interestingly, post-mortem immunohistochemical analysis on spinal cord tissue revealed no evidence of TDP-43 positively labelled inclusion bodies within the nuclear or cytoplasmic fractions of residual motor neurones which are normally a distinguishing feature of ALS pathology.

DAO encodes a universally expressed 39.4kDa peroxisomal flavin adenine dinucleotide (FAD)-dependent oxidase that is enriched in the neuronal and glial cell populations of the mammalian brainstem and spinal cord. The mutation results in the formation of an aberrant peptide product proposed to exert a dominant negative effect on the function of the wild type protein; *in vitro* work showed abnormal cellular morphology in cells over expressing the mutant protein, along with reduced cell viability, the presence of large intracellular ubiquitinated aggregates and an increased rate of apoptosis (Mitchell et al 2010).

3.2.6 Valosin containing protein (*VCP*)

Whole exome sequencing of two affected individuals in a large Italian pedigree identified a single heterozygous missense mutation in the *VCP* gene, located on chr9p13.3 (Johnson 2010). Screening of an additional cohort of ALS cases detected further *VCP* mutations at a frequency of 1.74%. There was no distinct phenotype associated with *VCP*-related ALS, with both limb and bulbar onset and an average age of onset of 49 years. Mutations in *VCP* have previously been linked to the autosomal dominant disorder inclusion body myopathy, Paget's disease and FTD (IBMPFD), which is characterised by muscle wasting, associated with osteolytic bone lesions and FTD (Watts et al 2004).

VCP is an evolutionarily conserved AAA+-ATPase that is known to be of importance in multiple biological processes including cell signalling, protein homeostasis, organelle biogenesis and autophagy (Ritson et al 2010), through its role in identifying ubiquitinated proteins in multimeric complexes and mediating their proteasomal degradation. It has been demonstrated both *in vitro* and *in vivo* that aberrant expression of VCP results in the cellular redistribution and mislocalisation of nuclear TDP-43 within the cytoplasm where neurotoxic ubiquitinated and phosphorylated aggregates form (Custer et al 2010; Gitcho et al 2009).

3.3 Genetic causes of autosomal dominant, juvenile onset ALS

3.3.1 ALS4: Senataxin (*SETX*)

The locus responsible for ALS4 was mapped to chr9q34 in an 11 generation pedigree affected by juvenile ALS and later confirmed by analysis of another two families with a similar phenotype (Chance et al 1998; De Jonghe et al 2002; Myrianthopoulos et al 1964). Sequence analysis of this region revealed disease associated mutations in the Senataxin (*SETX*) gene in all three affected families that were inherited in an autosomal dominant pattern (Chen et al 2004).   *SETX* mutations are rare, with only four FALS families discovered to date, although mutations in this gene are also associated with ataxia-oculomotor apraxia-2 (AOA2), an autosomal recessive cerebellar ataxia (Anheim et al 2009). ALS4 is characterised by young onset (below the age of 25 years), distal muscle weakness and atrophy, pyramidal signs, an absence of sensory abnormalities while bulbar and respiratory muscles are spared.   Disease progression is slow and patients have a normal life span (Chen et al 2004).

The *SETX* gene encodes a ubiquitously expressed DNA/RNA helicase that shares high homology to the yeast Sen1p protein and is suggested to play a role in DNA repair in response to oxidative stress (Suraweera et al 2007).   SETX interacts with several RNA processing proteins, including RNA polymerase II, and is proposed to regulate transcription and pre-mRNA processing (Suraweera et al 2009).

3.4 Genetic causes of autosomal recessive ALS
3.4.1 ALS2: Alsin (*ALS2*)

Linkage analysis in a large, inbred Tunisian family mapped the gene responsible for an autosomal recessive form of ALS to chr2p33-q35 (Hentati et al 1994). Subsequent sequencing in this family, and a Saudi pedigree with juvenile primary lateral sclerosis (PLS), revealed mutations in the previously uncharacterised gene now known as *ALS2* (Yang et al 2001). Thus, mutations cause a spectrum of early onset motor neurone disorders including infantile ascending hereditary spastic paraplegia (IAHSP), PLS and ALS (Bertini et al 1993). To date, 19 *ALS2* mutations have been identified in ALS patients, which are characterised by a juvenile onset of limb and facial spasticity with subsequent lower motor neurone signs (Hentati et al 1994; Lill et al 2011). The milder phenotypes of PLS and IAHSP are characterised by isolated upper motor neurone degeneration without lower motor neurone signs (Bertini et al 1993).

The *ALS2* gene is ubiquitously expressed and encodes the Alsin protein which contains three putative guanine-exchange factor (GEF) domains that activate small GTPases (Yang et al 2001). Evidence suggests that loss of Alsin is responsible for motor neurone damage and several groups have now generated *ALS2* knock-out mouse models, but only mild neurological changes have been reported in these animals to date (Cai et al 2008). The pathological mechanism of *ALS2* mutations remains unknown although evidence that Alsin has a role in endosomal transport and glutamate receptor targeting at the synapse offer interesting avenues for further study (Devon et al 2006; Hadano et al 2006; Lai et al 2006).

3.5 Genetic causes of ALS+FTD
3.5.1 Sigma non-opioid intracellular receptor 1 (*SIGMAR1*)

Following linkage analysis of a large multigenerational pedigree to chr9p, mutation screening of 34 genes in the candidate region identified a nucleotide substitution in the 3'UTR of the SIGMAR1 gene which co-segregated with the disease (Luty et al 2010). Two further FALS cases were also identified with 3'UTR substitutions, yet none of the 3 changes were present in controls. Pathological material was available from 2 individuals carrying one of the changes and both TDP-43 and FUS positive inclusions were observed. The SIGMAR1 protein functions as a subunit of the ligand-regulated potassium channel and regulates channel activity (Aydar et al 2002). It was suggested that the 3'UTR alterations alter the stability of the transcript, though how this subsequently causes motor neuronal cell death, is unknown (Luty et al 2010).

3.5.2 Microtubule associated protein tau (*MAPT*)

Pedigrees with clinical features of FTD, ALS and Parkinsonism have been identified with pathogenic mutations in the microtubule associated protein tau (*MAPT*) gene located on chr17 (Hutton et al 1998). Over 40 mutations have been identified to date that either affect the normal function of the tau protein to stabilise microtubules or disrupt alternative splicing leading to changes in the ratio of tau isoforms (Seelaar et al 2011). Affected individuals have a variable age of onset (25-65 years) with disease duration of 3-10 years and usually show symptoms of executive dysfunction, altered personality and behaviour. Many develop a Parkinsonism phenotype and/or other clinical features of 1 or 2 syndromes that may reflect an expansion of affected brain regions over time. Cases affected by an ALS phenotype are rare and so far mutations in *MAPT* have not been described in pure FALS (Boeve & Hutton 2008).

3.6 Genetic loci linked to ALS
3.6.1 ALS5: Spatacsin (*SPG11*)

The study of three consanguineous Tunisian pedigrees originally established linkage of chr15q15-q21 to an autosomal recessive form of ALS (Hentati et al 1998). A more recent study of 25 unrelated FALS families revealed 10 pedigrees with linkage to the same region and disease associated mutations in the spatacsin (*SPG11*) gene (Orlacchio et al 2010). Clinically, FALS patients with linkage to this region experience a juvenile onset, slowly progressive motor neuropathy associated with both upper and lower motor neurone signs. Disease duration is typically over 10-40 years without sensory symptoms and an absence of the feature of thin corpus callosum (Hentati et al 1998; Orlacchio et al 2010).

Mutations in this gene have been previously found to be the most common cause of autosomal recessive hereditary spastic paraplegia with thin corpus callosum (HSP-TCC), a condition characterised by progressive spasticity of lower limbs, mild cognitive impairment and a thin, but otherwise normally structured, corpus callosum (Abdel Aleem et al 2011). All but one of the mutations identified in FALS are also present in HSP-TCC pedigrees and the majority of these are truncating which may suggest a loss of function and a common pathological mechanism between the two conditions (Salinas et al 2008). The *SPG11* gene has 40 exons and encodes the highly conserved Spatacsin protein, which is ubiquitously expressed in the central nervous system (Salinas et al 2008). Although the function of Spatacsin remains unknown, neuropathological studies of HSP-TCC patients with *SPG11* mutations have revealed accumulations of membranous material in non-myelinated axons which are suggestive of axonal transport disturbance (Hehr et al 2007).

3.6.2 ALS7

To date, only one pedigree with ALS7 and linkage to chr20ptel-p13 has been identified (Sapp et al 2003). The family included 15 siblings, two of which were affected by an autosomal dominantly inherited form of ALS with mid-life onset and a rapid disease course of less than 2 years. The authors found probable linkage to a 6.25cM region of chr20 though more individuals from this pedigree are needed to confirm the findings (Sapp et al 2003).

3.6.3 ALS3

One large European kindred affected by an adult onset, autosomal dominant form of ALS has been linked to chr18q21 (Hand et al 2002). Patients in this family present with classical ALS involving progressive weakness in the limbs and bulbar regions with both upper and lower motor neurone signs. A candidate region of 7.5cM was identified on chr18, however, the pathogenic mutation is not yet known (Hand et al 2002).

3.6.4 ALSX

Linkage analysis of a 5-generation pedigree identified an adult onset, dominantly inherited locus on Xp11-q12. The causative gene has very recently been found to be ubiquilin 2 (*UBQLN2*), which encodes a cytosolic ubiquitin-like protein (Deng et al 2011). Mutation screening of additional cohorts of patients found a further 4 missense mutations in unrelated FALS cases, with all mutations affecting proline amino acids in the proline-x-x repeat region near the carboxyl end of the protein. Clinically, age of onset was variable (16-71 years) in the affected individuals, and although males were more likely to have an earlier age of onset, disease duration was similar. Some patients also showed symptoms of dementia. Post-mortem material from two unrelated FALS cases showed the classical skein like inclusions were positive for UBQLN2. The identified missense mutations lead to impairment of the protein degradation pathway in a cell model of *UBQLN2*-related ALS.

3.6.5 ALS-FTD1: 9p21-q22

A locus for FALS that arises in conjunction with FTD has been identified in 5 American families at chr9p21-q22 (Hosler et al 2000). Affected patients had adult onset of either: ALS and FTD, ALS alone or ALS with dementia. Disease duration was typically less than 4 years although one individual had a slow progression and survived for 15 years. No pathogenic mutations have been identified for this region to date (Hosler et al 2000).

3.6.6 ALS-FTD2: 9p13.2-p21.3

Linkage of autosomal dominant FALS and FTD to chr9p13.2-p21.3 has been established in two pedigrees, one large Dutch kindred and a Scandinavian family (Morita et al 2006; Vance et al 2006). Clinically, all members with ALS had definite or probable ALS by the El-Escorial Criteria with mid-life onset and a typical disease course of around 3 years. In the Scandinavian family ALS and FTD occurred separately, in contrast, affected individuals in the Dutch kindred all had features of both conditions. Linkage has been narrowed down to a 12cM (11Mb) region of chr9, however the pathogenic gene mutations have yet to be identified (Morita et al 2006; Vance et al 2006).

4. Conclusion

FALS accounts for 5% of ALS; an underlying mutation has been identified in approximately a third of these cases (Kiernan et al 2011). FALS causing mutations are used as a window into familial and the clinically indistinguishable sporadic disease; generating genetic models of ALS allows investigations into the mechanisms of motor neuronal degeneration, the identification of therapeutic targets and screening for candidate therapeutic agents (Van Damme & Robberecht 2009). However, the discovery of pathogenic mutations in ALS by linkage analysis is difficult because a relatively low prevalence and rapid disease course make large pedigrees difficult to obtain, therefore novel strategies to identify pathogenic mutations are essential (Hand & Rouleau 2002).

With the evolution of next generation sequencing technology, exhaustive sequencing of exonic regions of the genome has been used to identify pathogenic mutations in the *VCP* gene in ALS, and genetic mutations responsible for other diseases have also been identified from relatively few related or unrelated patients (Bowne et al 2011; Hoischen et al 2010; Johnson et al 2010a; Ng et al 2010; Ng et al 2009; Nikopoulos et al 2010; Simpson et al 2011). Exome sequencing, unlike a linkage analysis and positional cloning approach, is not targeted at a candidate region. Therefore it is likely that a large number of potential genetic variations will be discovered; the difficulty then is to determine which, if any, are pathogenic. However, next generation sequencing offers the potential for identifying at least some of the genes responsible for the remaining uncharacterised causes of FALS.

An expanded GGGGCC hexanucleotide repeat in *C9ORF72* has just been published as the cause of 9p-linked ALS-FTD, following next generation sequencing of the disease associated region (Renton et al 2011, DeJesus-Hernandez et al 2011). Expansions have been identified not only in ALS-FTD pedigrees, but also in familial FTD, familial ALS and sporadic ALS. Estimated frequencies vary from 23.5% to 46.4% for familial ALS and 4.1% to 21% for sporadic ALS. The expansion, which is non-coding, is therefore the most common genetic cause of ALS identified to date.

5. Acknowledgments

PJS and JK are funded by the European Community's Health Seventh Framework Programme (FP7/2007-2013) under grant agreement 259867 and by the Motor Neurone Disease Association (MNDA). EFG is also funded by the MNDA.

6. References

Abalkhail H, Mitchell J, Habgood J, Orrell R, de Belleroche J. 2003. A new familial amyotrophic lateral sclerosis locus on chromosome 16q12.1-16q12.2. *Am J Hum Genet* 73:383-9

Abdel Aleem A, Abu-Shahba N, Swistun D, Silhavy J, Bielas SL, et al. 2011. Expanding the clinical spectrum of SPG11 gene mutations in recessive hereditary spastic paraplegia with thin corpus callosum. *European journal of medical genetics* 54:82-5

Alexander MD, Traynor BJ, Miller N, Corr B, Frost E, et al. 2002. "True" sporadic ALS associated with a novel SOD-1 mutation. *Ann Neurol* 52:680-3

Anagnostou G, Akbar MT, Paul P, Angelinetta C, Steiner TJ, de Belleroche J. 2010. Vesicle associated membrane protein B (VAPB) is decreased in ALS spinal cord. *Neurobiol Aging* 31:969-85

Andersen PM. 2006. Amyotrophic lateral sclerosis associated with mutations in the CuZn superoxide dismutase gene. *Curr Neurol Neurosci Rep* 6:37-46

Andersen PM, Nilsson P, Ala-Hurula V, Keranen ML, Tarvainen I, et al. 1995. Amyotrophic lateral sclerosis associated with homozygosity for an Asp90Ala mutation in CuZn-superoxide dismutase. *Nat Genet* 10:61-6

Anheim M, Monga B, Fleury M, Charles P, Barbot C, et al. 2009. Ataxia with oculomotor apraxia type 2: clinical, biological and genotype/phenotype correlation study of a cohort of 90 patients. *Brain : a journal of neurology* 132:2688-98

Arai T, Hasegawa M, Akiyama H, Ikeda K, Nonaka T, et al. 2006. TDP-43 is a component of ubiquitin-positive tau-negative inclusions in frontotemporal lobar degeneration and amyotrophic lateral sclerosis. *Biochem Biophys Res Commun* 351:602-11

Aydar E, Palmer CP, Klyachko VA, Jackson MB. 2002. The sigma receptor as a ligand-regulated auxiliary potassium channel subunit. *Neuron* 34:399-410

Baumer D, Hilton D, Paine SM, Turner MR, Lowe J, et al. 2010. Juvenile ALS with basophilic inclusions is a FUS proteinopathy with FUS mutations. *Neurology* 75:611-8

Belzil VV, Daoud H, Desjarlais A, Bouchard JP, Dupre N, et al. 2011. Analysis of OPTN as a causative gene for amyotrophic lateral sclerosis. *Neurobiology of aging* 32:555 e13-4

Benatar M. 2007. Lost in translation: treatment trials in the SOD1 mouse and in human ALS. *Neurobiol Dis* 26:1-13

Bertini ES, Eymard-Pierre E, Boespflug-Tanguy O, Cleveland DW, Yamanaka K. 1993. In *GeneReviews*, ed. RA Pagon, TD Bird, CR Dolan, K Stephens. Seattle (WA)

Boeve BF, Hutton M. 2008. Refining frontotemporal dementia with parkinsonism linked to chromosome 17: introducing FTDP-17 (MAPT) and FTDP-17 (PGRN). *Arch Neurol* 65:460-4

Borroni B, Bonvicini C, Alberici A, Buratti E, Agosti C, et al. 2009. Mutation within TARDBP leads to frontotemporal dementia without motor neuron disease. *Hum Mutat* 30:E974-83

Bosco DA, Morfini G, Karabacak NM, Song Y, Gros-Louis F, et al. 2010. Wild-type and mutant SOD1 share an aberrant conformation and a common pathogenic pathway in ALS. *Nat Neurosci* 13:1396-403

Bowne SJ, Sullivan LS, Koboldt DC, Ding L, Fulton R, et al. 2011. Identification of Disease-Causing Mutations in Autosomal Dominant Retinitis Pigmentosa (adRP) Using Next-Generation DNA Sequencing. *Investigative Ophthalmology & Visual Science* 52:494-503

Budini M, Buratti E. 2011. TDP-43 Autoregulation: Implications for Disease. *J Mol Neurosci*

Byrne S, Walsh C, Lynch C, Bede P, Elamin M, et al. 2011. Rate of familial amyotrophic lateral sclerosis: a systematic review and meta-analysis. *J Neurol Neurosurg Psychiatry* 82:623-7

Cai H, Shim H, Lai C, Xie C, Lin X, et al. 2008. ALS2/alsin knockout mice and motor neuron diseases. *Neuro-degenerative diseases* 5:359-66

Chalasani ML, Balasubramanian D, Swarup G. 2008. Focus on molecules: optineurin. *Exp Eye Res* 87:1-2

Chance PF, Rabin BA, Ryan SG, Ding Y, Scavina M, et al. 1998. Linkage of the gene for an autosomal dominant form of juvenile amyotrophic lateral sclerosis to chromosome 9q34. *American journal of human genetics* 62:633-40

Chen HJ, Anagnostou G, Chai A, Withers J, Morris A, et al. 2010. Characterization of the properties of a novel mutation in VAPB in familial amyotrophic lateral sclerosis. *J Biol Chem* 285:40266-81

Chen YZ, Bennett CL, Huynh HM, Blair IP, Puls I, et al. 2004. DNA/RNA helicase gene mutations in a form of juvenile amyotrophic lateral sclerosis (ALS4). *American journal of human genetics* 74:1128-35

Chio A, Calvo A, Moglia C, Ossola I, Brunetti M, et al. 2010. A de novo missense mutation of the FUS gene in a "true" sporadic ALS case. *Neurobiology of aging*

Chow CY, Landers JE, Bergren SK, Sapp PC, Grant AE, et al. 2009. Deleterious variants of FIG4, a phosphoinositide phosphatase, in patients with ALS. *Am J Hum Genet* 84:85-8

Chow CY, Zhang Y, Dowling JJ, Jin N, Adamska M, et al. 2007. Mutation of FIG4 causes neurodegeneration in the pale tremor mouse and patients with CMT4J. *Nature* 448:68-72

Crabtree B, Thiyagarajan N, Prior SH, Wilson P, Iyer S, et al. 2007. Characterization of human angiogenin variants implicated in amyotrophic lateral sclerosis. *Biochemistry* 46:11810-8

Custer SK, Neumann M, Lu H, Wright AC, Taylor JP. 2010. Transgenic mice expressing mutant forms VCP/p97 recapitulate the full spectrum of IBMPFD including degeneration in muscle, brain and bone. *Hum Mol Genet* 19:1741-55

De Jonghe P, Auer-Grumbach M, Irobi J, Wagner K, Plecko B, et al. 2002. Autosomal dominant juvenile amyotrophic lateral sclerosis and distal hereditary motor neuronopathy with pyramidal tract signs: synonyms for the same disorder? *Brain : a journal of neurology* 125:1320-5

Del Bo R, Tiloca C, Pensato V, Corrado L, Ratti A, et al. 2011. Novel optineurin mutations in patients with familial and sporadic amyotrophic lateral sclerosis. *J Neurol Neurosurg Psychiatry*

Deng HX, Chen W, Hong ST, Boycott KM, Gorrie GH, et al. 2011. Mutations in UBQLN2 cause dominant X-linked juvenile and adult-onset ALS and ALS/dementia. *Nature*

DeJesus-Hernandez M, Mackenzie IR, Boeve BF, Boxer AL, Baker M, et al. 2011. Expanded GGGGCC Hexanucleotide Repeat in Noncoding Region of C9ORF72 Causes Chromosome 9p-Linked FTD and ALS. *Neuron*

Devon RS, Orban PC, Gerrow K, Barbieri MA, Schwab C, et al. 2006. Als2-deficient mice exhibit disturbances in endosome trafficking associated with motor behavioral abnormalities. *Proceedings of the National Academy of Sciences of the United States of America* 103:9595-600

Dormann D, Rodde R, Edbauer D, Bentmann E, Fischer I, et al. 2010. ALS-associated fused in sarcoma (FUS) mutations disrupt Transportin-mediated nuclear import. *Embo J* 29:2841-57

Ferguson CJ, Lenk GM, Meisler MH. 2010. PtdIns(3,5)P2 and autophagy in mouse models of neurodegeneration. *Autophagy* 6:170-1

Fernandez-Santiago R, Hoenig S, Lichtner P, Sperfeld AD, Sharma M, et al. 2009. Identification of novel Angiogenin (ANG) gene missense variants in German patients with amyotrophic lateral sclerosis. *J Neurol* 256:1337-42

Ferraiuolo L, Kirby J, Grierson AJ, Sendtner M, Shaw PJ. 2011. Molecular and cellular pathways of motor neuron injury in amyotrophic lateral sclerosis. *Nat Rev Neurology* (In Press)

Funke AD, Esser M, Kruttgen A, Weis J, Mitne-Neto M, et al. 2010. The p.P56S mutation in the VAPB gene is not due to a single founder: the first European case. *Clin Genet* 77:302-3

Gellera C, Colombrita C, Ticozzi N, Castellotti B, Bragato C, et al. 2008. Identification of new ANG gene mutations in a large cohort of Italian patients with amyotrophic lateral sclerosis. *Neurogenetics* 9:33-40

Geser F, Lee VM, Trojanowski JQ. 2010. Amyotrophic lateral sclerosis and frontotemporal lobar degeneration: a spectrum of TDP-43 proteinopathies. *Neuropathology* 30:103-12

Gitcho MA, Strider J, Carter D, Taylor-Reinwald L, Forman MS, et al. 2009. VCP mutations causing frontotemporal lobar degeneration disrupt localization of TDP-43 and induce cell death. *J Biol Chem* 284:12384-98

Gordon PH, Delgadillo D, Piquard A, Bruneteau G, Pradat PF, et al. 2011. The range and clinical impact of cognitive impairment in French patients with ALS: A cross-sectional study of neuropsychological test performance. *Amyotroph Lateral Scler*

Greenway MJ, Alexander MD, Ennis S, Traynor BJ, Corr B, et al. 2004. A novel candidate region for ALS on chromosome 14q11.2. *Neurology* 63:1936-8

Greenway MJ, Andersen PM, Russ C, Ennis S, Cashman S, et al. 2006. ANG mutations segregate with familial and 'sporadic' amyotrophic lateral sclerosis. *Nat Genet* 38:411-3

Hadano S, Benn SC, Kakuta S, Otomo A, Sudo K, et al. 2006. Mice deficient in the Rab5 guanine nucleotide exchange factor ALS2/alsin exhibit age-dependent neurological deficits and altered endosome trafficking. *Human molecular genetics* 15:233-50

Hand CK, Khoris J, Salachas F, Gros-Louis F, Lopes AA, et al. 2002. A novel locus for familial amyotrophic lateral sclerosis, on chromosome 18q. *Am J Hum Genet* 70:251-6

Hand CK, Rouleau GA. 2002. Familial amyotrophic lateral sclerosis. *Muscle & Nerve* 25:135-59

Hehr U, Bauer P, Winner B, Schule R, Olmez A, et al. 2007. Long-term course and mutational spectrum of spatacsin-linked spastic paraplegia. *Ann Neurol* 62:656-65

Hentati A, Bejaoui K, Pericak-Vance MA, Hentati F, Speer MC, et al. 1994. Linkage of recessive familial amyotrophic lateral sclerosis to chromosome 2q33-q35. *Nature genetics* 7:425-8

Hentati A, Ouahchi K, Pericak-Vance MA, Nijhawan D, Ahmad A, et al. 1998. Linkage of a commoner form of recessive amyotrophic lateral sclerosis to chromosome 15q15-q22 markers. *Neurogenetics* 2:55-60

Hewitt C, Kirby J, Highley JR, Hartley JA, Hibberd R, et al. 2010. Novel FUS/TLS mutations and pathology in familial and sporadic amyotrophic lateral sclerosis. *Arch Neurol* 67:455-61

Higashi S, Tsuchiya Y, Araki T, Wada K, Kabuta T. 2010. TDP-43 physically interacts with amyotrophic lateral sclerosis-linked mutant CuZn superoxide dismutase. *Neurochem Int* 57:906-13

Hoischen A, van Bon BWM, Gilissen C, Arts P, van Lier B, et al. 2010. De novo mutations of SETBP1 cause Schinzel-Giedion syndrome. *Nat Genet* 42:483-5

Hortobagyi T, Troakes C, Nishimura AL, Vance C, van Swieten JC, et al. 2011. Optineurin inclusions occur in a minority of TDP-43 positive ALS and FTLD-TDP cases and are rarely observed in other neurodegenerative disorders. *Acta Neuropathol* 121:519-27

Hosler BA, Siddique T, Sapp PC, Sailor W, Huang MC, et al. 2000. Linkage of familial amyotrophic lateral sclerosis with frontotemporal dementia to chromosome 9q21-q22. *JAMA : the journal of the American Medical Association* 284:1664-9

Huang C, Zhou H, Tong J, Chen H, Liu YJ, et al. 2011. FUS transgenic rats develop the phenotypes of amyotrophic lateral sclerosis and frontotemporal lobar degeneration. *PLoS genetics* 7:e1002011

Hutton M, Lendon CL, Rizzu P, Baker M, Froelich S, et al. 1998. Association of missense and 5'-splice-site mutations in tau with the inherited dementia FTDP-17. *Nature* 393:702-5

Ito D, Seki M, Tsunoda Y, Uchiyama H, Suzuki N. 2011a. Nuclear transport impairment of amyotrophic lateral sclerosis-linked mutations in FUS/TLS. *Ann Neurol* 69:152-62

Ito H, Nakamura M, Komure O, Ayaki T, Wate R, et al. 2011b. Clinicopathologic study on an ALS family with a heterozygous E478G optineurin mutation. *Acta Neuropathol*

Johnson JO, Mandrioli J, Benatar M, Abramzon Y, Van Deerlin VM, et al. 2010a. Exome Sequencing Reveals VCP Mutations as a Cause of Familial ALS. *Neuron* 68:857-64

Johnson JO, Mandrioli J, Benatar M, Abramzon Y, Van Deerlin VM, et al. 2010b. Exome sequencing reveals VCP mutations as a cause of familial ALS. *Neuron* 68:857-64

Joyce PI, Fratta P, Fisher EM, Acevedo-Arozena A. 2011. SOD1 and TDP-43 animal models of amyotrophic lateral sclerosis: recent advances in understanding disease toward the development of clinical treatments. *Mamm Genome*

Kabashi E, Valdmanis PN, Dion P, Spiegelman D, McConkey BJ, et al. 2008. TARDBP mutations in individuals with sporadic and familial amyotrophic lateral sclerosis. *Nat Genet* 40:572-4

Kiernan MC, Vucic S, Cheah BC, Turner MR, Eisen A, et al. 2011. Amyotrophic lateral sclerosis. *The Lancet* 377:942-55

Kim S, Leal SS, Ben Halevy D, Gomes CM, Lev S. 2010. Structural requirements for VAP-B oligomerization and their implication in amyotrophic lateral sclerosis-associated VAP-B(P56S) neurotoxicity. *J Biol Chem* 285:13839-49

Kirby J, Goodall EF, Smith W, Highley JR, Masanzu R, et al. 2010. Broad clinical phenotypes associated with TAR-DNA binding protein (TARDBP) mutations in amyotrophic lateral sclerosis. *Neurogenetics* 11:217-25

Kovacs GG, Murrell JR, Horvath S, Haraszti L, Majtenyi K, et al. 2009. TARDBP variation associated with frontotemporal dementia, supranuclear gaze palsy, and chorea. *Mov Disord* 24:1843-7

Kryndushkin D, Wickner RB, Shewmaker F. 2011. FUS/TLS forms cytoplasmic aggregates, inhibits cell growth and interacts with TDP-43 in a yeast model of amyotrophic lateral sclerosis. *Protein Cell* 2:223-36

Kwiatkowski TJ, Jr., Bosco DA, Leclerc AL, Tamrazian E, Vanderburg CR, et al. 2009. Mutations in the FUS/TLS gene on chromosome 16 cause familial amyotrophic lateral sclerosis. *Science* 323:1205-8

Lai C, Xie C, McCormack SG, Chiang HC, Michalak MK, et al. 2006. Amyotrophic lateral sclerosis 2-deficiency leads to neuronal degeneration in amyotrophic lateral sclerosis through altered AMPA receptor trafficking. *The Journal of neuroscience : the official journal of the Society for Neuroscience* 26:11798-806

Lambrechts D, Poesen K, Fernandez-Santiago R, Al-Chalabi A, Del Bo R, et al. 2009. Meta-analysis of vascular endothelial growth factor variations in amyotrophic lateral sclerosis: increased susceptibility in male carriers of the -2578AA genotype. *J Med Genet* 46:840-6

Landers JE, Leclerc AL, Shi L, Virkud A, Cho T, et al. 2008. New VAPB deletion variant and exclusion of VAPB mutations in familial ALS. *Neurology* 70:1179-85

Lanson NA, Jr., Maltare A, King H, Smith R, Kim JH, et al. 2011. A Drosophila model of FUS-related neurodegeneration reveals genetic interaction between FUS and TDP-43. *Hum Mol Genet* 20:2510-23

Lev S, Ben Halevy D, Peretti D, Dahan N. 2008. The VAP protein family: from cellular functions to motor neuron disease. *Trends Cell Biol* 18:282-90

Li S, Yu W, Hu GF. 2011. Angiogenin inhibits nuclear translocation of apoptosis inducing factor in a Bcl-2-dependent manner. *J Cell Physiol*

Lill CM, Abel O, Bertram L, Al-Chalabi A. 2011. Keeping up with genetic discoveries in amyotrophic lateral sclerosis: The ALSoD and ALSGene databases. *Amyotrophic lateral sclerosis : official publication of the World Federation of Neurology Research Group on Motor Neuron Diseases* 12:238-49

Lillo P, Mioshi E, Zoing MC, Kiernan MC, Hodges JR. 2011. How common are behavioural changes in amyotrophic lateral sclerosis? *Amyotroph Lateral Scler* 12:45-51

Lopate G, Baloh RH, Al-Lozi MT, Miller TM, Fernandes Filho JA, et al. 2010. Familial ALS with extreme phenotypic variability due to the I113T SOD1 mutation. *Amyotroph Lateral Scler* 11:232-6

Luty AA, Kwok JB, Dobson-Stone C, Loy CT, Coupland KG, et al. 2010. Sigma nonopioid intracellular receptor 1 mutations cause frontotemporal lobar degeneration-motor neuron disease. *Ann Neurol* 68:639-49

Mackenzie IR, Ansorge O, Strong M, Bilbao J, Zinman L, et al. 2011. Pathological heterogeneity in amyotrophic lateral sclerosis with FUS mutations: two distinct patterns correlating with disease severity and mutation. *Acta Neuropathol* 122:87-98

Mackenzie IR, Bigio EH, Ince PG, Geser F, Neumann M, et al. 2007. Pathological TDP-43 distinguishes sporadic amyotrophic lateral sclerosis from amyotrophic lateral sclerosis with SOD1 mutations. *Ann Neurol* 61:427-34

Mackenzie IR, Rademakers R, Neumann M. 2010. TDP-43 and FUS in amyotrophic lateral sclerosis and frontotemporal dementia. *Lancet Neurol* 9:995-1007

Maruyama H, Morino H, Ito H, Izumi Y, Kato H, et al. 2010. Mutations of optineurin in amyotrophic lateral sclerosis. *Nature* 465:223-6

Michell RH, Dove SK. 2009. A protein complex that regulates PtdIns(3,5)P2 levels. *EMBO J* 28:86-7

Millecamps S, Salachas F, Cazeneuve C, Gordon P, Bricka B, et al. 2010. SOD1, ANG, VAPB, TARDBP, and FUS mutations in familial amyotrophic lateral sclerosis: genotype-phenotype correlations. *J Med Genet* 47:554-60

Mitchell J, Paul P, Chen HJ, Morris A, Payling M, et al. 2010. Familial amyotrophic lateral sclerosis is associated with a mutation in D-amino acid oxidase. *Proc Natl Acad Sci U S A* 107:7556-61

Mitne-Neto M, Machado-Costa M, Marchetto MC, Bengtson MH, Joazeiro CA, et al. 2011. Downregulation of VAPB expression in motor neurons derived from induced pluripotent stem cells of ALS8 patients. *Hum Mol Genet*

Morita M, Al-Chalabi A, Andersen PM, Hosler B, Sapp P, et al. 2006. A locus on chromosome 9p confers susceptibility to ALS and frontotemporal dementia. *Neurology* 66:839-44

Myrianthopoulos NC, Lane MH, Silberberg DH, Vincent BL. 1964. Nerve Conduction and Other Studies in Families with Charcot-Marie-Tooth Disease. *Brain : a journal of neurology* 87:589-608

Neumann M, Sampathu DM, Kwong LK, Truax AC, Micsenyi MC, et al. 2006. Ubiquitinated TDP-43 in frontotemporal lobar degeneration and amyotrophic lateral sclerosis. *Science* 314:130-3

Ng SB, Bigham AW, Buckingham KJ, Hannibal MC, McMillin MJ, et al. 2010. Exome sequencing identifies MLL2 mutations as a cause of Kabuki syndrome. *Nat Genet* 42:790-3

Ng SB, Turner EH, Robertson PD, Flygare SD, Bigham AW, et al. 2009. Targeted capture and massively parallel sequencing of 12 human exomes. *Nature* 461:272-6

Nikopoulos K, Gilissen C, Hoischen A, Erik van Nouhuys C, Boonstra FN, et al. 2010. Next-Generation Sequencing of a 40 Mb Linkage Interval Reveals TSPAN12 Mutations in Patients with Familial Exudative Vitreoretinopathy. *The American Journal of Human Genetics* 86:240-7

Nishimura AL, Mitne-Neto M, Silva HC, Richieri-Costa A, Middleton S, et al. 2004. A mutation in the vesicle-trafficking protein VAPB causes late-onset spinal muscular atrophy and amyotrophic lateral sclerosis. *Am J Hum Genet* 75:822-31

Orlacchio A, Babalini C, Borreca A, Patrono C, Massa R, et al. 2010. SPATACSIN mutations cause autosomal recessive juvenile amyotrophic lateral sclerosis. *Brain : a journal of neurology* 133:591-8

Polymenidou M, Lagier-Tourenne C, Hutt KR, Huelga SC, Moran J, et al. 2011. Long pre-mRNA depletion and RNA missplicing contribute to neuronal vulnerability from loss of TDP-43. *Nat Neurosci* 14:459-68

Rakhit R, Chakrabartty A. 2006. Structure, folding, and misfolding of Cu,Zn superoxide dismutase in amyotrophic lateral sclerosis. *Biochim Biophys Acta* 1762:1025-37

Renton AE, Majounie E, Waite A, Simon-Sanchez J, Rollinson S, et al. 2011. A Hexanucleotide Repeat Expansion in C9ORF72 Is the Cause of Chromosome 9p21-Linked ALS-FTD. *Neuron*

Rezaie T, Child A, Hitchings R, Brice G, Miller L, et al. 2002. Adult-onset primary open-angle glaucoma caused by mutations in optineurin. *Science* 295:1077-9

Ringholz GM, Appel SH, Bradshaw M, Cooke NA, Mosnik DM, Schulz PE. 2005. Prevalence and patterns of cognitive impairment in sporadic ALS. *Neurology* 65:586-90

Ritson GP, Custer SK, Freibaum BD, Guinto JB, Geffel D, et al. 2010. TDP-43 mediates degeneration in a novel Drosophila model of disease caused by mutations in VCP/p97. *J Neurosci* 30:7729-39

Rosen DR, Siddique T, Patterson D, Figlewicz DA, Sapp P, et al. 1993. Mutations in Cu/Zn superoxide dismutase gene are associated with familial amyotrophic lateral sclerosis. *Nature* 362:59-62

Salinas S, Proukakis C, Crosby A, Warner TT. 2008. Hereditary spastic paraplegia: clinical features and pathogenetic mechanisms. *Lancet Neurol* 7:1127-38

Sapp PC, Hosler BA, McKenna-Yasek D, Chin W, Gann A, et al. 2003. Identification of two novel loci for dominantly inherited familial amyotrophic lateral sclerosis. *American journal of human genetics* 73:397-403

Seelaar H, Rohrer JD, Pijnenburg YA, Fox NC, van Swieten JC. 2011. Clinical, genetic and pathological heterogeneity of frontotemporal dementia: a review. *J Neurol Neurosurg Psychiatry* 82:476-86

Sephton CF, Cenik C, Kucukural A, Dammer EB, Cenik B, et al. 2011. Identification of neuronal RNA targets of TDP-43-containing ribonucleoprotein complexes. *J Biol Chem* 286:1204-15

Simpson CL, Al-Chalabi A. 2006. Amyotrophic lateral sclerosis as a complex genetic disease. *Biochimica et biophysica acta* 1762:973-85

Simpson MA, Irving MD, Asilmaz E, Gray MJ, Dafou D, et al. 2011. Mutations in NOTCH2 cause Hajdu-Cheney syndrome, a disorder of severe and progressive bone loss. *Nat Genet* 43:303-5

Sreedharan J, Blair IP, Tripathi VB, Hu X, Vance C, et al. 2008. TDP-43 mutations in familial and sporadic amyotrophic lateral sclerosis. *Science* 319:1668-72

Subramanian V, Crabtree B, Acharya KR. 2008. Human angiogenin is a neuroprotective factor and amyotrophic lateral sclerosis associated angiogenin variants affect neurite extension/pathfinding and survival of motor neurons. *Hum Mol Genet* 17:130-49

Sundar PD, Yu CE, Sieh W, Steinbart E, Garruto RM, et al. 2007. Two sites in the MAPT region confer genetic risk for Guam ALS/PDC and dementia. *Hum Mol Genet* 16:295-306

Suraweera A, Becherel OJ, Chen P, Rundle N, Woods R, et al. 2007. Senataxin, defective in ataxia oculomotor apraxia type 2, is involved in the defense against oxidative DNA damage. *The Journal of cell biology* 177:969-79

Suraweera A, Lim Y, Woods R, Birrell GW, Nasim T, et al. 2009. Functional role for senataxin, defective in ataxia oculomotor apraxia type 2, in transcriptional regulation. *Human molecular genetics* 18:3384-96

Suzuki H, Kanekura K, Levine TP, Kohno K, Olkkonen VM, et al. 2009. ALS-linked P56S-VAPB, an aggregated loss-of-function mutant of VAPB, predisposes motor neurons to ER stress-related death by inducing aggregation of co-expressed wild-type VAPB. *J Neurochem* 108:973-85

Tollervey JR, Curk T, Rogelj B, Briese M, Cereda M, et al. 2011. Characterizing the RNA targets and position-dependent splicing regulation by TDP-43. *Nat Neurosci* 14:452-8

Valdmanis PN, Rouleau GA. 2008. Genetics of familial amyotrophic lateral sclerosis. *Neurology* 70:144-52

Van Damme P, Robberecht W. 2009. Recent advances in motor neuron disease. *Current Opinion in Neurology* 22:486-92 10.1097/WCO.0b013e32832ffbe3

Vance C, Al-Chalabi A, Ruddy D, Smith BN, Hu X, et al. 2006. Familial amyotrophic lateral sclerosis with frontotemporal dementia is linked to a locus on chromosome 9p13.2-21.3. *Brain* 129:868-76

Vance C, Rogelj B, Hortobagyi T, De Vos KJ, Nishimura AL, et al. 2009. Mutations in FUS, an RNA processing protein, cause familial amyotrophic lateral sclerosis type 6. *Science* 323:1208-11

Watts GD, Wymer J, Kovach MJ, Mehta SG, Mumm S, et al. 2004. Inclusion body myopathy associated with Paget disease of bone and frontotemporal dementia is caused by mutant valosin-containing protein. *Nat Genet* 36:377-81

Worms PM. 2001. The epidemiology of motor neuron diseases: a review of recent studies. *J Neurol Sci* 191:3-9

Xiao S, Sanelli T, Dib S, Sheps D, Findlater J, et al. 2011. RNA targets of TDP-43 identified by UV-CLIP are deregulated in ALS. *Mol Cell Neurosci* 47:167-80

Yang Y, Hentati A, Deng HX, Dabbagh O, Sasaki T, et al. 2001. The gene encoding alsin, a protein with three guanine-nucleotide exchange factor domains, is mutated in a form of recessive amyotrophic lateral sclerosis. *Nature genetics* 29:160-5

Zhang X, Chow CY, Sahenk Z, Shy ME, Meisler MH, Li J. 2008. Mutation of FIG4 causes a rapidly progressive, asymmetric neuronal degeneration. *Brain* 131:1990-2001

7

Genetics of Amyotrophic Lateral Sclerosis

Max Koppers[1,2], Michael van Es[1], Leonard H. van den Berg[1],
Jan H. Veldink[1*] and R. Jeroen Pasterkamp[1,2*]
[1]Departments of Neurology, University Medical Center Utrecht,
[2]Deparment of Neuroscience and Pharmacology, University Medical Center Utrecht,
The Netherlands

1. Introduction

Amyotrophic lateral sclerosis (ALS) is a neurodegenerative disease characterized by progressive muscle weakness caused by loss of central and peripheral motor neurons. Symptoms typically have a localized limb or bulbar onset and progress to other muscle groups of the body. Denervation of respiratory muscles and dysphagia leading to respiratory complications are the most common causes of death. There is no cure for this rapidly progressive disease.

Approximately 5% of patients have a family history of ALS (fALS) (Byrne et al., 2011). All other cases are considered to have a sporadic form of the disease (sALS). A twin study of sALS patients has estimated hereditability to be considerable (0.38-0.76), indicating an important genetic component in disease etiology (Al-Chalabi et al., 2010). sALS, therefore, is considered to be a disease of complex etiology with both genetic and environmental factors contributing to disease susceptibility.

This chapter will provide an overview of the current knowledge of the genetics of both fALS and sALS. There will be, however, particular emphasis on two sALS associated regions identified in a large genome wide association study namely, chromosomal region 9p21.2 and 19p13.11. Evidence for the association with these regions as well as the function of the relevant genes in these regions will be discussed.

2. Genetics of familial amyotrophic lateral sclerosis

Familial ALS is a genetically heterogeneous group of diseases for which linkage has been found for over 13 different loci (Table 1). These loci account for approximately 25-30% of all fALS cases. In addition, variants in several other genes have been implicated in fALS but most of these data are still inconclusive. All currently known fALS loci and the genes involved will be briefly discussed in this section.

2.1 ALS1 (SOD1)

Linkage analysis in autosomal-dominant fALS pedigrees associated the copper-zinc superoxide dismutase (*SOD1*) gene on chromosome 21q to ALS. Several point mutations in

---

*Corresponding authors

Name of Disease	Locus	Gene	Protein	Inheritance	Clinical features
ALS1	21q22	SOD1	Cu/Zn superoxide dismutase	AD/AR	Typical ALS
ALS2	2q33	ALSin	ALSin	AR	Juvenile onset, slowly progressive, predominantly upper motor neuron signs
ALS3	18q21	N.K.	-	AD	Typical ALS, disease onset in legs
ALS4	9q34	SETX	Senataxin	AD	Childhood/Adolescent onset, slowly progressive, no respiratory and bulbar involvement
ALS5	15q15-21	SPG11	Spatacsin	AR	Juvenile onset, slowly progressive
ALS6	16p11.2	FUS	Fused in sarcoma	AD/AR	Typical ALS
ALS7	20p13	N.K.	-	AD	Typical ALS
ALS8	20q13	VAPB	VAMP-associated protein B	AD	Typical ALS, SMA and atypical ALS
ALS9	14q11	ANG	Angiogenin	AD	Typical ALS, frontotemporal dementia, Parkinson's disease
ALS10	1q36	TARDBP	TAR-DNA binding protein	AD	Typical ALS
ALS11	6q21	FIG4	PI(3,5)P(2)5-phosphatase	AD	Adult onset, prominent corticospinal tract signs
ALS12	10p13	OPTN	Optineurin	AD/AR	Adult onset
ALS14	9p13-p12	VCP	Valosin-containing protein	AD	Adult onset with or without FTD
ALS-FTD1	9q21-22	N.K.	-	AD	ALS, FTD
ALS-FTD2	9p13.2-21.3	C9ORF72	Chromosome 9 open reading frame 72	AD	ALS, FTD
ALS-FTDP	17q21.1	MAPT	Microtubule-associated protein tau	AD	Adult onset with FTD
ALS-X	Xcen	N.K.	-	XD	Adult onset

AD = Autosomal dominant, AR = Autosomal recessive, XD = X-linked dominant, FTD = frontotemporal dementia, SMA = spinal muscular atrophy, N.K. = not known, FTDP = frontotemporal dementia with parkinsonism

Table 1. Classification of familial ALS.

SOD1 that co-segregated with the disease were identified in several of these pedigrees (Rosen et al., 1993). To date, over 150 different mutations in *SOD1* have been identified (see http://alsod.iop.kcl.ac.uk). Mutations have been reported in ~20% of fALS patients and in 1-4% of sALS patients (Pasinelli and Brown, 2006; Valdmanis and Rouleau, 2008). The SOD1 protein is a cytoplasmic enzyme that converts superoxide radicals, a by-product of oxidative phosphorylation, to hydrogen peroxide and molecular oxygen. The exact mechanism by which *SOD1* mutations lead to ALS pathology is unknown although several toxic properties of mutant SOD1 such as aberrant oxidative stress, protein instability, and mitochondrial damage have been proposed to be causative (reviewed in Pasinelli and Brown, 2006). Interestingly, the presence of mutant SOD1 in non-neuronal cells contributes to pathogenesis and is needed for disease progression (Ilieva et al., 2009). *SOD1* mutations most likely result in a toxic gain of function pathology since *SOD1* knockout mice do not develop motor neuron degeneration whereas transgenic mice overexpressing mutant SOD1 show motor neuron degeneration and ALS-like pathology (Gurney et al., 1994; Reaume et al., 1996).

2.2 ALS2 (ALSin)

ALS2 is an autosomal recessive form of juvenile ALS that was first reported in a large consanguineous Tunisian kindred and linkage analysis in this family associated locus 2q33-q35 to ALS (Hentati et al., 1994). This led to the discovery of causal mutations in the gene encoding ALSin (Hadano et al., 2001; Yang et al., 2001). Mutations in *ALSin* have been scarcely reported and do not appear to be a common cause of ALS.

ALSin is a Rab5 and Rac1 guanine exchange factor that acts as a regulator of endosomal/membrane trafficking. The protein is able to promote neurite outgrowth in neuronal cultures through activation of the small GTPase Rac1 (Otomo et al., 2003; Topp et al., 2004). Overexpression of ALSin protects cultured motor neuronal cells from mutant SOD1 toxicity suggesting a neuroprotective role. Mutations in *ALSin* may induce a loss of this neuroprotective function (Kanekura et al., 2004). *ALSin* knockout mice do not develop overt motor neuron disease but degeneration of the corticospinal tract has been reported (Cai et al., 2008; Hadano et al., 2006).

2.3 ALS3 (18q21)

Linkage to chromosome 18q21 was identified in a large European family of which 20 members had autosomal-dominant ALS (Hand et al., 2002). This region contains 50 genes but the causal mutation at this locus remains to be identified.

2.4 ALS4 (SETX)

ALS4 is a rare, childhood- or adolescent-onset, autosomal dominant disease, which is also known as distal hereditary motor neuronopathy with pyramidal features. Linkage to chromosome 9q34 was found in a large family from the USA with 49 affected members (Chance et al., 1998). Sequencing of 19 genes in this locus revealed that missense mutations in the senataxin (*SETX*) gene were the cause of ALS4 in several families (Chen et al., 2004). Since then, mutations have been identified in additional ALS patients from China, Italy and the USA (Avemaria et al., 2011; Hirano et al., 2011; Zhao et al., 2009). Interestingly, mutations in *SETX* leading to a premature termination in the protein product have also been identified in ataxia oculomotor apraxia 2 (Moreira et al., 2004).

Senataxin contains a seven-motif domain characteristic for DNA/RNA helicases. It displays strong homology to several genes involved in RNA processing such as the immunoglobulin mu binding protein 2 gene (*IGHMBP2*), in which mutations are known to cause spinal muscular atrophy with respiratory distress type 1 (Grohmann et al., 2001). SETX was shown to be involved in the termination of RNA transcription (Skourti-Stathaki et al., 2011). It is therefore possible that mutations in *SETX* cause neuronal degeneration due to aberrant RNA processing. Overexpression of wild-type senataxin in primary hippocampal neurons is sufficient to trigger neuronal differentiation by protecting cells from apoptosis and promoting neuritogenesis (Vantaggiato et al., 2011).

2.5 ALS5 (SPG11)

This is the most common form of recessive fALS and is characterized by a juvenile onset. In seven families from Tunisia, Pakistan, and Germany, linkage to chromosome 15q15-21 was found (Hentati et al., 1998). Recently, 12 mutations in the spatacsin (*SPG11*) gene were identified in 10 unrelated pedigrees from Italy, Brazil, Canada, Turkey, and Japan (Orlacchio et al., 2010). Ten out of 12 mutations are frameshift or nonsense mutations. Mutations in *SPG11* are known to cause autosomal recessive hereditary spastic paraplegia with a thin corpus callosum (Stevanin et al., 2007).

Spatacsin contains four putative transmembrane domains, a leucine zipper and a coiled-coil domain. The exact function of spatacsin is unknown although it may play a role in axonal transport (Salinas et al., 2008).

2.6 ALS6 (FUS)

Linkage to a 42-Mb region containing more than 400 genes on chromosome 16 was reported in several families (Sapp et al. 2003). Recently, mutations in the fused in sarcoma/translated in liposarcoma (*FUS/TLS*) gene were shown to cause ALS6 (Kwiatkowski et al., 2009; Vance et al., 2009). Several subsequent studies have identified additional mutations in *FUS* in ALS cohorts from different populations with an overall frequency of ~4% in fALS and ~1% in sALS (Belzil et al., 2009; Corrado et al., 2010; Hewitt et al., 2010; Groen et al., 2010). *FUS* mutations have also been detected in fALS patients with frontemporal dementia (FTD) and patients with juvenile ALS with basophilic inclusions (Bäumer et al., 2010; Huang et al. 2010; Yan et al., 2010).

The *FUS* gene encodes for a DNA/RNA binding protein that is involved in several cellular pathways including the splicing, transport and maturation of RNA (Lagier-Tourenne et al., 2010). FUS positive ubiquitinated cytoplasmic inclusions have been observed in spinal cord tissue of sALS and fALS patients without *SOD1* and *FUS* mutations (Deng et al., 2010). The majority of *FUS* mutations identified reside in its C-terminal nuclear localization signal which results in an abnormal cytoplasmic localization of FUS and localization to stress granules (Bosco et al., 2010; Dormann et al., 2010; Ito et al., 2010). In yeast, overexpression of human FUS leads to toxicity, cytoplasmic inclusions and FUS localization to stress granules as can be seen in ALS patients (Ju et al., 2011; Sun et al., 2011). In addition, transgenic rats overexpressing ALS mutant FUS develop progressive paralysis due to motor axon degeneration as well as neuronal loss in the cortex and hippocampus which are phenotypes seen in ALS and FTD (Huang et al., 2011).

2.7 ALS7 (20p)

Linkage to chromosome 20p was found in a large autosomal dominant fALS pedigree from the USA. A 5-Mb segment was identified that was shared between two affected siblings (Sapp et al., 2003). This region contains 24 genes but no causal mutation has been identified.

2.8 ALS8 (VAPB)

In a large family from Brazil with 28 affected members across 4 generations, linkage was found at chromosome 20q13.3. Sequencing identified a mutation (P56S) in the vesicle associated membrane protein (VAMP)/synaptobrevin-associated membrane protein B (*VAPB*) gene in all affected members of this family (Nishimura et al., 2004). The same mutation was also identified in six additional families with different clinical courses including, ALS8, late-onset spinal muscular atrophy and typical severe ALS with rapid progression. A different mutation (T46I) was detected in a family from the UK (Chen et al., 2010).

The VAPB protein has been implicated in various cellular processes including the formation of the presynaptic terminal in neurons, vesicle trafficking and the unfolded protein response (Chen et al., 2010). Transgenic mice overexpressing ALS mutant VAPB or wild-type VAPB do not develop an overt motor neuron phenotype. However, transgenic mice overexpressing ALS mutant but not wild-type VAPB show TAR DNA-binding protein 43 (TDP-43) positive cytoplasmic inclusions, a pathological hallmark of ALS (Tudor et al., 2010). It has been suggested that mutant VAPB exerts a dominant-negative effect by forming dimeric complexes with wild-type VAPB thereby recruiting it into aggregates (Teuling et al., 2007).

2.9 ALS9 (ANG)

Angiogenin (*ANG*) was identified as a candidate gene for ALS because it is located 237kb downstream of apurinic endonuclease, multifunctional DNA repair enzyme (*APEX*) and because of its functional similarity to vascular endothelial growth factor (VEGF) (Greenway et al., 2004). Both *APEX* and *VEGF* are candidate genes for sALS and will be discussed in the next section. A single nucleotide polymorphism (SNP) in *ANG* was associated with ALS in patients from Ireland and Scotland (Greenway et al., 2004). Missense mutations in *ANG* were found in 4 fALS cases and 11 sALS cases (Greenway et al., 2006). Subsequent sequencing in populations from Europe and the USA identified additional mutations in approximately 2% of fALS cases and 1% of sALS cases (Conforti et al., 2008; Fernández-Santiago et al., 2009; Gellera et al., 2008; Paubel et al., 2008; Wu et al., 2007). However, *ANG* mutations have also been observed in healthy controls suggesting that not all mutations are pathogenic (Corrado et al., 2007). A K17I mutation was identified in a 4-generation family of which one patient presented with ALS, FTD, and Parkinsonism (Van Es et al., 2009a). An obligate carrier did not develop the disease suggesting incomplete penetrance. Two *ANG* mutations (K17I and K54E) were identified in two fALS cases from France who also had a mutation in FUS (Millecamps et al., 2010). An R145C mutation has been observed in a sALS patient with a G93D SOD1 mutation (Luigetti et al., 2011). A recent study showed a significantly higher frequency of *ANG* variants in both ALS and Parkinson's disease (PD) patients which could reflect a genetic susceptibility to widespread neurodegeneration (Van Es et al., 2011).

The ANG protein is a member of the pancreatic ribonuclease superfamily and a potent mediator of new blood vessel formation. In endothelial cells, the protein can promote ribosomal RNA (rRNA) production and cellular proliferation and is able to cleave transfer

RNA which results in inhibition of protein translation (Yamasaki et al., 2009). ANG is also expressed in spinal motor neurons (Sebastià et al., 2009). It is thought that *ANG* mutations cause ALS due to a loss of function and it has been shown that wild-type but not mutant angiogenin is neuroprotective and that mutant angiogenin impairs neurite outgrowth *in vitro* (Sebastià et al., 2009; Subramanian et al., 2008; Wu et al., 2007).

2.10 ALS10 (TARDBP)

TDP-43 was identified as one of the main components of ubiquitinated cytoplasmic inclusions in ALS and FTD (Neumann et al., 2006). Sequencing of the gene encoding this protein (*TARDBP*) identified mutations in ALS patients (Kabashi et al., 2008; Shreedharan et al., 2008). To date over 40 mutations in *TARDBP* have been identified in several different populations with a frequency of ~5% of fALS cases and up to 2% of sALS cases (Corrado et al., 2009; Iida et al., 2010; Millecamps et al., 2010; Ticozzi et al., 2009; Van Deerlin et al., 2008). *TARDBP* mutations have also been observed in ALS-FTD and FTD patients (Benajiba et al., 2009; Gitcho et al., 2009b). Despite the presence of *TARDBP* mutations in only a portion of ALS and FTD patients, TDP-43-positive cytoplasmic inclusions are found in almost all ALS patients but they are also seen in other neurodegenerative diseases such as FTD, Huntington's, Alzheimer's, and Parkinson's disease (Da Cruz and Cleveland, 2011).

TDP-43, like FUS, is a DNA/RNA binding protein that is part of the heterogeneous ribonucleoprotein family. It has a role in gene transcription, regulation of splicing, and mRNA transport and stabilization (Buratti and Baralle, 2010). Except for one truncation mutation, all *TARDBP* mutations identified in ALS patients are missense mutations clustered in the glycine-rich C-terminal region which is involved in protein-protein interactions (Lagier-Tourenne et al., 2010). *TARDBP* mutations lead to an abnormal distribution of the protein to the cytoplasm.

2.11 ALS11 (FIG4)

Mutations in the PI(3,5)P(2)5-phosphatase (*FIG4*) gene on chromosome 6q21 are known to cause a severe form of Charcot-Marie-Tooth (CMT) disease with early onset and loss of sensory and motor neurons, CMT4J (Chow et al., 2007). In a screen for *FIG4* mutations in a large cohort of sALS and fALS patients, several variants were detected that were unique to fALS and sALS patients (Chow et al., 2009). Two mutations were identified in patients diagnosed with primary lateral sclerosis. To date, no other studies have replicated the finding of ALS-associated FIG4 mutations in other cohorts and it is unclear whether *FIG4* mutations are pathogenic in ALS patients.

FIG4 is a phosphoinositide 5-phosphatase that regulates PI(3,5)P2 abundance. PI(3,5)P2 is a signalling lipid that mediates endosomal trafficking to the trans-Golgi network (Rutherford et al., 2006). Pale tremor mice, which are homozygous for null mutations in *FIG4*, show neurodegeneration in sensory and autonomic ganglia, motor cortex, striatum, and cerebellum. Motor neurons in the ventral spinal cord contain vacuoles (Chow et al., 2007). Mutant mice lacking *Vac14*, a gene encoding for a FIG4 interactor, show a similar neurodegeneration (Zhang et al., 2007).

2.12 ALS12 (OPTN)

Using homozygosity mapping in six ALS patients from consanguineous marriages, an overlapping region on chromosome 10 was identified as the candidate region. Screening of

17 genes in this region revealed a homozygous deletion in the gene for optineurin (*OPTN*), a gene known to cause primary open-angle glaucoma, in two siblings and an individual from a different family (Murayama et al., 2010; Rezaie et al., 2002). In addition, a homozygous nonsense (Q398X) mutation was identified in one fALS case (Murayama et al., 2010). Subsequent screening in a larger cohort of fALS and sALS patients identified a heterozygous missense mutation (E478G) in a four individuals with ALS from two families (Murayama et al., 2010). A homozygous E478G mutation was identified in a Japanese fALS case in a different study (Iida et al., 2011). One additional nonsense mutation and one missense mutation in *OPTN* were identified in fALS cases from Italy (Del Bo et al., 2011). Two separate studies identified novel variants in fALS patients but the authors state that these variants may be a genetic predisposition to glaucoma instead of causing ALS (Belzil et al., 2011; Millecamps et al., 2011). One study also detected mutations in sALS patients with a rapid disease progression (van Blitterswijk et al., 2011). Another study could not identify *OPTN* mutations in fALS and sALS patients (Sugihara et al., 2011).

OPTN is a multifunctional protein involved in membrane trafficking, maintainance of the Golgi complex, and exocytosis (Sahlender et al., 2005). OPTN can inhibit the activation of NFκB and it has been proposed that mutations in *OPTN* causing ALS may relieve this inhibition and cause neuronal death (Murayama et al., 2010).

2.13 ALS14 (VCP)

Recently an exome sequencing study detected a mutation in the gene encoding valosin-containing protein (*VCP*) in an Italian family. Subsequent screening in 210 ALS cases from unrelated families identified four mutations in *VCP* in four different families from Italy and the USA (Johnson et al., 2010). Mutations in the gene for *VCP*, located on chromosome 9p13.3, are a known cause for the multi-system degenerative disease inclusion body myopathy with Paget's disease and frontotemporal dementia (IBMPFD) (Watts et al. 2004). IBMPFD, like ALS, is characterized pathologically by TDP-43 inclusions (Weihl et al., 2008). VCP is an AAA+-ATPase that mediates ubiquitin-dependent extraction of substrates from multiprotein complexes for subsequent recycling or degradation by the proteasome. It plays a role in a variety of cellular functions including Golgi biogenesis, cell cycle regulation, DNA damage repair and protein homeostasis through the ubiquitin-proteasome system (Ju and Weihl, 2010). It is thought that *VCP* mutations result in the impairment of protein degradation trough both the ubiquitin-proteasome system and autophagy leading to the formation of inclusions. *VCP* mutations found in FTD and ALS have been shown to disrupt TDP-43 localization from the nucleus to the cytoplasm which could be caused by the disruption in protein homeostasis (Gitcho et al, 2009a; Ju and Weihl, 2010). In mice, a missense mutation in vacuolar sorting protein 54, the mouse homologue of VCP, causes motor neuron degeneration (Schmitt-John et al., 2005).

2.14 Other fALS associated genes

In addition to the genes listed in the previous sections, several other genes have been implicated in fALS.

Dynactin 1 (*DCTN1*) was discovered as a candidate gene for ALS when a G59S mutation in this gene was identified in a family with a slowly progressive, autosomal dominant form of lower motor neuron disease without sensory symptoms (Puls et al., 2003; Puls et al., 2005). Subsequent sequencing of the *DCNT1* gene in 250 ALS patients revealed the presence of three heterozygous missense mutations in one sALS and three fALS cases with typical ALS (Münch et al., 2004). An additional mutation was detected in a patient with ALS and his brother who had FTD (Münch et al., 2005). The pathogenicity of these variants has however not been established. Screening for *DCTN1* mutations in a cohort of ALS, FTD or ALS-FTD patients did not result in the identification of disease segregating variants (Vilariño-Güell et al., 2009). One of the missense variants identified in a sALS case was also found in controls in the same study (Vilariño-Güell et al., 2009). Interestingly, five mutations in *DCTN1* were found in eight families with Perry syndrome, a disease that is characterized by Parkinsonism and TDP-43- and ubiquitin- positive inclusions (Farrer et al., 2009).

In a 3-generation family with typical ALS, a mutation in the D-amino acid oxidase (*DAO*) gene was identified (Mitchell et al., 2010). However, screening of an additional 322 unrelated fALS cases did not reveal any other causal mutation in this gene (Mitchell et al., 2010). Additional screening will be needed but *DAO* mutations seem to be very rare in ALS.

Because of their structural and functional similarities to FUS, the genes encoding TAF15 RNA polymerase II, TATA box binding protein associated factor (*TAF15*) and Ewing sarcoma breakpoint region 1 (*EWS*) were screened in fALS cases (Ticozzi et al., 2010). Two missense mutations in *TAF15* (A31T and R395Q) were identified in three fALS cases and not in 1159 controls. However, one of the fALS cases with an R395Q mutation also carried a mutation in *TARDBP*. Moreover, the R395Q is in close proximity to two non-pathogenic variants, suggesting it is a benign polymorphism (Ticozzi et al., 2010).

Recently, a mutation in the sigma non-opioid intracellular receptor 1 (*SIGMAR1*) gene was identified in an autosomal recessive family with juvenile ALS (Al-Saif et al., 2011). Interestingly, variants in the 3'UTR of *SIGMAR1* were described in three ALS-FTD families (Luty et al., 2010).

An X-linked dominant ALS locus has been reported but has not been further described (Siddique et al., 1998). Recently, mutations in the gene encoding ubiquitin-like protein ubiquilin 2 (*UBQLN2*) were identified as the cause of dominantly inherited X-linked ALS and ALS/dementia (Deng et al., 2011).

Several family pedigrees contain individuals affected by ALS, FTD or both. The first linkage study performed in 16 of these ALS-FTD families found linkage to chromosome **9q21-q22**, designated as ALS-FTD1 (Hosler et al., 2000). This association has thus far not been replicated in other ALS-FTD families. Linkage to chromosome 9p in ALS-FTD families (ALS-FTD2) has also been reported. A hexanucleotide repeat expansion in the chromosome 9 open reading frame 72 (*C9ORF72*) gene was recently identified as the causal genetic defect of ALS-FTD2 and will be discussed in a next section (Dejesus-Hernandez et al., 2011; Renton et al., 2011). Mutations in the gene encoding microtubule-associated protein tau (*MAPT*) have been reported in patients with ALS or FTD (Hutton et al., 1998).

Finally, mutations in the neurofilament heavy (*NEFH*) gene and the paraoxonase genes (*PON1, 2, 3*) have been identified in fALS cases and these genes will be discussed in more detail in the following section.

3. Genetics of sporadic ALS

Sporadic ALS is considered to be a complex disease, where both genetic and environmental factors contribute to pathogenesis. Several association studies have been performed to identify the genetic contribution in sALS with mixed success, possibly due to the small sample sizes in many of these studies. Although their precise contribution to sALS is often unclear, a few of the risk factors identified to date have been consistently replicated. Furthermore, several of these associated genes have overlapping cellular functions such as in RNA metabolism, vesicle trafficking, and axonal transport. In this section, genes that have been associated with sALS will be discussed (Table 2). In addition to these genes, mutations in several fALS associated genes that were discussed in the previous section have been found in a portion of sALS cases.

Associated Gene	Protein	Positive studies	Negative studies	Type of association found	Additional information
APEX	Apurinic endonuclease, DNA repair enzyme	2	2	SNP association	Protein has a role in oxidative stress
ATXN2	Ataxin-2	6	0	PolyQ repeats	Intermediate polyQ repeats increase risk for sALS/interaction with TDP-43
CHMP2B	Chromatin modifying protein 2B	2	0	Mutations	Mutations are known to cause FTD. All patients have lower motor neuron signs consistent with PMA.
HFE	Haemo-chromatosis	5	1	SNP association	Mutations cause hereditary haemochromatosis
NEFH	Neurofilament-heavy	5	3	Deletions/ insertions/ mutations	Neurofilament-containing inclusions are a pathological hallmark of ALS
SMN1	Survival motor neuron 1	3	1	Abnormal copy number	SMN1 deletions cause SMA
SMN2	Survival motor neuron 2	1	5	Deletions	SMN2 copy number variation affects SMA disease severity
PON1, 2, 3	Paraoxonase	7	3	SNP association/ mutations	Possible gene-environment interaction
PRPH	Peripherin	3	0	Mutations	Peripherin-containing inclusions are a pathological hallmark of ALS. Possible involvement of abnormal splice forms.
VEGF	Vascular-endothelial growth factor	2	6	SNP association	Deletion of HRE in promoter results in an ALS phenotype in mice. Possible gender association.

Table 2. Genes associated with sporadic ALS

3.1 Apurinic endonuclease, multifunctional DNA repair enzyme (APEX1)

A study in 117 Scottish sALS patients showed association of a common SNP resulting in a D148E amino-acid change with ALS (Hayward et al., 1999). This finding was replicated in 169 Irish sALS patients (Greenway et al., 2004). In one study, DNA extracted from CNS tissue from 81 sALS patients was screened but the D184E SNP was not associated with ALS (Tomkins et al., 2000). A different study assessing 134 Italian sALS patients also failed to detect significant association between this SNP and ALS (Coppedè et al., 2010). These inconsistent association results might reflect a population-specific effect of the APEX1 D184E allele.

APEX1 is involved in DNA repair and maintains and stimulates the DNA binding activity of transcription factors (Fishel and Kelley, 2007). Frontal cortical levels and activity of APEX1 were significantly reduced in 11 ALS patients as compared to six controls (Kisby et al., 1997). However, in a different study, increased expression levels and activity in ALS brain and spinal cord motor neurons were observed (Shaikh and Martin, 2002).

3.2 Ataxin-2 (ATXN2)

In a screen for toxicity modifiers of TDP-43 in yeast, ataxin-2 (ATXN2) was identified (Elden et al., 2010). ATXN2 and TDP-43 form a RNA-dependent complex and are mislocalized in spinal cord motor neurons in ALS patients. *ATXN2* has a polyglutamine (polyQ) region which is normally 22-23 repeats long. Expansion of this region of the protein to 34 repeats causes spinocerebellar ataxia type 2 (SCA2) (Imbert et al., 1996; Pulst et al., 1996; Sanpei et al. 1996). The polyQ repeat length of *ATXN2* was determined in 915 ALS patients and 980 controls and intermediate length polyQ repeats (23-34) were found to be more common in ALS patients and thus may be a risk factor for ALS (Elden et al., 2010). This finding was replicated in several studies with ALS patients from different populations. Interestingly, the exact length of the polyQ repeat region seems to vary between populations (Chen et al., 2011; Daoud et al., 2011; Lee et al., 2011; Ross et al., 2011; Van Damme et al., 2011).

Longer polyQ repeats in ATXN2 possibly stabilize the protein and enhance its interaction with TDP-43. Under stress conditions, increased mislocalization of TDP-43 to the cytoplasm was observed in cells harbouring expanded polyQ repeats in ATXN2 (Elden et al., 2010). ATXN2 was shown to be part of stress granules and interacts with poly-A-binding-protein 1 (PABP), which is involved in poly(A) shortening and translation initiation (Ralser et al., 2005). ATXN2 was also shown to interact with endophilin A1 and A3, which are involved in synaptic vesicle endocytosis (Nonis et al., 2008).

3.3 Chromatin modifying protein 2B (CHMP2B)

A mutation in a splice-site of *CHMP2B* was first identified in a large Danish family with FTD and mutations have since been detected at low frequency in other FTD patients (Skibinski et al., 2005). Screening of the *CHMP2B* gene in ALS patients identified two mutations in two fALS patients. These patients displayed a predominant lower motor neuron phenotype and one of the patients showed signs of FTD (Parkinson et al., 2006). Sequencing of the *CHMP2B* gene in 433 ALS patients identified three missense mutations in one fALS case and three sALS cases (Cox et al., 2010).

The exact function of CHMP2B is unknown but its yeast homologue, vacuolar protein sorting 2 (VPS2), is a component of the ESCRTIII complex (Skibinski et al., 2005). This complex is involved in the trafficking of proteins between plasma membrane, trans-Golgi network, and lysosomes. The *CHMP2B* mutation identified in FTD results in dysmorphic endosomal structures similar to what is seen in ALSin overexpression (Skibinski et al., 2005). In cortical neurons, overexpression of the FTD related CHMP2B splice-site mutant leads to dendritic retraction prior to cell death and the accumulation of autophagosomes (Lee et al., 2007). In hippocampal neurons, the same FTD related CHMP2B mutant causes a decrease in large dendritic spines suggesting that CHMP2B is needed for dendritic spine growth and maturation (Belly et al., 2010).

3.4 Haemochromatosis (HFE)

Mutations in the *HFE* gene are a cause of hereditary haemochromatosis and have been associated with Alzheimer's disease and PD (reviewed by Nandar and Connor, 2011). The first report examining the presence of *HFE* mutations in ALS found no association between two mutations (H63D and C282Y) and ALS patients from the USA (Yen et al., 2004). However, several subsequent studies in a total of 1133 ALS patients and almost 7000 controls individuals from the USA, Ireland, UK, Italy, The Netherlands, and China reported association between the *HFE* H63D polymorphism and an increased risk for ALS (Goodall et al., 2005; He et al, 2011; Restagno et al., 2007; Sutedja et al., 2007; Wang et al., 2004). The most important function of HFE is the regulation of iron homeostasis by binding to the transferrin receptor and reducing the transport of iron molecules (Feder et al., 1998). When HFE with the H63D mutation binds to the transferrin receptor, iron transport is reduced leading to iron accumulation and increased oxidative stress. In addition, it has been shown that in neuronal cell lines the H63D mutation induces increased oxidative stress, altered glutamate regulation and prolonged ER stress, all cellular processes affected in ALS (Liu et al., 2011; Mitchell et al. 2011).

3.5 Neurofilaments (NEFL, NEFM, NEFH)

One of the pathological hallmarks of ALS is the presence of neurofilament-containing inclusions in the cell body and proximal axon of spinal motor neurons (Delisle and Carpenter, 1984). Neurofilaments are intermediate filaments that constitute the most abundant cytoskeletal element in large myelinated axons. Neurofilaments are formed by the co-polymerization of light (NEFL), medium (NEFM), and heavy (NEFH) subunits, which are each encoded by different genes.

Several lines of evidence suggest a role for neurofilaments in neurodegeneration. Initial evidence came from mouse models overexpressing or deficient for neurofilaments (reviewed in Lariviere and Julien, 2004). Overexpression of NEFL or NEFH resulted in an abnormal accumulation of neurofilaments, as seen in ALS patients, and in axonal atrophy and motor dysfunction but not degeneration. Surprisingly, both overexpression and knockout of neurofilaments in transgenic mutant SOD1 mice increases life span (Couillard-Després et al., 1998; Williamson et al., 1998). This indicates that the role of neurofilaments in ALS is complex and more research is needed to examine the possible contribution of neurofilaments to ALS pathogenesis.

Additional evidence for a role for neurofilaments in ALS comes from genetic studies. Mutations in *NEFL* have been identified in some forms of the sensory and motor neuropathy Charcot-Marie-Tooth disease (Mersiyanova et al., 2000; Shin et al., 2008). The C-terminal tail region of NEFH contains phosphorylation motifs known as KSP repeats. In humans there are two common polymorphic variants of 44 (short) or 45 (long) repeats. Homozygosity for the short repeat allele is associated with Russian sporadic motor neuron disease patients (Skvortsova et al., 2004). Deletions and insertions in the KSP repeats of *NEFH* were detected in ALS patients (Al-Chalabi et al., 1999; Figlewicz et al., 1994; Tomkins et al., 1998). However, another study in 117 unrelated fALS patients could not identify deletions or insertions in the KSP repeats of *NEFH* (Rooke et al., 1996). A missense mutation in the *NEFH* gene was identified in a sALS case and not in controls (Garcia et al., 2006). Moreover, in a recent candidate gene sequencing study, three missense mutations were identified in the *NEFH* gene in two sALS and one fALS case. However, co-segregation of the mutation in the fALS case could not be tested and none of the missense mutations were predicted to be deleterious (Daoud et al., 2011). One study did not identify ALS specific variation in the *NEFH* gene in fALS and sALS samples (Vechio et al., 1996).

3.6 Paraoxonase genes (PON)

The paraoxonase gene cluster consists of 3 genes (*PON1, PON2,* and *PON3*) and is located in an 80-kb block on chromosome 7q21.3-22.1. PON1 and PON3 are primarily expressed in liver where they are associated with high-density lipoproteins, whereas PON2 is ubiquitously expressed (Costa et al., 2005; Draganov et al., 2000; Ng et al., 2002). Both PON1 and PON2 expression has been shown in mouse brain (Giordano et al., 2011). All PON proteins are able to hydrolyze lactones and PON1 is able to detoxify organophosphate pesticides and neurotoxins. Since neurotoxins are not normally present in the body the biological function of PON1 is thought to be protection of low-density lipoproteins from oxidation (Mackness et al., 1991). PON2 and PON3 share this function (Draganov et al., 2000; Ng et al., 2001). A higher incidence of ALS among Gulf war veterans and farmers suggested that chemical exposure may be a risk factor for ALS (Chió et al., 1991; Horner et al., 2003). Because PON proteins reduce oxidation and are able to detoxify neurotoxins these proteins have been investigated for association with ALS.

Polymorphisms in *PON1* and *PON2* as well as a haploblock spanning *PON2* and *PON3* were found to be associated with sALS (Saeed et al., 2006; Slowik et al., 2006). Since then several other studies in different populations have reported association of SNPs in the *PON* genes with sALS (Cronin et al., 2007; Landers et al., 2008; Morahan et al., 2007; Valdmanis et al., 2008). However, a meta-analysis including 4037 cases and 4609 controls from five case-control studies and several genome-wide association studies showed no significant association between *PON* polymorphisms and ALS (Wills et al., 2009). More recently, two other studies failed to detect association between *PON* polymorphisms and ALS (Ricci et al. 2011; Zawislak et al., 2010). In a recent sequencing study, eight mutations in all three *PON* genes were identified in fALS and sALS patients (Ticozzi et al., 2010). Mutations in the *PON* genes might play a role in ALS but additional sequencing is needed to confirm this.

Interestingly, PON1 activity can vary greatly depending on polymorphisms in its coding region (Costa et al., 2005). Thus, mutations in the *PON* genes could affect PON activity and thereby contribute to ALS pathogenesis. Toxicity in neurons caused by oxidative stress was higher in cells from PON2 knockout mice than in wild-type mice, suggesting that PON2 has a protective effect against neurotoxicity caused by oxidative stress (Giordano et al., 2011).

3.7 Peripherin (PRPH)

Peripherin is an intermediate filament similar to neurofilaments and is also associated with axonal spheroids in the proximal axon of spinal cord motor neurons of ALS patients (Corbo and Hays, 1992). It is also present in Lewy body-like inclusions and Bunina bodies that are seen in a portion of ALS patients (He and Hays, 2004; Mizuno et al., 2011). Peripherin is predominantly expressed in the peripheral nervous system and in spinal motor neurons in the central nervous system. After neuronal injury, peripherin expression is upregulated in spinal motor neurons and this upregulation has been linked to axonal regeneration (Troy et al., 1990). However, transgenic mice with wild-type overexpression of peripherin develop a late-onset and selective motor neuron disease characterized by intermediate filament inclusions (Beaulieu et al., 1999). For these reasons, the possibility of *PRPH* mutations in

ALS patients was investigated. Two missense mutations and a frameshift deletion in the PRPH gene have been identified in sALS patients (Corrado et al., 2011; Gros-Louis et al., 2004; Leung et al., 2004). Additional screening of the *PRPH* gene for mutations in larger cohorts of ALS patients and controls is needed to determine the frequency and pathogenecity of *PRPH* mutations.

Expression of abnormal peripherin splice variants has also been suggested to play a role in ALS pathogenesis. A toxic splice variant of peripherin (Per61) was found in motor neurons of mutant SOD1 transgenic mice but not wild-type mice (Robertson et al., 2003). Expression of Per61 has more recently also been observed in mutant TDP-43 transgenic mice but not in wild-type TDP-43 transgenic mice (Swarup et al., 2011). In addition, Per61 specific antibodies stain aggregates in human ALS but not in control spinal cord (Swarup et al., 2011). The presence of abnormal peripherin splice variants (Per28) has also been shown in humans (Xiao et al., 2008). Per28 overexpression results in peripherin aggregation and an upregulation of peripherin expression at the mRNA and protein levels in ALS patients as compared to controls (Xiao et al., 2008). A different study showed expression of Per28 in lumbar spinal cord lysates of ALS patients but not control cases (McLean et al., 2010). Although the functional significance of these abnormal splice forms is unknown they seem to play a role in the development ALS.

3.8 Survival motor neuron (SMN) 1 and 2

Two highly homologous copies of the survival motor neuron gene exist in humans, telomeric *SMN1* and centromeric *SMN2*. *SMN2*, which lacks exon 7 due to a nucleotide difference in a splice enhancer site, produces a less stable SMN protein and has only 20% of the biological function of SMN1 (Lorson et al., 1998). It has been shown that TDP-43 overexpression regulates the inclusion of exon 7 during pre-mRNA splicing of *SMN2* (Bose et al., 2008).

Deletions or mutations in *SMN1* cause the autosomal recessive disorder spinal muscular atrophy (SMA), whereas variation in *SMN2* copy number affects SMA disease severity (Lefebvre et al., 1997). SMA patients with a higher copy number of *SMN2* generally have a milder form of the disease (Gavrilov et al., 1998). SMN1 is widely expressed and functions in the assembly of the spliceosome as part of the SMN complex. SMN1 also interacts with several proteins involved in mRNA editing, transport, splicing, transcriptional regulation, and post-transcriptional processing and modification of rRNA (Eggert et al., 2006). The impaired assembly of the spliceosome could lead to neuronal degeneration.

Thus far, five different studies have failed to detect homozygous *SMN1* deletions in ALS patients (Gamez et al., 2002; Jackson et al., 1996; Moulard et al., 1998; Orrell et al., 1997; Parboosingh et al., 1999). However, an increased frequency of abnormal copy number (one or three copies) of *SMN1* was found in ALS patients compared to controls (Corcia et al., 2002). However, these results were inconsistent with other reports (Corcia et al., 2006; Veldink et al., 2001; Veldink et al., 2005). Recently, a large study was published including new samples of 847 sALS patients and 984 controls, showing that *SMN1* duplications were associated with ALS susceptibility (odds ratio [OR] = 2.07, 95% confidence interval [CI] = 1.34 - 3.20. (Blauw et al, 2011)). A meta-analysis of all previously published data, taking possible heterogeneity between studies into account, confirmed this association with *SMN1* duplications. Other work has shown that homozygous deletions of *SMN2* are associated with sporadic adult-onset lower motor neuron disease (Echaniz-Laguna et al., 2002; Moulard et al., 1998). Homozygous deletions of *SMN2* were also found to be overrepresented in 110 ALS patients (16%) compared to 100 controls (4%) (Veldink et al., 2001). *SMN2* deletions were associated with shorter survival in this study. However, a study by the same group using more ALS and control samples and several other studies did not find a higher frequency of *SMN2* deletions in ALS patients versus controls (Corcia et al., 2006; Gamez et al., 2002; Moulard et al., 1998; Parboosingh et al., 1999; Veldink et al., 2005). The recent meta-analysis showed that there is no increased frequency of homozygous *SMN2* deletions in ALS patients, and that neither *SMN1* nor *SMN2* appear to influence survival or age at onset of disease (Blauw et al. 2011).

Homozygous deletions in *SMN1* or *SMN2* do not play a role in ALS but an abnormal copy number in *SMN1* could increase risk for ALS and it is important to study the consequences on protein level in brain and spinal cord of having three copies of *SMN1* in order to determine the potential damaging effect.

3.9 Vascular endothelial growth factor (VEGF)

VEGF, a protein that stimulates angiogenesis in response to hypoxia, was identified as a candidate gene for ALS based on the finding that a deletion in the hypoxia response element (HRE) in the promoter of this gene in mice, resulting in decreased VEGF expression, led to progressive motor neuron degeneration (Oosthuyse et al., 2001). In addition, *VEGF* gene delivery in muscle and VEGF overexpression prolongs survival in mutant SOD1 transgenic mice. Furthermore, intracerebroventricular VEGF administration prolongs survival in mutant SOD1 transgenic rats (Azzouz et al., 2004; Storkebaum et al., 2005; Wang et al., 2007). Finally, decreased expression of VEGF and its receptor VEGFR2 is observed in spinal cords of ALS patients (Brockington et al., 2006).

Sequencing of the *VEGF* gene and its promotor in ALS patients failed to identify ALS specific mutations (Brockington et al., 2005; Gros-Luois et al., 2003; Lambrechts et al., 2003). However, a large study in 750 ALS patients and over 1200 controls from Sweden, Belgium, and England found association between two haplotypes determined by three SNPs and an increased risk for ALS (Lambrechts et al., 2003). These haplotypes lowered the circulating levels of VEGF and *VEGF* transcription (Lambrechts et al., 2003). This association was replicated in a study with small sample size (Terry et al., 2004). In contrast, subsequent studies could not confirm the association between *VEGF* and ALS in Dutch, British, American, Italian, Polish and Chinese populations (Brockington et al., 2005; Chen et al., 2006; Del Bo et al., 2008a; Golenia et al., 2010; Van Vught et al., 2005; Zhang et al., 2006). Furthermore, a meta-analysis on several of these studies found no association between *VEGF* polymorphisms and ALS (Lambrechts et al., 2009). A study in German ALS patients identified an association of a *VEGF* SNP with sALS in women (Fernández-Santiago et al., 2006). A different SNP was associated with ALS in male patients in a large meta-analysis (Lambrechts et al., 2009). This suggests that the role of *VEGF* in ALS may be gender dependent. An association of *VEGF* SNPs with age of onset in ALS was also reported although no such association was observed in the meta-analysis (Chen et al., 2007; Lambrechts et al., 2009).

In summary, studies in rodent models suggest a role for VEGF in ALS, possibly as a therapeutic target. However, genetic studies do not yet provide conclusive evidence for a genetic role for VEGF in ALS, although gender dependent effects may exist.

3.10 Genome wide association studies in sporadic ALS

Several genome-wide association studies (GWAS) have been performed in sALS patients. These studies have generated association results that have been replicated in the same study but rarely in independent studies. Although several of the associated genes discussed below are plausible to contribute to ALS considering their functional roles, the lack of consistent replication results makes it difficult to firmly establish their role in sALS.

A GWAS in 276 ALS patients and 271 healthy controls identified 34 possible associated SNPs but none of these reached genome-wide significance after Bonferroni correction (Schymick et al., 2007). A SNP near the gene FGGY carbohydrate kinase domain containing (*FGGY*) was reported to be associated in a GWAS in 1152 ALS patients with an odds ratio of 1.35 (Dunckley et al., 2007). However, two replication studies in a total of 2478 sALS patients and 2744 controls did not detect this association (Fernández-Santiago et al., 2011; Van Es et al., 2009b). No mutations in *FGGY* were found by sequencing in 190 ALS patients (Daoud et al., 2010).

A GWAS in 461 ALS patients and 450 controls found a variant in the inositol 1, 4, 5-triphosphate receptor 2 gene (*ITPR2*) to be associated with ALS. This association was replicated in the same study in a cohort of 876 patients and 906 controls and in the combined analysis (Van Es et al., 2007). ITPR2 has a role in glutamate-mediated neurotransmission, regulation of calcium concentration and apoptosis. However, the *ITPR2* association has not been found in a replication study and in subsequent GWAS (Chiò et al., 2009; Cronin et al., 2008; Fernández-Santiago et al., 2011; Laaksovirta et al., 2010; Shatunov et al., 2010; Van Es et al., 2009c).

Variation in the dipeptidyl-peptidase 6 (*DPP6*) gene was found to be significantly associated with sALS in a GWAS performed in a combined GWA data set from the USA and the Netherlands (Van Es et al., 2008). This association was replicated in three additional independent populations from The Netherlands, Sweden, and Belgium (Van Es et al., 2008). The same variant was the top hit in a joint analysis of GWA data sets in an Irish population and the same Dutch and American populations, although it did not reach genome-wide significance (Cronin et al., 2008). Upon addition of a Polish data set the association could not be replicated which could point to a population-specific effect (Cronin et al., 2009). In an Italian cohort of 266 ALS patients association of the same SNP was replicated (Del Bo et al., 2008b). However, subsequent replication studies and GWAS could not find evidence for a role of *DPP6* in ALS (Chiò et al., 2009; Daoud et al., 2010; Fogh et al., 2011; Laaksovirta et al., 2010; Li et al., 2009; Shatunov et al., 2010; Van Es et al., 2009c). Interestingly, in a genome scan for copy number variations, including 4434 ALS patients and over 14000 controls, a suggestive association was found for the *DPP6* locus (Blauw et al., 2010). Not much data is available on the function of DPP6, but it is expressed in brain and able to regulate the activity of neuropeptides and to bind A-type neuronal potassium channels (Nadal et al., 2003).

Another two-stage GWAS in sALS patients was unable to find any associated SNPs that reached genome-wide significance, although suggestive association was found on **chromosome 7p13.3** (Chiò et al., 2009).

Survival analysis in a GWAS using samples from the USA and Europe revealed that a CC genotype of a SNP in the kinesin-associated protein 3 (*KIFAP3*) gene conferred a 14-month survival advantage on ALS patients (Landers et al., 2009). Expression data using RNA from brain tissue and lymphoblasts of patients showed that the favorable genotype significantly decreased KIFAP3 expression (Landers et al., 2009). However, two subsequent studies in two Italian cohorts could not replicate the finding that the CC genotype had a beneficial effect on survival or decreased KIFAP3 expression in ALS patients (Orsetti et al., 2011; Traynor et al., 2010). KIFAP3 is part of the trimeric kinesin 2 motor complex KIF3 which mediates binding between proteins and their cargo. It serves multiple functions including a role in mitosis and intracellular transport of organelles and proteins in various tissues including neurons (Haraguchi et al., 2006; Takeda et al., 2000).

The largest GWAS to date identified two loci, on **chromosome 9p21.2** and **19p13.11**, to be associated with sALS. The genetic variant in 19p13.11 maps to a haplotype within the boundaries of the *UNC13A* gene. Two studies failed to replicate this finding, but were underpowered, and more studies are needed to firmly establish genetic variation in *UNC13A* as being causative to sALS.

The association to chromosome 9p21.2 will be discussed in more detail in the following sections.

4. ALS-FTD2 (9p13.2-21.3)

Several linkage studies associated **chromosome 9p** to ALS-FTD, designated as ALS-FTD2 (Table 3). The first two independent studies found linkage to locus 9p13.2-21.3 in a Dutch and a Scandinavian family (Morita et al., 2006; Vance et al., 2006). Subsequently, eight other linkage studies in families from Canada, France, Belgium, North-America, Australia and Wales showed association to regions on chromosome 9p13.1-q21 (Boxer et al., 2010; Gijselinck et al., 2010; Le Ber et al., 2009; Luty et al., 2009; Momeni et al., 2006; Pearson et al., 2011; Valdmanis et al., 2007; Yan et al., 2006). Individuals in these families were diagnosed with ALS, FTD, and ALS-FTD. However, dementia, psychosis and Parkinsonism were also seen. Besides the co-occurrence of ALS and FTD in families, there is also considerable clinical overlap between ALS and FTD, i.e. mild cognitive abnormalities occur in up to 50% of ALS patients and in approximately 5% of ALS patients FTD is present with marked behavioral changes and language impairment (Elamin et al., 2011; Ringholz et al., 2005). Furthermore, ALS and FTD are both characterized by TDP-43 positive ubiquitinated cytoplasmic inclusions (Neumann et al., 2006). This strongly supports the idea that there is a common genetic contribution to the pathogenesis of both diseases.

A total of 41 genes, four micro RNAs, two pseudogenes, and a non-coding RNA in the associated chromosome 9p region have been screened for mutations but only in one study a premature stop codon in the intraflagellar transport 74 gene (*IFT-74*) was identified in two brothers from one family (Momeni et al., 2006). However, no mutations in *IFT-74* were identified in any of the other ALS-FTD families that were linked to chromosome 9p and it is therefore unlikely that this mutation is the underlying cause in these families.

Interestingly, a recent GWAS in sALS patients found association between ALS and chromosome 9p21.2. 2323 ALS patients and 9013 controls were genotyped and genome-wide significance was found for SNPs on these two loci (van Es et al., 2009c). This finding was replicated in a second, independent cohort of 2532 ALS patients and 5940 controls. The associated SNPs are in a 80-kb linkage disequilibrium (LD) block on chromosome 9 which overlaps with the common region found in the ALS-FTD linkage studies (Figure 1).

Study	Linkage region	Families	Country/ Region	fALS	FTD	ALS- FTD	Genes screened	Mutatio ns
Yan et al. 2006	9p13.3-p22.1 (D9S1684- D9S1678)	15	N.K.	N.K.	N.K.	N.K.	27	None
Morita et al. 2006	9p13.2-p21.3 (D9S1870- D9S1791)	1	Scandinavia	5	9	-	2	None
Vance et al. 2006	9p13.2-p21.2 (D9S2154- D9S1874)	1	The Netherlands	7	2	3	3	None
Momeni et al. 2006	9p13.2-p22.2 (D9S157-D9S1874)	2	North- America	1	-	9	14	p.Q342X in IFT-74
Valdmanis et al. 2007	9p13.3-p22.2 (D9S157-D9S1805)	2	Canada/ France	14	3	4	4	None
Le Ber et al. 2009	9p11.2-p21.2 (AFM218xg11- D9S301)	6	France	9	10	12	29 + 4 miRNAs	None
Luty et al. 2008	9p21.2-q21 (D9S169-D9S167)	1	Australia	2	5	2	11	None
Gijselinck et al. 2010	9p22.3-q21 (D9S235-D9S257)	1	Belgium	1	8	-	17	None
Boxer et al. 2010	9p21.2-p23 (D9S1808-D9S251)	1	USA	2	5	3	10	None
Pearson et al. 2011	9p21.2-p21.2	1	Wales	2	5	1	8	None

Table 3. Overview of linkage studies in ALS-FTD families. N.K. = not known

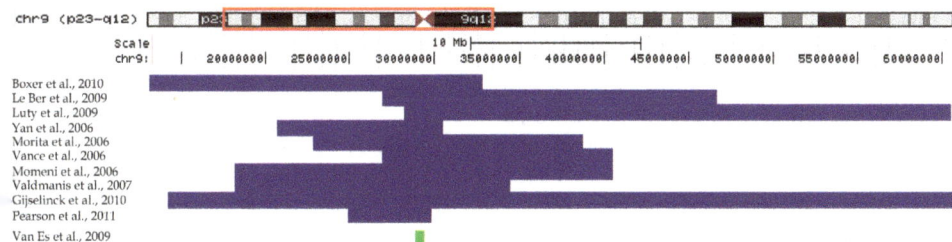

Fig. 1. Schematic overview of the associated regions found by linkage studies and GWAS.

Since this initial report several other GWAS in ALS patients have replicated the association to chromosome 9p21.2. In a GWAS performed on 405 Finnish ALS patients, of whom 93 patients had fALS, and 497 control individuals two association peaks were identified (Laaksovirta et al., 2010). One peak corresponded to the autosomal recessive D90A allele of the SOD1 gene. The other was identified in a 232-kb LD block on chromosome 9p21.2. The association signals in this study were mainly driven by the 93 fALS patients. A 42-SNP risk haplotype across the chromosome 9p21 locus was shared between 41 fALS cases with an odds ratio of 21.0 (Laaksovirta et al., 2010). In another GWAS in an ALS cohort from the UK consisting of 599 ALS patients and 4144 control individuals two SNPs on chromosome 9p21.2 were found to be associated with ALS (Shatunov et al., 2010). A joint analysis including 4132 ALS patients and 8425 controls from this UK cohort and from previously published data from the UK, USA, Netherlands, Ireland, Italy, France, Sweden, and Belgium also showed significant association to the locus on chromosome 9p21.2 (Shatunov et al., 2010). In addition, replication of one of the associated SNPs on chromosome 9p21.2 was found in a GWAS performed in FTD patients when analyzing the ALS-FTD patients only. A different SNP in this locus was significantly associated with FTD (Rollinson et al., 2011). A trend towards significant genome-wide association between chromosome 9p21.2 and FTD was found when analyzing 426 FTD patients with TDP-43 pathology without mutations in the progranulin gene and 2509 control individuals (Van Deerlin et al., 2009). A replication study in Chinese and Japanese sALS patients failed to find association to one of the previously associated SNPs on chromosome 9p21.2 but this might be due to a lack of power (Iida et al., 2011).

In summary, linkage studies in ALS-FTD families and GWAS in sALS, ALS-FTD and FTD patients provide compelling evidence for a role of chromosome 9p21.2 in ALS and/or FTD.

As mentioned, recently two studies identified a GGGGCC hexanucleotide repeat expansion in intron 1 of the *C9ORF72* gene as the cause of chromosome 9p-linked ALS-FTD (Dejesus-Hernandez et al., 2011; Renton et al., 2011).

5. Gene function

A hexanucleotide repeat expansion in the *C9ORF72* gene has recently been identified as the cause of chromosome 9p-linked ALS-FTD. The mechanism as to how this expanded repeat causes ALS is unknown. No causal mutations in *UNC13a* have been identified in ALS patients to date. Close examination of the reported function(s) of the proteins encoded by the *C9ORF72* and *UNC13a* gene may help to design strategies for determining the functional role of these loci in ALS and/or FTD.

In this section the current knowledge of the function of these genes will be discussed in light of a possible contribution to ALS pathogenesis.

5.1 Chromosome 9 open reading frame 72

The *C9ORF72* gene encodes a protein of 481 amino acids. Alternative splicing of this gene is thought to produce five isoforms of which three are protein coding. Isoform 1 contains the entire sequence and consists of 481 amino acids, while isoform 2 and 3 have an asparagine to lysine change at amino acid 222 which results in the truncation of amino acids 223 to 481. Thus far, no C9ORF72 protein has been detected and nothing is known about the function of C9ORF72.

The *C9ORF72* gene has been sequenced in four linkage studies in 39 patients from different families, but no mutations have been identified. No changes in splicing, small deletions or duplications were detected in patients from an ALS-FTD family (Boxer et al., 2010). The gene has been sequenced in 16 sALS patients and 16 controls but no variants specific for sALS were identified (Laaksovirta et al., 2010). Hexanucleotide repeat expansions were recently found to be the most common cause of fALS and familial FTD and were also identified in sALS patients (Dejesus-Hernandez et al., 2011; Renton et al., 2011). The functional consequence of these repeat expansions are however unknown.

Further studies will be needed to characterize the C9ORF72 protein and to establish the consequences of the intronic repeat on ALS pathogenesis.

5.2 UNCoordinated 13 homolog A (UNC13a)

UNC13a is a member of UNC13 family of presynaptic proteins. The protein consists of 1791 amino acids but several isoforms exist. It contains a zinc-finger like C1 domain that is homologous to a diacylglycerol and phorbol ester binding region of protein kinase C (PKC), three C2 domains that are similar to the calcium binding regulatory regions of PKC and synaptotagmin, a calmodulin binding domain and two Munc homology domains (Basu et al., 2005).

In mammals, the Munc13 family comprises four homologous members, Munc13-1, Munc13-2, Munc13-3, and Munc13-4. Deletion mutants of Munc13-1 in mice, the murine homologue of UNC13a, shows that the protein is needed for presynaptic vesicle maturation and fusion competence in glutamergic hippocampal neurons (Augustin et al., 1999). GABA-ergic neurons in the hippocampus show no spontaneous or evoked synaptic transmission in absence of both Munc13-1 and Munc13-2 (Varoqueaux et al., 2002). Neuromuscular junction (NMJ) axon terminals contain Munc13-1 and a splice variant of Munc13-2 (Varoqueaux et al., 2005). Mice deficient in Munc13 due to a double knockout of Munc13-1 and Munc13-2 form specialized neuromuscular endplates. However, the distribution, size and shape of these synapses are altered. Also, muscle morphology is abnormal and a larger number of motor neurons is present in the spinal cord in Munc13-1/2 knockout mice, probably as a result of defective apoptosis. Furthermore, evoked synaptic transmission is impaired in these mutants but spontaneous transmission is unchanged (Varoqueaux et al., 2005). This indicates that vesicle priming in NMJs is partially independent of Munc13-1 or Munc13-2. However, despite the unchanged spontaneous transmission, muscle innervation is aberrant in Munc13-1/2 knockout mice (Varoqueaux et al., 2005).

As exemplified by the defects observed in Munc13-1 and Munc13-1/2 knockout mice, it is plausible that a disruption in UNC13a expression affects motor neurons and muscle innervation. The effect of UNC13a on glutamate exocytosis is also interesting since Riluzole, the only drug with a proven effect on ALS, is a glutamate release inhibitor. Therefore, *UNC13a* is an interesting candidate gene to be investigated further for a role in ALS pathogenesis.

6. Conclusion and future research

The use of linkage analysis, candidate gene studies, and GWAS has led to the identification of several causal loci and genes for fALS and sALS. The overview above clearly shows the extent of heterogeneity in genes that underlie fALS, let alone sALS, illustrating the complex molecular basis of this disease. There is not one dominant biological process that is represented by these genes, although RNA-processing, axonal transport and synaptic dysfunction appear to emerge as being relevant in ALS etiology. Interestingly, several of the genes implicated in these processes are already known to be causal or have been implicated in other neurodegenerative diseases which suggests that there is, at least in part, a common underlying mechanism.

Since these findings explain only about a third of the genetic variability in fALS and a small percentage of the genetic contribution to sALS, there is a clear need for the identification of additional causal loci. This would require the collection of large family pedigrees with many affected individuals, which is difficult in ALS considering the adult onset with rapid disease progression. However, the development of next generation sequencing techniques provides a possible solution to this problem. Using exome and whole-genome sequencing, causal genes can be identified with a small number of affected and unaffected individuals as has been shown in several, mostly autosomal recessive disorders (Choi et al., 2009; Ng et al., 2009). Recently, exome sequencing in two affected individuals from the same family identified *VCP* as a causal gene for fALS, illustrating that this technique is a promising tool for gene identification in ALS as well (Johnson et al., 2010). In addition, the repeat expansion in C9ORF72 was also discovered with the use of whole-genome sequencing (Renton et al., 2011).

The identification of causal genes for ALS has broadened our understanding of this motor neuron degenerative disease. Studying the function of associated genes in neurons and animal models has revealed several possible processes underlying ALS such as RNA processing, axonal transport, glutamate regulation, oxidative stress and synaptic dysfunction. However, the contribution of most genes to ALS pathogenesis has not been resolved. SOD1 and TDP-43 transgenic animal models have provided valuable insights into ALS pathogenesis. Further research using existing animal models of ALS associated genes and the generation of new animal models are needed to further determine their role in the disease. Generation of animal models harbouring repeat expansions in C9ORF72 and ATXN2 could help to reveal the pathogenic mechanisms behind these repeats. The effect of overexpression or knockdown of ALS associated genes and the expression of repeat expansions in motor neurons or motor neuron-like cell lines on protein aggregation and cell survival could also help to unravel the contribution of these genes to ALS. In addition, some associated genes (e.g. *DCTN1*, *PON1/2/3*, *TAF15*, and *VCP*) remain to be sequenced in larger cohorts from different populations in order to determine the actual contribution of these genes to ALS.

Additional new strategies in sALS include a more network oriented approach to gene identification. It is possible to detect networks of genes, proteins and metabolites that are misregulated in ALS, or that determine disease progression. By searching for subtle genetic variation that drives these network perturbations, new genes might be identified that are hard to detect with GWAS. Also, the focus in ALS genetics thus far has been on common variation in exonic DNA. The regulatory part of the genome is challenging to study, but might be relevant as well. This also requires the combined analysis of gene-expression and protein data with data on genetic variation. In addition, recent studies show that tandem repeats in DNA might be also relevant, as exemplified by the ATXN2 and C9ORF72 findings. Typically, this type of variation is hard to detect by current high-throughput methods. Lastly, the type of copy number variation that has not yet been covered very well to date, including variation in microRNAs or inversions, deserves more attention.

In summary, impressive progress in the understanding of the genetics of ALS has been made over the past several years with the identification of several causal genes. However, most of the genetic variability underlying ALS remains to be identified. The use of deep sequencing techniques and functional research will be needed to further broaden our understanding of ALS pathogenesis.

7. Acknowledgements

This work has received funding from the European Community's Health Seventh Framework Programme (FP7/2007-2013) under grant agreement n° 259867, VSB fonds, EURO-MOTOR FP7, The Netherlands ALS Foundation (J.H.V, and L.H.v.d.B.), Neuroscience and Cognition Utrecht (NCU), the Prinses Beatrix Fonds (Kersten Foundation) and the Adessium Foundation (R.J.P., J.H.V. and L.H.v.d.B.). J.H.V. is supported by the Brain Foundation of The Netherlands and J.H.V, R.J.P., and M.K are supported by the Thierry Latran Foundation.

8. References

Al-Chalabi A., et al. (2010). An estimate of amyotrophic lateral sclerosis heritability using twin data. *Journal of Neurology, Neurosurgery, and Psychiatry*, Vol. 81, No. 12, (December 2010), pp. 1342-1346, ISSN 0022-3050

Al-Saif A., Al-Mohanna F. & Bohlega S. (2011). A mutation in Sigma-1 receptor causes juvenile amyotrophic lateral sclerosis. *Annals of Neurology*, 2011, Ahead of print, ISSN 0364-5134

Augustin I., et al. (1999). Munc13-1 is essential for fusion competence of glutamergic synaptic vesicles. *Nature*, Vol. 400, No. 29, (July 2009), pp. 457-461, ISSN 0028-0836

Avemaria F., et al. (2011). Mutation in the senataxin gene found in a patients affected by familial ALS with juvenile onset and slow progression. *Amyotrophic Lateral Sclerosis*, Vol. 12, No. 3, (May 2011), pp. 228-230, ISSN 1748-2968

Azzouz M., et al. (2004). VEGF delivery with retrogradely transported lentivector prolongs survival in a mouse ALS model. *Nature*, Vol. 429, No. 6990, (May 2004), pp. 413-417, ISSN 0028-0836

Badouel C & McNeill H. (2011). Snapshot: The hippo signaling pathway. *Cell*, Vol. 145, No. 3, (April 2011), pp. 484-484.e1, ISSN 1097-4172

Bandyopadhyay S., et al. (2010). A human MAP kinase interactome. *Nature Methods*, Vol. 7, No. 10, (October 2010), pp. 801-805, ISSN 1548-7091

Basu J., et al. (2005). A minimal domain responsible for Munc13 activity. *Nature Structural & Molecular Biology*, Vol. 12, No. 11, (November 2005), pp. 1017-1018, ISSN 1545-9993

Bäumer D., et al. (2010). Juvenile ALS with basophilic inclusions is a FUS proteinopathy with FUS mutations. *Neurology*, Vol. 75, No. 7, (August 2010), pp. 611-618, ISSN 0028-3878

Beaulieu JM, Nguyen MD & Julien JP. (1999). Late onset of motor neurons in mice overexpressing wild-type peripherin. *Journal of Cell Biology*, Vol. 147, No. 3, (November 1999), pp. 531-544, ISSN 0021-9525

Belly A., et al. (2010). CHMP2B mutants linked to frontotemporal dementia impair maturation of dendritic spines. *Journal of Cell Science*, Vol. 123, Pt. 17, (September 2010), pp. 2943-2954, ISSN 0021-9533

Belzil VV., et al. (2009). Mutations in FUS cause FALS and SALS in French and French Canadian populations. *Neurology*, Vol. 73, No. 15, (October 2009), pp. 1176-1179, ISSN 0028-3878

Belzil VV., et al. (2010). Analysis of OPTN as a causative gene for amyotrophic lateral sclerosis. *Neurobiology of Aging*, Vol. 32, No. 3, (March 2011), pp. 555.e13-4, ISSN 1558-1497

Benajiba L., et al. (2009). TARDBP mutations in motoneuron disease with frontotemporal lobar degeneration. *Annals of Neurology*, Vol. 65, No. 4, (April 2009), pp. 470-473, ISSN 0364-5134

Blauw HM., et al. (2010). A large genome scan for rare CNVs in amyotrophic lateral sclerosis. *Human Molecular Genetics*, Vol. 19, No. 20, (October 2010), pp. 4091-4099, ISSN 0964-6906

Blauw HM., et al. *Neurology*, 2011;in press

Bosco DA., et al. (2010). Mutant FUS proteins that cause amyotrophic lateral sclerosis incorporate into stress granules. *Human Molecular Genetics*, Vol. 19, No. 21, (November 2010), pp. 4160-4175, ISSN 0964-6906

Bose JK., et al. (2008). TDP-43 overexpression enhances exon 7 inclusion during the survival of motor neuron pre-mRNA splicing. *Journal of Biological Chemistry*, Vol. 283, No. 43, (October 2008), pp. 28852-28859, ISSN 0021-9258

Boxer AL., et al. (2010). Clinical, neuroimaging and neuropathological features of a new chromosome 9p-linked FTD-ALS family. *Journal of Neurology, Neurosurgery and Psychiatry*, Vol.82, No.2, (February 2011), pp.196-203, ISSN 0022-3050

Brockington A., et al. (2005). Screening of the regulatoy and coding regions of vascular endothelial growth factor in amyotrophic lateral sclerosis. *Neurogenetics*, Vol. 6, No. 2, (May 2005), pp. 101-104, ISSN 1364-6745

Brockington A., et al. (2006). Expression of vascular endothelial growth factor and its receptors in the central nervous system in amyotrophic lateral sclerosis. *Journal of Neuropathology and Experimental Neurology*, Vol. 65, No. 1, (January 2006), pp. 26-36, ISSN 0022-3069

Broeke JHP., et al. (2010). Munc18 and Munc13 regulate early neurite outgrowth. *Biology of the Cell*, Vol. 102, No. 8, (June 2010), pp. 479-488, ISSN 0248-4900

Buratti E & Baralle FE. (2010). The multiple roles of TDP-43 in pre-mRNA processing and gene expression regulation. *RNA Biology*, Vol. 7, No. 4, (July-August 2010), pp. 420-429, ISSN 1547-6286

Byrne S., et al. (2010). Rate of familial amyotrophic lateral sclerosis: a systematic review and meta-analysis. *Journal of Neurology, Neurosurgery, and Psychiatry*, Vol. 82, No. 6, (June 2011), pp. 623-627, ISSN 0022-3050

Cai H., et al. (2008). ALS2/alsin knockout mice and motor neuron diseases. *Neurodegenerative diseases*, Vol. 5, No. 6, (2008), pp. 359-366, ISSN 1660-2854

Calvo A., et al. (2010). Involvement of immune response in the pathogenesis of amyotrophic lateral sclerosis: a therapeutic opportunity? *CNS & Neurological Disorders Drug Targets*, Vol. 9, No. 3, (July 2010), pp. 325-330, ISSN 1871-5273

Chance PF., et al. (1998). Linkage of the gene for an autosomal dominant form of juvenile amyotrophic lateral sclerosis to chromosome 9q34. *American Journal of Human Genetics*, Vol. 62, No. 3, (March 1998), pp. 633-640, ISSN 0002-9297

Chen D., et al. (2007). Association of polymorphisms in vascular endothelial growth factor gene with the age of onset of amyotrophic lateral sclerosis. *Amyotrophic Lateral Sclerosis*, Vol. 8, No. 3, (June 2007), pp. 144-149, ISSN 1748-2968

Chen HJ., et al. (2010). Characterization of the properties of a novel mutation in VAPB in familial amyotrophic lateral sclerosis. *Journal of Biological Chemistry*, Vol. 285, No. 51, (December 2010), pp. 40266-40281, ISSN 0021-9258

Chen W., et al. (2006). Lack of association of VEGF promoter polymorphisms with sporadic ALS. *Neurology*, Vol. 67, No. 3, (August 2006), pp. 508-510, ISSN 0028-3878

Chen Y., et al. (2011). Ataxin-2 intermediate-length polyglutamine: a possible risk factor for Chinese patients with amyotrophic lateral sclerosis. *Neurobiology of Aging*, 2011, Ahead of print, ISSN 0197-4580

Chen YZ., et al. (2004). DNA/RNA helicase gene mutations in a form of juvenile amyotrophic lateral sclerosis (ALS4). *American Journal of Human Genetics*, Vol. 74, No. 6, (June 2004), pp. 1128-1135, ISSN 0002-9297

Chió A., et al. (1991). Risk factors in motor neuron disease: a case-control study. *Neuroepidemiology*, Vol. 10, No. 4, (1991), pp 174-184, ISSN 0251-5350

Chió A., et al. (2009). A two-stage genome-wide association study of sporadic amyotrophic lateral sclerosis. *Human Molecular Genetics*, Vol. 18, No. 8, (April 2009), pp. 1524-1532, ISSN 0964-6906

Choi M., et al. (2009). Genetic diagnosis by whole exome capture and massively parallel DNA sequencing. *Proceedings of the National Academy of Sciences of the USA*, Vol. 106, No. 45, (November 2009), pp. 19096-19101, ISSN 0027-8424

Chow CY., et al. (2007). Mutation of FIG4 causes neurodegeneration in the pale tremor mouse and patients with CMT4J. *Nature*, Vol. 448, No. 7149, (July 2007), pp. 68-73, ISSN 0028-0836

Chow CY., et al. (2009). Deleterious variants of FIG4, a phosphoinositide phosphatase, in patients with ALS. *American Journal of Human Genetics*, Vol. 84, No. 1, (January 2009), pp. 85-88, ISSN 0002-9297

Conforti FL., et al. (2007). A novel angiogenin gene mutation in a sporadic patient with amyotrophic lateral sclerosis from southern Italy. *Neuromuscular Disorders*, Vol. 18, No. 1, (January 2008), pp. 68-70, ISSN 0960-8966

Coppedè F., et al. (2008). Lack of association between the APEX1 Asp184Glu polymorphism and sporadic amyotrophic lateral sclerosis. *Neurobiology of Aging*, Vol. 31, No. 2, (February 2010), pp. 353-355, ISSN 0197-4580

Corbo M & Hays AP. (1992). Peripherin and neurofilament protein coexist in spinal spheroids of motor neuron disease. *Journal of Neuropathology and Experimental Neurology*, Vol. 51, No. 5, (September 1992), pp. 531-537, ISSN 0022-3069

Corcia P., et al. (2002). Abnormal SMN1 gene copy number is a susceptibility factor for amyotrophic lateral sclerosis. *Annals of Neurology*, Vol. 51, No. 2, (February 2002), pp. 243-246, ISSN 0364-5134

Corcia P., et al. (2006). SMN1 gene, but not SMN2, is a risk factor for sporadic ALS. *Neurology*, Vol. 67, No. 7, (October 2006), pp. 1147-1150, ISSN 0028-3878

Corcia P., et al. (2009). The importance of the SMN genes in the genetics of sporadic ALS. *Amyotrophic Lateral Sclerosis*, Vol. 10, No. 5-6, (October-December 2009), pp. 436-440, ISSN 1748-2968

Corrado L., et al. (2007). Variations in the coding and regulatory sequences of the angiogenin (ANG) gene are not associated to ALS (amyotrophic lateral sclerosis) in the Italian population. *Journal of Neurological Sciences*, Vol. 258, No. 1-2, (July 2007), pp. 123-127, ISSN 0022-510X

Corrado L., et al. (2009). High frequency of TARDBP gene mutations in Italian patients with amyotrophic lateral sclerosis. *Human Mutation*, Vol. 30, No. 4, (April 2009), pp. 688-694, ISSN 1059-7794

Corrado L., et al. (2009). Mutations of FUS gene in sporadic amyotrophic lateral sclerosis. *Journal of Medical Genetics*, Vol. 47, No. 3, (March 2010), pp. 190-194, ISSN 0022-2593

Corrado L., et al. (2010). A novel peripherin gene (PRPH) mutation identified in one sporadic amyotrophic lateral sclerosis patients. *Neurobiology of Aging*, Vol. 32, No. 3, (March 2011), pp. 552.e1-6, ISSN 0197-4580

Costa LG., et al. (2005). Modulation of paraoxonase (PON1) activity. *Biochemical Pharmacology*, Vol. 69, No. 4, (February 2005), pp. 541-550, ISSN 0006-2952

Couillard-Després S., et al. (1998). Protective effect of neurofilament heavy gene overexpression in motor neuron disease induced by mutant superoxide dismutase. *Proceedings of the National Academy of Sciences of the USA*, Vol. 95, No. 16, (August 1998), pp. 9626-9630, ISSN 0027-8424

Cox LE., et al. (2010). Mutations in CHMP2B in lower motor neuron predominant amyotrophic lateral sclerosis (ALS). *PLoS One*, Vol. 5, No. 3, (March 2010), e9872, ISSN 1932-6203

Cronin S., et al. (2007). Paraoxonase promoter and intronic variants modify risk of sporadic amytrophic lateral sclerosis. *Journal of Neurology, Neurosurgery, and Psychiatry*, Vol. 78, No. 9, (September 2007), pp. 984-986, ISSN 0022-3050

Cronin S,. et al. (2007). A genome-wide association study of sporadic ALS in a homogenous Irish population. *Human Molecular Genetics*, Vol. 17, No. 5, (March 2008), pp. 768-774, ISSN 0964-6906

Cronin S., et al. (2008). Screening for replication of genome-wide SNP associations in sporadic ALS. *European Journal of Human Genetics*, Vol. 17, No. 2, (February 2009), pp. 213-218, ISSN 1018-4813

Crow MK. (2010). Type I interferon in organ-targeted autoimmune and inflammatory diseases. *Artrhitis Research and Therapy*, Vol.12, (2010), Suppl.1:S5, ISSN 1478-6354

Da Cruz S & Cleveland DW. (2011). Understanding the role of TDP-43 and FUS/TLS in ALS and beyond. *Current Opinion in Neurobiology*, 2011:Ahead of print

Daoud H., et al. (2010). Analysis of DPP6 and FGGY as candidate genes for amyotrophic lateral sclerosis. *Amyotrophic Lateral Sclerosis*, Vol. 11, No. 4, (August 2011), pp. 389-391, ISSN 1748-2968

Daoud H., et al. (2011). Association of long ATXN2 CAG repeat sizes with increased risk of amyotrophic lateral sclerosis. *Archives of Neurology*, Vol. 68, No. 6, (June 2011), pp. 739-742, ISSN 0003-9942

Dedoni S, Olianas MC & Onali P. (2010). Interferon-β induces apoptosis in human SH-Sy5Y neuroblasto cells through activation of JAK-STAT signaling and down-regulation of PI3K/Akt pathway. *Journal of Neurochemistry*, Vol. 115, No. 6, (December 2010), pp. 1421-1433, ISSN 0022-3042

Dejesus-Hernandez M et al. (2011). Expanded GGGGCC hexanucleotide repeat in noncoding region of C9ORF72 causes chromosome 9p-linked FTD and ALS. *Neuron*, September 2011, Ahead of print.

Del Bo R., et al. (2006). Absence of angiogenic genes modification in Italian ALS patients. *Neurobiology of Aging*, Vol. 29, No. 2, (February 2008), pp. 314-316, ISSN 0197-4580

Del Bo R., et al. (2008). DPP6 gene variability confers increate risk of developing sporadic amyotrophic lateral sclerosis in Italian patients. *Journal of Neurology, Neurosurgery, and Psychiatry*, Vol. 79, No. 9, (September 2008), pp. 1085, ISSN 0022-3050

Del Bo R., et al. (2011). Novel optineurin mutations in patients with familial and sporadic amyotrophic lateral sclerosis. *Journal of Neurology, Neurosurgery, and Psychiatry,* 2001, Ahead of print, ISSN 0022-3050

Delisle MB & Carpenter S. (1984). Neurofibrillary axonal swellings and amyotrophic lateral sclerosis. *Journal of the Neurological Sciences,* Vol. 63, No. 2, (February 1984), pp. 241-250, ISSN 0022-510X

Deng HX., et al. (2010). FUS-immunoreactive inclusions are a common feature in sporadic and non-SOD1 familial amyotrophic lateral sclerosis. *Annals of Neurology,* Vol. 67, No. 6, (June 2010), pp. 739-748, ISSN 0364-5134

Deng HX., et al. (2011). Mutations in UBQLN2 cause dominant X-linked juvenile and adult-onset ALS and ALS/dementia. *Nature,* Vol. 477, No. 7363, (August 2011), pp. 211-215, ISSN 0028-0836

De Weerd NA, Samarajiwa SA & Hertzog PJ. (2007). Type I interferon receptors: biochemistry and biological functions. *Journal of Biological Chemistry,* Vol. 282, No. 28, (July 2007), pp. 20053-20057, ISSN 0021-9258

Dickson SP., et al. (2010). Rare variants create synthetic genome-wide associations. *PLoS Biology,* Vol. 8, No. 1, (January 2010), e1000294, ISSN 1544-9173

Dion PA, Daoud H & Rouleau GA. (2009). Genetics of motor neuron disorders: new insights into pathogenic mechanisms. *Nature Reviews. Genetics,* Vol. 10, No. 11, (November 2009), pp. 769-782, ISSN 1471-0056

Dormann D., et al. (2010). ALS-associated fused in sarcoma (FUS) mutations disrupt Transportin-mediated nuclear import. *EMBO Journal,* Vol. 29, No. 16, (August 2010), pp. 2841-2857, ISSN 0261-4189

Draganov DI., et al. (2000). Rabbit serum paraoxonase 3 (PON3) is a high density lipoprotein-associated lactonase and protects low density lipoprotein against oxidation. *Journal of Biological Chemistry,* Vol. 275, No. 43, (October 2000), pp. 33435-33442, ISSN 0021-9258

Dunckley T., et al. (2007). Whole-genome analysis of sporadic amyotrophic lateral sclerosis. *New England Journal of Medicine,* Vol. 357, No. 8, (August 2007), pp. 775-788, ISSN 0028-4793

Echaniz-Laguna A., et al. (2002). Homozygous exon 7 deletion of the SMN centromeric gene (SMN2): a potential susceptibility factor for adult-onset lower motor neuron disease. *Journal of Neurology,* Vol. 249, No. 3, (March 2002), pp. 290-293, ISSN 0340-5354

Eggert C., et al. (2006). Spinal muscular atrophy: the RNP connection. *Trends in Molecular Medicine,* Vol. 12, No. 3, (March 2006), pp. 113-121, ISSN 1471-4914

Elamin M., et al. (2011). Executive dysfunction is a negative prognostic indicator in patients with ALS without dementia. *Neurology,* Vol. 76, No. 14, (April 2011), pp. 1263-1269, ISSN 0028-3878

Elden AC., et al. (2010). Ataxin-2 intermediate-length polyglutamine expansions are associated with increased risk for ALS. *Nature,* Vol. 466, No.7310, (August 2010), pp.1069-1075, ISSN 0028-0836

Ewing RM., et al. (2007). Large-scale mapping of human protein-protein interactions by mass spectrometry. *Molecular Systems Biology,* Vol. 3, (2007), pp. 89, ISSN 1744-4292

Farrer MJ., et al. (2009). DCTN1 mutations in Perry syndrome. *Nature Genetics,* Vol. 41, No. 2, (February 2009), pp. 163-165, ISSN 1061-4036

Feder JN., et al. (1998). The hemochromatosis gene product complexes with the transferrin receptor and lowers its affinity for ligand binding. *Proceedings of the National Academy of Sciences of the United States of America*, Vol. 95, No. 4, (February 1998), pp.1472-1477, ISSN 0027-8424

Fernández-Santiago R., et al. (2006). Possible gender-dependent association of vascular endothelial growth factor (VEGF) gene and ALS. *Neurology*, Vol. 66, No. 12, (June 2006), pp. 1929-1931, ISSN 0028-3878

Fernández-Santiago R., et al. (2009). Identification of novel Angiogenin (ANG) gene missense variants in German patients with amyotrophic lateral sclerosis. *Journal of Neurology*, Vol. 256, No. 8, (August 2009), pp. 1337-1342, ISSN 1351-5101

Fernández-Santiago R., et al. (2009). No evidence of association of FLJ10986 and ITPR2 with ALS in a large German cohort. *Neurobiology of Aging*, Vol. 32, No. 3, (March 2011), pp. 551.e1-4, ISSN 0197-4580

Figlewicz DA., et al. (1994). Variants of the heavy neurofilament subunit are associated with the development of amyotrophic lateral sclerosis. *Human Molecular Genetics*, Vol. 3, No. 10, (October 1994), pp. 1757-1761, ISSN 0964-6906

Fishel ML & Kelley MR. (2007). The DNA base excision repair protein Ape1/Ref-1 as a therapeutic and chemopreventive target. *Molecular Aspects of Medicine*, Vol. 28, No. 3-4, (June-August 2007), pp. 375-395, ISSN 0098-2997

Fogh I., et al. (2009) No association of DPP6 with amyotrophic lateral sclerosis in an Italian population. *Neurobiology of Aging*, Vol. 32, No. 5, (May 2011), pp. 966-967, ISSN 0197-4580

Gamez J., et al. (2002). Survival and respiratory decline are not related to homozygous SMN2 deletions in ALS patients. *Neurology*, Vol. 59, No. 9, (November 2002), pp. 1456-1460, ISSN 0028-3878

Gavrilov DK., et al. (1998). Differential SMN2 expression associated with SMA severity. *Nature Genetics*, Vol. 20, No. 3, (November 1998), pp. 230-231, ISSN 1061-4036

Gellera C., et al. (2007). Identification of new ANG gene mutations in a large color of Italian patients with amyotrophic lateral sclerosis. *Neurogenetics*, Vol. 9, No. 1, (February 2008), pp. 33-40, ISSN 1364-6745

Gijselinck I., et al. (2010). Identification of 2 loci at chromosome 9 and 14 in a multiplex family with frontotemporal lobar degeneration and amyotrophic lateral sclerosis. *Archives of Neurology*, Vol. 67, No. 5, (May 2010), pp. 606-616, ISSN 0003-9942

Giordano G., et al. (2011). Paraoxonase 2 (PON2) in the mouse central nervous system: A neuroprotective role? *Toxicology and Applied Pharmacology*, (February 2011), Ahead of print, ISSN 0041-008X

Gitcho MA., et al. (2009). VCP mutations causing frontotemporal lobar degeneration disrupt localization of TDP-43 and induce cell death. *Journal of Biological Chemistry*, Vol. 284, No. 18, (May 2009), pp. 12384-12398, ISSN 0021-9258

Gitcho MA., et al. (2009). TARDBP 3´UTR variant in autopsy-confirmed frontotemporal lobar degeneration with TDP-43 proteinopathy. *Acta Neuropathologica*, Vol. 118, No. 5, (November 2009), pp. 633-645, ISSN 0001-6322

Goodall EF., et al. (2005). Association of the H63D polymorphism in the hemochromatosis gene with sporadic ALS. *Neurology*, Vol. 65, No. 6, (September 2005), pp. 934-937, ISSN 0028-3878

Golenia A., et al. (2010). Lack of association between VEGF gene polymorphisms and plasma VEGF levels and sporadic ALS. *Neurology*, Vol. 75, No. 22, (November 2010), pp. 2035-2037, ISSN 0028-3878

Greenway MJ., et al. (2004). A novel candidate region for ALS on chromosome 14q11.2. *Neurology*, Vol. 63, No. 10, (November 2004), pp. 1936-1938, ISSN 0028-3878

Greenway MJ., et al. (2006). ANG mutations segregate with familial and 'sporadic' amyotrophic lateral sclerosis. *Nature Genetics*, Vol. 38, No. 4, (April 2006), pp. 411-413, ISSN 1061-4036

Groen EJ., et al. (2010). FUS mutations in amyotrophic lateral sclerosis in the Netherlands. *Archives of Neurology*, Vol. 67, No. 2, (February 2010), pp. 224-230, ISSN 0003-9942

Grohmann K., et al. (2011). Mutations in the gene encoding immunoglobulin mu-binding protein 2 cause spinal muscular atrophy with respiratory distress type 1. *Nature Genetics*, Vol. 29, No. 1, (September 2001), pp. 75-77, ISSN 1061-4036

Gurney ME., et al. (1994). Motor neuron degeneration in mice that express a human Cu,Zn superoxide dismutase mutation. *Science*, Vol. 264, No. 5166, (June 1994), pp. 1772-1775, ISSN 0036-8075

Hadano S., et al. (2001. A gene encoding a putative GTPase regulator is mutated in familial amyotrophic lateral sclerosis 2. *Nature Genetics*, Vol.29, No.2, (October 2001), pp.166-173, ISSN 1061-4036

Hadano S., et al. (2005). Mice deficient in the Rab5 guanine nucleotide exchange factor ALS2/alsin exhibit age-dependent neurological deficits and altered endosome trafficking. *Human Molecular Genetics*, Vol. 15, No. 2, (January 2006), pp. 233-250, ISSN 0964-6906

Hand CK., et al. (2001). A novel locus for familial amyotrophic lateral sclerosis on chromosome 18q. *The American Journal of Human Genetics*, Vol. 70, No.1, (January 2002), pp.251-256, ISSN 0002-9297

Haraguchi K., et al. (2005). Role of the kinesin-2 family protein, KIF3, during mitosis. *Journal of Biological Chemistry*, Vol. 281, No. 7, (February 2006), pp. 4094-4099, ISSN 0021-9258

Harley IT., et al. (2010). The role of genetic variation near interferon-kappa in systemic lupus erythematosus. *Journal of Biomedicine and Biotechnology*, 2010, ISSN 1110-7243

Hayward C., et al. (1999). Molecular genetic analysis of the APEX nuclease gene in amyotrophic lateral sclerosis. *Neurology*, Vol. 52, No. 9, (June 1999), pp. 1899-1901, ISSN 0028-3878

He X., et al. (2011). H63D polymorphism in the hemochromatosis gene is associated with sporadic amyotrophic lateral sclerosis in China. *European Journal of Neurology*, Vol. 18, No. 2, (February 2011), pp. 359-361, ISSN 1351-5101

He CZ & Hays AP. (2004). Expression of peripherin in ubiquitinated inclusions of amyotrophic lateral sclerosis. *Journal of Neurological Sciences*, Vol. 217, No. 1, (January 2004), pp. 47-54, ISSN 0022-510X

Hentati A., et al. (1994). Linkage of recessive familial amyotrophic lateral sclerosis to chromosome 2q33-q35. *Nature Genetics*, Vol. 7, No. 3, (July 1994), pp. 425-428, ISSN 1061-4036

Hentati A., et al. (1998). Linkage of a commoner form of recessive amyotrophic lateral sclerosis to chromosome 15q15-q22 markers. *Neurogenetics*, Vol. 2, No. 1, (December 1998), pp. 55-60, ISSN 1364-6745

Hergovich A. (2011). MOB control: reviewing a conserved family of kinase regulators. *Cellular Signaling*, Vol. 23, No.9, (September 2011), pp.1433-1440, ISSN 0898-6568

Hervas-Stubss S., et al. (2011). Direct effects of type I interferons on cells of the immune system. *Clinical Cancer Research*, Vol. 17, No. 9, (May 2011), pp. 2619-2627, ISSN 1078-0432

Hewitt C., et al. (2010). Novel FUS/TLS mutations and pathology in familial and sporadic amyotrophic lateral sclerosis. *Archives of Neurology*, Vol. 67, No. 4, (April 2010), pp. 455-461, ISSN 0003-9942

Hirano M., et al. (2010). Senataxin mutations in amyotrophic lateral sclerosis. *Amyotrophic Lateral Sclerosis*, Vol. 12, No. 3, (May 2011), pp. 223-227, ISSN 1748-2968

Horner RD., et al. (2003). Occurrence of amyotrophic lateral sclerosis among Gulf War veterans. *Neurology*, Vol. 61, No. 6, (September 2003), pp. 742-749, ISSN 0028-3878

Hosler BA., et al. (2000). Linkage of familial amyotrophic lateral sclerosis with frontotemporal dementia to chromosome 9q21-q22. *Journal of the American Medical Association*, Vol. 284, No. 13, (October 2000), pp. 1664-1669, ISSN 0098-7484

Huang C., et al. (2011). FUS transgenic rats develop the phenotypes of amyotrophic lateral sclerosis and frontotemporal lobar degeneration. *PLoS Genetics*, Vol. 7, No. 3, (March 2011), pp. e1002011, ISSN 1553-7404

Huang EJ., et al. (2010). Extensive FUS-immunoreactive pathology in juvenile amyotrophic lateral sclerosis with basophilic inclusions. *Brain Pathology*, Vol. 20, No. 6, (November 2010), pp. 1069-1076, ISSN 1015-6305

Hutton M., et al. (1998). Association of missense and 5'-splice-site mutations in tau with the inherited dementia FTDP-17. *Nature*, Vol. 393, No. 6686, (June 1998), pp. 702-705, ISSN 0028-0836

Iida A., et al. (2010). Large-scale screening of TARDBP mutation in amyotrophic lateral sclerosis. *Neurobiology of Aging*, 2010, Ahead of print

Iida A., et al. (2011). Optineurin mutations in Japanese amyotrophic lateral sclerosis. *Journal of Neurology, Neurosurgery and Psychiatry*, (January 2011), ISSN 0022-3050

Iida A., et al. (2011). Replication analysis of SNPs on 9p21.2 and 19p13.11 with amyotrophic lateral sclerosis in East Asians. *Neurobiology of Aging*, Vol. 32, No. 4, (April 2011), pp. 757.e13-4, ISSN 0197-4580

Ilieva H, Polymenidou M & Cleveland DW. (2009). Non-cell autonomous toxicity in neurodegenerative disorders: ALS and beyond. *Journal of Cell Biology*, Vol. 187, No. 6, (December 2009), pp. 761-772, ISSN 0021-9525

Imbert G., et al. (1996). Cloning of the gene for spinocerebellar ataxia 2 reveals a locus with high sensitivity to expanded CAG/glutamine repeats. *Nature Genetics*, Vol. 14, No. 3, (November 1996), pp. 285-291, ISSN 1061-4036

Ito D., et al. (201). Nuclear transport impairment of amyotrophic lateral sclerosis-linked mutations in FUS/TLS. *Annals of Neurology*, 2010, Ahead of print

Jackson M., et al. (1996). Analysis of chromosome 5q13 genes in amyotrophic lateral sclerosis: homozygous NAIP deletion in a sporadic case. *Annals of Neurology*, Vol. 39, No. 6, (June 1996), pp. 796-800, ISSN 0364-5134

Johnson JO., et al. (2010). Exome sequencing reveals VCP mutations as a cause of familial ALS. *Neuron*, Vol. 68, No. 5, (December 2010), pp. 857-864, ISSN 0896-6273

Ju JS & Weihl CC. (2010). Inclusion body myopathy, Paget's disease of the bone and frontotemporal dementia: a disorder of autophagy. *Human Molecular Genetics*, Vol. 19, No. R1, (April 2010), pp. R38-45, ISSN 0964-6906

Ju S., et al. (2011). A yeast model of FUS/TLS-dependent cytotoxicity. *PLoS Biology*, Vol. 9, No. 4, (April 2011), pp. e1001052, ISSN 1545-7885

Kabashi E., et al. (2008). TARDBP mutations in individuals with sporadic and familial amyotrophic lateral sclerosis. *Nature Genetics*, Vol. 40, No. 5, (May 2008), pp. 572-574, ISSN 1061-4036

Kanekura K., et al. (2004). Alsin, the product of ALS2 gene, suppresses SOD1 mutant neurotoxicity through RhoGEF domain by interacting with SOD1 mutants. *Journal of Biological Chemistry*, Vol. 279, No. 18, (April 2004), pp. 19247-19256, ISSN 0021-9258

Kiernan MC., et al. (2011). Amyotrophic lateral sclerosis. *Lancet*, Vol. 377, No. 9769, (March 2011), pp. 942-955, ISSN 0140-6736

Kisby GE, Milne J & Sweatt C. (1997). Evidence of reduced DNA repair in amyotrophic lateral sclerosis brain tissue. *Neuroreport*, Vol. 8, No. 6, (April 1997), pp. 1337-1340, ISSN 0959-4965

Kohler RS., et al. (2010). Differential NDR/LATS interactions with the human MOB family reveal a negative role for human MOB2 in the regulation of human NDR kinases. *Molecular and Cellular Biology*, Vol. 30, No. 18, (September 2010), pp. 4507-4520, ISSN 1098-5549

Kwiatkowski TJ Jr., et al. (2009). Mutations in the FUS/TLS gene on chromosome 16 cause familial amyotrophic lateral sclerosis. *Science*, Vol. 323, No. 5918, (February 2009), pp. 1205-1208, ISSN 1095-9203

Laaksovirta H., et al. (2010). Chromosome 9p21 in amyotrophic lateral sclerosis in Finland: a genome-wide association study. *Lancet Neurology*, Vol. 9, No. 10, (October 2010), pp. 978-985, ISSN 1474-4422

LaFleur DW., et al. (2001). Interferon-κ, a novel type I interferon expressed in human keratinocytes. *Journal of Biological Chemistry*, Vol. 276, No. 43, (October 2001), pp. 39765-39771, ISSN 0021-9258

Lagier-Tourenne C, Polymenidou M & Cleveland DW. (2010). TDP-43 and FUS/TLS: emerging roles in RNA processing and neurodegeneration. *Human Molecular Genetics*, Vol. 19, No. R1, (April 2010), pp. R46-R64, ISSN 0964-6906

Lambrechts D., et al. (2003). VEGF is a modifier of amyotrophic lateral sclerosis in mice and humans and protects motoneuron against ischemic death. *Nature Genetics*, Vol. 34, No. 4, (August 2003), pp. 383-394, ISSN 1061-4036

Lambrechts D., et al. (2009). Meta-analysis of vascular endothelial growth factor variations in amyotrophic lateral sclerosis: increased susceptibility in male carriers of the -2578AA genotype. *Journal of Medical Genetics*, Vol. 46, No. 12, (December 2009), pp. 840-846, ISSN 0022-2593

Landers JE., et al. (2008). A common haplotype within the PON1 promoter region is associated with sporadic ALS. *Amyotrophic Lateral Sclerosis*, Vol. 9, No. 5, (October 2008), pp. 306-314, ISSN 1748-2968

Lariviere RC & Julien JP. (2004). Functions of intermediate filaments in neuronal development and disease. *Journal of Neurobiology*, Vol. 58, No. 1, (January 2004), pp. 131-148, ISSN 0022-3034

Le Ber I., et al. (2009). Chromosome 9p-linked families with frontotemporal dementia associated with motor neuron disease. *Neurology*, Vol. 72, No. 19, (May 2009), pp. 1669-1676, ISSN 0028-3878

Lee JA., et al. (2007). ESCRT-III dysfunction causes autophagosomes accumulation and neurodegeneration. *Current Biology*, Vol. 17, No. 18, (September 2007), pp. 1561-1567, ISSN 0960-9822

Lee T., et al. Ataxin-2 intermediate-length polyglutamine expansions in European ALS patients. *Human Molecular Genetics*, Vol. 20, No. 9, (May 2011), pp. 1697-1700, ISSN 0964-6906

Lefebvre S., et al. (1997). Correlation between severity and SMN protein level in spinal muscular atrophy. *Nature Genetics*, Vol. 16, No. 3, (July 1997), pp. 265-269, ISSN 1061-4036

Li XG., et al. (2009). Association between DPP6 polymorphism and the risk of sporadic amyotrophic lateral sclerosis in Chinese patients. *Chinese Medical Journal*, Vol. 122, No. 24, (December 2009), pp. 2989-2992, ISSN 0366-6999

Lorson CL., et al. (1998). SMN oligomerization defect correlates with spinal muscular atrophy severity. *Nature Genetics*, Vol. 19, No. 1, (May 1998), pp. 63-66, ISSN 1061-4036

Liu Y., et al. (2011). Mutant HFE H63D protein is associated with prolonged endoplasmic reticulum stress and increased neuronal vulnerability. *Journal of Biological Chemistry*, Vol. 286, No. 15, (April 2011), pp. 13161-13170, ISSN 0021-9258

Luty AA., et al. (2008). Pedigree with frontotemporal lobar degeneration – motor neuron disease and Tar DNA binding protein-43 positive neuropathology: genetic linkage to chromosome 9. *BMC Neurology*, Vol. 8, (August 2008), pp. 32, ISSN 1471-2377

Luty AA., et al. (2010). Sigma nonopioid intracellular receptor 1 mutations cause frontotemporal lobar degeneration-motor neuron disease. *Annals of Neurology*, Vol. 68, No. 5, (November 2010), pp. 639-649, ISSN 0364-5134

Mackness MI, Arrol S & Durrington PN. (1991). Paraoxonase prevents accumulation of lipoperoxides in low-density lipoprotein. *FEBS Letters*, Vol. 286, No. 1-2, (July 1991), pp. 151-154, ISSN 0014-5793

McLean J., et al. (2010). Distinct biochemical signatures characterize peripherin isoform expression in both traumatic neuronal injury and motor neuron disease. *Journal of Neurochemistry*, Vol. 114, No. 4, (August 2010), pp. 1177-1192, ISSN 0022-3042

Mersiyanova IV., et al. (2000). A new variant of Charchot-Marie-Tooth disease type 2 is probably the result of a mutation in the neurofilaments-light gene. *American Journal of Human Genetics*, Vol. 67, No. 1, (July 2000), pp. 37-46, ISSN 0002-9297

Millecamps S., et al. (2010). SOD1, ANG, VAPB, TARDBP, and FUS mutations in familial amyotrophic lateral sclerosis: genotype-phenotype correlations. *Journal of Medical Genetics*, Vol. 47, No. 8, (August 2010), pp. 554-560, ISSN 0022-2593

Millecamps S., et al. (2011). Screening of OPTN in French familial amyotrophic lateral sclerosis. *Neurobiology of Aging*, Vol. 32, No. 3, (March 2011), pp. 557.e11-3, ISSN 1558-1497

Mitchell J., et al. (2010). Familial amytrophic lateral sclerosis is associated with a mutation in D-amino acid oxidase. *Proceedings of the National Academy of Sciences of the USA*, Vol. 107, No. 16, (April 2010), pp. 7556-7561, ISSN 0027-8424

Mitchell RM., et al. (2009). HFE polymorphisms affect cellular glutamate regulation. *Neurobiology of Aging*, Vol. 32, No. 6, (June 2011), pp. 1114-1123, ISSN 0197-4580

Mizuno Y., et al. (2011). Peripherin partially localizes in Bunina bodies in amyotrophic lateral sclerosis. *Journal of Neurological Sciences*, Vol. 301, No. 1-2, (March 2011), pp. 14-18, ISSN 0022-510X

Morahan JM., et al. (2006). A gene-environment study of the paraoxonase 1 gene and pesticides in amyotrophic lateral sclerosis. *Neurotoxicology*, Vol. 28, No. 3, (May 2007), pp. 532-540, ISSN 0161-813X

Moreira MC., et al. (2004). Senataxin, the ortholog of a yeast RNA helicase, is mutant in ataxia-ocular apraxia 2. *Nature Genetics*, Vol. 36, No. 3, (March 2004), pp. 225-227, ISSN 1061-4036

Morita M., et al. (2006). A locus on chromosome 9p confers susceptibility to ALS and frontotemporal dementia. *Neurology*, Vol. 66, No. 6, (March 2006), pp. 839-844, ISSN 0028-3878

Moulard B., et al. (1998). Association between centromeric deletions of the SMN gene and sporadic adult-onset lower motor neuron disease. *Annals of Neurology*, Vol. 43, No. 5, (May 1998), pp. 640-644, ISSN 0364-5134

Münch C., et al. (2004). Point mutations of the p150 subunit of dynactin (DCTN1) gene in ALS. *Neurology*, Vol. 63, No. 4, (August 2004), pp. 724-726, ISSN 0028-3878

Münch C., et al. (2005). Heterozygous R1101K mutation of the DCTN1 gene in a family with ALS and FTD. *Annals of Neurology*, Vol. 58, No. 5, (November 2005), pp. 777-780, ISSN 0364-5134

Murayama H., et al. (2010). Mutations of optineurin in amyotrophic lateral sclerosis. *Nature*, Vol. 465, No. 7295, (May 2010), pp. 223-226, ISSN 0028-0836

Nadal MS., et al. (2003). The CD26-related dipeptidyl aminopeptidase-like protein DPPX is a critical component of neuronal A-type K+ channels. *Neuron*, Vol. 37, No. 3, (February 2003), pp. 449-461, ISSN 0896-6273

Nandar W & Connor JR. (2011). HFE gene variants affect iron in the brain. *Journal of Nutrition*, Vol. 141, No. 4, (April 2011), pp. 729S-739S, ISSN 0022-3166

Nardelli B., et al. (2002). Regulatory effect of IFN-κ, a novel type I IFN, on cytokine production by cells of the innate immune system. *Journal of Immunology*, Vol. 169, No. 9, (November 2002), pp. 4822-4830, ISSN 0022-1767

Neumann M., et al. (2006). Ubiquitinated TDP-43 in frontotemporal lobar degeneration and amyotrophic lateral sclerosis. *Science*, Vol. 314, No. 5796, (October 2006), pp. 130-133, ISSN 1095-9203

Nishimura AL., et al. (2004). A mutation in the vesicle-trafficking protein VAPB causes late-onset spinal muscular atrophy and amyotrophic lateral sclerosis. *American Journal of Human Genetics*, Vol. 75, No. 5, (November 2004), pp. 822-831, ISSN 0002-9297

Nonis D., et al. (2008). Ataxin-2 associates with the endocytosis complex and affects EGF receptor trafficking. *Cellular Signalling*, Vol. 20, No. 10, (October 2008), pp. 1725-1739, ISSN

Ng CJ., et al. (2001). Paraoxonase-2 is a ubiquitously expressed protein with antioxidant properties and is capable of preventing cell-mediated oxidative modification of low density lipoprotein. *Journal of Biological Chemistry*, Vol. 276, No. 48, (November 2001), pp. 44444-44449, ISSN 0021-9258

Ng SB., et al. (2009). Targeted capture and massively parallel sequencing of 12 human exomes. *Nature*, Vol. 461, No. 7261, (September 2009), pp. 272-276, ISSN 0028-0836

Oosthuyse B., et al. (2001). Deletion of the hypoxia-response element in the vascular endothelial growth factor promoter causes motor neuron degeneration. *Nature Genetics*, Vol. 28, No. 2, (June 2001), pp. 131-138, ISSN 1061-4036

Orlacchio A., et al. (2010). SPATACSIN mutations cause autosomal recessive juvenile amyotrophic lateral sclerosis. *Brain*, Vol. 133, Pt. 2, (February 2010), pp. 591-598, ISSN 0006-8950

Orozco G, Barrett JC & Zeggini E. (2010). Synthetic associations in the context of genome-wide association scan signals. *Human Molecular Genetics*, Vol. 19, No. R2, (October 2010), pp. R137-R144, ISSN 0964-6906

Orrell RW., et al. (1997). The relationship of spinal muscular atrophy to motor neuron disease: investigation of SMN and NAIP gene deletions in sporadic and familial ALS. *Journal of Neurological Sciences*, Vol. 145, No. 1, (January 1997), pp. 55-61, ISSN 0022-510X

Otomo A., et al. (2003). ALS2, a novel guanine nucleotide exchange factor for the small GTPase Rab5, is implicated in endosomal dynamics. *Human Molecular Genetics*, Vol. 12, No. 14, (July 2003), pp. 1671-1687, ISSN 0964-6906

Parboosingh JS., et al. (1999). Deletions causing spinal muscular atrophy do not predispose to amyotrophic lateral sclerosis. *Archives of Neurology*, Vol. 56, No. 6, (June 1999), pp. 710-712, ISSN 0003-9942

Parkinson N., et al. (2006). ALS phenotypes with mutations in CHMP2B (charged multivesicular body protein 2B). *Neurology*, Vol. 67, No. 6, (September 2006), pp. 1074-1077, ISSN 0028-3878

Pasinelli P & Brown RH. (2006). Molecular biology of amyotrophic lateral sclerosis: insights from genetics. *Nature Reviews Neuroscience*, Vol. 7, No. 9, (September 2006), pp. 710-723, ISSN 1471-003X

Paubel A., et al. (2008). Mutations of the ANG gene in French patients with amyotrophic lateral sclerosis. *Archives of Neurology*, Vol. 65, No. 10, (October 2008), pp. 1333-1336, ISSN 0003-9942

Pearson JP., et al. (2010). Familial frontotemporal dementia with amyotrophic lateral sclerosis and a shared haplotype on chromosome 9p. *Journal of Neurology*, Vol. 258, No. 4, (April 2011), pp. 647-655, ISSN 0340-5354

Pestka S, Krause CD & Walter MR. (2004). Interferons, interferon-like cytokines, and their receptors. *Immunological reviews*, Vol. 202, (December 2004), pp. 8-32, ISSN 0105-2896

Phillips T & Robberecht W. (2010). Neuroinflammation in amyotrophic lateral sclerosis: role of glial activation in motor neuron disease. *Lancet Neurology*, Vol. 10, No. 3, (March 2010), pp. 253-263, ISSN 1474-4422

Puls I., et al. (2003). Mutant dynactin in motor neuron disease. *Nature Genetics*, Vol. 33, No. 4, (April 2003), pp. 455-456, ISSN 1061-4036

Puls I., et al. (2005). Distal spinal and bulbar muscular atrophy caused by dynactin mutation. *Annals of Neurology*, Vol. 57, No. 5, (May 2005), pp. 687-694, ISSN 0364-5134

Pulst SM., et al. (1996). Moderate expansion of a normally biallelic trinucleotide repeat in spinocerebellar ataxia type 2. *Nature Genetics*, Vol. 14, No. 3, (November 1996), pp. 269-276, ISSN 1061-4036

Ralser M., et al. (2004). An integrative approach to gain insights into the cellular function of human ataxin-2. *Journal of Molecular Biology*, Vol. 346, No. 1, (February 2005), pp. 203-214, ISSN 0022-2836

Reaume AG., et al. (1996). Motor neurons in Cu/Zn superoxide dismutase-deficient mice develop normally but exhibit enhanced cell death after axonal injury. *Nature Genetics*, Vol. 13, No. 1, (May 1996), pp. 43-47, ISSN 1061-4036

Renton AE et al. (2011). A hexanucleotide repeat expansion in C9ORF72 is the cause of chromosome 9p21-linked ALS-FTD. *Neuron*, September 2011, Ahead of print

Restagno G., et al. (2007). HFE H63D polymorphism is increate in patients with amyotrophic lateral sclerosis of Italian origin. *Journal of Neurology, Neurosurgery and Psychiatry*, Vol. 78, No. 3, (March 2007), pp. 327, ISSN 0022-3050

Rezaie T., et al. (2002). Adult-onset primary open-angle glaucoma caused by mutations in optineurin. *Science*, Vol. 295, No. 5557, (February 2002), pp.1077-1079, ISSN 1095-9203

Ricci C., et al. (2010). Lack of association of PON polymorphisms with sporadic ALS in an Italian population. *Neurobiology of Aging*, Vol. 32, No. 3, (March 2011), pp. 552.e7-13, ISSN 1558-1497

Ringholz GM., et al. (2005). Prevalence and patterns of cognitive impairment in sporadic ALS. *Neurology*, Vol. 65, No. 4, (August 2005), pp. 586-590, ISSN 0028-3878

Robertson J., et al. (2003). A neurotoxic peripherin splice variant in a mouse model of ALS. *Journal of Cell Biology*, Vol. 160, No. 6, (March 2003), pp. 939-949, ISSN 0021-9525

Rollinson S., et al. (2011). Frontotemporal lobar degeneration genome wide association study replication confirms a risk locus shared with amyotrophic lateral sclerosis. *Neurobiology of Aging*, Vol. 32, No. 4, (April 2011), pp. 758.e1-7, ISSN 0197-4580

Rooke K., et al. (1996). Analysis of the KSP repeat of the neurofilament heavy subunit in familial amyotrophic lateral sclerosis. *Neurology*, Vol. 46, No. 3, (March 1996), pp. 789-790, ISSN 0028-3878

Rosen DR., et al. (1993). Mutations in Cu/Zn superoxide dismutase gene are associated with familial amyotrophic lateral sclerosis. *Nature*, Vol. 362, No. 6415, (March 1993), pp. 59-62, ISSN 0028-0836

Ross OA., et al. (2011). Ataxin-2 repeat-length variation and neurodegeneration. *Human Molecular Genetics*, Vol. 20, No. 16, (August 2011), pp. 3207-3212, ISSN 0964-6906

Rual JF., et al. (2005). Towards a proteome-scale map of the human protein-protein interaction network. *Nature*, Vol. 437, No. 7062, (October 2005), pp. 1173-1178, ISSN 0028-0836

Rutherford AC., et al. (2006). The mammalian phosphatidylinositol 3-phosphate 5-kinase (PIKfyve) regulates endosome-to-TGN retrograde transport. *Journal of Cell Science*, Vol. 119, Pt. 19, (October 2006), pp. 3944-3957, ISSN 0021-9533

Saeed M., et al. (2006). Paraoxonase cluster polymorphisms are associated with sporadic ALS. *Neurology*, Vol. 67, No. 5, (September 2006), pp. 771-776, ISSN 0028-3878

Sahlender DA., et al. (2005). Optineurin links myosin VI to the Golgi complex and is involved in Golgi organization and exocytosis. *Journal of Cell Biology*, Vol. 169, No. 2, (April 2005), pp. 285-295, ISSN 0021-9525

Salinas S., et al. (2008). Heriditary spastic paraplegia: clinical features and pathogenic mechanisms. *Lancet Neurology*, Vol. 7, No. 12, (December 2008), pp. 1127-1138, ISSN 1474-4422

Sanpei K., et al. (1996). Identification of the spinocerebellar ataxia type 2 gene using a direct identification of repeat expansion and cloning technique, DIRECT. *Nature Genetics*, Vol. 14, No. 3, (November 1996), pp. 277-284, ISSN 1061-4036

Sapp PC., et al. (2003). Identification of two novel loci for dominantly inherited familial amyotrophic lateral sclerosis. *American Journal of Human Genetics*, Vol. 73, No. 2, (August 2003), pp. 397-403, ISSN 0002-9297

Schmitt-John T., et al. (2005). Mutation of Vps54 causes motor neuron disease and defective spermiogenesis in the wobbler mouse. *Nature Genetics*, Vol. 37, No. 11, (November 2005), pp. 1213-1215, ISSN 1061-4036

Schymick JC., et al. (2007). Genome-wide genotyping in amyotrophic lateral sclerosis and neurologically normal controls: first stage analysis and public release of data. *Lancet Neurology*, Vol. 6, No. 4, (April 2007), pp. 322-328, ISSN 1474-4422

Sebastià J., et al. (2009). Angiogenin protects motoneurons against hypoxic injury. *Cell Death and Differentiation*, Vol. 16, No. 9, (September 2009), pp. 1238-1247, ISSN 1350-9047

Shaikh AY & Martin LJ. (2002). DNA base-excision repair enzyme apurinic/apyrimidinic endonuclease/redox factor-1 is increased and competent in the brain and spinal cord of individuals with amyotrophic lateral sclerosis. *Neuromolecular Medicine*, Vol. 2, No. 1, (2002), pp. 47-60, ISSN 1535-1084

Shatunov A., et al. (2010). Chromosome 9p21 in sporadic amyotrophic lateral sclerosis in the UK and seven other countries: a genome-wide association study. *Lancet Neurology*, Vol. 9, No. 10, (October 2010), pp. 986-994, ISSN 1474-4422

Shin JS., et al. (2008). NEFL Pro22Arg mutation in Charcot-Marie-Tooth disease type 1. *Journal of Human Genetics*, Vol. 53, No. 10, (2008), pp. 936-940, ISSN 1434-5161

Siddique T., et al. (1998). X-linked dominant locus for late-onset familial amyotrophic lateral sclerosis. *American Journal of Human Genetics*, Vol. 63, Suppl. A308.

Skibinski G., et al. (2005). Mutations in the endosomal ESCRTIII-complex subunit CHMP2B in frontotemporal dementia. *Nature Genetics*, Vol. 37, No. 8, (August 2005), pp. 806-808, ISSN 1061-4036

Skourti-Stathaki K, Proudfoot NJ & Gromak N. (2011). Human senataxin resolves RNA/DNA hybrids formed at transcriptional pause sites to promote Xrn2-dependent termination. *Molecular Cell*, Vol. 42, No. 6, (June 2011), pp. 794-805, ISSN 1097-2765

Skvortsova V., et al. (2004). Analysis of heavy neurofilament subunit gene polymorphism in Russian patients with sporadic motor neuron disease (MND). *European Journal of Human Genetics*, Vol. 12, No. 3, (March 2004), pp. 241-244, ISSN 1018-4813

Slowik A., et al. (2006). Paraoxonase gene polymorphisms and sporadic ALS. *Neurology*, Vol. 67, No. 5, (September 2006), pp. 766-770, ISSN 0028-3878

Sreedharan J., et al. (2008). TDP-43 mutations in familial and sporadic amytrophic lateral sclerosis. *Science*, Vol. 319, No. 5870, (March 2008), pp. 1668-1672, ISSN 1095-9203

Stevanin G., et al. (2007). Mutations in SPG11, encoding spatacsin, are a major cause of spastic paraplegia with thin corpus callosum. *Nature Genetics*, Vol. 39, No. 3, (March 2007), pp. 366-372, ISSN 1061-4036

Storkebaum E., et al. (2005). Treatment of motoneuron degeneration by intracerebroventricular delivery of VEGF in a rat model of ALS. *Nature Neuroscience*, Vol. 8, No. 1, (January 2005), pp. 85-92, ISSN 1097-6256

Subramanian V, Crabtree B & Acharya KR. (2007). Human angiogenin is a neuroprotective factor and amyotrophic lateral sclerosis associated angiogenin variants affect neurite extension/pathfinding and survival of motor neurons. *Human Molecular Genetics*, Vol. 17, No. 1, (January 2008), pp. 130-149, ISSN 0964-6906

Sugihara K., et al. (2011). Screening for OPTN mutations in amyotrophic lateral sclerosis in a mainly Caucasian population. *Neurobioloy of Aging*, Vol. 32, No. 10, (October 2011), pp. 1923.e9-1923.e10, ISSN 1558-1497

Sun Z., et al. (2011). Molecular determinants and genetic modifiers of aggregation and toxicity for the ALS disease proten FUS/TLS. *PLoS Biology*, Vol. 9, No. 4, (April 2011), pp. e1000614, ISSN 1545-7885

Sutedja NA., et al. (2007). The association between H63D mutations in HFE and amyotrophic lateral sclerosis in a Dutch population. *Archives of Neurology*, Vol. 64, No. 1, (January 2007), pp. 63-67, ISSN 0003-9942

Swarup V., et al. (2011). Pathological hallmarks of amyotrophic lateral sclerosis/frontotemporal lobar degeneration in transgenic mice produced with TDP-43 genomic fragments. *Brain*, 2011, Ahead of print.

Takeda S., et al. (2000). Kinesin superfamily protein 3 (KIF3) motor transports fodrin-associating vesicles important for neurite building. *Journal of Cell Biology*, Vol. 148, No. 6, (March 2000), pp. 1255-1265, ISSN 0021-9525

Terry PD., et al. (2004). VEGF promoter haplotype and amyotrophic lateral sclerosis (ALS). *Journal of Neurogenetics*, Vol. 18, No. 2, (April-June 2004), pp. 429-434, ISSN 0167-7063

Teuling E., et al. (2007). Motor neuron disease-associated mutant vesicle-associated membrane protein-associated protein (VAP) B recruits wild-type VAPs into endoplasmatic reticulum-derived tubular aggregates. *Journal of Neuroscience*, Vol. 27, No. 36, (September 2007), pp. 9801-9815, ISSN 0270-6474

Ticozzi N., et al. (2009). Mutational analysis of TARDBP in neurodegenerative disease. *Neurobiology of Aging*, 2009, Ahead of print.

Ticozzi N., et al. (2011). Mutational analysis reveals the FUS homolog TAF15 as a candidate gene for familial amyotrophic lateral sclerosis. *American Journal of Medical Genetics B: Neuropsychiatric Genetics*, Vol. 156B, No. 3, (April 2011), pp. 285-290, ISSN 1552-485X

Tomkins J., et al. (2000). Screening of AP endonuclease as a candidate gene for amyotrophic lateral sclerosis (ALS). *Neuroreport*, Vol.11, No. 8 (June 2000), pp. 1695-1697, ISSN 0959-4965

Topp JD., et al. (2004). Alsin is a Rab5 and Rac1 guanine nucleotide exchange factor. *Journal of Biological Chemistry*, Vol. 279, No. 23, (June 2004), pp. 24612-24623, ISSN 0021-9258

Troy CM., et al. (1990). Regulation of peripherin and neurofilaments expression in regenerating rat motor neurons. *Brain Research*, Vol. 529, No. 1-2, (October 1990), pp. 232-238, ISSN 0006-8993

Tudor EL., et al. (2010). Amyotrophic lateral sclerosis mutant vesicle-associated membrane protein-associated protein-B transgenic mice develop TAR-DNA-binding protein-43 pathology. *Neuroscience*, Vol. 167, No. 3, (May 2010), pp. 774-785, ISSN 0306-4522

Valdmanis PN., et al. (2007). Three families with amyotrophic lateral sclerosis and frontotemporal dementia with evidence of linkage to chromosome 9p. *Archives of Neurology*, Vol. 64, No. 2, (February 2007), pp. 240-245, ISSN 0003-9942

Valdmanis PN., et al. (2008). Association of paraoxonase gene cluster polymorphisms with ALS in France, Quebec, and Sweden. *Neurology*, Vol. 71, No. 7, (August 2008), pp. 514-520, ISSN 0028-3878

Valdmanis PN & Rouleau GA. (2008). Genetics of familial amyotrophic lateral sclerosis. *Neurology*, Vol. 70, No. 2, (January 2008), pp. 144-152, ISSN 0028-3878

Van Blitterswijk M., et al. (2011). Novel optineurin mutations in sporadic amyotrophic lateral sclerosis patients. *Neurobiology of Aging*, Ahead of print, ISSN 0197-4580

Vance C., et al. (2006). Familial amyotrophic lateral sclerosis with frontotemporal dementia is linked to a locus on chromosome 9p13.2-21.3. *Brain*, Vol. 129, No. 4, (April 2006), pp. 868-876, ISSN 0006-8950

Vance C., et al. (2009). Mutations in FUS, an RNA processing protein, cause familial amyotrophic lateral sclerosis type 6. *Science*, Vol. 323, No. 5918, (February 2009), pp. 1208-1211, ISSN 1095-9203

Van Damme P., et al. (2011). Expanded ATXN2 CAG repeat size in ALS identifies genetic overlap between ALS and SCA2. *Neurology*, Vol. 76, No. 24, (June 2011), pp. 2066-2072, ISSN 0028-3878

Van Deerlin VM., et al. (2008). TARDBP mutations in amyotrophic lateral sclerosis with TDP-43 neuropathology: a genetic and histopathological analysis. *Lancet Neurology*, Vol. 7, No. 5, (May 2008), pp. 409-416, ISSN 1474-4422

Van Deerlin VM., et al. (2010) Common variants at 7p21 are associated with frontotemporal lobar degeneration with TDP-43 inclusions. *Nature Genetics*, Vol. 42, No. 3, (March 2010), pp. 234-239, ISSN 1061-4036

Van Es MA., et al. (2007). ITPR2 as a susceptibility gene in sporadic amyotrophic lateral sclerosis: a genome-wide association study. *Lancet Neurology*, Vol. 6, No. 10, (October 2007), pp. 869-877, ISSN 1474-4422

Van Es MA., et al. (2008). Genetic variation in DPP6 is associated with susceptibility to amyotrophic lateral sclerosis. *Nature Genetics*, Vol. 40, No. 1, (January 2008), pp. 29-31, ISSN 1061-4036

Van Es MA., et al. (2009). A case of ALS-FTD in a large FALS pedigree with a K17I ANG mutation. *Neurology*, Vol. 72, No. 3, (January 2009), pp. 287-288, ISSN 0028-3878

Van Es MA., et al. (2009). Analysis of FGGY as a risk factor for sporadic amyotrophic lateral sclerosis. *Amyotrophic Lateral Sclerosis*, Vol. 10, No. 5-6, (October-December 2009), pp 441-447, ISSN 1748-2968

Van Es MA., et al. (2009). Genome-wide association study identifies 19p13.11 (UNC13A) and 9p21.2 as susceptibility loci for sporadic amyotrophic lateral sclerosis. *Nature Genetics*, Vol. 41, No. 10 (October 2009), pp. 1083-1087, ISSN 1061-4036

Van Es MA., et al. (2011). Angiogenin variants in Parkinson's disease and amyotrophic lateral sclerosis. *Annals of Neurology*, 2011:Ahead of print

Van Vught PW., et al. (2005). Lack of association between VEGF polymorphisms and ALS in a Dutch population. *Neurology*, Vol. 65, No. 10, (November 2005), pp. 1643-1645, ISSN 0028-3878

Vantaggiato C., et al. (2011). Senataaxin modulates neurite growth through fibroblast growth factor 8 signalling. *Brain*, Vol. 134, Pt. 6, (June 2011), pp. 1808-1828, ISSN 0006-8950

Varoqueaux F., et al. (2002). Total arrest of spontaneous and evoked synaptic transmission but normal synaptogenesis in the absence of Munc13-mediated vesicle priming. *Proceedings of the National Academy of Sciences of the United States of America*, Vol. 99, No. 13, (June 2002), pp. 9037-9042, ISSN 0027-8424

Varoqueaux F., et al. (2005). Aberrant morphology and residual transmitter release at the Munc13-deficient mouse neuromuscular synapse. *Molecular and Cellular Biology*, Vol. 25, No. 14, (July 2005), pp. 5973-5984, ISSN 0270-7306

Veldink JH., et al. (2001). Homozygous deletion of the survival motor neuron 2 gene is a prognostic factor in sporadic ALS. *Neurology*, Vol. 56, No. 6, (March 2001), pp. 749-752, ISSN 0028-3878

Veldink JH., et al. (2005). SMN genotypes producing less SMN protein increase susceptibility to and severity of sporadic ALS. *Neurology*, Vol. 65, No. 6, (September 2005), pp. 820-825, ISSN 0028-3878

Vilariño-Güell C., et al. (2009). Characterization of DCTN1 genetic variability in neurodegeneration. *Neurology*, Vol. 72, No. 23, (June 2009), pp. 2024-2028, ISSN 0028-3878

Wang XS., et al. (2004). Increased incidence of the Hfe mutation in amyotrophic lateral sclerosis and related cellular consequences. *Journal of the Neurological Sciences*, Vol. 227, No. 1 (December 2004), pp. 27-33, ISSN 0022-510X

Wang Y., et al. (2007). Vascular endothelial growth factor overexpression delays neurodegeneration and prolongs survival in amyotrophic lateral sclerosis mice. *Journal of Neuroscience*, Vol. 27, No. 2, (January 2007), pp. 304-307, ISSN 0270-6474

Wang J, Campbell IL & Zhang H. (2007). Systemic interferon-alpha regulates interferon-stimulated genes in the central nervous system. *Molecular Psychiatry*, Vol. 13, No. 3, (March 2008), pp. 293-301, ISSN 1359-4184

Watts GD., et al. (2004). Inclusion body myopathy associated with Paget disease of bone and frontotemporal dementia is caused by mutant valosin-containing protein. *Nature Genetics*, Vol. 36, No. 4, (April 2004), pp. 377-381, ISSN 1061-4036

Weihl CC., et al. (2008). TDP-43 accumulation in inclusion body myopathy muscle suggests a common pathogenic mechanism with frontotemporal dementia. *Journal of Neurology, Neurosurgery and Psychiatry*, Vol. 79, No. 10, (October 2008), pp. 1186-1189, ISSN 0022-3050

Williamson TL., et al. (1998). Absence of neurofilaments reduce the selective vulnerability of motor neurons and slows disease caused by a familial amyotrophic lateral sclerosis-linked superoxide dismutase 1 mutant. *Proceedings of the National Academy of Sciences of the USA*, Vol. 95, No. 16, (August 1998), pp. 9631-9636, ISSN 0027-8424

Wills AM., et al. (2009). A large-scale international meta-analysis of paraoxonase gene polymorphisms in sporadic ALS. *Neurology*, Vol. 73, No. 1, (July 2009), pp. 16-24, ISSN 0028-3878

Wu D., et al. (2007). Angiongenin loss-of-function mutations in amyotrophic lateral sclerosis. *Annals of Neurology*, Vol. 62, No. 6, (December 2007), pp. 609-617, ISSN 0364-5134

Xiao S., et al. (2008). An aggregate-inducing peripherin isoform generated through intron retention is upregulated in amyotrophic lateral sclerosis and associated with disease pathology. *Journal of Neuroscience*, Vol. 28, No. 8, (February 2008), pp. 1833-1840, ISSN 0270-6474

Yamasaki S., et al. (2009). Angiogenin cleaves tRNA and promotes stress-induced translational repression. *Journal of Cell Biology*, Vol. 185, No. 1, (April 2009), pp. 35-42, ISSN 0021-9525

Yan J., et al. (2006). A major novel locus for ALS/FTD on chromosome 9p21 and its pathological correlates. *Neurology*, Vol. 67, No. 1, (July 2006), pp. 186-186b, ISSN 0028-3878

Yan J., et al. (2010). Frameshift and novel mutations in FUS in familial amyotrophic lateral sclerosis and ALS/dementia. *Neurology*, Vol. 75, No. 9, (August 2010), pp. 807-814, ISSN 0028-3878

Yang Y., et al. (2001). The gene encoding alsin, a protein with three guanine-nucleotide exchange factor domains, is mutated in a form of recessive amyotrophic lateral sclerosis. *Nature Genetics*, Vol. 29, No. 2, (October 2001), pp. 160-165, ISSN 1061-4036

Yen AA., et al. (2004). HFE mutations are not strongly associated with sporadic ALS. *Neurology*, Vol. 62, No. 9, (May 2004), pp. 1611-1612, ISSN 0028-3878

Zawiślak D., et al. (2010). The −A162G polymorphism of the PON1 gene and the risk of sporadic amyotrophic lateral sclerosis. *Neurologia I Neurochirurgia Polska*, Vol. 44, No. 3, (May 2010), pp. 246-250, ISSN 0028-3843 (Abstract)

Zhang Y., et al. (2006). VEGF C2578A polymorphism does not contribute to amyotrophic lateral sclerosis susceptibility in sporadic Chinese patients. *Amyotrophic Lateral Sclerosis*, Vol. 7, No. 2, (June 2006), pp. 119-122, ISSN 1748-2968

Zhang Y., et al. (2007). Loss of Vac14, a regulator of the signaling lipid phosphatidylinositol 3,5-biphosphate, results in neurodegeneration in mice. *Proceedings of the National Academy of Sciences of the USA*, Vol. 104, No. 44, (October 2007), pp. 17518-17523, ISSN 0027-8424

Zhao ZH., et al. (2009). A novel mutation in the senataxin gene identified in a Chinese patient with sporadic amyotrophic lateral sclerosis. *Amyotrophic Lateral Sclerosis*, Vol. 10, No. 2, (April 2009), pp. 118-122, ISSN 1748-2968

8

A Major Genetic Factor at Chromosome 9p Implicated in Amyotrophic Lateral Sclerosis (ALS) and Frontotemporal Lobar Degeneration (FTLD)

Ilse Gijselinck[1,2], Kristel Sleegers[1,2],
Christine Van Broeckhoven[1,2] and Marc Cruts[1,2]
[1]Department of Molecular Genetics, VIB, Antwerpen
[2]University of Antwerp, Antwerpen
Belgium

1. Introduction

Amyotrophic lateral sclerosis (ALS) and frontotemporal lobar degeneration (FTLD) are two fatal neurodegenerative diseases for which effective therapies aiming at delaying, halting or preventing the disease are lacking. ALS is the most common motor neuron disorder (Rowland & Shneider, 2001) and FTLD has a prevalence close to that of Alzheimer disease in the population below age 65 years (Rosso et al., 2003). They are considered as both extremes of a spectrum of clinically and pathologically overlapping disorders (Lillo & Hodges, 2009). In addition, there is emerging evidence that FTLD and ALS also share common genetic aetiologies, suggesting that overlapping disease mechanisms are involved in both diseases. Clinically, ALS patients show reduced control of voluntary muscle movement expressed in increased muscle weakness, disturbances of speech, swallowing or breathing, as a result of progressive upper and lower motor neuron degeneration in motor cortex, brainstem and spinal cord, and up to 50% of ALS patients shows mild disturbances in executive functions while a minority also develop overt FTLD (Lomen-Hoerth et al., 2003; Ringholz et al., 2005). FTLD symptoms include behavioural, personality and language disturbances, and also cognitive dysfunctions, due to affected frontal and temporal cortical neurons in the brain. FTLD patients may additionally present with typical clinical signs of ALS in a later stage of the disease (Neary et al., 1998). Pathologically, although in different neuronal cells, TAR DNA-binding protein-43 (TDP-43) is a major constituent of neuronal deposits in both ALS and TDP-43 positive FTLD (FTLD-TDP), the most common pathological FTLD subtype (Arai et al., 2006; Neumann et al., 2006). Five to 10% of ALS patients and up to 50% of FTLD patients has a positive familial history of disease with a Mendelian mode of inheritance indicating a significant contribution of genetic factors in disease aetiology. Although the exact biochemical pathways involved in ALS or FTLD are still unknown, several molecular components were identified in the last twenty years through molecular genetic studies in familial and sporadic patients, which are most likely part of a complex network of cellular mechanisms. Since these genes explain only a minority of patients, further unraveling the genetic heterogeneity is necessary to identify new therapeutic targets. Mutations causing ALS were observed in genes encoding Cu/Zn superoxide dismutase 1 (*SOD1*) (Rosen et al., 1993), TDP-43 (*TARDBP*) (Gitcho et al., 2008; Kabashi et al., 2008; Sreedharan et al., 2008; Van Deerlin et al., 2008; Yokoseki et al., 2008), fused in sarcoma (*FUS*) (Kwiatkowski, Jr. et al., 2009; Vance et al., 2009) and angiogenin (*ANG*) (Greenway et al., 2006), among other genes, while in familial FTLD patients mutations in the genes encoding granulin (*GRN*) (Baker et al., 2006; Cruts et al., 2006), the microtubule-associated protein tau (*MAPT*) (Hutton et al., 1998), the valosin-containing protein (*VCP*) (Watts et al., 2004) and the charged multivesicular body protein 2B (*CHMP2B*) (Skibinski et al., 2005) were found. Recent family-based linkage and population-based association studies identified genetic factors overlapping between ALS and FTLD. For example, mutations in the ALS genes *TARDBP* and *FUS* are occasionally found in FTLD patients (Kovacs et al., 2009; Van Langenhove et al., 2010) and mutations in the FTLD gene *VCP* were also detected in ALS (Johnson et al., 2010). However, most convincing evidence for the genetic overlap comes from the observation that both ALS and FTLD can occur within the same family or within a single patient of a family. More than 15 autosomal dominant families with ALS and FTLD worldwide are causally linked with a major disease locus at chromosome 9p13-p21 (ALSFTD2 locus) (Boxer et al., 2010; Gijselinck et al., 2010; Le Ber et al., 2009; Luty et al., 2008; Momeni et al., 2006; Morita et al., 2006; Pearson et al., 2011; Valdmanis et al., 2007; Vance et al., 2006). The minimally linked region in all these families is about 3.6 Mb in size containing five known protein-coding genes. Moreover, several recent genome-wide association studies (GWAS) in ALS populations from different European origins showed the presence of a major genetic risk factor for ALS at the same chromosome 9p region (Laaksovirta et al., 2010; Shatunov et al., 2010; van Es et al., 2009). The Finnish study narrowed the associated region to a 232 kb linkage disequilibrium (LD) block containing three known genes (*MOBKL2B*, *IFNK*, *C9orf72*) and suggested the presence of a major risk gene with high penetrance (Laaksovirta et al., 2010). Likewise, a GWAS in FTLD has implicated the same region (Van Deerlin et al., 2010). This finding was further confirmed in other FTLD and ALS-FTLD cohorts (Rollinson et al., 2011). Together, these data demonstrate that ALS and FTLD share a major common genetic factor on chromosome 9p, most likely showing high mutation frequencies. Despite all attempts of several research groups, the genetic defect(s) underlying both genetic linkage and association to this region have not been identified yet.

In this book chapter we will report and discuss the latest findings in the studies aiming at identifying the chromosome 9 gene defect.

2. Family-based linkage to ALSFTD2 locus on chromosome 9p

Since the original reports of a Dutch and a Scandinavian ALS-FTLD family linked with chromosome 9p21 (Morita et al., 2006; Vance et al., 2006), a growing number of families with inherited ALS and FTLD are reported with significant linkage to the ALSFTD2 locus on chromosome 9p21 (Boxer et al., 2010; Gijselinck et al., 2010; Le Ber et al., 2009; Luty et al., 2008; Valdmanis et al., 2007) (table 1). In all these families patients show similar clinical and pathological characteristics. Clinically, individuals may present with symptoms of both ALS and FTLD, or with ALS or FTLD alone. Pathologically, autopsied patients have TDP-43 positive type 2 (Sampathu et al., 2006) brain inclusions (Boxer et al., 2010; Gijselinck et al., 2010; Le Ber et al., 2009; Luty et al., 2008; Morita et al., 2006; Vance et al., 2006). (table 1)

The minimal candidate region was previously defined by D9S169 (Luty et al., 2008) and D9S1805 (Valdmanis et al., 2007) spanning 7 Mb and was recently reduced to 3.6 Mb between D9S169 (Luty et al., 2008) and D9S251 by Boxer and colleagues (2010) (figure 1). Therefore, several parts of this study were still investigated in the 7 Mb region.

Family	Origin	Max LOD score at 9p21	Mean onset age in years (range)	Mean disease duration in years (range)	TDP-43+	# ALS	# ALS + FTLD	# FTLD	References
Luty	Australian	3.41	53 (43-68)	9 (1-16)	+	2	2	7	(Luty et al., 2008)
DR14	Belgian	3.38	58.1 (51-65)	6.4 (1-17)	+	1	0	10	(Gijselinck et al., 2010)
F2	Dutch	3.02	60.3 (39-72)	3.0 (1-8)	ND	7	3	2	(Vance et al., 2006)
Que23	Canadian	3.01	55.8 (46-58)	2.4 (1.5-3)	ND	5	0	3	(Valdmanis et al., 2007)
VSM20	Irish	3.01	45.7 (35-57)	5.4 (3-10)	+	2	3	5	(Boxer et al., 2010)
F438	Scandinavian	3.00	55.3 (45-64)	4.3 (1-9)	ND	5	0	9	(Morita et al., 2006)
6 families	French	8.0[1]	57.9 (40-84)	3.6 (1-8)	+	9	12	10	(Le Ber et al., 2009)
Que1	French-Canadian	2.51	54.3 (45-63)	4.8 (2-9)	ND	5	3	0	(Valdmanis et al., 2007)
Fr104	Spanish	1.55	ND	ND	ND	4	1	0	(Valdmanis et al., 2007)
F2	North-American	1.5	ND	ND	ND	0	7	0	(Momeni et al., 2006)
Gwent	Brittish	ND	42.2 (31-52)	3.6 (1-13)	+	3	6	0	(Pearson et al., 2011)
F476	North-American	ND	ND	ND	ND	2	3	0	(Momeni et al., 2006)
ALS_A	American	ND	? (35-73)	? (0.5-5)	ND	6	0	0	(Krueger et al., 2009)

Table 1. Genetic, clinical and pathological characteristics of ALS-FTLD families linked or associated with chromosome 9p21 (ND: not determined; [1]summed LODscore in 6 small families, not linked separately)

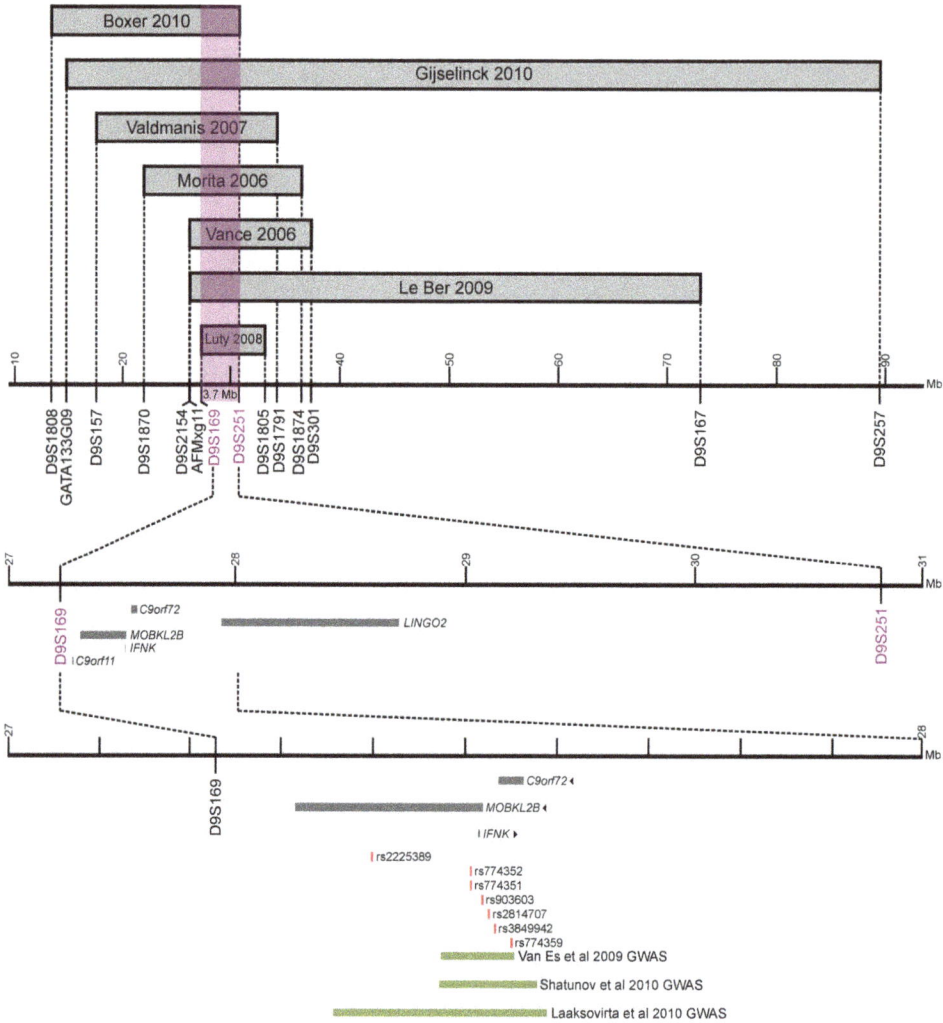

Fig. 1. Schematic representation of the chromosome 9p21 ALS-FTLD locus. Upper panel: grey bars indicate the minimal candidate regions in all reported significantly linked ALS-FTLD families, defining a minimal interval of 3.7 Mb between D9S169 and D9S251 containing five protein coding genes, illustrated with grey lines. Lower panel: associated SNPs in ALS and FTLD GWAS are shown in red and LD blocks or finemapped regions of these GWAS are indicated with green lines. Three genes are located in the associated region.

2.1 Family DR14

We studied a Belgian 4-generation family (family DR14) with autosomal dominant transmission of ALS and FTLD. We collected DNA from 29 family members of whom 3 patients in generation III and 11 at-risk individuals in generation III and IV each (figure 1). Two patients (III.2 and III.12) were diagnosed with FTLD (subtype FTD), while patient III.10 was diagnosed with ALS (figure 2). The mean age at onset was 58.1 ± 4.2 years (N = 9, range 51-65 years) and mean disease duration was 6.4 ± 4.9 years (range 1-17 years). The index patient was clinically diagnosed with familial FTLD (subtype FTD) and pathological TDP-43 positive inclusions were observed in the brain (FTLD-TDP type 2 (Sampathu et al., 2006)). Mutations in the known genes for ALS and dementia were excluded. (Gijselinck et al., 2010)

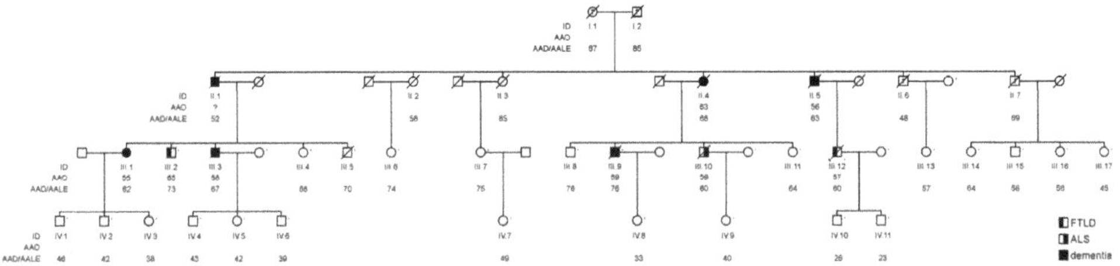

Fig. 2. The pedigree of DR14 consists of four generations. Left-filled and right-filled symbols represent patients with FTLD and ALS respectively. Patients with unspecified dementia are indicated with filled symbols. Open symbols represent unaffected individuals or at-risk individuals with unknown phenotype. Individuals with unclear phenotype are designated with a question mark (?). The arrow indicates index patient III.12. Numbers below the symbols denote age at onset and age at death (AAD) for patients and either age at last examination (AALE) or AAD for unaffected individuals or individuals with unknown phenotype. An asterisk (*) indicates individuals of whom DNA was available.

2.2 Mutation analyses of known genes and conserved regions, and CNV analysis

We performed a genome-wide scan using an in-house developed mapping set of 425 microsatellite markers in 30 multiplex panels with an average distance of 8 cM. Multipoint LOD scores were calculated revealing two loci on chromosome 9 and 14: one at chromosome 9 with a maximal LOD score of 2.71 between D9S1121 and D9S270 and one at chromosome 14 with the highest LOD score of 2.61 between D14S302 and D14S611. Finemapping of the chromosome 9 locus resulted in a significant maximal multipoint LOD score of 3.38 between D9S1833 and D9S1121 at 9p21 and segregation analysis defined a candidate region of 64.6 cM (74.7 Mb) between markers D9S235 and D9S257 on chromosome 9p23-9q21, based on two obligate recombinants (figure 3), harboring 271 protein coding genes (Gijselinck et al., 2010). This region overlaps with the ALSFTD2 locus at chromosome 9p21 but did not reduce the minimally linked region. Therefore, we analyzed the 7 Mb overlap region, including the minimal locus of 3.6 Mb, for mutations. We sequenced all 27 protein-coding genes, either the complete coding sequence of cDNA (N=17) including *MOBKL2B, C9orf72, ACO1, DDX58, TOPORS, NDUFB6, DNAJA1, SMU1, B4GALT1, BAG1, CHMP5, AQP3, NOL6, UBE2R2, UBAP2, WDR40A* and *UBAP1,* or the exons and exon-intron boundaries on gDNA using classical sequencing (N=10). cDNA was prepared from lymphoblasts of two patients and two healthy control individuals of the family not carrying the disease haplotype, treated with or without cycloheximide allowing also the detection of degraded aberrant transcripts.

Mutation analysis on cDNA allows not only detecting simple point mutations and small insertions/deletions but also exon deletions/duplications and alternative transcripts. Similar to other chr9-linked ALS-FTLD families, this mutation analysis did not reveal patient-specific novel variants segregating with disease.

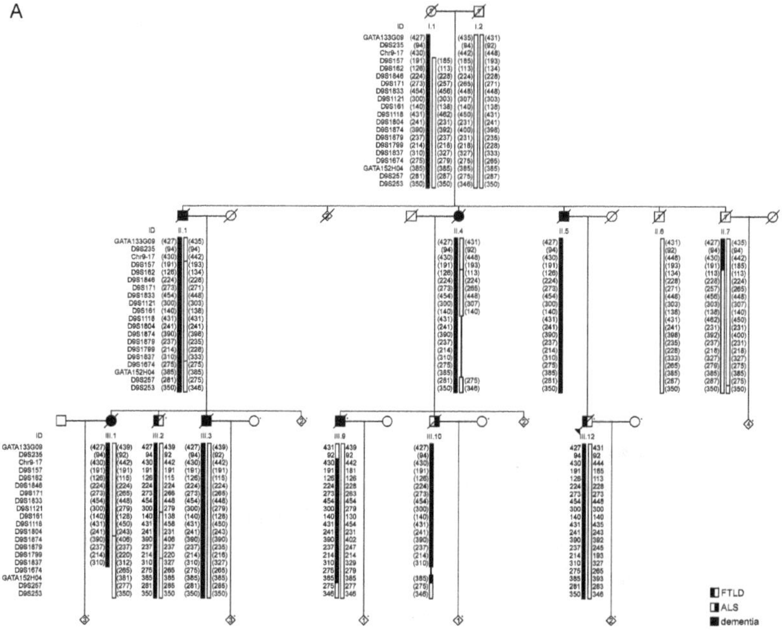

Fig. 3. Segregation of the 9p23-q21 haplotype in family DR14. Haplotypes are based on a selection of 20 informative STR markers at chromosome 9. The black haplotype represents the disease haplotype. Haplotypes for deceased individuals were inferred based on genotype data obtained in their offspring (between brackets). The disease haplotype was arbitrarily set for I.1, and numbers in diamonds indicate the number of genotyped at-risk individuals. An asterisk (*) indicates individuals of whom DNA was available.

Since all coding exons of known genes were excluded for mutations, we selected other evolutionary conserved regions and investigated these sequences for the presence of non-coding variants in evolutionary constrained regulatory elements, e.g. promoters and distant regulatory elements or conserved epigenetic sequence motifs, or coding variants in unknown novel genes (protein coding or non-coding RNA genes). Using the UCSC-PhastCons-mammalian-28way track predicting and scoring the presence of conserved elements in the genome by comparing the sequence between 28 mammalian species, we defined 149 kb of conserved elements throughout the ALSFTD2 locus of 7 Mb. These elements were grouped in 1108 clusters with a total sequence of 465 kb and ranked according to conservation strength. We performed sanger sequencing in two patients and two healthy control individuals of the family not carrying the disease haplotype. In total we sequenced 95 kb of highest conserved elements (total of 260 kb clusters) in the 7 Mb region, not revealing patient-specific novel variants segregating with disease. Of these, 61 kb of conserved regions are located in the minimal candidate region of 3.6 Mb. Using this approach, we excluded mutations in highly conserved regions. However, we did not exclude variants in regions with no or low conservation in mammalian species because it is well known that a substantial number of primate/human-specific exons exist (e.g. Sela et al., 2007) and that the location of regulatory elements is not always highly conserved, even not in mammals e.g. between human and mouse (Ravasi et al., 2010).

In addition, we performed chromosome-specific oligo-based array-comparative genomic hybridization (array-CGH, Nimblegen) at chromosome 9 with a resolution of about 1kb, on the index patient and an independent control individual not carrying the disease haplotype to detect copy number variations (CNVs). The CGH data were analyzed by Signalmap software (Nimblegen) and the scoring program CGHcall, revealing one large CNV (chr9:29082732-29087816) covered by 20 CGH probes. This deletion was confirmed in the index patient by six qPCR fragments demonstrating a deleted region of at least 5273 bp (chr9:29082677-29087949) (data not shown). It did not segregate with disease in DR14 and represented a polymorphism since it was also present in individuals not carrying the disease haplotype and since a frequent CNV had previously been reported at this position (chr9:29082445-29088195) (Cooper et al., 2008). Consequently, these experiments failed to identify a copy number mutation (deletion or insertion) of more than 1 kb (Gijselinck et al., 2010). Cytogenetics excluded large chromosomal rearrangements.

Since all these mutation analyses did not reveal the causal mutation, we hypothesized that the mutation is most likely unusual with respect to location (extragenic or intronic) and/or type (small indel, inversion or other complex rearrangement). Therefore, we performed whole genome sequencing in family DR14 and subsequently analyzed sequences or variants in the linked region.

2.3 Whole genome sequencing

The complete genome sequence of four chromosome 9p disease haplotype carriers of family DR14, including two patients and two asymptomatic individuals was determined using next generation sequencing technology. These family members were selected such that they have a different unaffected haplotype. The sequencing was done with the company Complete Genomics (Mountain View CA, USA, www.completegenomics.com) who provides 35 bp paired-end sequence reads at a high sequence coverage obtained with high-accuracy combinatorial probe anchor ligation (cPAL) sequencing technology (Drmanac et al., 2010; Roach et al., 2010). Also, the paired-end sequencing data enable the identification of copy number variations (CNVs) and other structural variants (SV) including inversions, in addition to single nucleotide polymorphisms (SNPs).

In the 4 genomes, we obtained an average coverage of 62-fold genome sequence and captured both alleles at 95.4% of the genomes. All sequence variants, including SNPs and small indels, were mapped to the human reference genome sequence (NCBI Build 36/hg18). We initially focused on the 3.6 Mb candidate region on chromosome 9p21. We filtered and prioritized variants according to several criteria. First, variants must be present heterozygously in all 4 patients since the disease is segregating in an autosomal dominant manner. As a heterozygous variant might be rarely missed using NGS technology, depending on local sequence coverage and quality, variants detected in three of four patients were also considered. Second, variants were selected that were not catalogued in the dbSNP database (http://www.ncbi.nlm.nih.gov/projects/SNP) and were not found as common polymorphisms (allele frequency ≥ 1%) in the 1000 Genomes

Project (http://www.1000genomes.org). Third, variants in nucleotide stretches were filtered out because they are known to be error-prone in NGS data. This resulted in a total of 189 variants, all located outside coding regions of known genes confirming gene-based mutation analyses. These variants were genotyped in all 29 individuals of the DR14 family using Sanger sequencing and tested for segregation. 120 variants were located on the disease haplotype and were analyzed in a series of 300 neurologically healthy control individuals collected in Flanders, Belgium, i.e. the geographical region of which family DR14 originates, using multiplex Sequenom MassARRAY technology. 37 of these variants were completely absent in 300 control individuals and are all located in untranslated regions or introns of genes, or intergenic. We are currently prioritizing these variants based on evolutionary conservation, regulatory potential, location compatible with cis-acting function on functional candidate genes, etc. Also, we are determining the presence of these variants in a Belgian population of unrelated patients with ALS (N=124), ALS-FTLD (N=21) and FTLD (N=203), aiming to find a possible founder mutation. We already showed evidence for the presence of founder mutations in the Flanders-Belgian FTLD collection, by the *GRN* IVS1+5 G>C founder mutation identified in 19% of familial FTLD (Cruts et al., 2006). We have investigated the patient population for chromosome 9p STR markers and did not find evidence for haplotype sharing with family DR14; however, we cannot exclude the presence of a small, previously undetected founder haplotype.

3. Population-based association for ALS and FTLD to chromosome 9p

In 2009, the first ALS GWAS showing association with a locus at chromosome 9p21 was reported by Van Es and colleagues. They identified genome-wide significance with two SNPs, rs2814707 and rs3849942, almost in complete linkage disequilibrium (LD) with each other and located in an LD block of ~80 kb. Also a third SNP in this LD block (rs774359) showed suggestive association (figure 1). This LD block is situated at the telomeric end of the minimally linked candidate region found in the ALS-FTLD families and contains only three genes: part of *MOBKL2B*, *IFNK* and *C9orf72* (figure 1). Next, data of the first GWAS in FTLD-TDP were suggestive for association of five SNPs (rs774352, rs774351, rs3849942, rs2814707, rs774359) on chromosome 9p21, in the same LD block (Van Deerlin et al., 2010). Subsequently, a Finnish and a British independent ALS GWAS identified genome-wide significance with SNPs rs3849942, rs2814707, rs774359, rs2225389 (Laaksovirta et al., 2010) and with SNPs rs3849942, rs2814707, rs903603 (Shatunov et al., 2010) respectively, all in the same locus at chromosome 9p21. The Finnish study defined a 42-SNP haplotype associated with increased risk of ALS in the Finnish population, located in a 232 kb LD block which overlaps with the previously reported 80 kb LD block (van Es et al., 2009) and the 106.5 kb LD block of the UK study (Shatunov et al., 2010). Because of the unique homogeneous genetic structure of the Finnish isolated population, the extent and structure of LD is different than in other European countries. To date, one study replicated the association of the chr9p21 locus in an ALS-FTLD subpopulation (Rollinson et al., 2011).

To assess the contribution of the chr9p21 risk factor to disease etiology in Belgium, we replicated one of the top SNPs associated in all GWAS reports, rs2814707, in a Belgian population of ALS, ALS-FTLD and FTLD patients. In addition, we performed a meta-analysis of the different published association studies with inclusion of our study.

A Major Genetic Factor at Chromosome 9p Implicated in Amyotrophic Lateral Sclerosis (ALS) and Frontotemporal Lobar Degeneration (FTLD)

171

3.1 Replication study chr9p21 GWAS

We investigated association of the most widely studied GWAS top SNP at chr9p21, rs2814707, in a Flanders-Belgian population of genealogically unrelated patients clinically diagnosed with ALS (N=124), ALS-FTLD (N=21) or FTLD (N=203) according to established consensus criteria (Brooks et al., 2000; Neary et al., 1998), compared to a group of 510 unrelated neurologically healthy control individuals from the same region in Belgium. We genotyped rs2814707 and showed that this SNP is in Hardy-Weinberg Equilibrium. Allelic and genotypic single SNP association was calculated using logistic regression analysis. The SNP showed significant allelic and genotypic association in the total population and highly significant association in the ALS and ALS-FTLD subpopulation reaching a maximal odds ratio of 3.27 in ALS patients homozygous for the minor allele (table 2). In the FTLD subpopulation no association was found, demonstrating that the effect in the total population can entirely be explained by the effect in patients with an ALS phenotype. When we include 21 ALS samples of Bulgarian origin, the relative risk became even higher, compared to Belgians only, indicating that the associated allele is the same between different populations.

SNP ID	Genotype	Controls	ALS, ALS-FTLD and FTLD			ALS and ALS-FTLD		
		N=510	N=348			N=145		
		freq (%)	freq (%)	p-value	OR (95%CI)	freq (%)	p-value	OR (95%CI)
rs2814707	C	77.9	71.3	0.006	1.39 (1.10-1.75)	67.0	0.001	1.69 (1.25-2.29)
	T	22.1	28.7			33.0		
	CC	59.7	50.4	ref	ref	43.1	ref	ref
	CT	36.5	41.8	0.08	1.31 (0.97-1.77)	47.9	0.007	1.76 (1.17-2.64)
	TT	3.8	7.8	0.008	2.41 (1.26-4.62)	9.0	0.005	3.27 (1.44-7.41)

Table 2. Allelic and genotypic association of a GWAS top SNP in the total population and the ALS/ALS-FTLD subpopulation. P-values are corrected for age at onset or inclusion and gender. (OR: odds ratio; CI: confidence interval)

3.2 Meta analysis on chromosome 9p21

We combined the data from the different GWA studies and our study to determine the relative risk of carrying the risk allele on chromosome 9p21. A meta-analysis of the most widely studied SNP on chromosome 9p21 (rs2814707) underscores the presence of a genetic risk factor for ALS and/or FTLD at this locus. Carriers of the rs2814707 minor allele are at increased risk to develop ALS or FTLD (OR_{meta} 1.29 (95% CI 1.18-1.41), p-value $2.3*10^{-8}$ (Figure 4)). When excluding the GWAS cohorts in which the association was first reported (van Es et al., 2009) to exclude bias because of winner's curse, the strength of the association remains similar (OR_{meta} 1.32 (95%CI 1.17-1.49; p-value $3.5*10^{-6}$). Exclusion of three studies, including our own, which combine FTLD and ALS phenotypes would have resulted in an OR_{meta} 1.24 (95%CI 1.13-1.36); p-value $3.3*10^{-6}$).

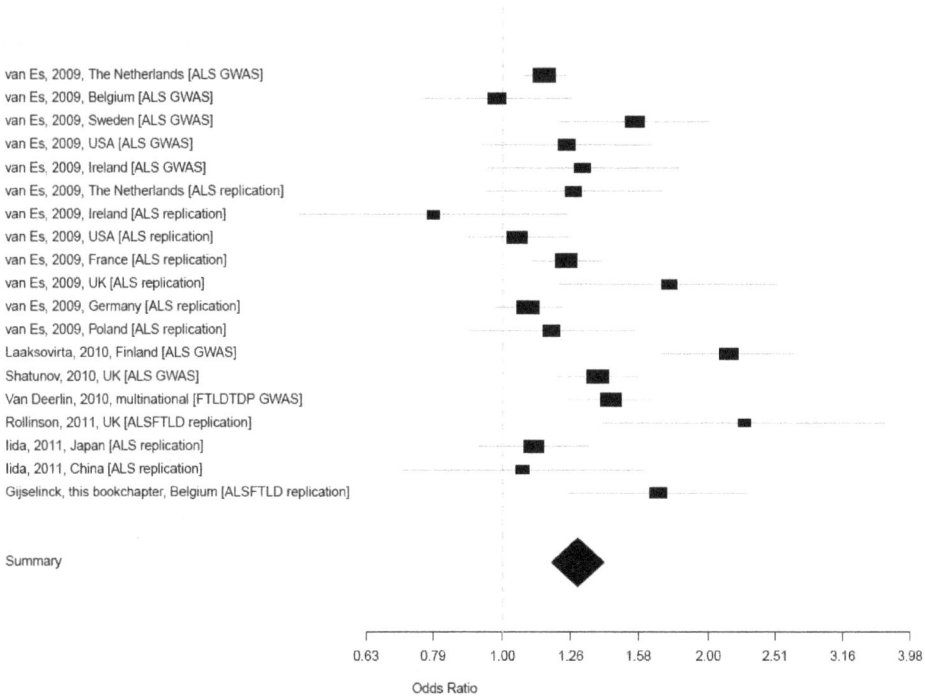

Fig. 4. Forest plot of a random effects meta-analysis of rs2814707. Meta-analysis was conducted in rmeta v2.16, and based on effect estimates and standard errors for the minor allele reported in each individual publication. Odds Ratios and 95% Confidence Intervals are given for each study separately along with a summary Odds Ratio, of the minor allele relative to the major allele. All 9p21 association studies on ALS, ALS-FTLD and FTLD published until July 2011 were included, in addition to our own unpublished data. For the study of Shatunov and colleagues we only included data on the independent UK cohort, to avoid overlap of datasets with previous studies. From Rollinson et al, only data on the Manchester ALS-FTLD cohort are included.

4. Discussion and conclusion

Family-based linkage and population-based association studies in Belgian patients with ALS and/or FTLD provided further evidence for the presence of a major genetic factor on chromosome 9p21 for these diseases.

In the Belgian family DR14 we analyzed the minimally linked region shared in all linked families. We excluded mutations in exons of all known protein-coding genes, in the highest conserved sequences and also copy number mutations of more than 1 kb were excluded. Further we used next generation sequencing technology to sequence the whole genome of four disease haplotype carriers. We are currently analyzing the first selection of variants. If we are left with only a very small number of putative disease-associated variants, we will analyze the complete sequence of the functional unit in which the remaining variants are located in the complete set of ALS, ALS-FTLD and FTLD patients. `Functional unit' in this context means the gene, regulatory element, conserved element or, in the absence of recognizable elements, 1 kb flanking each side of the putative mutation. This might identify additional mutations resulting in the same functional defect as the mutations detected in DR14 and further enhance the likelihood of the variant(s) to be disease-related. Finding such variants will provide strong genetic evidence of a disease causing effect of the variants. Alternatively, in case we do not find a mutation in this first selection of variants, we can use more relaxing filters. Taking into account that dbSNP may include rare clinical variants, rare or non-validated dbSNP SNPs will also be considered (N=91). Also the candidate region can be extended to the next recombinant or to the large DR14 candidate region. Further, regions that are not covered in more than one genome, will be completed using classical sanger sequencing. Finally, structural variants and copy number mutations will be investigated.

More than five years of research in the ALSFTD2 locus in different ALS-FTLD families worldwide did not identify pathogenic mutations yet (table 1), although mutations in two different genes on chromosome 9 outside the minimal candidate region, *IFT74* and *SIGMAR1*, were suggested (Luty et al., 2010; Momeni et al., 2006) but without further confirmation in other families. The fact that the culprit gene is still not found may in part be explained by the fact that families linked with chromosome 9p21 do not all have the same disease haplotype so that different mutations, probably with the same effect on the same gene, are most likely involved. Also, the causal mutations are most likely unusual with respect to position or type. For example, deep intronic mutations or mutations in a distant regulatory element might cause the disease but assessing their effect is rather complicated. Also, identification of small insertions/deletions or inversions is challenging.

In addition, we replicated association in a Belgian cohort of ALS, ALS-FTLD and FTLD patients of two major top SNPs on chromosome 9p21 previously associated in several ALS and FTLD GWA studies. More specifically, we found that the risk haplotype at chromosome 9p21 is most substantially increased in patients with ALS or ALS-FTLD compared to control individuals. The lack of association in the FTLD subpopulation is similar to what was observed in a previous replication study in which association was only found in ALS-FTLD patients (Rollinson et al., 2011). Also, the weakest association signal was found in the FTLD GWAS compared to ALS GWAS. This is the first time that a susceptibility locus for ALS is replicated in different GWA studies and replication studies, underlining the importance of the chromosome 9p21 locus harbouring a risk increasing factor for ALS (and ALS-FTLD) across multiple populations with a high relative risk of disease susceptibility. We are further characterizing this genetic association to reduce the associated region in the Belgian population. We are finemapping the chromosome 9p risk haplotype in great detail in our ALS, FTLD, ALS-FTLD patient cohorts by making a high density SNP map of the complete LD block and using extended association analyses of series of known and newly identified variants in the LD block. These variants were identified in previous publications, hapmap, 1000 Genomes Project and extended genomic sequencing efforts of the linkage disequilibrium block in a selection of ALS and ALS-FTLD patients carrying the associated allele of the GWAS SNPs in a homozygous or heterozygous state. This will finally result in the identification of the functional variant explaining the strong association in the chromosome 9p21 region.

The observation that the chromosome 9p21 region is harboring both disease-causing variants and susceptibility factors with high penetrance, might suggest that different genetic variants with variable degree of biological consequences might be involved. Alternatively, one genetic defect might act as high penetrant susceptibility factor in sporadic patients and as disease-causing factor with reduced penetrance in ALS-FTLD families, carrying also other disease modifying factors. In this respect it is interesting to note that in our studied belgian family DR14 all patients carry in addition to the disease haplotype at chromosome 9p21 also a haplotype in a novel locus at chromosome 14q32, possibly harboring a disease modifying gene (Gijselinck et al., 2010) and of which the sequences are present in the whole genome sequencing data of the family. Combining the family-based and the population-based approach to ultimately find the gene with one or more genetic defects would be of great value. For example, prioritizing the associated LD block in the whole genome sequence analysis of the family could be useful. Further, since in the associated LD block only three genes are located (*IFNK*, *C9orf72*, *MOBKL2B*) (figure 1), we could focus on these genes with respect to expression and dosage studies (eg. single exon deletions or duplications) in the family. Also, the region in and around the associated LD block can be saturated with STR markers for sharing studies with the DR14 family to detect a small founder haplotype. Combining all these comprehensive data will bring us closer to the identification of the chromosome 9 gene. As long as the genetic defect underlying linkage and association is not known, the full epidemiological impact of the chromosome 9p gene in familial and non-familial forms of ALS, ALS-FTLD and FTLD cannot be determined. However, the combined evidence emerging from all molecular genetic studies in chromosome 9p21-linked families and in chromosome 9p21 associated ALS/FTLD populations, suggests it is the most important genetic factor contributing to disease in the center of the disease spectrum linking ALS and FTLD (table 1). Moreover, next to the chr9p21 conclusively linked ALS-FTLD families, several other (smaller) families were also reported without conclusive linkage but with several indications pointing towards the presence of a segregating haplotype in the ALSFTD2 locus (Krueger et al., 2009; Le Ber et al., 2009; Momeni et al., 2006; Pearson et al., 2011; Valdmanis et al., 2007; Yan et al., 2008) (table 1). Identification of this major gene will undoubtedly be a steppingstone for subsequent cell biological studies aiming at better understanding of the pathobiology of neurodegenerative processes leading to ALS and FTLD.

5. Acknowledgment

We are grateful to the patients for their cooperation. We further acknowledge the contribution of personnel of the VIB Genetic Service Facility (www.vibgeneticservicefacility.be). This research of the authors was in part funded by the Special Research Fund of the University of Antwerp, the Research Foundation Flanders (FWO-F), the Institute for Science and Technology - Flanders (IWT-F), the Methusalem excellence grant of the Flemish Government, the Interuniversity Attraction Poles program (IUAP) P6/43 of the Belgian Science Policy Office, the Stichting Alzheimer Onderzoek (SAO-FRMA). I.G. is holding a postdoctoral fellowship of FWO-F.

6. References

Arai, T., Hasegawa, M., Akiyama, H., Ikeda, K., Nonaka, T., Mori, H., Mann, D., Tsuchiya, K., Yoshida, M., Hashizume, Y. & Oda, T. (2006). TDP-43 is a component of ubiquitin-positive tau-negative inclusions in frontotemporal lobar degeneration and amyotrophic lateral sclerosis. *Biochem Biophys Res Commun*, 351, 3, 602-611

Baker, M., Mackenzie, I.R., Pickering-Brown, S.M., Gass, J., Rademakers, R., Lindholm, C., Snowden, J., Adamson, J., Sadovnick, A.D., Rollinson, S., Cannon, A., Dwosh, E., Neary, D., Melquist, S., Richardson, A., Dickson, D., Berger, Z., Eriksen, J., Robinson, T., Zehr, C., Dickey, C.A., Crook, R., McGowan, E., Mann, D., Boeve, B., Feldman, H. & Hutton, M. (2006). Mutations in progranulin cause tau-negative frontotemporal dementia linked to chromosome 17. *Nature*, 442, 7105, 916-919

Boxer, A.L., Mackenzie, I.R., Boeve, B.F., Baker, M., Seeley, W.W., Crook, R., Feldman, H., Hsiung, G.Y., Rutherford, N., Laluz, V., Whitwell, J., Foti, D., McDade, E., Molano, J., Karydas, A., Wojtas, A., Goldman, J., Mirsky, J., Sengdy, P., Dearmond, S., Miller, B.L. & Rademakers, R. (2010). Clinical, neuroimaging and neuropathological features of a new chromosome 9p-linked FTD-ALS family. *J Neurol Neurosurg Psychiatry*

Brooks, B.R., Miller, R.G., Swash, M. & Munsat, T.L. (2000). El Escorial revisited: revised criteria for the diagnosis of amyotrophic lateral sclerosis. *Amyotroph Lateral Scler Other Motor Neuron Disord*, 1, 5, 293-299

Cooper, G.M., Zerr, T., Kidd, J.M., Eichler, E.E. & Nickerson, D.A. (2008). Systematic assessment of copy number variant detection via genome-wide SNP genotyping. *Nat Genet*, 40, 10, 1199-1203

Cruts, M., Gijselinck, I., van der Zee, J., Engelborghs, S., Wils, H., Pirici, D., Rademakers, R., Vandenberghe, R., Dermaut, B., Martin, J.J., van Duijn, C., Peeters, K., Sciot, R., Santens, P., de Pooter, T., Mattheijssens, M., Van den Broeck, M., Cuijt, I., Vennekens, K., De Deyn, P.P., Kumar-Singh, S. & Van Broeckhoven, C. (2006). Null mutations in progranulin cause ubiquitin-positive frontotemporal dementia linked to chromosome 17q21. *Nature*, 442, 7105, 920-924

Drmanac, R., Sparks, A.B., Callow, M.J., Halpern, A.L., Burns, N.L., Kermani, B.G., Carnevali, P., Nazarenko, I., Nilsen, G.B., Yeung, G., Dahl, F., Fernandez, A., Staker, B., Pant, K.P., Baccash, J., Borcherding, A.P., Brownley, A., Cedeno, R., Chen, L., Chernikoff, D., Cheung, A., Chirita, R., Curson, B., Ebert, J.C., Hacker, C.R., Hartlage, R., Hauser, B., Huang, S., Jiang, Y., Karpinchyk, V., Koenig, M., Kong, C., Landers, T., Le, C., Liu, J., McBride, C.E., Morenzoni, M., Morey, R.E., Mutch, K., Perazich, H., Perry, K., Peters, B.A., Peterson, J., Pethiyagoda, C.L., Pothuraju, K., Richter, C., Rosenbaum, A.M., Roy, S., Shafto, J., Sharanhovich, U., Shannon, K.W., Sheppy, C.G., Sun, M., Thakuria, J.V., Tran, A., Vu, D., Zaranek, A.W., Wu, X., Drmanac, S., Oliphant, A.R., Banyai, W.C., Martin, B., Ballinger, D.G., Church, G.M. & Reid, C.A. (2010). Human genome sequencing using unchained base reads on self-assembling DNA nanoarrays. *Science*, 327, 5961, 78-81

Gijselinck, I., Engelborghs, S., Maes, G., Cuijt, I., Peeters, K., Mattheijssens, M., Joris, G., Cras, P., Martin, J.J., De Deyn, P.P., Kumar-Singh, S., Van Broeckhoven, C. & Cruts, M. (2010). Identification of 2 Loci at chromosomes 9 and 14 in a multiplex family with frontotemporal lobar degeneration and amyotrophic lateral sclerosis. *Arch Neurol*, 67, 5, 606-616

Gitcho, M.A., Baloh, R.H., Chakraverty, S., Mayo, K., Norton, J.B., Levitch, D., Hatanpaa, K.J., White, C.L., III, Bigio, E.H., Caselli, R., Baker, M., Al Lozi, M.T., Morris, J.C., Pestronk, A., Rademakers, R., Goate, A.M. & Cairns, N.J. (2008). TDP-43 A315T mutation in familial motor neuron disease. *Ann Neurol*, 63, 4, 535-538

Greenway, M.J., Andersen, P.M., Russ, C., Ennis, S., Cashman, S., Donaghy, C., Patterson, V., Swingler, R., Kieran, D., Prehn, J., Morrison, K.E., Green, A., Acharya, K.R., Brown, R.H., Jr. & Hardiman, O. (2006). ANG mutations segregate with familial and 'sporadic' amyotrophic lateral sclerosis. *Nat Genet*, 38, 4, 411-413

Hutton, M., Lendon, C.L., Rizzu, P., Baker, M., Froelich, S., Houlden, H., Pickering-Brown, S., Chakraverty, S., Isaacs, A., Grover, A., Hackett, J., Adamson, J., Lincoln, S., Dickson, D., Davies, P., Petersen, R.C., Stevens, M., de Graaff, E., Wauters, E., van Baren, J., Hillebrand, M., Joosse, M., Kwon, J.M., Nowotny, P., Che, L.K., Norton, J., Morris, J.C., Reed, L.A., Trojanowski, J., Basun, H., Lannfelt, L., Neystat, M., Fahn, S., Dark, F., Tannenberg, T., Dodd, P.R., Hayward, N., Kwok, J.B., Schofield, P.R., Andreadis, A., Snowden, J., Craufurd, D., Neary, D., Owen, F., Oostra, B.A., Hardy, J., Goate, A., van Swieten, J., Mann, D., Lynch, T. & Heutink, P. (1998). Association of missense and 5'-splice-site mutations in tau with the inherited dementia FTDP-17. *Nature*, 393, 6686, 702-705

Johnson, J.O., Mandrioli, J., Benatar, M., Abramzon, Y., Van Deerlin, V.M., Trojanowski, J.Q., Gibbs, J.R., Brunetti, M., Gronka, S., Wuu, J., Ding, J., McCluskey, L., Martinez-Lage, M., Falcone, D., Hernandez, D.G., Arepalli, S., Chong, S., Schymick, J.C., Rothstein, J., Landi, F., Wang, Y.D., Calvo, A., Mora, G., Sabatelli, M., Monsurro, M.R., Battistini, S., Salvi, F., Spataro, R., Sola, P., Borghero, G., Galassi, G., Scholz, S.W., Taylor, J.P., Restagno, G., Chio, A. & Traynor, B.J. (2010). Exome sequencing reveals VCP mutations as a cause of familial ALS. *Neuron*, 68, 5, 857-864

Kabashi, E., Valdmanis, P.N., Dion, P., Spiegelman, D., McConkey, B.J., Vande, V.C., Bouchard, J.P., Lacomblez, L., Pochigaeva, K., Salachas, F., Pradat, P.F., Camu, W., Meininger, V., Dupre, N. & Rouleau, G.A. (2008). TARDBP mutations in individuals with sporadic and familial amyotrophic lateral sclerosis. *Nat Genet*, 40, 5, 572-574

Kovacs, G.G., Murrell, J.R., Horvath, S., Haraszti, L., Majtenyi, K., Molnar, M.J., Budka, H., Ghetti, B. & Spina, S. (2009). TARDBP variation associated with frontotemporal dementia, supranuclear gaze palsy, and chorea. *Mov Disord*, 24, 12, 1843-1847

Krueger, K.A., Tsuji, S., Fukuda, Y., Takahashi, Y., Goto, J., Mitsui, J., Ishiura, H., Dalton, J.C., Miller, M.B., Day, J.W. & Ranum, L.P. (2009). SNP haplotype mapping in a small ALS family. *PLoS One*, 4, 5, e5687

Kwiatkowski, T.J., Jr., Bosco, D.A., Leclerc, A.L., Tamrazian, E., Vanderburg, C.R., Russ, C., Davis, A., Gilchrist, J., Kasarskis, E.J., Munsat, T., Valdmanis, P., Rouleau, G.A., Hosler, B.A., Cortelli, P., de Jong, P.J., Yoshinaga, Y., Haines, J.L., Pericak-Vance, M.A., Yan, J., Ticozzi, N., Siddique, T., McKenna-Yasek, D., Sapp, P.C., Horvitz, H.R., Landers, J.E. & Brown, R.H., Jr. (2009). Mutations in the FUS/TLS gene on chromosome 16 cause familial amyotrophic lateral sclerosis. *Science*, 323, 5918, 1205-1208

Laaksovirta, H., Peuralinna, T., Schymick, J.C., Scholz, S.W., Lai, S.L., Myllykangas, L., Sulkava, R., Jansson, L., Hernandez, D.G., Gibbs, J.R., Nalls, M.A., Heckerman, D., Tienari, P.J. & Traynor, B.J. (2010). Chromosome 9p21 in amyotrophic lateral sclerosis in Finland: a genome-wide association study. *Lancet Neurol*, 9, 10, 978-985

Le Ber, I., Camuzat, A., Berger, E., Hannequin, D., Laquerriere, A., Golfier, V., Seilhean, D., Viennet, G., Couratier, P., Verpillat, P., Heath, S., Camu, W., Martinaud, O., Lacomblez, L., Vercelletto, M., Salachas, F., Sellal, F., Didic, M., Thomas-Anterion,

C., Puel, M., Michel, B.F., Besse, C., Duyckaerts, C., Meininger, V., Campion, D., Dubois, B. & Brice, A. (2009). Chromosome 9p-linked families with frontotemporal dementia associated with motor neuron disease. *Neurology*, 72, 19, 1669-1676

Lillo, P. & Hodges, J.R. (2009). Frontotemporal dementia and motor neurone disease: overlapping clinic-pathological disorders. *J Clin Neurosci*, 16, 9, 1131-1135

Lomen-Hoerth, C., Murphy, J., Langmore, S., Kramer, J.H., Olney, R.K. & Miller, B. (2003). Are amyotrophic lateral sclerosis patients cognitively normal? *Neurology*, 60, 7, 1094-1097

Luty, A.A., Kwok, J.B., Dobson-Stone, C., Loy, C.T., Coupland, K.G., Karlstrom, H., Sobow, T., Tchorzewska, J., Maruszak, A., Barcikowska, M., Panegyres, P.K., Zekanowski, C., Brooks, W.S., Williams, K.L., Blair, I.P., Mather, K.A., Sachdev, P.S., Halliday, G.M. & Schofield, P.R. (2010). Sigma nonopioid intracellular receptor 1 mutations cause frontotemporal lobar degeneration-motor neuron disease. *Ann Neurol*, 68, 5, 639-649

Luty, A.A., Kwok, J.B., Thompson, E.M., Blumbergs, P., Brooks, W.S., Loy, C.T., Dobson-Stone, C., Panegyres, P.K., Hecker, J., Nicholson, G.A., Halliday, G.M. & Schofield, P.R. (2008). Pedigree with frontotemporal lobar degeneration--motor neuron disease and Tar DNA binding protein-43 positive neuropathology: genetic linkage to chromosome 9. *BMC Neurol*, 8, 32

Momeni, P., Schymick, J., Jain, S., Cookson, M.R., Cairns, N.J., Greggio, E., Greenway, M.J., Berger, S., Pickering-Brown, S., Chio, A., Fung, H.C., Holtzman, D.M., Huey, E.D., Wassermann, E.M., Adamson, J., Hutton, M.L., Rogaeva, E., George-Hyslop, P., Rothstein, J.D., Hardiman, O., Grafman, J., Singleton, A., Hardy, J. & Traynor, B.J. (2006). Analysis of IFT74 as a candidate gene for chromosome 9p-linked ALS-FTD. *BMC Neurol*, 6, 44

Morita, M., Al Chalabi, A., Andersen, P.M., Hosler, B., Sapp, P., Englund, E., Mitchell, J.E., Habgood, J.J., de Belleroche, J., Xi, J., Jongjaroenprasert, W., Horvitz, H.R., Gunnarsson, L.G. & Brown, R.H., Jr. (2006). A locus on chromosome 9p confers susceptibility to ALS and frontotemporal dementia. *Neurology*, 66, 6, 839-844

Neary, D., Snowden, J.S., Gustafson, L., Passant, U., Stuss, D., Black, S., Freedman, M., Kertesz, A., Robert, P.H., Albert, M., Boone, K., Miller, B.L., Cummings, J. & Benson, D.F. (1998). Frontotemporal lobar degeneration: a consensus on clinical diagnostic criteria. *Neurology*, 51, 6, 1546-1554

Neumann, M., Sampathu, D.M., Kwong, L.K., Truax, A.C., Micsenyi, M.C., Chou, T.T., Bruce, J., Schuck, T., Grossman, M., Clark, C.M., McCluskey, L.F., Miller, B.L., Masliah, E., Mackenzie, I.R., Feldman, H., Feiden, W., Kretzschmar, H.A., Trojanowski, J.Q. & Lee, V.M. (2006). Ubiquitinated TDP-43 in frontotemporal lobar degeneration and amyotrophic lateral sclerosis. *Science*, 314, 5796, 130-133

Pearson, J.P., Williams, N.M., Majounie, E., Waite, A., Stott, J., Newsway, V., Murray, A., Hernandez, D., Guerreiro, R., Singleton, A.B., Neal, J. & Morris, H.R. (2011). Familial frontotemporal dementia with amyotrophic lateral sclerosis and a shared haplotype on chromosome 9p. *J Neurol*, 258, 4, 647-655

Ravasi, T., Suzuki, H., Cannistraci, C.V., Katayama, S., Bajic, V.B., Tan, K., Akalin, A., Schmeier, S., Kanamori-Katayama, M., Bertin, N., Carninci, P., Daub, C.O., Forrest, A.R., Gough, J., Grimmond, S., Han, J.H., Hashimoto, T., Hide, W., Hofmann, O., Kamburov, A., Kaur, M., Kawaji, H., Kubosaki, A., Lassmann, T., van, N.E.,

MacPherson, C.R., Ogawa, C., Radovanovic, A., Schwartz, A., Teasdale, R.D., Tegner, J., Lenhard, B., Teichmann, S.A., Arakawa, T., Ninomiya, N., Murakami, K., Tagami, M., Fukuda, S., Imamura, K., Kai, C., Ishihara, R., Kitazume, Y., Kawai, J., Hume, D.A., Ideker, T. & Hayashizaki, Y. (2010). An atlas of combinatorial transcriptional regulation in mouse and man. *Cell*, 140, 5, 744-752

Ringholz, G.M., Appel, S.H., Bradshaw, M., Cooke, N.A., Mosnik, D.M. & Schulz, P.E. (2005). Prevalence and patterns of cognitive impairment in sporadic ALS. *Neurology*, 65, 4, 586-590

Roach, J.C., Glusman, G., Smit, A.F., Huff, C.D., Hubley, R., Shannon, P.T., Rowen, L., Pant, K.P., Goodman, N., Bamshad, M., Shendure, J., Drmanac, R., Jorde, L.B., Hood, L. & Galas, D.J. (2010). Analysis of Genetic Inheritance in a Family Quartet by Whole-Genome Sequencing. *Science*

Rollinson, S., Mead, S., Snowden, J., Richardson, A., Rohrer, J., Halliwell, N., Usher, S., Neary, D., Mann, D., Hardy, J. & Pickering-Brown, S. (2011). Frontotemporal lobar degeneration genome wide association study replication confirms a risk locus shared with amyotrophic lateral sclerosis. *Neurobiol Aging*, 32, 4, 758-7

Rosen, D.R., Siddique, T., Patterson, D., Figlewicz, D.A., Sapp, P., Hentati, A., Donaldson, D., Goto, J., O'Regan, J.P., Deng, H.X. & . (1993). Mutations in Cu/Zn superoxide dismutase gene are associated with familial amyotrophic lateral sclerosis. *Nature*, 362, 6415, 59-62

Rosso, S.M., Donker, K.L., Baks, T., Joosse, M., de, K., I, Pijnenburg, Y., de Jong, D., Dooijes, D., Kamphorst, W., Ravid, R., Niermeijer, M.F., Verheij, F., Kremer, H.P., Scheltens, P., van Duijn, C.M., Heutink, P. & van Swieten, J.C. (2003). Frontotemporal dementia in The Netherlands: patient characteristics and prevalence estimates from a population-based study. *Brain*, 126, Pt 9, 2016-2022

Rowland, L.P. & Shneider, N.A. (2001). Amyotrophic lateral sclerosis. *N Engl J Med*, 344, 22, 1688-1700

Sampathu, D.M., Neumann, M., Kwong, L.K., Chou, T.T., Micsenyi, M., Truax, A., Bruce, J., Grossman, M., Trojanowski, J.Q. & Lee, V.M. (2006). Pathological heterogeneity of frontotemporal lobar degeneration with ubiquitin-positive inclusions delineated by ubiquitin immunohistochemistry and novel monoclonal antibodies. *Am J Pathol*, 169, 4, 1343-1352

Sela, N., Mersch, B., Gal-Mark, N., Lev-Maor, G., Hotz-Wagenblatt, A. & Ast, G. (2007). Comparative analysis of transposed element insertion within human and mouse genomes reveals Alu's unique role in shaping the human transcriptome. *Genome Biol*, 8, 6, R127

Shatunov, A., Mok, K., Newhouse, S., Weale, M.E., Smith, B., Vance, C., Johnson, L., Veldink, J.H., van Es, M.A., van den Berg, L.H., Robberecht, W., Van, D.P., Hardiman, O., Farmer, A.E., Lewis, C.M., Butler, A.W., Abel, O., Andersen, P.M., Fogh, I., Silani, V., Chio, A., Traynor, B.J., Melki, J., Meininger, V., Landers, J.E., McGuffin, P., Glass, J.D., Pall, H., Leigh, P.N., Hardy, J., Brown, R.H., Jr., Powell, J.F., Orrell, R.W., Morrison, K.E., Shaw, P.J., Shaw, C.E. & Al-Chalabi, A. (2010). Chromosome 9p21 in sporadic amyotrophic lateral sclerosis in the UK and seven other countries: a genome-wide association study. *Lancet Neurol*, 9, 10, 986-994

Skibinski, G., Parkinson, N.J., Brown, J.M., Chakrabarti, L., Lloyd, S.L., Hummerich, H., Nielsen, J.E., Hodges, J.R., Spillantini, M.G., Thusgaard, T., Brandner, S., Brun, A.,

Rossor, M.N., Gade, A., Johannsen, P., Sorensen, S.A., Gydesen, S., Fisher, E.M. &
Collinge, J. (2005). Mutations in the endosomal ESCRTIII-complex subunit
CHMP2B in frontotemporal dementia. *Nat Genet*, 37, 8, 806-808
Sreedharan, J., Blair, I.P., Tripathi, V.B., Hu, X., Vance, C., Rogelj, B., Ackerley, S., Durnall,
J.C., Williams, K.L., Buratti, E., Baralle, F., de Belleroche, J., Mitchell, J.D., Leigh,
P.N., Al Chalabi, A., Miller, C.C., Nicholson, G. & Shaw, C.E. (2008). TDP-43
mutations in familial and sporadic amyotrophic lateral sclerosis. *Science*, 319, 5870,
1668-1672
Valdmanis, P.N., Dupre, N., Bouchard, J.P., Camu, W., Salachas, F., Meininger, V., Strong,
M. & Rouleau, G.A. (2007). Three families with amyotrophic lateral sclerosis and
frontotemporal dementia with evidence of linkage to chromosome 9p. *Arch Neurol*,
64, 2, 240-245
Van Deerlin, V.M., Leverenz, J.B., Bekris, L.M., Bird, T.D., Yuan, W., Elman, L.B., Clay, D.,
Wood, E.M., Chen-Plotkin, A.S., Martinez-Lage, M., Steinbart, E., McCluskey, L.,
Grossman, M., Neumann, M., Wu, I.L., Yang, W.S., Kalb, R., Galasko, D.R.,
Montine, T.J., Trojanowski, J.Q., Lee, V.M., Schellenberg, G.D. & Yu, C.E. (2008).
TARDBP mutations in amyotrophic lateral sclerosis with TDP-43 neuropathology: a
genetic and histopathological analysis. *Lancet Neurol*, 7, 5, 409-416
Van Deerlin, V.M., Sleiman, P.M., Martinez-Lage, M., Chen-Plotkin, A., Wang, L.S., Graff-
Radford, N.R., Dickson, D.W., Rademakers, R., Boeve, B.F., Grossman, M., Arnold,
S.E., Mann, D.M., Pickering-Brown, S.M., Seelaar, H., Heutink, P., van Swieten, J.C.,
Murrell, J.R., Ghetti, B., Spina, S., Grafman, J., Hodges, J., Spillantini, M.G., Gilman,
S., Lieberman, A.P., Kaye, J.A., Woltjer, R.L., Bigio, E.H., Mesulam, M., Al-Sarraj, S.,
Troakes, C., Rosenberg, R.N., White, C.L., III, Ferrer, I., Llado, A., Neumann, M.,
Kretzschmar, H.A., Hulette, C.M., Welsh-Bohmer, K.A., Miller, B.L., Alzualde, A.,
de Munain, A.L., McKee, A.C., Gearing, M., Levey, A.I., Lah, J.J., Hardy, J., Rohrer,
J.D., Lashley, T., Mackenzie, I.R., Feldman, H.H., Hamilton, R.L., Dekosky, S.T., van
der Zee, J., Kumar-Singh, S., Van, B.C., Mayeux, R., Vonsattel, J.P., Troncoso, J.C.,
Kril, J.J., Kwok, J.B., Halliday, G.M., Bird, T.D., Ince, P.G., Shaw, P.J., Cairns, N.J.,
Morris, J.C., McLean, C.A., DeCarli, C., Ellis, W.G., Freeman, S.H., Frosch, M.P.,
Growdon, J.H., Perl, D.P., Sano, M., Bennett, D.A., Schneider, J.A., Beach, T.G.,
Reiman, E.M., Woodruff, B.K., Cummings, J., Vinters, H.V., Miller, C.A., Chui,
H.C., Alafuzoff, I., Hartikainen, P., Seilhean, D., Galasko, D., Masliah, E., Cotman,
C.W., Tunon, M.T., Martinez, M.C., Munoz, D.G., Carroll, S.L., Marson, D.,
Riederer, P.F., Bogdanovic, N., Schellenberg, G.D., Hakonarson, H., Trojanowski,
J.Q. & Lee, V.M. (2010). Common variants at 7p21 are associated with
frontotemporal lobar degeneration with TDP-43 inclusions. *Nat Genet*, 42, 3, 234-239
van Es, M.A., Veldink, J.H., Saris, C.G., Blauw, H.M., van Vught, P.W., Birve, A., Lemmens,
R., Schelhaas, H.J., Groen, E.J., Huisman, M.H., Van Der Kooi, A.J., De, V.M.,
Dahlberg, C., Estrada, K., Rivadeneira, F., Hofman, A., Zwarts, M.J., van Doormaal,
P.T., Rujescu, D., Strengman, E., Giegling, I., Muglia, P., Tomik, B., Slowik, A.,
Uitterlinden, A.G., Hendrich, C., Waibel, S., Meyer, T., Ludolph, A.C., Glass, J.D.,
Purcell, S., Cichon, S., Nothen, M.M., Wichmann, H.E., Schreiber, S., Vermeulen,
S.H., Kiemeney, L.A., Wokke, J.H., Cronin, S., McLaughlin, R.L., Hardiman, O.,
Fumoto, K., Pasterkamp, R.J., Meininger, V., Melki, J., Leigh, P.N., Shaw, C.E.,
Landers, J.E., Al-Chalabi, A., Brown, R.H., Jr., Robberecht, W., Andersen, P.M.,

Ophoff, R.A. & van den Berg, L.H. (2009). Genome-wide association study identifies 19p13.3 (UNC13A) and 9p21.2 as susceptibility loci for sporadic amyotrophic lateral sclerosis. *Nat Genet*, 41, 10, 1083-1087

Van Langenhove, T., van der Zee, J., Sleegers, K., Engelborghs, S., Vandenberghe, R., Gijselinck, I., Van den Broeck, M., Mattheijssens, M., Peeters, K., De Deyn, P.P., Cruts, M. & Van, B.C. (2010). Genetic contribution of FUS to frontotemporal lobar degeneration. *Neurology*, 74, 5, 366-371

Vance, C., Al Chalabi, A., Ruddy, D., Smith, B.N., Hu, X., Sreedharan, J., Siddique, T., Schelhaas, H.J., Kusters, B., Troost, D., Baas, F., de, J., V & Shaw, C.E. (2006). Familial amyotrophic lateral sclerosis with frontotemporal dementia is linked to a locus on chromosome 9p13.2-21.3. *Brain*, 129, Pt 4, 868-876

Vance, C., Rogelj, B., Hortobagyi, T., De Vos, K.J., Nishimura, A.L., Sreedharan, J., Hu, X., Smith, B., Ruddy, D., Wright, P., Ganesalingam, J., Williams, K.L., Tripathi, V., Al Saraj, S., Al Chalabi, A., Leigh, P.N., Blair, I.P., Nicholson, G., de Belleroche, J., Gallo, J.M., Miller, C.C. & Shaw, C.E. (2009). Mutations in FUS, an RNA processing protein, cause familial amyotrophic lateral sclerosis type 6. *Science*, 323, 5918, 1208-1211

Watts, G.D., Wymer, J., Kovach, M.J., Mehta, S.G., Mumm, S., Darvish, D., Pestronk, A., Whyte, M.P. & Kimonis, V.E. (2004). Inclusion body myopathy associated with Paget disease of bone and frontotemporal dementia is caused by mutant valosin-containing protein. *Nat Genet*, 36, 4, 377-381

Yan J, Slifer S, Siddique N, Chen W, Yong S, Erdong L, Haines JL, Pericak-Vance M, Siddique T. 2008. Fine-Mapping and Candidate Gene Sequencing of the Chromosome 9p Locus of ALS/FTD.

Yokoseki, A., Shiga, A., Tan, C.F., Tagawa, A., Kaneko, H., Koyama, A., Eguchi, H., Tsujino, A., Ikeuchi, T., Kakita, A., Okamoto, K., Nishizawa, M., Takahashi, H. & Onodera, O. (2008). TDP-43 mutation in familial amyotrophic lateral sclerosis. *Ann Neurol*, 63, 4, 538-542

Part 3

Clinical Research in ALS

9

Assessment and Management of Respiratory Dysfunction in Patients with Amyotrophic Lateral Sclerosis

Daniele Lo Coco et al.*
ALS Clinical Research Center, Dipartimento di Biomedicina Sperimentale e Neuroscienze Cliniche (BioNeC), University of Palermo, Palermo, Italy

1. Introduction

Amyotrophic Lateral Sclerosis (ALS) is a relatively rare neurodegenerative disorder that causes progressive dysfunction of voluntary muscle groups secondary to motor neurons death. The relentless involvement of all skeletal muscles of the body, characterized by weakness and atrophy to complete paralysis, invariably involves respiratory muscles (particularly the diaphragm) resulting in a failure to deliver adequate amounts of oxygen to, and remove carbon dioxide from blood. As a result, respiratory failure, frequently complicated by pneumonia related to respiratory muscle weakness and ineffective cough, is the most frequent cause of death in these patients (Lo Coco et al., 2008).

Considering the natural history of ALS, only a few number of patients shows respiratory muscle dysfunction at the onset of the disease (Marti-Fabregas et al., 1995; De Carvalho et al., 1996), and the majority of patients maintains an almost normal pulmonary function for months or years. Patients thus need to be regularly and progressively evaluated to identify early signs of respiratory muscle weakness so that adequate treatment can be implemented. Indeed, in the last few years it has been repeatedly shown that non-invasive positive-pressure ventilation (NIPPV), the treatment of choice for chronic hypoventilation and respiratory failure in ALS, allows a significant improvement in survival and quality of life (Heiman-Patterson & Miller, 2006). Many tests are available to objectively assess the performances of the respiratory system, and there is increasing interest toward those able to sensitively detect mild impairment. Moreover, great attention has to be put on monitoring of cough effectiveness, management of respiratory secretions and prevention of respiratory infections. For all these reasons the management of respiratory dysfunction has become a

*Paolo Volanti[2], Domenico De Cicco[2], Antonio Spanevello[3], Gianluca Battaglia[2], Santino Marchese[4], Alfonsa Claudia Taiello[1], Rossella Spataro[1] and Vincenzo La Bella[1]
[1]ALS Clinical Research Center, Dipartimento di Biomedicina Sperimentale e Neuroscienze Cliniche (BioNeC), University of Palermo, Palermo, Italy
[2]Neurorehabilitation Unit, Fondazione Salvatore Maugeri, Mistretta (ME), Italy
[3]Università Degli Studi dell'Insubria, Varese, Italy
[4]Respiratory Intensive Care Unit, Ospedale Civico ARNAS, Palermo, Italy*

major issue in the multidisciplinary assessment of patients with ALS, and the pulmonologist has gained an increasing role in this process. However, there is still little consensus on pulmonary care worldwide, and clinical practice varies widely from country to country, especially when NIPPV becomes inadequate to support respiratory muscle failure. It is, then, good practice to discuss respiratory issues in advance with the patients and their carers in order to avoid emergency interventions or unwanted treatments, and frequently review these decisions during the course of the disease.

This chapter focuses on the recent advances that have emerged in the management of pulmonary dysfunction in patients with ALS with emphasis on respiratory evaluation and mechanical ventilation.

2. Evaluation of pulmonary function

As already mentioned, when patients with ALS seek medical attention, they do not usually display signs of pulmonary involvement, and do not refer respiratory complaints. However, during the progression of the disease all patients eventually complain of dyspnea with exertion, orthopnea, and poor sleep quality with frequent awakenings, nightmares, early morning headaches or excessive daytime sleepiness (Heffernan et al., 2006; Beneditt & Boitano, 2008). A clinical examination at this point might show respiratory paradox, rapid shallow breathing or accessory muscle contraction. Nevertheless, the observation that many patients may remain asymptomatic even when there is a marked reduction of vital capacity limits the reliability of these signs and symptoms. There are, however, several dyspnea rating scales, such as the Borg dyspnoea score, the baseline dyspnea index and the transition dyspnea index, that have been recently reconsidered and their implementation has been encouraged (Lechtzin et al., 2007a; Just et al., 2010).

In addition to respiratory symptoms and signs, many exams are used in the evaluation of pulmonary function in patients with ALS (Heffernan et al., 2006; Beneditt & Boitano, 2008; Lo Coco et al., 2008; Miller et al., 2009a).

The most widely available measure for detecting respiratory decline is forced vital capacity (FVC) sitting and/or supine. FVC is correlated with survival, and usually presents an almost linear decrease during the course of the disease, but with a marked variability from patient to patient (within 2% to 4% of predicted value per month) (Fallat et al., 1979; Munsat et al., 1988; Schiffman & Belsh, 1993; Stembler et al., 1998; Czaplinski et al., 2006; Lo Coco et al., 2006a).

FVC, however, has some well known limitations, such as low sensitiveness in patients with bulbar involvement, because of reduced buccal strength, or cognitive involvement, and a relative insensitiveness to detect mild or moderate diaphragmatic dysfunction. According to many specialists, supine FVC, although more difficult to perform, has superior sensitivity over seated FVC in predicting survival, is closely correlated with transdiaphragmatic pressure, and then should be always executed in the evaluation of patients with ALS (Varrato et al., 2001; Schmidt et al., 2006; Baumann et al., 2010).

Maximal inspiratory and expiratory pressure (MIP and MEP) are other sensitive measurements, and it has been shown that many patients with an FVC > 70% had abnormal MIP (< -60 cm) (Jackson et al., 2001). However, since many patients are unable to perform the test with the progression of disease, in many centres these two tests are not routinely executed.

Arterial blood gas analysis may also be of help in the evaluation of patients with ALS, especially in those with severe bulbar involvement, since it could reveal resting hypercapnia ($PaCO_2$ > 6.5 kPa) and/or hypoxemia (PaO_2 < 80 mmHg). However, these are usually very late signs of respiratory failure in ALS.

Sniff nasal inspiratory pressure (SNIP) is regarded as a good measure of diaphragmatic strength, and is probably more accurate than FVC, especially at later stages, although even SNIP may underestimate respiratory function in patients with bulbar involvement, because of upper airway collapse. However, a sniff nasal pressure test < 40% of predicted value (or < 60 cmH_2O) is a significant predictor of sleep disordered breathing, nocturnal hypoxemia, hypercapnia and mortality (Fitting et al., 1999; Lyall et al., 2001b; Carrat et al., 2011).

Finally, nocturnal hypoventilation and sleep-disordered breathing are common problems in ALS with the progression of the disease, and can occur even when respiratory muscle function is only mildly affected and in the presence of normal daytime gas exchange (Gay et al., 1991; Ferguson et al., 1996; Arnulf et al., 2000). Nocturnal hypoventilation is particularly severe during rapid eye movements (REM) sleep, when all postural and accessory muscles are physiologically atonic, and only the diaphragm, which may itself be impaired, is left to sustain ventilation and overcome any upper airway resistance (Ferguson et al., 1996). Then, since nocturnal oximetry is easily performed and can be executed domiciliary, it has become frequently used in clinical practice for the evaluation of respiratory involvement in patients with ALS and as a guide to initiate mechanical ventilation. Nocturnal oximetry correlated with survival (mean SaO_2 < 93 mmHg was associated with mean survival of 7 months vs 18 months when mean SaO_2 > 93 mmHg) (Velasco et al., 2002), and nocturnal desaturations < 90% for 1 cumulative minute was a more sensitive indicator of nocturnal hypoventilation than either FVC or MIP (Jackson et al., 2001). Polysomnography is not routinely performed, because is costly and demanding, although it can reveal causes of poor sleep quality different from disordered breathing, such as motor activity during sleep (Lo Coco et al., 2011).

3. Non-invasive mechanical ventilation

Long-term mechanical ventilation in patients with neuromuscular problems was first introduced between 1950 and 1960 in France and Sweden as a consequence of the poliomyelitis epidemics. During the following decades, the concept of home mechanical ventilation expanded rapidly, and long-term non-invasive positive-pressure ventilation (NIPPV) was implemented in many other countries and for many other conditions, including ALS, to treat chronic alveolar hypoventilation.

Chronic alveolar hypoventilation is a state characterized by reduced arterial oxygen tension and increased carbon dioxide tension, which the patient may correct at least partially by voluntary hyperventilation. The underlying mechanisms are not yet fully understood and may involve impairment of lung mechanics or airway function and cough, ventilation-perfusion mismatch, blunted central ventilatory drive, or respiratory muscle fatigue. Abnormalities may occur while awake or during sleep. In most cases, chronic alveolar hypoventilation leads to daytime fatigue, hypersomnia, and changes in psychological function.

The application of ventilatory assistance in ALS, most frequently non-invasively, has led in the last fifteen years to a revolution in respiratory assistance and ventilatory support in these patients, with a significant impact on the natural history of the disorder. Indeed, NIPPV has been shown to alleviate respiratory symptoms, to extend survival considerably, and to improve quality of life and cognitive functions in most patients (Miller et al., 2009a). At present time, NIV, usually via nasal mask with Bi-level Positive Airway Pressure (BiPAP) machines, is the most effective treatment available for ALS patients (Heiman-Patterson & Miller, 2006).

The first study that investigated the effects of NIPPV in patients with ALS dates back to 1995. In a non-randomized trial of NIPPV, Pinto and colleagues showed that survival was significantly longer in the nine patients that received NIPPV compared to the nine patients that received standard care (Pinto et al., 1995). In the following years, many cohort and retrospective studies, and a single randomized trial confirmed these results in those patients that used the ventilatory device for more than 4 hours/night (defined as tolerant patients) (Aboussouan et al., 1997, 2001; Kleopa et al., 1999; Bourke et al., 2003, 2006; Farrero et al., 2005; Gruis et al., 2005; Lo Coco et al., 2006b). In general, these studies demonstrated a median survival of 10 to 15 months in those who were able to tolerate NIPPV. It was also pointed out that NIPPV treatment could slow the rate of respiratory impairment, while severe bulbar impairment could affect NIPPV tolerance (Pinto et al., 1995; Aboussouan et al., 1997, 2001; Kleopa et al., 1999; Bourke et al., 2003, 2006; Farrero et al., 2005; Gruis et al., 2005; Lo Coco et al., 2006b). Furthermore, many recent studies showed that NIPPV therapy could improve quality of life of patients with ALS (Gelinas et al., 1998; Lyall et al., 2001a; Kaub-Wittemer et al., 2003; Bourke et al., 2003, 2006; Mustfa et al., 2006), although some suggested that the caregivers' burden could become heavier (Gelinas et al., 1998; Kaub-Wittemer et al., 2003). Finally, it has been reported that mechanical ventilation could improve cognitive function after some months of treatment (Newson-Davis et al., 2001).

Notwithstanding the aforementioned effects on respiratory symptoms, quality of life, and survival many studies suggest that the employment of NIPPV in ALS is poor worldwide (Bourke et al., 2002; Lechtzin et al., 2004), with a need for more education of clinicians and patients regarding the benefits of mechanical ventilation earlier in the course of the disease (Bradley et al., 2001). The reasons for such low uptake of NIPPV treatment are multifactorial but are influenced by differences in the experience of physicians, its availability and cost, uncertainty of the benefits and timing for starting ventilation, and concerns that ventilatory support might prolong suffering, render home care less feasible, and lead to dependency or ventilator entrapment (Radunović et al., 2007).

Moreover, there is still debate about the optimal timing to introduce ventilation in these patients and whether early NIPPV initiation could actually lead to increased survival rates. With regard to the first aspect, as previously discussed, there are at present many different guidelines that suggest numerous exams to be performed, including upright and supine spirometry, nocturnal oximetry, blood gas analysis and MIP (Andersen et al., 2005, 2007; Miller et al., 2009a).

Concerning to the effects of early NIPPV introduction in patients with ALS, there are some studies that reported increased compliance, quality of life and survival in those patients that received earlier treatment (mainly defined by the evidence of significant desaturations at nocturnal oximetry) (Velasco et al., 2002; Jackson et al., 2001; Pinto et al., 2003; Lechtzin et al., 2007b; Carratù et al., 2009), encouraging earlier use of NIPPV or the use of more sensitive tests to detect chronic alveolar hypoventilation.

According to recently published guidelines, all patients with ALS could benefit from NIPPV therapy, and a trial with this appliance should never be discouraged, although marked bulbar involvement could be associated with reduced tolerance and maybe survival (Miller et al., 2009a). Indeed, the increased risk of aspiration in patients with bulbar onset and problems because of difficulties in clearing secretions or obstructions, such as those related to abnormal function of the vocal cords, should be considered.

In our experience NIPPV can be well tolerated by both patients and caregivers, even in patients with bulbar involvement, especially if an intensive educational training and adaptation on NIPPV can be performed (Volanti et al., 2011). Special importance, then, should be deserved to adaptation and compliance during the first few weeks of NIPPV use, since this could be a crucial step in determining the efficacy of the treatment.

Factors predicting survival following NIPPV include advanced age, airway mucus accumulation and lower body mass index (Peysson et al., 2008; Lo Coco et al., 2006). Noncompliance with NIPPV has been related to frontotemporal dysfunction and severe bulbar involvement, whereas compliance with the treatment was associated with young age, preserved upper limb function, symptoms of orthopnea and dyspnea, use of percutaneous endoscopic gastrostomy (PEG), speech devices, and riluzole (Bourke et al., 2003, 2006; Gruis et al., 2005; Olney et al., 2005; Jackson et al., 2006). Nocturnal hypercapnea has also been recently indicated as a predictor of good compliance with subsequent NIPPV treatment (Kim et al., 2011). Oxygen supplementation should be avoided unless provided with mechanical ventilation or to treat dyspnea as a palliative, periodically monitoring CO_2 levels. In fact oxygen therapy may reduce respiratory drive particularly during sleep and has been associated with CO_2 retention and a less favourable outcome than ventilation (Bach et al., 1998; Gay & Edmonds, 1995).

At present, worldwide accepted guidelines propose NIPPV initiation in the presence of respiratory symptoms, and/or evidence of respiratory muscles weakness (FVC ≤ 80% of predicted or SNIP ≤ 40 cmH$_2$O), evidence of significant nocturnal desaturation on overnight oximetry (< 90% for > 5% of the time asleep) or a morning arterial PaCO$_2$ > 6.5 kPa (Radunović et al., 2007; Miller et al., 2009a).

4. Physiotherapy and management of airway secretions

Physiotherapy is a useful palliative adjunction in the treatment on ALS, in particular in the management of respiratory secretions (Lo Coco et al., 2008). Indeed, during the course of the disease progressive inspiratory and expiratory muscle weakness and bulbar innervated muscle dysfunction result in ineffective cough reflex. Coughing, an important part of the airway defence aiding in the removal of secretions, consists of three components: an inspiratory phase, a compressive phase with glottic closure, and an expulsive phase resulting from sudden glottic opening. Patients with ALS may develop impairment of any of these three phases, and as a result, clearance of respiratory secretions may become problematic, leading to further pulmonary complications.

The effectiveness of mucus clearance is largely dependent on the magnitude of peak cough flows (PCFs) (King et al., 1985), which can be measured using a standard peak flow meter adapted to an anesthesia face mask. A PCF of < 2.7 L/s has been suggested to indicate an ineffective cough (Bach & Saporito, 1996; Tzeng & Bach, 2000). However, since PCF decreases during respiratory tract infections, when the pressure generated by expiratory muscles is reduced (Poponick et al., 1997), it has been suggested that once a patient's PCF is < 4.5 L/s, particularly in the presence of bulbar dysfunction, there is a risk for pulmonary complications (Bach et al., 1997; Sancho et al., 2007). That threshold could be an appropriate time to implement assisted cough techniques. Moreover, patients with a mean PCF above

337 L/min had a significantly greater chance of being alive at 18 months (Chaudri et al., 2002).

Methods of treatment include breathing exercises, postural drainage, exercise regimens and the use of assisted cough techniques (Lo Coco et al., 2008).

Medications with mucolytics like guaifenesin or N-acetylcysteine, a β-receptor antagonist (such as metoprolol and propanolol), nebulized saline, or an anticholinergic bronchodilator such as ipratropium are widely used, although no controlled studies exist in ALS (Miller et al., 2009a).

The benefit of breathing exercises is difficult to evaluate but their main aims can be summarized as: to promote a normal breathing pattern; to teach controlled breathing for use during attacks of dyspnoea; in conjunction with forced expiration technique and postural drainage to assist the removal of secretions; and to maintain the mobility of the chest wall. Patients must be carefully instructed by a physiotherapist and should practise these exercises regularly.

Patients who have excess secretions in the bronchial tree or difficulties in secretions removal may benefit from postural drainage. Postural drainage can be defined as the placement of a patient in various positions so that, with the aid of gravity, secretions may drain from the peripheral to the more central areas of the lung and thus become more easily expectorated. The positions to be used and also the length of time spent in each position must be determined for each patient by a skilled physiotherapist. Clearance of bronchial secretions by postural drainage may be further assisted by the use of deep breathing, percussion and chest vibration, which may be combined with compression of the chest wall and also with the use of the forced expiration technique. However, patients with limited mobility and muscle weakness have difficulty with postural drainage and generally do not benefit from chest physical therapy (Kirilloff et al., 1985). Moreover, intensive cycles of physiotherapy may be exhausting for many patients, particularly those with advanced disease, and may cause arterial desaturation.

Interestingly, a recent double-blind, randomized-controlled trial showed that inspiratory muscle training may potentially strengthen the inspiratory muscles and slow the decline in respiratory function in patients with ALS (Cheah et al., 2009).

Among non-invasive expiratory aids, manually assisted coughing techniques, such as anterior chest compression and abdominal trust, have been shown to be effective in facilitating the elimination of airway secretions in patients with neuromuscular diseases (Massery & Frownfelter, 1990; Bach, 1993a). Nevertheless, manually assisted coughing is labour intensive and often difficult for non-professional caregivers, both during outpatient and in-hospital management, and it depends on precise care provider-patient coordination (Vianello et al., 2005).

The mechanical in-exsufflator (MI-E) is a device that assists patients in clearing bronchial secretions. It consists of a two-stage axial compressor that provides positive pressure (that causes a deep insufflation), thereby generating a forced expiration in which high expiratory flow rates and a high expiratory pressure gradient are generated between the mouth and the alveoli. It is usually applied via a facemask. The use of MI-E has been described to be simple and safe enough for application by non-professional caregivers (Bach, 1993a, 1994), and has been proposed as a complement to manually assisted coughing in the prevention of pulmonary morbidity in neuromuscular patients (Tzeng & Bach, 2000; Bach et al., 1993b). MI-E has also been shown to be helpful in the management of patients with ALS (Sancho et al., 2004) and to be effective in prolonging non-invasive respiratory aids delaying the need for tracheostomy (Bach, 2002). However, this device seems to be ineffective in patients with severe bulbar dysfunction (Bach, 2002; Sancho et al., 2004), perhaps because the application of the exsufflation cycle of MI-E for those patients with weakness of the genioglossus activity due to bulbar dysfunction might produce a dynamic, total, or partial collapse of the upper airway (Sancho et al., 2004).

It is useful to remember that for patients whose vital capacities are less than normal, manually assisted coughing is not optimally effective unless preceded by a maximal lung insufflation, and MI-E is not optimal unless an abdominal trust is applied during the exsufflation (Goncalves & Bach, 2005). Then abdominal trusts and MI-E should be combined together for effective prevention of lower respiratory tract infection and respiratory insufficiency. Failure to correctly administer physical medicine aids continues to make respiratory failure inevitable for the great majority of people with neuromuscular diseases (Goncalves & Bach, 2005).

Finally, high-frequency chest-wall oscillation (HFCWO), another airway-clearance technique, has been recently evaluated in a 12-week randomized, controlled trial on 46 patients with ALS (Lange et al., 2006). HFCWO is a technique that, through generation of high flow in the small airways, is thought to mobilize secretions from the distal airways to the larger airways, from where they can be more easily removed. It has been reported that HFCWO is well tolerated, considered to be helpful by a majority of patients, and decreases symptoms of breathlessness, suggesting that the intervention was useful in the clearance of airway secretions in patients with ALS (Lange et al., 2006). Another study, however, failed to show any benefit in loss of lung function or mortality in 9 patients with ALS (Chaisson et al., 2006).

A part from sustaining respiration with mechanical devices, special consideration should be given to prevention of aspiration and development of pneumonia (Radunović et al., 2007; Miller et al, 2009 a,b). In this regard, it is of fundamental importance the reduction of the amount of salivary secretions through the use of several medications (such as amitriptyline and botulinum toxin injections), devoting adequate amount of time in teaching proper swallowing technique, and maintaining hydration. It is also useful to provide a portable mechanical home suction device. In addition, when dysphagia worsens, placement of a PEG tube should be the preferred option, especially when the respiratory function is not too much compromised. Smoking cessation advice should be offered to all patients who are current smokers. Influenza and pneumococcal immunization should be encouraged during the progression of the disease, although ALS has not been included in specific risk-group recommendations available so far. In case of acute pneumonia, adequacy and length of treatment, proper dosages and intervals of administration, and reduction of delay of initial antibiotic treatment are all important issues (American Thoracic Society, 2005; Lim et al., 2009).

Antibiotic prophylaxis strategies are especially useful to prevent ventilator-associated pneumonia, whereas passive humidifiers or heat–moisture exchangers decrease ventilator circuit colonization, but have not consistently reduced the incidence of ventilator-associated pneumonia, and thus they cannot be regarded as a pneumonia prevention tool (American Thoracic Society, 2005).

5. Invasive mechanical ventilation

ALS is a relentless pathology that causes progressive muscle dysfunction. Therefore respiratory capacity eventually fails, despite NIPPV treatment. Indeed, at first, NIPPV is generally used for intermittent nocturnal support to alleviate symptoms of nocturnal hypoventilation, although as respiratory function worsens, patients tend to require increasing daytime support and eventually continuous support. When all the respiratory aids fail to maintain adequate blood oxygen saturation, the only intervention that allows survival of these patients is invasive mechanical ventilation through a tracheostomy tube. Treatment failure seems not to be dependent on lung or respiratory muscle function but on bulbar dysfunction (Bach et al., 2004).

When placed on invasive ventilation patients are supported from a respiratory point of view; however, the loss of motor neurons goes on progressively, leading to complete paralysis and muscular atrophy. Some patients may eventually reach a "locked in" state in which they cannot communicate at all, because there is also total paralysis of the extraocular muscles. When connected to tracheostomy tubes patients may survive for many years, with respiratory tract infections the most frequent cause of death (Bradley et al., 2002; Hayashi & Oppenheimer, 2003; Lo Coco et al., 2007; Marchese et al., 2008; Vianello et al., 2011). Median survival time usually ranges from 2 to 4 years. Interestingly, the amyotrophic lateral sclerosis functional rating scale (ALSFRS), a disease-specific rating scale that assesses functional impairment, has been shown to predict both length of hospital stay as a result of acute respiratory failure and survival after initiation of invasive ventilation in these patients (Lo Coco et al., 2007).

Notwithstanding its effect on survival, only a minority of patients with ALS receive invasive mechanical ventilation, at least in the western Countries (Moss et al., 1993; Miller et al., 2000; Neudert et al., 2001). On the contrary, in Japan the frequency of invasive ventilation is considerably higher. Many patients are treated in emergency without advance planning, because of a respiratory crisis, whereas the number of patients that electively choose this treatment is low (Moss et al., 1993, 1996; Cazzoli & Oppenheimer, 1996; Lo Coco et al., 2007). Socio-economic reasons may be one of the possible explanations for the low prevalence of invasive ventilation in ALS, given the relatively high costs of this treatment. Moreover there is a need for 24-hour-caregiving, which could be perceived by caregivers and relatives as extremely burdensome. A recent study suggested that the choice of invasive ventilation was consistent with a sustained sense that life was worth living in any way possible, at least for some time and within certain boundaries, although it may involve unrealistic expectations of cure by some (Rabkin et al., 2006). Moreover, the attitudes of the treating physician have also a great influence (Moss et al., 1993), and there is concern that tracheostomy will prolong life beyond the point that the patient can communicate or interact with others.

Despite these many doubts and concerns, the majority of patients that underwent invasive ventilation were positive about their choice (Moss et al., 1993), reporting a satisfying quality of life (Cazzoli & Oppenheimer, 1996; Kaub-Wittemer et al., 2003), and indicating that they would repeat the choice again in the same situation. Caregivers were more frequently burdened and distressed by this intervention and they frequently witnessed a marked reduction of social life activities (Cazzoli & Oppenheimer, 1996; Gelinas et al., 1998; Kaub-Wittemer et al., 2003; Rabkin et al., 2006).

It is good practice that patients together with their families discuss end-of-life issues and preferences with the physician, so that advance directives and patient's wishes are well known in advance of a respiratory crisis (Silverstein et al., 1991; Andersen et al., 2005, 2007). Indeed, once intubated, patients can rarely get free from the ventilator. These preferences should also be reviewed periodically during the course of the disease, since patients' desires concerning life-sustaining interventions might change with disease progression. Ideally, emergency intubation and tracheostomy should be avoided (Andersen et al., 2005, 2007), but this is a much debated question, since there is not universal consent from public authorities. As a result, the percentage of patients that had been tracheotomized without informed consent is very high across studies (Moss et al., 1993, 1996; Cazzoli & Oppenheimer, 1996; Lo Coco et al., 2007).

Symptomatic treatment of severe dyspnea includes use of opioids (morphine) alone or in combination with benzodiazepines (such as lorazepam, diazepam or midazolam), if significant anxiety is present (Voltz & Borasio, 1997; Miller et al., 1999; Andersen et al., 2007; Clemens et al., 2008). Relief of dyspnea using opioids was rated as good by 81% of hospice patients with ALS. (O'Brien et al., 1992). Dose titration against clinical symptoms is recommended and rarely results in life-threatening respiratory depression. Anxiety of choking correlated highly significantly with the intensity of dyspnea (Clemens et al., 2008).

Terminal relentlessness and confusion secondary to hypecapnia could be relieved by administration of neuroleptic drugs (Voltz & Borasio, 1997; Miller et al., 1999; Andersen et al., 2007).

There are some case series offering practical advice for withdrawing both invasive and non-invasive ventilation, including frequent and repeated discussions and counseling with the patient and his family, assessment for discomfort, such as dyspnea, agitation, or anxiety, and symptom management during the withdrawal process with morphine and benzodiazepines (such as diazepam) (Borasio &, Voltz, 1998; Ankrom et al., 2001; O'Mahony et al., 2003). However, there are no controlled studies specifically examining withdrawal of ventilation in ALS (Miller et al., 2009b).

6. Conclusion

Recent publications provided important contributions to many aspects of respiratory care for patients with ALS, such as non-invasive ventilation and assisted cough. There is a need for regular assessment and follow up of respiratory function, and investigations should include daytime assessment of respiratory function (including FVC and SNIP) as well as sleep studies in order to ensure early recognition of patients with respiratory muscle impairment (Lo Coco et al., 2008).

At present time the only approved pharmacological treatment for ALS is riluzole, which extends survival by about 2 months (Miller et al., 2007). On the other hand, NIPPV treatment allows survival for longer periods of time, improves quality of life, and may probably alter the disease course. As a consequence, NIPPV should be considered a major treatment option in patients with chronic hypoventilation or in whom respiratory impairment has become evident during sleep despite normal diurnal respiratory function. Every effort, then, should be made to improve NIPPV implementation in the management of patients with ALS worldwide, since it is still underutilized. The degree of hypoventilation that should prompt introduction of NIPPV must be defined further, even if there is a general tendency toward earlier intervention. Nocturnal hypoventilation could be particularly useful for this purpose.

Prevention of aspiration and pneumonia, and adequate management of bronchial secretions are two other important issues. Adequate treatment of sialorrhea and dysphagia are important in the reduction of pneumonia risk. Insufficient cough is a condition that can be diagnosed by measuring peak cough flow and should, whenever present, be treated in patients with ALS. There is some evidence that the MI-E device could be of help in cough assistance, except for patients with severe bulbar dysfunction, but further research is needed, as well as randomized trials that compare the MI-E with other techniques of assisted coughing.

7. References

Aboussouan, LS; Khan, SU; Meeker, DP; Stelmach, K; Mitsumoto, H. (1997). Effect of noninvasive positive pressure ventilation on survival in ALS. *Ann. Intern. Med.*, vol.127:450-453.

Aboussouan, LS; Khan, Su; Banerjee, M; Arroliga, AC; Mitsumoto, H. (2001). Objective measures of the efficacy of non-invasive positive-pressure ventilation in ALS. *Muscle Nerve*, vol.24:403-409.

American Thoracic Society. (2005). Guidelines for the management of adults with hospital-acquired, ventilator-associated, and healthcare-associated pneumonia. *Am. J. Respir. Crit. Care Med.*, vol.171:388-416.

Andersen, PM; Borasio, GD; Dengler, R; Hardiman, O; Kollewe, K; Leigh, PN; Pradat, PF; Silani, V; Tomik, B; EFNS Task Force on Diagnosis and Management of Amyotrophic Lateral Sclerosis. (2005). EFNS Task Force on managment of amyotrophic lateral sclerosis: guidelines for diagnosing and clinical care of patients and relatives. *Eur. J. Neurol.*, vol.12:921-938.

Andersen, PM; Borasio, GD; Dengler, R; Hardiman, O; Kollewe, K; Leigh, PN; Pradat, PF; Silani, V; Tomik, B; EALSC Working Group. (2007). Good practice in the management of amyotrophic lateral sclerosis: clinical guidelines. An evidence-based review with good practice points. EALSC Working Group. *Amyotroph. Lateral Scler.*, vol.8:195-213.

Ankrom, M; Zelesnick, L; Barofsky, I; Georas, S; Finucane, TE; Greenough, WB 3rd. (2001). Elective discontinuation of life-sustaining mechanical ventilation on a chronic ventilator unit. *J. Am. Geriatr. Soc.*, vol.49:1549-1554.

Arnulf, I; Similowski, T; Salachas, F; Garma, L; Mehiri, S; Attali, V; Behin-Bellhesen, V; Meininger, V; Derenne, JP. (2000). Sleep disorders and diaphragmatic function in patients with ALS. *Am. J. Respir. Crit. Care Med.*, vol.161:849-856.

Bach, JR. (1993). Mechanical insufflation-exsufflation: Comparison of peak expiratory flow with manually assisted and unassisted coughing techniques. *Chest*, vol.104:1553-1562.

Bach, JR; Smith, WH; Michaels, J; Saporito, L; Alba, AS; Dayal, R; Pan, J. (1993). Airway secretion clearance by mechanical exsufflation for post-poliomyelitis ventilator assisted individuals. *Arch. Phys. Med. Rehabil.*, vol.74:170-177.

Bach, JR. (1994). Update and perspective on noninvasive respiratory muscle aids: Part 2. The expiratory aids. *Chest*, vol.105:1538-1544.

Bach, JR & Saporito, LR. (1996). Criteria for extubation and tracheostomy tube removal for patients with ventilatory failure: a different approach to weaning. *Chest*, vol.110:1566-1571.

Bach, JR; Ishikama Y; Kim, H. (1997). Prevention of pulmonary morbidity for patients with Duchenne muscular dystrophy. *Chest*, vol.112:1024-1028.

Bach, JR; Rajaraman, R; Ballanger, F; Tzeng, AC; Ishikawa, Y; Kulessa, R; Bansal, T. (1998). Neuromuscular ventilatory insufficiency: effect of home mechanical ventilator use v oxygen therapy on pneumonia and hospitalization rates. *Am. J. Phys. Med. Rehabil.*, vol.77:8-19.

Bach, JR. (2002). Amyotrophic lateral sclerosis: prolongation of life by noninvasive respiratory aids. *Chest*, vol.122:92-98.

Bach, JR; Bianchi, C; Aufiero, E. (2004). Oximetry and indications for tracheostomy for amyotrophic lateral sclerosis. *Chest*, vol.126:1502-1507.

Baumann, F; Henderson, RD; Morrison, SC; Brown, M; Hutchinson, N; Douglas, JA; Robinson, PJ; McCombe, PA. (2010). Use of respiratory function tests to predict survival in amyotrophic lateral sclerosis. *Amyotroph. Lateral Scler.*, vol.11:194-202.

Beneditt, JO & Boitano L. (2008). Respiratory treatment of amyotrophic lateral sclerosis. *Phys. Med. Rehabil. Clin. N. Am.*, vol.19:559-572.

Borasio, GD & Voltz, R. (1998). Discontinuation of mechanical ventilation in patients with amyotrophic lateral sclerosis. *J. Neurol.*, vol.245:717-722.

Bourke, SC; Williams, TL; Bullock, RE; Gibson, GJ; Shaw, PJ. (2002). Non-invasive ventilation in motor neuron disease: current UK practice. *Amyotroph. Lateral Scler.*, vol.3:145-149.

Bourke, SC; Bullock, RE; Williams, TL; Shaw, PJ; and Gibson, GJ. (2003). Noninvasive ventilation in ALS. Indications and effect on quality of life. *Neurology*, vol.61:171-177.

Bourke, SC; Tomlinson, M; Williams, TL; Bullock, RE; Shaw, PJ; Gibson, GJ. (2006). Effects of non-invasive ventilation on survival and quality of life in patients with amyotrophic lateral sclerosis: a randomised controlled trial. *Lancet Neurol.*, vol.5:140-147.

Bradley, WG; Anderson, F; Bromberg, M; Gutmann, L; Harati, Y; Ross, M; Miller, RG; ALS CARE Study Group. (2001). Current management of ALS: comparison of the ALS CARE Database and the AAN Practice Parameter. *Neurology*, vol.57:500-504.

Bradley, MD; Orrell, RW; Clarke, J; Davidson, AC; Williams, AJ; Kullmann, DM; Hirsch, N; Howard, RS. (2002). Outcome of ventilatory support for acute respiratory failure in motor neuron disease. *J. Neurol. Neurosurg. Psychiatry*, vol.72:752-756.

Carrat, P; Cassano, A; Gadaleta, F; Tedone, M; Dongiovanni, S; Fanfulla, F; Resta, O. (July 2011). Association between low sniff nasal-inspiratory pressure (SNIP) and sleep disordered breathing in amyotrophic lateral sclerosis: Preliminary results. *Amyotroph. Lateral Scler.*, [Epub ahead of print].

Carratù, P; Spicuzza, L; Cassano, A; Maniscalco, M; Gadaleta, F; Lacedonia, D; Scoditti, C; Boniello, E; Di Maria, G; Resta, O. (2009). Early treatment with non invasive positive pressure ventilation prolongs survival in Amyotrophic Lateral Sclerosis patients with nocturnal respiratory insufficiency. *Orphanet J. Rare Dis.*, vol.4:10.

Cazzoli, PA & Oppenheimer, EA. (1996). Home mechanical ventilation for ALS: Nasal compared to tracheostomy-intermittent positive pressure ventilation. *J. Neurol. Sci.*, vol.139(suppl):123-128.

Chaisson, KM; Walsh, S; Simmons, Z; Vender, RL. (2006). A clinical pilot study: high frequency chest wall oscillation airway clearance in patients with amyotrophic lateral sclerosis. *Amyotroph. Lateral Scler.,* vol.7:107-11.

Chaudri, MB; Liu, C; Watson, L; Jefferson, D; Kinnear, WJ. (2000). Sniff nasal inspiratory pressure as a marker of respiratory function in motor neuron disease. *Eur. Respir. J.,* vol.15:539-542.

Chaudri, MB; Liu, C; Hubbard, R; Jefferson, D; Kinnear, WJ. (2002). Relationship between supramaximal flow during cough and mortality in motor neuron disease. *Eur. Respir. J.,* vol.19:434-438.

Cheah, BC; Boland, RA; Brodaty, NE; Zoing, MC; Jeffery, SE; McKenzie, DK; Kiernan, MC. (2009). INSPIRATIonAL - INSPIRAtory muscle Training In Amyotrophic Lateral sclerosis. *Amyotroph. Lateral Scler.,* vol.28:1-9.

Clemens, KE & Klaschik, E. (2008). Morphine in the management of dyspnoea in ALS. A pilot study. *Eur. J. Neurol.,* vol.15:445-450.

Czaplinski, A; Yen, AA; Appel, SH. (2006). Forced vital capacity (FVC) as an indicator of survival and disease progression in an ALS clinic population. *J. Neurol. Neurosurg. Psychiatry,* vol.77:390-392.

De Carvalho, M ; Matias, T ; Coelho, F ; Evangelista, T ; Pinto, A ; Luis, ML. (1996). Motor neuron disease presenting with respiratory failure. *J. Neurol. Sci.,* vol.139(Suppl.):117-122.

Fallat, RJ; Jewitt, B, Bass, M; Kamm, B; Norris, F. (1979). Spirometry in amyotrophic lateral sclerosis. *Arch. Neurol.,* vol.36:74-80.

Farrero, E; Prats, E; Povedano, M; Martinez-Matos, JA; Manresa, F; Escabrill, J. (2005). Survival in amyotrophic lateral sclerosis with home mechanical ventilation. The impact of systematic respiratory assessment and bulbar involvement. *Chest,* vol.127:2132-2138.

Ferguson, KA; Strong, MJ; Ahmad, D; George, FP. (1996). Sleep-disordered breathing in amyotrophic lateral sclerosis. *Chest,* vol.110:664-669.

Fitting, JW; Paillex, R; Hirt, L; Aebischer, P; Schluep, M. (1999). Sniff nasal pressure: A sensitive respiratory test to assess progression of amyotrophic lateral sclerosis. *Ann. Neurol.,* vol.46:887-893.

Gay, PC; Westbrook, PR; Daube, JR; Litchy, WJ; Windebank, AJ; Iverson, R. (1991). Effects of alterations in pulmonary function and sleep variables on survival in patients with ALS. *Mayo Clin. Proc.,* vol.66:686-694.

Gay, PC & Edmonds, LC. (1995). Severe hypercapnia after low-flow oxygen therapy in patients with neuromuscular disease and diaphragmatic dysfunction. *Mayo Clin. Proc.,* vol.70:327-330.

Gelinas, DF; O'Connor, P; Miller, RG. (1998). Quality of life for ventilator-dependent ALS patients and their caregivers. *J. Neurol. Sci.,* vol.160(Suppl. 1):S134-S136.

Goncalves, MR & Bach, JR. (2005). Mechanical insullation.exsufflation improves outcomes for neuromuscular disease patients with respiratory tract infections. A step in the right direction (Commentary). *Am. J. Phys. Med. Rehabil.,* vol.84:89-91.

Gruis, KL; Brown, DL; Schoennemann, A; Zebarah, VA; Feldman, EL. (2005). Predictors of noninvasive ventilation tolerance in patients with amyotrophic lateral sclerosis. *Muscle Nerve,* vol.32:808-811.

Hayashi, H & Oppenheimer, EA. (2003). ALS patients on TPPV. Totally locked-in state, neurologic findings and ethical implications. *Neurology*, vol.61:135-137.

Heffernan, C; Jenkinson, C; Holmes, T; Macleod, H; Kinnear, W; Oliver, D; Leigh, N; Ampong, MA. (2006). Management of respiration in MND/ALS patients: an evidence based review. *Amyotroph. Lateral Scler.*, vol.7:5-15.

Heiman-Patterson, TD & Miller, RG. (2006). NIPPV: A treatment for ALS whose time has come. *Neurology*, vol.67:736-737.

Jackson, CE; Rosenfeld, J; Moore, DH; Bryan, WW; Barohn, RJ; Wrench, M; Myers, D; Heberlin, L; King, R; Smith, J; Gelinas, D; Miller, RG. (2001). A preliminary evaluation of a prospective study of pulmonary function studies and symptoms of hypoventilation in ALS/MND patients. *J. Neurol. Sci.*, vol.191:75-78.

Just, N; Bautin, N; Danel-Brunaud, V; Debroucker, V; Matran, R; Perez, T. (2010). The Borg dyspnoea score: a relevant clinical marker of inspiratory muscle weakness in amyotrophic lateral sclerosis. *Eur. Respir. J.*, vol.35:353-360.

Kaub-Wittemer, D; von Steinbüchel, N; Wasner, M; Laier-Groenveld, G; and Borasio, GD. (2003). Quality of life and psychososcial issues in ventilated patients with amyotrophic lateral sclerosis and their caregivers. *J. Pain and Symptom Manage.*, vol.26:890-896.

Kim, SM; Lee, KM; Hong, YH; Park, KS; Yang, JH; Nam, HW; Sung, JJ; Lee, KW. (2007). Relationship between cognitive dysfunction and reduced vital capacity in ALS. *J. Neurol. Neurosurg. Psychiatry*, vol.78:1387-1389.

Kim, SM; Park, KS; Nam, H; Ahn, SW; Kim, S; Sung, JJ; Lee, KW. (March 2011). Capnography for assessing nocturnal hypoventilation and predicting compliance with subsequent noninvasive ventilation in patients with ALS. *PLoS One*, vol.6(3):e17893. [Epub ahead of print].

King, M; Brock, G; Lundell, C. (1985). Clearance of mucus by simulated cough. *J. Appl. Physiol.*, vol.58:1776-1782.

Kirilloff, LH; Owens, GR; Rogers, RM; Mazzocco, MC. (1985). Does chest physical therapy work? *Chest*, vol.88:436-444.

Kleopa, KA; Sherman, M; Bettle, N; Romano, CJ; Heiman-Patterson, T. (1999). BiPap improves survival and rate of pulmonary function decline in patients with ALS. *J. Neurol. Sci.*, vol.164:82-88.

Lange, DJ; Lechtzin, N; Davey, C; David, W; Heiman-Patterson, T; Gelinas, D; Becker, B; Mitsumoto, H; HFCWO Study Group. (2006). High-frequency chest wall oscillation in ALS: an exploratory randomized, controlled trial. *Neurology*, vol.67:991-997.

Lechtzin, N; Wiener, CM; Clawson, L; Davidson, MC; Anderson, F; Gowda, N; Diette, GB; and the ALS CARE Study Group. (2004). Use of noninvasive ventilation in patients with amyotrophic lateral sclerosis. *Amyotroph. Lateral Scler.*, vol.5:9-15.

Lechtzin, N; Lange, DJ; Davey, C; Becker, B; Mitsumoto, H. (2007). Measures of dyspnea in patients with amyotrophic lateral sclerosis. *Muscle Nerve*, vol.35:98-102.

Lechtzin, N; Scott, Y; Busse, AM; Clawson, LL; Kimball, R; Wiener, CM. (2007). Early use of non-invasive ventilation prolongs survival in subjects with ALS. *Amyotroph. Lateral Scler.*, vol.8:185-188.

Lim WS, Baudouin SV, George RC, *et al.* (2009). BTS guidelines for the management of community acquired pneumonia in adults: update 2009. *Thorax*, vol.64(Suppl. 3):iii1-55.

Lo Coco, D; Marchese, S; Corrao, S; Pesco, MC; La Bella, V; Piccoli, F; Lo Coco, A. (2006). Development of chronic hypoventilation in Amyotrophic Lateral Sclerosis patients. *Respir. Med.,* vol.100:1028-1036.

Lo Coco, D; Marchese, S; Pesco, MC; La Bella, V; Piccoli, F; Lo Coco, A. (2006). Noninvasive positive-pressure ventilation in ALS. Predictors of tolerance and survival. *Neurology,* vol.67:761-765.

Lo Coco, D; Marchese, S; La Bella, V; Piccoli, T; Lo Coco, A. (2007). The amyotrophic lateral sclerosis functional rating scale predicts survival time in amyotrophic lateral sclerosis patients on invasive mechanical ventilation. *Chest,* vol.132:64-69.

Lo Coco, D; Marchese, S; Lo Coco, A. (2008). Recent advances in respiratory care for Motor Neuron Disease, In: *Motor Neuron Disease Research Progress,* R.L. Mancini, (Ed.), 253-269, Nova Science Publishers, Inc., ISBN 978-60456-155-5, New York, U.S.A.

Lo Coco, D; Mattaliano, P; Spataro, R; Mattaliano, A; La Bella, V. (2011). Sleep-wake disturbances in patients with amyotrophic lateral sclerosis. *J. Neurol. Neurosurg. Psychiatry,* vol.82:839-842.

Lomen-Hoerth, C. (2005). The effects of executive and behavioral dysfunction on the course of ALS. *Neurology,* vol.65:1774-1777.

Lyall, RA; Donaldson, N; Fleming, T; Wood, C; Newsom-Davis, I; Polkey, MI; Leigh, PN; Moxham, J. (2001). A prospective study of quality of life in ALS patients treated with noninvasive ventilation. *Neurology,* vol.57:153-156.

Lyall, RA; Donaldson, N; Polkey, MI; Leigh, PN; Moxham, J. (2001). Respiratory muscle strength and ventilatory failure in amyotrophic lateral sclerosis. *Brain,* vol.124:2000-2013.

Marchese, S; Lo Coco, D; Lo Coco, A. (2008). Outcome and attitudes toward home tracheostomy ventilation of consecutive patients: a 10-year experience. *Respir. Med.,* vol.102:430-436.

Marti-Fabregas, J; Dourado, M; Sanchis, J; Miralda, R; Pradas, J; Illa, I. (1995). Respiratory function deterioration is not time-linked with upper-limb onset in amyotrophic lateral sclerosis. *Acta Neurol. Scand.,* vol.92:261-264.

Massery, M & Frownfelter, D. (1990). Assisted cough techniques: There's more than one way to cough. *Phys. Ther. Forum.,* vol.9:1-4.

Miller, RG; Rosenberg, JA; Gelinas, DF; Mitsumoto, H; Newman, D; Sufit, R; Borasio, GD; Bradley, WG; Bromberg, MB; Brooks, BR; Kasarskis, EJ; Munsat, TL; Oppenheimer, EA. (1999). Practice parameter. The care of the patient with ALS (an evidence based review). *Neurology,* vol.52:1311-1323.

Miller, RG; Anderson, FA Jr; Bradley, WG; Brooks, BR; Mitsumoto, H; Munsat, TL; Ringel, SP. (2000). The ALS patient care database: goals, design, and early results. ALS C.A.R.E. Study Group. *Neurology,* vol.54:53-57.

Miller, RG; Mitchell, JD; Lyon, M, Moore, DH. (2007). Riluzole for amyotrophic lateral sclerosis (ALS)/motor neuron disease (MND). *Cochrane Database Syst. Rev.,* vol.1:CD001447.

Miller, RG; Jackson, CE; Kasarskis, EJ; England, JD; Forshew, D; Johnston, W; Kalra, S; Katz, JS; Mitsumoto, H; Rosenfeld, J; Shoesmith, C; Strong, MJ; Woolley, SC; Quality Standards Subcommittee of the American Academy of Neurology. (2009). Practice parameter update: The care of the patient with amyotrophic lateral sclerosis: drug, nutritional, and respiratory therapies (an evidence-based review): report of the

Quality Standards Subcommittee of the American Academy of Neurology. *Neurology*, vol.73:1218-1226.

Miller, RG; Jackson, CE; Kasarskis, EJ; England, JD; Forshew, D; Johnston, W; Kalra, S; Katz, JS; Mitsumoto, H; Rosenfeld, J; Shoesmith, C; Strong, MJ; Woolley, SC; Quality Standards Subcommittee of the American Academy of Neurology. (2009). Practice parameter update: The care of the patient with amyotrophic lateral sclerosis: multidisciplinary care, symptom management, and cognitive/behavioral impairment (an evidence-based review): report of the Quality Standards Subcommittee of the American Academy of Neurology. *Neurology*, vol.73:1227-1233.

Morgan, RK; McNally, S; Alexander, M; Conroy, R; Hardiman, O; Costello, RW. (2005). Use of Sniff nasal-inspiratory force to predict survival in amyotrophic lateral sclerosis. *Am. J. Respir. Crit. Care Med.*, vol.171:269-274.

Moss, AH; Casey, P; Stocking, CB; Roos, RP; Brooks, BR; Siegler, M. (1993). Home ventilation for ALS patients: outcomes, costs, and patient, family, and physician attitudes. *Neurology*, vol.43:438-443.

Moss, AH; Oppenheimer, EA; Casey, P; Cazzolli, PA; Roos, RP; Stocking, CB; Siegler, M. (1996). Patients with amyotrophic lateral sclerosis receiving long-term mechanical ventilation: advance care planning and outcomes. *Chest*, vol.110:249-255.

Munsat, TL; Andres, PL; Finison, L; Conlon, T; Thibodeau, L. (1988). The natural history of motorneuron loss in amyotrophic lateral sclerosis. *Neurology*, vol.38:409-413.

Mustfa, N; Walsh, E; Bryant, V; Lyall, RA; Addington-Hall, J; Goldstein, LH; Donaldson, N; Polkey, MI; Moxham, J; Leigh, PN. (2006). The effect of noninvasive ventilation on ALS patients and their caregivers. *Neurology*, vol.66:1211-1217.

Neudert, C; Oliver, D; Wasner, M; Borasio, G. (2001). The course of the terminal phase in patients with amyotrophic lateral sclerosis. *J. Neurol.*, vol.248:612-616.

Newson-Davis, IC; Lyall, RA; Leigh, PN; Morham, J; Goldstein, LH. (2001). The effect of NIPPV on cognitive function in ALS: a prospective study. *J. Neurol. Neurosur. Psychiatry*, vol.71:482-487.

O'Brien, T; Kelly, M; Saunders, C. (1992). Motor neuron disease: a hospice perspective. *BMJ*, vol.304:471-473.

Olney, RK; Murphy, J; Forshew, D; Garwood, E; Miller, BL; Langmore, S; Kohn, MA; Lomen-Hoerth, C. (2005). The effects of executive and behavioral dysfunction on the course of ALS. *Neurology*, vol.65:1774-1777.

O'Mahony, S; McHugh, M; Zallman, L; Selwyn, P. (2003). Ventilator withdrawal: procedures and outcomes. Report of a collaboration between a critical care division and a palliative care service. *J. Pain Symptom Manage.*, vol.26:954-961.

Peysson, S; Vandenberghe, N; Philit, F; Vial, C; Petitjean, T; Bouhour, F; Bayle, JY; Broussolle E. (2008). Factors predicting survival following noninvasive ventilation in amyotrophic lateral sclerosis. *Eur. Neurol.*, vol.59:164-171.

Pinto, A; de Carvalho, M; Evangelista, T; Lopes, A; Sales-Luis, L. (2003). Nocturnal pulse oximetry: a new approach to estabilish the appropriate time for non-invasive ventilation in ALS patients. *Amyotroph. Lateral Scler.*, vol.4:31-35.

Pinto, AC; Evangelista, T; Carvalho, M; Alves, MA; Sales Luis, ML. (1995). Respiratory assistance with a non-invasive ventilator (BiPaP) in motor neuron disease/ALS patients: survival rates in a controlled trial. *J. Neurol. Sci.*, vol.129(Suppl.):19-26.

Poponick, JM; Jacobs, I; Supinski, G; Di Marco AF. (1997). Effect of upper respiratory tract infection in patients with neuromuscular disease. *Am. J. Resp. Crit. Care Med.,* vol.156.659-664.

Rabkin, JG; Albert, SM; Tider, T; Del Bene, ML; O'Sullivan, I; Rowland, LP; Mitsumoto, H. (2006). Predictors and course of elective long-term mechanical ventilation: A prospective study of ALS patients. *Amyotroph. Lateral Scler.,* vol.7:86-95.

Radunović, A; Mitsumoto, H; Leigh, PN. (2007). Clinical care of patients with amyotrophic lateral sclerosis. *Lancet Neurol.,* vol.6:913-25.

Sancho, J; Servera, E; Diaz, J; Marin J. (2004). Efficacy of mechanical insufflation-exsufflation in medically stable patients with amyotrophic lateral sclerosis. *Chest,* vol.125:1400-1405.

Sancho, J; Servera, E; Diaz, J; Marin J. (2007). Predictors of ineffective cough during a chest infection in stable ALS patients. *Am. J. Resp. Crit. Care Med.,* vol.175:1266-1271.

Schiffman, PL & Belsh, JM. (1993). Pulmonary function at diagnosis of ALS. Rate of deterioration. *Chest,* vol.103:508-513.

Schmidt, EP; Drachman, DB; Wiener, CM; Clawson, L; Kimball, R; Lechtzin, N. (2006). Pulmonary predictors of survival in amyotrophic lateral sclerosis: Use in clinical trial design. *Muscle Nerve,* vol.33:127-132.

Silverstein, MD; Stocking, CB; Antel, JP; Beckwith, J; Roos, RP; Siegler, M. (1991). Amyotrophic lateral sclerosis and life-sustaining therapy: patients' desires for information, participation in decision making, and life-sustaining therapy. *Mayo Clin. Proc.,* vol.66:906-913.

Stembler, N; Charatan, M; Cederbaum, JM; and the ALS CNTF Treatment Study Croup. (1998). Prognostic indicators of survival in ALS. *Neurology,* vol.50:66-72.

Tzeng, AC & Bach, JR. (2000). Prevention of pulmonary morbidity for patients with neuromuscular disease. *Chest,* vol.118:1390-1396.

Varrato, J; Siderowf, A; Damiano, P; Gregory, S; Feinberg, D; McCluskey, L. (2001). Postural change of forced vital capacity predicts some respiratory symptoms in ALS. *Neurology,* vol.57:357-359.

Velasco, R; Salachas, F; Munerati, E; Le Forestier, N; Pradat, PF; Lacomblez, L; Orvoen Frija, E; Meininger, V. (2002). Nocturnal oximetry in patients with amyotrophic lateral sclerosis: role in predicting survival. *Rev. Neurol.,* vol.158:575-578.

Vianello, A; Corrado, A; Arcaro, G; Gallan, F; Ori, C; Minuzzo, M; Bevilacqua, M. (2005). Mechanical insullation.exsufflation improves outcomes for neuromuscular disease patients with respiratory tract infections. *Am. J. Phys. Med. Rehabil.,* vol.84:83-88.

Vianello, A; Arcaro, G; Palmieri, A; Ermani, M; Braccioni, F; Gallan, F; Sorarù, G; Pegoraro, E. (2011). Survival and quality of life after tracheostomy for acute respiratory failure in patients with amyotrophic lateral sclerosis. *J. Crit. Care,* vol.26:329.e7-14.

Volanti, P; Cibella, F; Sarvà, M; De Cicco, D; Spanevello, A; Mora, G; La Bella, V. (2011). Predictors of non-invasive ventilation tolerance in amyotrophic lateral sclerosis. *J. Neurol. Sci.,* vol.303:114-118.

Voltz, R & Borasio, GD. (1997). Palliative therapy in the terminal stage of neurological disease. *J. Neurol.,* vol.244(Suppl. 4):S2-10.

10

Multidisciplinary Rehabilitation in Amyotrophic Lateral Sclerosis

Louisa Ng and Fary Khan
Royal Melbourne Hospital and University of Melbourne
Australia

1. Introduction

Amyotrophic Lateral Sclerosis (ALS) is the most common chronic neurodegenerative disorder of the motor system in adults. It is a relatively rare disease with a reported population incidence of between 1.5 and 2.5 per 100,000 per year worldwide and a gender ratio of 3:2 men: women. Amyotrophic Lateral Sclerosis is characterized by the loss of motor neurons in the cortex, brain stem, and spinal cord, manifested by upper and lower motor neuron signs and symptoms affecting bulbar, limb, and respiratory muscles. Death usually results from respiratory failure and follows on average two to four years after onset, but some may survive for a decade or more.

Amyotrophic Lateral Sclerosis is a devastating condition with unknown aetiology and no current cure. The symptoms in ALS are diverse and challenging and include weakness, spasticity, limitations in mobility and activities of daily living, communication deficits and dysphagia, and in those with bulbar involvement, respiratory compromise, fatigue and sleep disorders, pain and psychosocial distress. The International Classification of Functioning, Disability and Health (ICF) (World Health Organization, 2001), defines a common language for describing the impact of disease at different levels: impairment (body structure and function), limitation in activity and participation (see Figure 1). Within this framework ALS related impairments (weakness, spasticity), can limit "activity" or function (decreased mobility, self-care, pain) and "participation" (driving, employment, family, social reintegration). "Contextual factors", such as environmental (extrinsic) and personal factors (intrinsic) interact with all the other constructs to shape the impact of ALS on patients and their families. The impact of ALS upon patients, their caregivers (often family members) and on society is substantial, often beginning long before the actual diagnosis is made, and increasing with increasing disability and the need for medical equipment and assisted care (Klein and Forshew, 1996).

Given the broad spectrum of needs, current management spans from diagnosis (acute neurological needs) through to symptomatic and supportive rehabilitation and palliative care. The interface between neurology, rehabilitation and palliative care is of utmost importance to ensure co-ordinated care for persons with ALS rather than duplicating services (Royal College of Physicians National Council for Palliative Care and British Society of Rehabilitation Medicine, 2008). It should be noted however that the focus of this chapter is on the rehabilitation phases, hence discussion of acute neurological and palliative care aspects are limited.

Rehabilitation is defined as "a problem solving educational process aimed at reducing disability and increasing participation experienced by someone as a result of disease or injury" (Wade, 1992). Although it is sometimes effective in reducing impairment, its principal focus is to reduce symptoms and limitations at the level of activity and participation, through holistic interventions, which incorporate personal and environmental factors. The multidisciplinary rehabilitation team (see Figure 2) comprises of a group of clinical professionals with expertise in ALS, directed by a physician, who work as an integrated unit to provide seamless care which is patient-centred, flexible and responsive to the evolving nature of the condition (Hardiman, 2007). The role of multidisciplinary rehabilitation in ALS is supported by a recent Cochrane review (Ng et al., 2009) which suggested some advantage for quality of life without increasing healthcare costs, reduced hospitalisation and improved disability with conflicting evidence for survival.

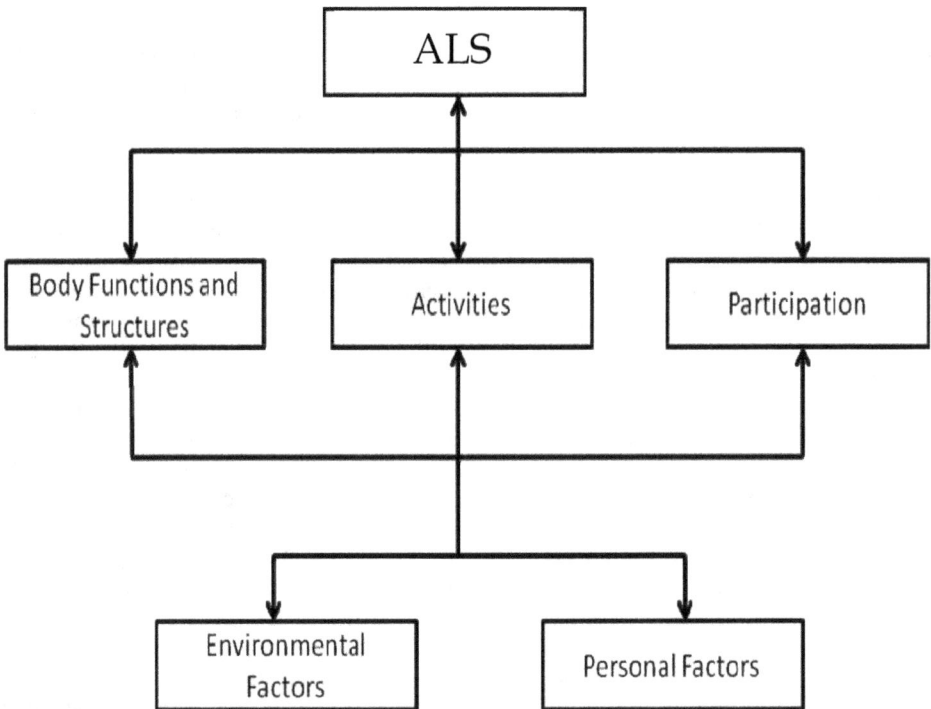

Fig. 1. The interaction between the various domains of the International Classification of Functioning, Disability and Health (adapted from (World Health Organization, 2001))

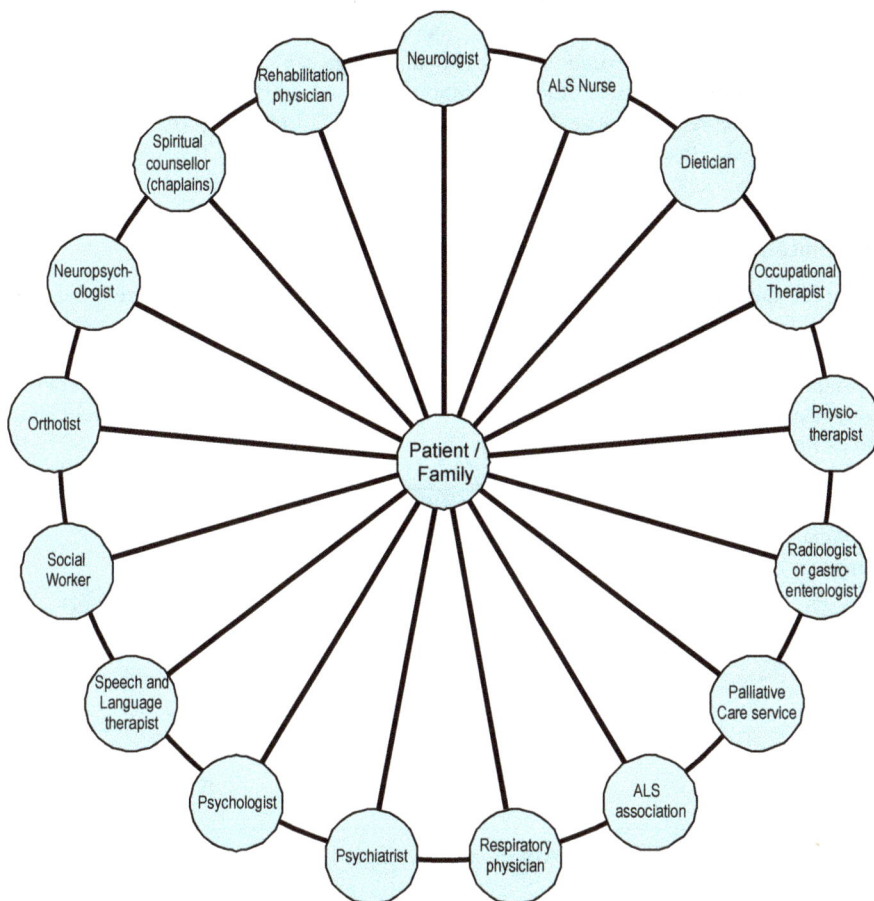

Fig. 2. The multidisciplinary rehabilitation team in ALS (adapted from (Hardiman, 2007))

A proposed model for service interaction in caring for persons with ALS shows involvement of neurologists and palliative care teams in the acute and terminal phases of care, with a relatively smaller role for rehabilitation physicians. However rehabilitation plays a major role in long-term care and support (over years) in the more slowly progressive phase (Royal College of Physicians National Council for Palliative Care and British Society of Rehabilitation Medicine, 2008). Early rehabilitation intervention and treatment has much to contribute to improve health and quality of life prior to accumulation of disability through symptomatic and supportive therapies to enhance functional independence and community integration and reduce barriers (such as lack of knowledge about treatment, economic constraints) (Kemp, 2005). Disability management in ALS should also be planned, with deficits should be anticipated (over time) to avoid "crisis management". As patients deteriorate the rehabilitation and palliative care approaches can overlap, i.e. "neuropalliative rehabilitation". Key skills in neuropalliative rehabilitation include: understanding disease progression, symptom control, managing expectations, issues relating to communication, addressing end of life issues, legal issues (mental capacity, wills), specialist interventions (ventilation), equipment needs, counselling and support, and welfare advice (Royal College of Physicians National Council for Palliative Care and British Society of Rehabilitation Medicine, 2008).

The literature presented in this review includes all levels of evidence for multidisciplinary rehabilitation of ALS (including randomised and clinical controlled trials, case studies and expert opinion).

2. Rehabilitation issues in ALS

Amyotrophic Lateral Sclerosis is a fatal disease with a challenging progressive course that results in a broad and ever-changing spectrum of care needs. Symptoms are varied (see Table 1) and need to be carefully assessed and managed. The timing of provision of appropriate care is important as whilst information needs to be provided when patients are psychologically in the right frame of mind, the options of certain interventions may be time-limited as the disease continues to progress.

Weakness	94%
Dysphagia	90%
Dyspnoea	85%
Pain	73%
Weight loss	71%
Speech issues	71%
Constipation	54%
Cough	48%
Sleep issues	29%
Emotional lability	27%
Drooling	25%

Table 1. Symptoms experienced by ALS patients (adapted from (Oliver, 1996))

2.1 Respiratory dysfunction

Most deaths in ALS are due to respiratory failure from respiratory muscle weakness, hence the diagnosis and management of respiratory symptoms is important (Figure 3) (Miller et al., 2009a). Counselling may be initiated at the time of diagnosis especially if respiratory symptoms are present and/or forced vital capacity (FVC) is <60% of predicted. Early symptoms may be suggestive of nocturnal hypoventilation (eg. frequent arousals, morning headaches, excessive daytime sleepiness, vivid dreams) rather than overt dyspnoea (Miller et al., 2009a). It is important to discuss the options of respiratory choices, including tracheostomy and ventilatory support well before these are clinically indicated to enable advance planning or directives. It is also important to offer patients information about the terminal stages of ALS and reassure regarding terminal hypercapnoeic coma and resulting peaceful death, as many may fear "choking to death" (Borasio et al., 2001b).

Respiratory function should be evaluated every three months from the time of diagnosis. Whilst FVC is the most commonly used (Melo et al., 1999) and significantly predicts survival (Czaplinski et al., 2006), it can be insensitive to slight changes in muscle strength (Fitting et al., 1999). The maximal sniff nasal inspiratory force (sniff nasal pressure) may be more appropriate especially in those with bulbar weakness (no mouthpiece) and may be more sensitive to changes in diaphragmatic and respiratory muscle strength (Stefanutti et al., 2000;Lyall et al., 2001). It is also more reliably recorded in the later stages of ALS (Morgan et al., 2005).

Initial management can include chest physiotherapy and postural drainage, especially if the patient has difficulty clearing secretions from the chest (Shaw, 2003). A suction machine may also be helpful. Preventing respiratory infections is a primary goal and pneumococcal and influenza vaccines should be administered. Respiratory muscle exercise can be instituted and may delay the onset of ventilatory failure (Schiffman, 1996).

Non-invasive ventilation (NIV) should be considered in respiratory dysfunction (see Figure 3) especially for nocturnal symptomatic respiratory compromise. A recent Cochrane review concluded that NIV significantly improves quality of life when tolerated and may prolong survival in those with normal to moderately impaired bulbar function especially if used for ≥ 4 hours/day (Radunovic et al., 2009). Successful use of NIV is dependent on respiratory therapists and patients working closely and patiently through the adjustment phase of NIV, especially with selection and tolerance of face masks. A small dose of anxiolytic may assist with the process in select patients. Bulbar involvement and executive dysfunction may also reduce compliance (Miller et al., 2009a).

Invasive ventilation should be offered when longer-term survival is the goal. Counselling is necessary with regards to benefits and burden (expense, intensive physical support with suctioning and nursing care, high caregiver burden) as many may not be able to manage invasive ventilation at home, thus requiring nursing home placement (Kaub-Wittemer et al., 2003;Miller et al., 2009a). There is evidence however that the 10-20% of persons with ALS who undergo invasive ventilation (including those administered at the time of acute respiratory failure without advance discussion) appear to have good acceptance and satisfactory quality of life (Vianello et al., 2010).

2.2 Communication

Dysarthria is common as a result of bulbar involvement and is often a source of significant frustration to the persons with ALS and their families. Early changes include nasality or reduced vocal volume and changes in oral movement rates and speech rates (Yorkston et al., 1993). As weakness and spasticity of the oral and laryngeal muscles increase, imprecise consonant production, hypernasality, harsh vocal quality, slowed rate of speech and breath volumes affect intelligibility (Hillel and Miller, 1989). Speech pathologists can teach the patient to slow speech rate, exaggerate articulation and improve respiratory efficiency through phrasing (Francis et al., 1999). Palatal lift and palatal augmentation prostheses may also be of some use to reduce the hypernasal aspect of dysarthria (Esposito et al., 2000).

As intelligibility in ALS worsens, Augmentative and Alternative Communication (AAC) is required. AACs can improve quality of life by optimising function and assisting with decision making (Brownlee and Palovcak, 2007). AACs range from no or low technology (gestures, communication boards with letters) to high-tech electronic communication devices that allow the user to have voice output (Brownlee and Palovcak, 2007). For example, speech-generating devices such as LightWRITERs are commonly used. These devices can be used as long as there is voluntary motor movement (including eye gaze). The specific access method depends on the abilities of the patient – for example, pointing with a body part or pointer, adapted mice or joysticks or switches and scanning technology can be used. For those who have no voluntary motor control for communication, a recent case study using a brain-computer interface system has been reported and appears promising (Sellers et al., 2010). The emotional aspect of using an alternative form of communication however can result in significant patient resistance and acceptance as the ability to speak and use language is what distinguishes us from all other species (Pinker and Jackendoff, 2005;Brownlee and Palovcak, 2007). Hence, acceptance of an AAC may take weeks to months.

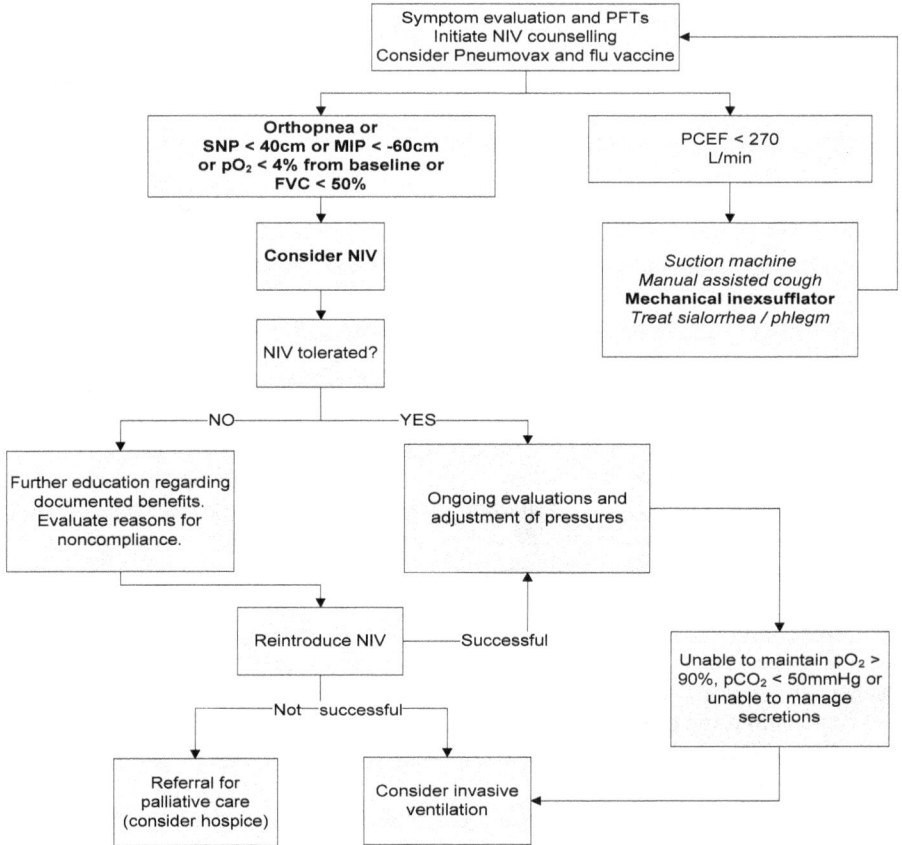

Symptom evaluation and PFTs
Initiate NIV counselling
Consider Pneumovax and flu vaccine

Orthopnea or
SNP < 40cm or MIP < -60cm
or pO₂ < 4% from baseline or
FVC < 50%

PCEF < 270
L/min

Consider NIV

Suction machine
Manual assisted cough
Mechanical inexsufflator
Treat sialorrhea / phlegm

NIV tolerated?

NO   YES

Further education regarding documented benefits. Evaluate reasons for noncompliance.

Ongoing evaluations and adjustment of pressures

Reintroduce NIV ———— Successful

Unable to maintain pO₂ > 90%, pCO₂ < 50mmHg or unable to manage secretions

Not—successful

Referral for palliative care (consider hospice)

Consider invasive ventilation

Text in bold = evidence-based
Text in italics = consensus-based

PFT = pulmonary function tests; PCEF = peak cough expiratory flow; NIV = noninvasive ventilation; SNP = sniff nasal pressure; MIP = maximal inspiratory pressure; FVC = forced vital capacity (supine or erect)

Fig. 3. Respiratory management algorithm in ALS (adapted from (Miller et al., 2009a))

A source of significant frustration for those with speech difficulties is use of the telephone. Technology is available and varies from country to country. In the United States, "Speech to Speech" technology can be used, where trained communication assistants are used by the patient to complete phone calls. They are trained to use superior equipment to hear the caller and place the call, then repeat verbatim what the caller says so the call is completed successfully .

2.3 Swallowing and nutrition

Dysphagia affects a third of persons with ALS at onset and the majority by late disease (Higo et al., 2004). It increases the risk of suboptimal caloric and fluid intake and can worsen weakness and fatigue (Borasio, 2001). Aspiration pneumonia (13%) is a contributor to respiratory complications and is associated with increased mortality with mean survival time post-infection of 2 months (Sorenson et al., 2007).

Difficulties in the oral preparatory stage of swallowing (preparation of food for propulsion to the pharynx) is common (Mayberry and Atkinson, 1986). Symptoms include jaw weakness, fatigue, drooling, choking on food and slow eating. In addition, loss of upper limb function and fear of choking or depression can further impact on self-feeding abilities and oral intake (Slowie et al., 1983). A speech pathologist can evaluate the degree of dysphagia through bed-side assessments and/or further imaging (eg videofluroscopy). Mild dysphagia can be managed with specific interventions such a alteration of food consistency, upright positioning, small bolus size, soft collar for neck extensor weakness and the chin-tuck technique, in which the person flexes their neck to the anterior chest wall as they swallow, narrowing the inlet to the larynx and reducing the chance of food aspiration. Dieticians monitor nutritional status through body weight, percentage weight loss and body mass index. Common advice includes high calorie diets, texture modification and prescription of nutritional supplements (Rio and Cawadias, 2007). Patients may show nutritional compromise even before bulbar symptoms become significant (Slowie et al., 1983) as in addition to muscle wasting, persons with ALS at all stages of disease often do not meet their energy requirements (Kasarskis and Neville, 1996). Dehydration is also a common and important problem contributing to fatigue and thickened secretions (Francis et al., 1999).

As dysphagia progresses, evidence (Level B) suggests a percutaneous endoscopic gastrostomy (PEG) or equivalent (eg. radiologically inserted gastrostomy) is indicated to supplement oral intake (as long as this remains safe) for weight maintenance (Loser et al., 2005). PEGs prolong survival but there is currently little evidence regarding the impact of PEG on quality of life (Langmore et al., 2006). Timing of a PEG can be challenging. Indicators may include weight loss (5-10% of body weight loss implies nutritional risk (Francis et al., 1999)) and reduced FVC. If FVC falls below 50% of predicted (Kasarskis et al., 1999), risks of largyngeal spasm, localised infection, gastric haemorrhage, technical difficulties of PEG placement and respiratory arrest increase (Mazzini et al., 1995;Mathus-Vliegen et al., 1994)).

Sialorrhoea can be a significant issue in ALS and is generally not related to increased saliva production but rather to impaired ability to swallow saliva, combined with facial weakness causing labial incompetence and neck weakness causing the head to tip forward (Francis et al., 1999). Improved positioning, use of a cervical collar and orolingual exercises may be helpful. Medications such as anticholinergics and tricyclics can also be trialled (Schiffman and Belsh, 1996), as can suction machines. In the US, most commonly used medications are amitriptyline, glycopyrrolate, atropine and propantheline (Forshew and Bromberg, 2003). However, medications may further thicken secretions, hence should be used with caution in those with respiratory insufficiency or poor cough. More recently, botulinum toxin injected into the salivary glands (parotid, submandibular) appears to be safe and has been used to treat sialorrhea with beneficial effects lasting approximately 3 months (Verma and Steele, 2006;Contarino et al., 2007). Thick oropharyngeal secretions may be treated with increased fluid intake, humidification of air, cough augmentation, suction machines and guaifenesin (Forshew and Bromberg, 2003).

2.4 Exercise

The effects of exercise and safe therapeutic range in ALS are poorly understood. It is generally thought that weakness and muscle fibre degeneration may be accelerated by overwork or heavy exercise as it is already functioning close to its maximal limits (Johnson and Braddom, 1971). However, inactivity leads to deconditioning and disuse weakness. In addition, muscle and joint spasticity can cause pain, contractures and further loss of function. A recent Cochrane review (Dalbello-Haas et al., 2008) identified two trials (n = 52), which addressed therapeutic exercise in ALS. The trials examined the effects of moderate intensity, endurance type exercise on spasticity, and effects of moderate intensity resistance type exercises in ALS. Although one of the trials reported improvement in function and quality of life, both trials were too small to determine to what extent strengthening exercises were beneficial or harmful in this population (Dalbello-Haas et al., 2008). A more recent pilot study demonstrated that repetitive rhythmic exercise – supported treadmill ambulation training was feasible, tolerated and safe for patients with ALS and appeared to improve work capacity and gait functioning in patients with ALS who were dependent on assistive devices for ambulation (Sanjak et al., 2010). In view of the paucity of evidence to guide exercise prescription, the current recommendations are (Chen et al., 2008):

- Stretching exercise to improve flexibility to maintain muscle length and joint mobility and prevent contractures.
- Strengthening exercise of sub-maximal (low, non-fatiguing) intensity, with degree of resistance tailored to muscle strength.
- Aerobic/endurance exercise may improve cardio-respiratory fitness and is probably safe but adequate oxygenation, aeration and carbohydrate load is important to reduce oxidative stress load. Supported treadmill ambulation training can be considered if available.

2.5 Mobility and activities of daily living

In early stages of disease, rehabilitation aims to prolong independence in mobility and activities of daily living, prevent complications such as falls, contractures, and musculoskeletal pain, maintain strength, range of movement and conditioning through an appropriate exercise program, educate the patient and family about the disease, provide psychological support, evaluate the home for safety and teach energy conservation techniques (Khanna et al., 2007).

As weakness worsens, the physiotherapist can instruct the patient and family in safe transfer techniques (eg. between bed and chair, in and out of cars), optimise gait pattern and provide gait re-training with appropriate gait aids (eg. walking frame, sticks) and orthoses (ankle-foot orthosis to facilitate foot clearance during gait and stabilise knee to prevent falls). Occupational therapists can fabricate with upper limb orthoses to assist with fine motor function. For example, patients with distal weakness can improve hand function with wrists braced in 30° extension which improves efficiency of grip and addition of a universal cuff can assist those with weak grasp in feeding and typing (Francis et al., 1999). Other adaptive equipment is also provided, such as built-up cutlery for eating, Velcro fasteners for dressing, long-handled aids, and bathroom equipment (rails, over-the-toilet frames, bath boards, shower chairs, commodes). Wheelchairs are generally eventually required although introduction of a wheelchair whilst a patient is still ambulant, for intermittent community use, is important to enhance energy conservation. Future needs should be anticipated and considered when prescribing a powered wheelchair (eg. reclining, tilt-in-space, custom seating, and modifiable control system) to optimise independence and social interaction whilst preventing contractures, compression nerve palsies, skin breakdown and aspiration. A motorised scooter may be more appropriate for some patients (Francis et al., 1999). Other equipment such as hospital beds with pressure-relieving mattress and hoists for lifting might also be required. Caregiver training in the use of hoists is important to prevent injury.

A recent study (n=44) (Ng et al., 2011) showed that a small but significant gap exists from the perspective of persons with ALS with regards to advice and assistance relating to continued employment and driving. Healthcare providers may underestimate the importance of maintaining employment as a priority in a fatal condition such as ALS and hence under treat this issue. For these persons, the use of assistive technology may be particularly useful, especially in employment where computer use is crucial. Computer technology is fast advancing and options include different types of keyboards, mouse alternatives, switches, interfaces, mounting systems, integrated communication/computer access packages, software and systems. For those who have some proximal arm control, track balls, type writing sticks and forearm supports may be useful. In persons with ALS who have more severe upper limb weakness, head tracking systems, on-screen keyboards and voice recognition software may be required. Text-entry software such as Dasher (which is free) can be used whenever a full-size keyboard cannot be used such as on a palmtop computer or with a joystick, touchscreen, trackball, headpointer, or eyetracker . There are also many mouse alternatives available -- eyegaze system, foot control mouse, head tracking mouse, joysticks and switch-adapted mouse.

Assistive technology can have a dramatic effect on restoring and maintaining independence, a sense of control and quality of life. Apart from technologies that assist with mobility and communication which have already been discussed, other forms of assistive technology such as environmental control units (ECU) should be considered. Environmental control systems offer sophisticated electronics to enable people with a range of impairments and severe disability to use a wide variety of electrical devices. Aids may include unobtrusive control units (eg. remote control for TV), home security (door intercoms, door release and alarms), adapted telephones (such as hands-free control) and lighting and heating/cooling systems (Wellings and Unsworth, 1997). These environmental control units may be used to facilitate function and decrease reliance on carers, improve family dynamics and improve patients' self-esteem (Wellings and Unsworth, 1997). It is important for patients, families and therapists to work closely together when prescribing and using assistive technology to ensure the correct, safe and optimal use of such aids and equipment; and to anticipate future needs especially with the expense of such technology. Close collaboration with specialised providers of assistive technology that can provide back-up technical support is also crucial.

2.6 Bladder, bowel and sexuality

Although bowel and bladder sphincters are generally spared, bowel, bladder and sexual dysfunction may be much more common (30%) than reported to health professionals by persons with ALS (Ng et al., 2011). These areas are in general poorly studied in ALS. Constipation is common with inactivity and poor nutritional intake, and can be treated with a regular bowel program with intake of fibre/bulking agents and adequate fluids. Suppositories, stool softeners and enemas should be considered. In one of the few studies addressing bladder function in ALS (n=38), 47% had micturition symptoms and urodynamics studies found a range of UMN abnormalities (Hattori et al., 1983). Where urinary urgency is an issue, oxybutinin may be helpful. Contributory factors to incontinence, such as urinary tract infections, drinking large amount of fluids late in the day and dependent oedema causing nocturia when the legs are elevated overnight should be considered and treated. Wasner et al (Wasner et al., 2004) suggested a prevalence of 62% (n=62) in sexual dysfunction with issues including decreased libido and passivity of the patient and partner due to physical weakness and the body image changes. The wide variation in reported prevalence in bowel, bladder and sexual dysfunction suggests that patients may not volunteer this information; hence its inclusion in routine enquiries might help to encourage reporting and thus the facilitation of appropriate treatment, such as sexual counselling and suggestion of specific techniques.

2.7 Pain

Pain is common in ALS (50% in a recent study (Ng et al., 2011)), especially in the later stages. Fatigue and depressive symptoms may also worsen a patient's experience of pain.

Spasticity and muscle spasms are not an uncommon source of pain and with the current paucity of supporting evidence, this is often treated with stretching exercises in combination with a muscle relaxant (baclofen is the drug of choice) (Ashworth et al., 2006). Baclofen should be started at low doses (5mg twice to three times daily) and slowly increased (up to 100mg a day in divided doses). Baclofen however can be associated with muscle weakness. Tizanidine (2mg twice daily up to 24 mg a day) is likely as efficacious but it is associated with dry mouth. Other options include clonidine (25 µg twice a day) which can cause hypotension, drowsiness and bradycardia and benzodiazepines which can cause sedation and habituation and respiratory depression. Dantrolene is not recommended as it can cause excessive muscle weakness in ALS (Krivickas and Carter, 2005). Intrathecal baclofen is rarely required but may be indicated in those with intractable spasticity, needing more than the maximum oral dose (Marquardt and Seifert, 2002). There are few reports of use of botulinum toxin for spasticity in ALS in literature. Caution is advised as persons with ALS may be more prone to developing generalised weakness after being injected with botulinum toxin A to treat spasticity (Mezaki et al., 1996).

Muscle cramps can cause severe pain and discomfort and are a result of spontaneous activity of motor units induced by contraction of shortened muscles (Norris et al., 1957). The list of potentially useful drugs for cramps is extensive, implying efficacy of individual agents is low and variable and the evidence base weak. In the US, quinine (35%), baclofen (19%), phenytoin (10%), and gabapentin (7%) were the preferred agents (Forshew and Bromberg, 2003); in Europe, choices were quinine (58%), benzodiazepines (40%), magnesium (25%) and carbamazepine (23%) (Borasio et al., 2001a). In 2006 however, the US Food and Drug administration restricted the use of quinine sulfate in the US to treatment of malaria falciparum because of concerns regarding severe adverse events, including cardioarthymias, thrombocytopaenia, severe hypersentivity reactions and serious drug interaction (U.S. Food and Drug Administration, 2006).

In advanced disease, pain often results due to immobility. Musculoskeletal pain from weakness and resulting postural changes can be ameliorated with range of motion exercises, adequate support in sitting and supine positions and proper lifting and transfer techniques to prevent undue traction on weakened joints. Equipment such as motorised beds that slowly rotate from the side to side can be useful for reducing caregiver burden (Francis et al., 1999). Analgesia such as nonsteroidal anti-inflammatory drugs or narcotics (oral or sublingual) may also be required (with careful respiratory status monitoring in the latter). Intramuscular delivery of medications should be avoided due to muscle wasting (Mayadev et al., 2008).

2.8 Fatigue and sleep disorders

Fatigue is a common disability in ALS – 77-83% in recent studies (Ng et al., 2011;Ramirez et al., 2008) but understudied and often overlooked by clinicians (Lou, 2008). It is unrelated to clinical strength as a large component of fatigue in ALS has a central origin (Kent-Braun and Miller, 2000). Fatigue in ALS does not correlate directly with gender, educational level, disease duration, physical function, quality of life, dyspnoea, depression or sleepiness (Ramirez et al., 2008). However, contributory factors may include sepsis (including aspiration), depression and/or anxiety, pain, hypoventilation, positioning, sleep disruption and effortful activity and these should be treated where possible. It may manifest as reduced energy, difficulty in maintaining sustained attention and increased motor weakness, incoordination and gait difficulties. No double-blind, placebo-controlled trials have been performed for treatment of fatigue. Physostigmine is sometimes prescribed but not necessarily effective (Norris et al., 1993). Modafinil appears to be well-tolerated in a recent small open-label study (n=15) and may reduce symptoms of fatigue (Carter et al., 2005). Rehabilitation strategies involve pacing activities (regular rest breaks), energy conservation and fatigue management strategies, addressing sleep disorders, consideration of exercise to improve fitness if appropriate and treating other exacerbating factors.

High incidence of sleep disturbance in ALS has been reported with pain, micturition, and choking listed by patients as the most common causes for awakening (Kinnear et al., 1997 Nov 3-5). Other contributors to poor sleep include abnormal nocturnal movements such as periodic leg movements or fragmentary myoclonus, which was demonstrated on polysomnography in almost all patients with fatigue (Kinnear et al., 1997 Nov 3-5). Such movements may be treated with controlled release carbidopa-levodopa (Sinemet CR) (Sufit, 1997). Antihistamines (eg. diphenhydramine) and other sedatives (eg. Chloral hydrate 250-500mg, benzodiazepines) can also be considered once respiratory causes for sleep disturbance have been ruled out.

2.9 Cognition and behavioural impairment

Cognitive impairment is increasingly recognised in ALS -- 50% are thought to have frontal executive deficits (see Table 2) (Lomen-Hoerth et al., 2003). Visuospatial function, praxis and memory storage are usually spared (Massman et al., 1996;Abrahams et al., 2005;Ringholz et al., 2005). Use of memory aids such as diaries, planners and structured daily routine is encouraged. Other conditions (depression, anxiety, fatigue) and medications (anticholinergics, benzodiazepines) should be monitored as they can worsen cognitive function.

Behavioural changes unrelated to mood or cognition has also been noted although estimates of prevalence vary widely (Woolley and Jonathan, 2008). Marked apathy occurs in an estimated 55% of persons with ALS (Grossman et al., 2007).This correlates with deficits in verbal fluency but not depression, disease duration, FVC or ALSFRS scores and may be related to fatigue, respiratory weakness, impaired sleep, anxiety or medication (Woolley and Jonathan, 2008). It may also be a psychological coping mechanism (Woolley and Jonathan, 2008).

In a subset of persons with ALS (approximately 5%), clear fronto-temporal dementia (also known as fronto-temporal lobar degeneration) is the presenting picture with severe behavioural dysfunction (insidious onset with gradual progression, altered social conduct, impaired regulation of personal conduct, emotional blunting, loss of insight) that begins before motor weakness becomes obvious (Woolley and Jonathan, 2008). In addition, those with fronto-temporal dementia may exhibit disinhibition, restlessness, reduced empathy, lack of foresight, impulsiveness, social withdrawal, verbal stereotypes, verbal or motor perseveration and/or sexual hyperactivity (Neary et al., 1998).

Management of behavioural and cognitive deficits can be challenging and begins with the identification of these issues. An assessment by a neuropsychologist is often helpful in terms of defining the deficits and provision of cognitive and behavioural remediation strategies. Education and counselling of the patient and family is important. No trials have been conducted in efficacy of pharmacological interventions in this area; however the use of antidepressants and antipsychotics may be considered.

Attention and concentration
Working memory
Cognitive flexibility (rigidity)
Response inhibition
"Executive function" - Planning/problem/solving/abstract reasoning
Visual-perceptual skills
Memory
Word generation (fluency)

Table 2 Cognitive deficits in ALS (adapted from (Woolley and Jonathan, 2008))

2.10 Pseudobulbar affect

Pseudobulbar affect describes sudden uncontrollable outbursts of laughter or tearfulness and is a result of bilateral corticobulbar tract degeneration (Rosen and Cummings, 2007). It is common, affecting between 50-70% of persons with ALS (Palmieri et al., 2009) especially those with the bulbar form of ALS. Pseudobulbar affect can have a significant impact on anxiety and emotional frailty (Palmieri et al., 2009), social functioning and relationships in persons with ALS as these sudden, frequent, extreme, uncontrollable emotional outbursts may lead to severe embarrassment and social withdrawal (Moore et al., 1997).

Despite the prevalence of this issue, less than 15% ask for treatment (Meininger, 2005). Education of the persons with ALS and their family and friends assists with understanding and acceptance of these pathological and involuntary outbursts and is an important component of the appropriate treatment of pseudobulbar affect. Crying associated with pseudobulbar affect is easily incorrectly interpreted as depression; laughter may be embarrassing. Pharmacological treatment can include amitryiptiline (10-150mg nocte, starting with 10mg and slowly increasing the dose) which also has the positive benefit on weight loss and loss of appetite (Meininger, 2005) or fluvoxamine (100-200mg daily). A more recent study (n=140) showed that dextromethorphan and quinidine in combination appears to be more effective in reducing the frequency and severity of psudobulbar affect and to improve quality of life) (Brooks et al., 2004). However, side effects are also more common (nausea, dizziness, gastrointestinal complaints) (Brooks et al., 2004).

2.11 Psychosocial issues

ALS is a devastating condition, which takes its toll on the patient and family especially as the disease progresses, and loss of independence occurs. Rates of depression and anxiety are reported to be 0-44% and 0-30% respectively in persons with ALS (Kurt et al., 2007) and depression does not appear to increase in more advanced disease (Rabkin et al., 2005). Quality of life also appears to be more dependent on psychological and existential factors than physical factors (Goldstein et al., 2006b;Simmons et al., 2000). Amongst caregivers, 23% are depressed (Rabkin et al., 2009) and caregiver strain is often significant as a result of increased caregiving time, cognitive impairments in persons with ALS, emotional labour and socio-economic considerations (Chio et al., 2006;Goldstein et al., 2006a;Ray and Street, 2006). Hence, referrals to support groups and counselling and education of patients and their families (often their caregivers) are essential. Frank discussions facilitate understanding of the disease and improve coping skills. Carer support (both physical and emotional) and respite care should be discussed. Referrals to the local ALS associations are also recommended as these provide patients and families with ongoing support, resources and equipment needs. Psychotherapy should also be considered to assist with coping strategies (Matuz et al., 2010). Antidepressants such as amitriptyline and selective serotonin reuptake inhibitors may be used, the former being also useful for other symptoms such as drooling, pseudobulbar affect and insomnia. Anxiety is difficult to measure due to physical confounding symptoms such as shortness of breath, muscle cramps and restlessness. Anxiety can be treated with psychotherapy and training in relaxation and breathing techniques, as well as participation in support groups. It is generally thought that the rates of anxiety increase in the pre-terminal stage (Kurt et al., 2007), hence anxiolytics at this time such as benzodiazepines should be offered. With good support, mental health and quality of life can remain stable despite deteriorating physical health (De Groot et al., 2007).

2.12 End of life issues

It is important to establish an open environment of communication with persons with ALS and their families from the time of diagnosis. Specialist palliative care providers should be involved as early as possible. Discussions should take place early, well before specific decisions need to be made. The actual timing of when to introduce these discussions however can be challenging and will depend on a number of factors including coping skills, depression and anxiety, cultural issues and functional status (Mitsumoto et al., 2005). Some triggers may include the patient or family initiation of discussion, severe psychosocial distress, pain requiring high dosages of analgesia, dysphagia, dyspnoea and functional loss in two body regions (Mitsumoto et al., 2005). Given the progressive nature of the disease, the patient eventually has to choose between life-sustaining therapies (respiratory assistance, feeding tubes) and terminal palliative care whilst considering issues relating to quality of life, burden of therapies, their own wishes and those of their family. It is important that clinicians caring for ALS patients and their families appreciate and communicate the significance of life-threatening symptoms, monitor decision-making capacity, ensure that multiple possible end of life scenarios are anticipated and managed with all options provided (including hospice care), review advance care directives and comprehensively consider and aggressively manage symptoms (McCluskey, 2007).

Medications should be available for all patients who are deteriorating and may be approaching the terminal phase, although the terminal phase may be difficult to recognise as there is usually slow deterioration until a quicker change leads to death within a few days or less (Oliver, 2007). Medications should include morphine to relieve dyspnoea and pain, midazolam to relieve distress and agitation and glycopyrronium bromide or hyoscine hydrobromide to reduce chest secretions, delivered parenterally (Oliver, 2007). Cultural and spiritual issues should also be addressed (Mitsumoto et al., 2005;Albert et al., 2007). Although many persons with ALS fear the terminal stages of ALS, with good palliative care, the later stages can be a time of fulfilment and peace for both persons with ALS and their families (Oliver, 2007).

Bereavement in ALS occurs in both the patient and their family and continues, in families, after the death of the patient. Some families feel relieved of their caregiver burden and the burden of losses for the patient but also have feelings of guilt that they feel these emotions; hence support is vital in this area (Skyes, 2006).

3. Conclusion

ALS is a complex and challenging condition with no cure. Current "gold-standard" management is "multidisciplinary care"which includes neurological, rehabilitative and palliative care. As consistent with the guidelines from the American Academy of Neurology (Miller et al., 2009b) and the World Federation of Neurology (Andersen et al., 2007), multidisciplinary care should be available to all persons with ALS. Where multidisciplinary care is currently available, it should be delivered with a high level of coordination and integration, with evidence-based intervention to ensure holistic and seamless care for persons with ALS and their caregivers. Many areas in ALS are poorly understood, with research often further hindered by the logistical and ethical difficulties. Much more work is needed in the area of evidence-based interventions. At present, much of the evidence has been concentrated in areas such as respiratory and nutritional management. There is paucity of information on effective rehabilitation interventions and very little is understood with regards to the "black box of rehabilitation". For example, evidence to guide exercise prescription (such as strengthening, stretching, aerobic/endurance exercises) is much needed. The use and development of assistive technology is another area that warrants much more attention, as is a better understanding of bowel, bladder and sexuality issues. Further research is also needed into appropriate study designs; outcome measurement; the evaluation of optimal settings, type, intensity or frequency and cost-effectiveness of multidisciplinary care; and the different phases of ALS, covering the spectrum of care required for this patient population. The interface between neurological, rehabilitative and palliative components of care, and caregiver needs should be explored and developed to provide long-term support for this population. Last but not least, national and international guidelines incorporating evidence-based practice in rehabilitation should be further developed to enable optimisation of clinical care and practice.

4. References

The Family Center on Technology and Disability, [Accessed January 2011], Available from: http://www.fctd.info/resources?on=disability&tag=Neurological+Disorders

Abrahams, S.;Leigh P.N. & Goldstein L.H. (2005). Cognitive change in ALS: a prospective study. *Neurology*, Vol. 64, No. 7, pp. 1222-6, 1526-632X (Electronic) 0028-3878 (Linking)

Albert, S.M.;Wasner M.;Tider T.;Drory V.E. & Borasio G.D. (2007). Cross-cultural variation in mental health at end of life in patients with ALS. *Neurology*, Vol. 68, No. 13, pp. 1058-61, 1526-632X (Electronic) 0028-3878 (Linking)

Andersen, P.M.;Borasio G.D.;Dengler R., et al. (2007). Good practice in the management of amyotrophic lateral sclerosis: clinical guidelines. An evidence-based review with good practice points. EALSC Working Group. *Amyotroph Lateral Scler*, Vol. 8, No. 4, pp. 195-213, 1748-2968 (Print) 1471-180X (Linking)

Ashworth, N.L.;Satkunam L.E. & Deforge D. (2006). Treatment for spasticity in amyotrophic lateral sclerosis/motor neuron disease. *Cochrane Database Syst Rev*, Issue 1, pp. CD004156, 1469-493X (Electronic) 1361-6137 (Linking)

Borasio, G.D. (2001). Palliative care in ALS: searching for the evidence base. *Amyotroph Lateral Scler Other Motor Neuron Disord*, Vol. 2 Suppl 1, pp. S31-5, 1466-0822 (Print) 1466-0822 (Linking)

Borasio, G.D.;Shaw P.J.;Hardiman O.;Ludolph A.C.;Sales Luis M.L. & Silani V. (2001a). Standards of palliative care for patients with amyotrophic lateral sclerosis: results of a European survey. *Amyotroph Lateral Scler Other Motor Neuron Disord*, Vol. 2, No. 3, pp. 159-64, 1466-0822 (Print) 1466-0822 (Linking)

Borasio, G.D.;Voltz R. & Miller R.G. (2001b). Palliative care in amyotrophic lateral sclerosis. *Neurol Clin*, Vol. 19, No. 4, pp. 829-47, 0733-8619 (Print) 0733-8619 (Linking)

Brooks, B.R.;Thisted R.A.;Appel S.H., et al. (2004). Treatment of pseudobulbar affect in ALS with dextromethorphan/quinidine: a randomized trial. *Neurology*, Vol. 63, No. 8, pp. 1364-70, 1526-632X (Electronic) 0028-3878 (Linking)

Brownlee, A. & Palovcak M. (2007). The role of augmentative communication devices in the medical management of ALS. *NeuroRehabilitation*, Vol. 22, No. 6, pp. 445-50, 1053-8135 (Print) 1053-8135 (Linking)

Carter, G.T.;Weiss M.D.;Lou J.S., et al. (2005). Modafinil to treat fatigue in amyotrophic lateral sclerosis: an open label pilot study. *Am J Hosp Palliat Care*, Vol. 22, No. 1, pp. 55-9, 1049-9091 (Print) 1049-9091 (Linking)

Chen, A.;Montes J. & Mitsumoto H. (2008). The role of exercise in amyotrophic lateral sclerosis. *Phys Med Rehabil Clin N Am*, Vol. 19, No. 3, pp. 545-57, ix-x, 1047-9651 (Print) 1047-9651 (Linking)

Chio, A.;Gauthier A.;Vignola A., et al. (2006). Caregiver time use in ALS. *Neurology*, Vol. 67, No. 5, pp. 902-4, 1526-632X (Electronic) 0028-3878 (Linking)

Contarino, M.F.;Pompili M.;Tittoto P., et al. (2007). Botulinum toxin B ultrasound-guided injections for sialorrhea in amyotrophic lateral sclerosis and Parkinson's disease. *Parkinsonism Relat Disord*, Vol. 13, No. 5, pp. 299-303, 1353-8020 (Print) 1353-8020 (Linking)

Czaplinski, A.;Yen A.A. & Appel S.H. (2006). Forced vital capacity (FVC) as an indicator of survival and disease progression in an ALS clinic population. *J Neurol Neurosurg Psychiatry*, Vol. 77, No. 3, pp. 390-2, 0022-3050 (Print) 0022-3050 (Linking)

Dalbello-Haas, V.;Florence J.M. & Krivickas L.S. (2008). Therapeutic exercise for people with amyotrophic lateral sclerosis or motor neuron disease. *Cochrane Database Syst Rev*, Issue. 2, pp. CD005229, 1469-493X (Electronic) 1361-6137 (Linking)

De Groot, I.J.;Post M.W.;van Heuveln T.;Van den Berg L.H. & Lindeman E. (2007). Cross-sectional and longitudinal correlations between disease progression and different health-related quality of life domains in persons with amyotrophic lateral sclerosis. *Amyotroph Lateral Scler*, Vol. 8, No. 6, pp. 356-61, 1471-180X (Electronic) 1471-180X (Linking)

Esposito, S.J.;Mitsumoto H. & Shanks M. (2000). Use of palatal lift and palatal augmentation prostheses to improve dysarthria in patients with amyotrophic lateral sclerosis: a case series. *J Prosthet Dent*, Vol. 83, No. 1, pp. 90-8, 0022-3913 (Print) 0022-3913 (Linking)

Fitting, J.W.;Paillex R.;Hirt L.;Aebischer P. & Schluep M. (1999). Sniff nasal pressure: a sensitive respiratory test to assess progression of amyotrophic lateral sclerosis. *Ann Neurol*, Vol. 46, No. 6, pp. 887-93, 0364-5134 (Print) 0364-5134 (Linking)

Forshew, D.A. & Bromberg M.B. (2003). A survey of clinicians' practice in the symptomatic treatment of ALS. *Amyotroph Lateral Scler Other Motor Neuron Disord*, Vol. 4, No. 4, pp. 258-63, 1466-0822 (Print) 1466-0822 (Linking)

Francis, K.;Bach J.R. & DeLisa J.A. (1999). Evaluation and rehabilitation of patients with adult motor neuron disease. *Arch Phys Med Rehabil*, Vol. 80, No. 8, pp. 951-63, 0003-9993 (Print) 0003-9993 (Linking)

Goldstein, L.H.;Atkins L.;Landau S.;Brown R. & Leigh P.N. (2006a). Predictors of psychological distress in carers of people with amyotrophic lateral sclerosis: a longitudinal study. *Psychol Med*, Vol. 36, No. 6, pp. 865-75, 0033-2917 (Print) 0033-2917 (Linking)

Goldstein, L.H.;Atkins L.;Landau S.;Brown R.G. & Leigh P.N. (2006b). Longitudinal predictors of psychological distress and self-esteem in people with ALS. *Neurology*, Vol. 67, No. 9, pp. 1652-8, 1526-632X (Electronic) 0028-3878 (Linking)

Grossman, A.B.;Woolley-Levine S.;Bradley W.G. & Miller R.G. (2007). Detecting neurobehavioral changes in amyotrophic lateral sclerosis. *Amyotroph Lateral Scler*, Vol. 8, No. 1, pp. 56-61, 1748-2968 (Print) 1471-180X (Linking)

Hardiman, O. (2007). Multidisciplinary care in motor neurone disease, In: *The Motor Neurone Disease Handbook*, M. Kiernan, (Ed.), pp. (164), Australasian Medical Publishing Company Limited, Prymont

Hattori, T.;Hirayama K.;Yasuda K. & Shimazaki J. (1983). [Disturbance of micturition in amyotrophic lateral sclerosis]. *Rinsho Shinkeigaku*, Vol. 23, No. 3, pp. 224-7, 0009-918X (Print) 0009-918X (Linking)

Higo, R.;Tayama N. & Nito T. (2004). Longitudinal analysis of progression of dysphagia in amyotrophic lateral sclerosis. *Auris Nasus Larynx*, Vol. 31, No. 3, pp. 247-54, 0385-8146 (Print) 0385-8146 (Linking)

Hillel, A.D. & Miller R. (1989). Bulbar amyotrophic lateral sclerosis: patterns of progression and clinical management. *Head Neck,* Vol. 11, No. 1, pp. 51-9, 1043-3074 (Print) 1043-3074 (Linking)

Johnson, E.W. & Braddom R. (1971). Over-work weakness in facioscapulohuumeral muscular dystrophy. *Arch Phys Med Rehabil,* Vol. 52, No. 7, pp. 333-6, 0003-9993 (Print) 0003-9993 (Linking)

Kasarskis, E.J. & Neville H.E. (1996). Management of ALS: nutritional care. *Neurology,* Vol. 47, No. 4 Suppl 2, pp. S118-20, 0028-3878 (Print) 0028-3878 (Linking)

Kasarskis, E.J.;Scarlata D.;Hill R.;Fuller C.;Stambler N. & Cedarbaum J.M. (1999). A retrospective study of percutaneous endoscopic gastrostomy in ALS patients during the BDNF and CNTF trials. *J Neurol Sci,* Vol. 169, No. 1-2, pp. 118-25, 0022-510X (Print) 0022-510X (Linking)

Kaub-Wittemer, D.;Steinbuchel N.;Wasner M.;Laier-Groeneveld G. & Borasio G.D. (2003). Quality of life and psychosocial issues in ventilated patients with amyotrophic lateral sclerosis and their caregivers. *J Pain Symptom Manage,* Vol. 26, No. 4, pp. 890-6, 0885-3924 (Print) 0885-3924 (Linking)

Kemp, B.J. (2005). What the rehabilitation professional and the consumer need to know. *Phys Med Rehabil Clin N Am,* Vol. 16, No. 1, pp. 1-18, vii, 1047-9651 (Print) 1047-9651 (Linking)

Kent-Braun, J.A. & Miller R.G. (2000). Central fatigue during isometric exercise in amyotrophic lateral sclerosis. *Muscle Nerve,* Vol. 23, No. 6, pp. 909-14, 0148-639X (Print) 0148-639X (Linking)

Khanna, P.;Nations S.P. & Trivedi J.R. (2007). Motor Neuron Diseases, In: *Physical Medicine & Rehabilitation,* R. Braddom, (Ed.), 3rd ed. Saunders Elsevier, Philadelphia

Kinnear, W.;Scriven N.;Orpe V. & Jefferson D. (1997 Nov 3-5). Prevalence of symptoms of sleep disturbance in patients with motor neurone disease [abstract]. *Proceedings of 8th International Symposium on ALS/MND,* Glasgow, Nov 1997

Klein, L.M. & Forshew D.A. (1996). The economic impact of ALS. *Neurology,* Vol. 47, No. 4 Suppl 2, pp. S126-9, 0028-3878 (Print) 0028-3878 (Linking)

Krivickas, L.S. & Carter G.T. (2005). Motor neuron disease, In: *Physical medicine and rehabilitation: principles and practice,* D. J.A., Gans, B.M. & Walsh, N.E., (Eds.), 4th ed. Lippincott Williams & Wilkins, Philadelphia

Kurt, A.;Nijboer F.;Matuz T. & Kubler A. (2007). Depression and anxiety in individuals with amyotrophic lateral sclerosis: epidemiology and management. *CNS Drugs,* Vol. 21, No. 4, pp. 279-91, 1172-7047 (Print) 1172-7047 (Linking)

Langmore, S.E.;Kasarskis E.J.;Manca M.L. & Olney R.K. (2006). Enteral tube feeding for amyotrophic lateral sclerosis/motor neuron disease. *Cochrane Database Syst Rev,* Issue. 4, pp. CD004030, 1469-493X (Electronic) 1361-6137 (Linking)

Lomen-Hoerth, C.;Murphy J.;Langmore S.;Kramer J.H.;Olney R.K. & Miller B. (2003). Are amyotrophic lateral sclerosis patients cognitively normal? *Neurology,* Vol. 60, No. 7, pp. 1094-7, 1526-632X (Electronic) 0028-3878 (Linking)

Loser, C.;Aschl G.;Hebuterne X., et al. (2005). ESPEN guidelines on artificial enteral nutrition--percutaneous endoscopic gastrostomy (PEG). *Clin Nutr,* Vol. 24, No. 5, pp. 848-61, 0261-5614 (Print) 0261-5614 (Linking)

Lou, J.S. (2008). Fatigue in amyotrophic lateral sclerosis. *Phys Med Rehabil Clin N Am*, Vol. 19, No. 3, pp. 533-43, ix, 1047-9651 (Print) 1047-9651 (Linking)

Lyall, R.A.;Donaldson N.;Polkey M.I.;Leigh P.N. & Moxham J. (2001). Respiratory muscle strength and ventilatory failure in amyotrophic lateral sclerosis. *Brain*, Vol. 124, No. Pt 10, pp. 2000-13, 0006-8950 (Print) 0006-8950 (Linking)

Marquardt, G. & Seifert V. (2002). Use of intrathecal baclofen for treatment of spasticity in amyotrophic lateral sclerosis. *J Neurol Neurosurg Psychiatry*, Vol. 72, No. pp. 275-276

Massman, P.J.;Sims J.;Cooke N.;Haverkamp L.J.;Appel V. & Appel S.H. (1996). Prevalence and correlates of neuropsychological deficits in amyotrophic lateral sclerosis. *J Neurol Neurosurg Psychiatry*, Vol. 61, No. 5, pp. 450-5, 0022-3050 (Print) 0022-3050 (Linking)

Mathus-Vliegen, L.M.;Louwerse L.S.;Merkus M.P.;Tytgat G.N. & Vianney de Jong J.M. (1994). Percutaneous endoscopic gastrostomy in patients with amyotrophic lateral sclerosis and impaired pulmonary function. *Gastrointest Endosc*, Vol. 40, No. 4, pp. 463-9, 0016-5107 (Print) 0016-5107 (Linking)

Matuz, T.;Birbaumer N.;Hautzinger M. & Kubler A. (2010). Coping with amyotrophic lateral sclerosis: an integrative view. *J Neurol Neurosurg Psychiatry*, Vol. 81, No. 8, pp. 893-8, 1468-330X (Electronic) 0022-3050 (Linking)

Mayadev, A.S.;Weiss M.D.;Distad B.J.;Krivickas L.S. & Carter G.T. (2008). The amyotrophic lateral sclerosis center: a model of multidisciplinary management. *Phys Med Rehabil Clin N Am*, Vol. 19, No. 3, pp. 619-31, xi, 1047-9651 (Print) 1047-9651 (Linking)

Mayberry, J.F. & Atkinson M. (1986). Swallowing problems in patients with motor neuron disease. *J Clin Gastroenterol*, Vol. 8, No. 3 Pt 1, pp. 233-4, 0192-0790 (Print) 0192-0790 (Linking)

Mazzini, L.;Corra T.;Zaccala M.;Mora G.;Del Piano M. & Galante M. (1995). Percutaneous endoscopic gastrostomy and enteral nutrition in amyotrophic lateral sclerosis. *J Neurol*, Vol. 242, No. 10, pp. 695-8, 0340-5354 (Print) 0340-5354 (Linking)

McCluskey, L. (2007). Amyotrophic Lateral Sclerosis: ethical issues from diagnosis to end of life. *NeuroRehabilitation*, Vol. 22, No. 6, pp. 463-72, 1053-8135 (Print) 1053-8135 (Linking)

Meininger, V. (2005). Treatment of emotional lability in ALS. *Lancet Neurol*, Vol. 4, No. 2, pp. 70, 1474-4422 (Print) 1474-4422 (Linking)

Melo, J.;Homma A.;Iturriaga E., et al. (1999). Pulmonary evaluation and prevalence of non-invasive ventilation in patients with amyotrophic lateral sclerosis: a multicenter survey and proposal of a pulmonary protocol. *J Neurol Sci*, Vol. 169, No. 1-2, pp. 114-7, 0022-510X (Print) 0022-510X (Linking)

Mezaki, T.;Kaji R.;Kohara N. & Kimura J. (1996). Development of general weakness in a patient with amyotrophic lateral sclerosis after focal botulinum toxin injection. *Neurology*, Vol. 46, No. 3, pp. 845-6, 0028-3878 (Print) 0028-3878 (Linking)

Miller, R.G.;Jackson C.E.;Kasarskis E.J., et al. (2009a). Practice parameter update: The care of the patient with amyotrophic lateral sclerosis: drug, nutritional, and respiratory therapies (an evidence-based review): report of the Quality Standards Subcommittee of the American Academy of Neurology. *Neurology*, Vol. 73, No. 15, pp. 1218-26, 1526-632X (Electronic) 0028-3878 (Linking)

Miller, R.G.;Jackson C.E.;Kasarskis E.J., et al. (2009b). Practice parameter update: The care of the patient with amyotrophic lateral sclerosis: multidisciplinary care, symptom management, and cognitive/behavioral impairment (an evidence-based review): report of the Quality Standards Subcommittee of the American Academy of Neurology. *Neurology*, Vol. 73, No. 15, pp. 1227-33, 1526-632X (Electronic) 0028-3878 (Linking)

Mitsumoto, H.;Bromberg M.;Johnston W., et al. (2005). Promoting excellence in end-of-life care in ALS. *Amyotroph Lateral Scler Other Motor Neuron Disord*, Vol. 6, No. 3, pp. 145-54, 1466-0822 (Print) 1466-0822 (Linking)

Moore, S.R.;Gresham L.S.;Bromberg M.B.;Kasarkis E.J. & Smith R.A. (1997). A self report measure of affective lability. *J Neurol Neurosurg Psychiatry*, Vol. 63, No. 1, pp. 89-93, 0022-3050 (Print) 0022-3050 (Linking)

Morgan, R.K.;McNally S.;Alexander M.;Conroy R.;Hardiman O. & Costello R.W. (2005). Use of Sniff nasal-inspiratory force to predict survival in amyotrophic lateral sclerosis. *Am J Respir Crit Care Med*, Vol. 171, No. 3, pp. 269-74, 1073-449X (Print) 1073-449X (Linking)

Neary, D.;Snowden J.S.;Gustafson L., et al. (1998). Frontotemporal lobar degeneration: a consensus on clinical diagnostic criteria. *Neurology*, Vol. 51, No. 6, pp. 1546-54, 0028-3878 (Print) 0028-3878 (Linking)

Ng, L.;Khan F. & Mathers S. (2009). Multidisciplinary care for adults with amyotrophic lateral sclerosis or motor neuron disease. *Cochrane Database Syst Rev*, Issue. 4, pp. CD007425, 1469-493X (Electronic) 1361-6137 (Linking)

Ng, L.; Talman, P. & Khan F. (2011). Motor Neurone Disease: Disability profile and service needs in an Australian cohort. *Int J Rehabil Res*, Vol 34, No. 2, pp.151-9.

Norris, F.H., Jr.;Gasteiger E.L. & Chatfield P.O. (1957). An electromyographic study of induced and spontaneous muscle cramps. *Electroencephalogr Clin Neurophysiol*, Vol. 9, No. 1, pp. 139-47, 0013-4694 (Print) 0013-4694 (Linking)

Norris, F.H.;Tan Y.;Fallat R.J. & Elias L. (1993). Trial of oral physostigmine in amyotrophic lateral sclerosis. *Clin Pharmacol Ther*, Vol. 54, No. 6, pp. 680-2, 0009-9236 (Print) 0009-9236 (Linking)

Oliver, D. (1996). The quality of care and symptom control--the effects on the terminal phase of ALS/MND. *J Neurol Sci*, Vol. 139 Suppl, pp. 134-6, 0022-510X (Print) 0022-510X (Linking)

Oliver, D. (2007). Palliative care, In: *The motor neurone disease handbook*, M. Kiernan, (Ed.), pp. (186-195), Australasian Medical Publishing Company Limited, Prymont

Palmieri, A.;Abrahams S.;Soraru G., et al. (2009). Emotional Lability in MND: Relationship to cognition and psychopathology and impact on caregivers.*J Neurol Sci*, Vol. 278, No. 1-2, pp. 16-20, 0022-510X (Print) 0022-510X (Linking)

Pinker, S. & Jackendoff R. (2005). The faculty of language: what's special about it? *Cognition*, Vol. 95, No. 2, pp. 201-36, 0010-0277 (Print) 0010-0277 (Linking)

Rabkin, J.G.;Albert S.M.;Del Bene M.L., et al. (2005). Prevalence of depressive disorders and change over time in late-stage ALS. *Neurology*, Vol. 65, No. 1, pp. 62-7, 1526-632X (Electronic) 0028-3878 (Linking)

Rabkin, J.G.;Albert S.M.;Rowland L.P. & Mitsumoto H. (2009). How common is depression among ALS caregivers? A longitudinal study. *Amyotroph Lateral Scler*, Vol. 10, No. 5-6, pp. 448-55, 1471-180X (Electronic) 1471-180X (Linking)

Radunovic, A.;Annane D.;Jewitt K. & Mustfa N. (2009). Mechanical ventilation for amyotrophic lateral sclerosis/motor neuron disease. *Cochrane Database Syst Rev*, Issue. 4, pp. CD004427, 1469-493X (Electronic) 1361-6137 (Linking)

Ramirez, C.;Piemonte M.E.;Callegaro D. & Da Silva H.C. (2008). Fatigue in amyotrophic lateral sclerosis: frequency and associated factors. *Amyotroph Lateral Scler*, Vol. 9, No. 2, pp. 75-80, 1471-180X (Electronic) 1471-180X (Linking)

Ray, R.A. & Street A.F. (2006). Caregiver bodywork: family members' experiences of caring for a person with motor neurone disease. *J Adv Nurs*, Vol. 56, No. 1, pp. 35-43, 0309-2402 (Print) 0309-2402 (Linking)

Ringholz, G.M.;Appel S.H.;Bradshaw M.;Cooke N.A.;Mosnik D.M. & Schulz P.E. (2005). Prevalence and patterns of cognitive impairment in sporadic ALS. *Neurology*, Vol. 65, No. 4, pp. 586-90, 1526-632X (Electronic) 0028-3878 (Linking)

Rio, A. & Cawadias E. (2007). Nutritional advice and treatment by dietitians to patients with amyotrophic lateral sclerosis/motor neurone disease: a survey of current practice in England, Wales, Northern Ireland and Canada. *J Hum Nutr Diet*, Vol. 20, No. 1, pp. 3-13, 0952-3871 (Print) 0952-3871 (Linking)

Rosen, H.J. & Cummings J. (2007). A real reason for patients with pseudobulbar affect to smile. *Ann Neurol*, Vol. 61, No. 2, pp. 92-6, 0364-5134 (Print) 0364-5134 (Linking)

Royal College of Physicians National Council for Palliative Care and British Society of Rehabilitation Medicine (2008). Long Term Neurological Conditions: Management at the interface between neurology, rehabilitation and palliative care. *Concise guidance to good practice series*, Royal College of Physicians, London

Sanjak, M.;Bravver E.;Bockenek W.L.;Norton H.J. & Brooks B.R. (2010). Supported treadmill ambulation for amyotrophic lateral sclerosis: a pilot study. *Arch Phys Med Rehabil*, Vol. 91, No. 12, pp. 1920-9, 1532-821X (Electronic) 0003-9993 (Linking)

Schiffman, P.L. (1996). Pulmonary function and respiratory management of the ALS patient, In: *Amyotrophic Lateral Sclerosis: diagnosis and management for the clinician*, J.M. Belsh & Schiffman, P.L., (Eds.), pp. (333-355), Futura Publishing Company, Armonk (NY)

Schiffman, P.L. & Belsh J.M. (1996). Overall management of the ALS patient, In: *Amyotrophic lateral sclerosis: diagnosis and management for the clinician*, J.M. Belsh & Schiffman, P.L., (Eds.), pp. (271-301), Futura Publishing Company, Armonk (NY)

Sellers, E.W.;Vaughan T.M. & Wolpaw J.R. (2010). A brain-computer interface for long-term independent home use. *Amyotroph Lateral Scler*, Vol. 11, No. 5, pp. 449-55, 1471-180X (Electronic) 1471-180X (Linking)

Shaw, P. (2003). Motor neurone disease, In: *Handbook of neurological rehabilitation*, R.J. Greenwood, Barnes, M.P., McMillan, T.M. & al, (Eds.), 2nd ed, pp. (641-661), Psychology Press, New York

Simmons, Z.;Bremer B.A.;Robbins R.A.;Walsh S.M. & Fischer S. (2000). Quality of life in ALS depends on factors other than strength and physical function. *Neurology*, Vol. 55, No. 3, pp. 388-92, 0028-3878 (Print) 0028-3878 (Linking)

Skyes, N.P. (2006). End of life care, In: *Palliative care in amyotrophic lateral sclerosis - from diagnosis to bereavement*, D. Oliver, Borasio, G.D. & Walsh, D. (Eds.), Oxford University Press, Oxford

Slowie, L.A.;Paige M.S. & Antel J.P. (1983). Nutritional considerations in the management of patients with amyotrophic lateral sclerosis (ALS). *J Am Diet Assoc*, Vol. 83, No. 1, pp. 44-7, 0002-8223 (Print) 0002-8223 (Linking)

Sorenson, E.J.;Crum B. & Stevens J.C. (2007). Incidence of aspiration pneumonia in ALS in Olmsted County, MN. *Amyotroph Lateral Scler*, Vol. 8, No. 2, pp. 87-9, 1748-2968 (Print) 1471-180X (Linking)

Stefanutti, D.;Benoist M.R.;Scheinmann P.;Chaussain M. & Fitting J.W. (2000). Usefulness of sniff nasal pressure in patients with neuromuscular or skeletal disorders. *Am J Respir Crit Care Med*, Vol. 162, No. 4 Pt 1, pp. 1507-11, 1073-449X (Print) 1073-449X (Linking)

Sufit, R. (1997). Symptomatic treatment of ALS *Neurology*, Vol. 48, No. pp. 15S-22S

U.S. Food and Drug Administration. (2006). FDA advances effort against marketed unapproved drugs. FDA orders unapproved quinine drugs from the market and cautions consumers about "off-label" use of quinine to treat leg cramps, [Accessed January 2011], Available from: http://www.fda.gov/NewsEvents/Newsroom/PressAnnouncements/2006/ucm108799.htm

Verma, A. & Steele J. (2006). Botulinum toxin improves sialorrhea and quality of living in bulbar amyotrophic lateral sclerosis. *Muscle Nerve*, Vol. 34, No. 2, pp. 235-7, 0148-639X (Print) 0148-639X (Linking)

Vianello, A.;Arcaro G.;Palmieri A., et al. (2010). Survival and quality of life after tracheostomy for acute respiratory failure in patients with amyotrophic lateral sclerosis. *J Crit Care*, Vol., No. pp., 1557-8615 (Electronic) 0883-9441 (Linking)

Wade, D.T. (1992). *Measurement in Neurology Rehabilitation*, Oxford University Press, Oxford

Wasner, M.;Bold U.;Vollmer T.C. & Borasio G.D. (2004). Sexuality in patients with amyotrophic lateral sclerosis and their partners. *J Neurol*, Vol. 251, No. 4, pp. 445-8, 0340-5354 (Print) 0340-5354 (Linking)

Wellings, D.J. & Unsworth J. (1997). Fortnightly review. Environmental control systems for people with a disability: an update. *BMJ*, Vol. 315, No. 7105, pp. 409-12, 0959-8138 (Print) 0959-535X (Linking)

Woolley, S.C. & Jonathan S.K. (2008). Cognitive and behavioral impairment in amyotrophic lateral sclerosis. *Phys Med Rehabil Clin N Am*, Vol. 19, No. 3, pp. 607-17, xi, 1047-9651 (Print) 1047-9651 (Linking)

World Health Organization (2001). International Classification of Functioning, Disability and Health (ICF). Geneva: World Health Organization

Yorkston, K.M.;Strand E.;Miller R.;Hillel A. & Smith K. (1993). Speech deterioration in amyotrophic lateral sclerosis: implications for the timing of intervention. *J Med Speech-Language Pathol*, Vol. 1, pp. 35-46

11

Nutritional Care in Amyotrophic Lateral Sclerosis: An Alternative for the Maximization of the Nutritional State

Luciano Bruno de Carvalho-Silva

Federal University of Alfenas- MG (UNIFAL-MG); Center for Food Security Studies
(NEPA), State University of Campinas (UNICAMP)
Brazil

1. Introduction

Amyotrophic lateral sclerosis (ALS) is characterized by progressive paralysis secondary to the impairment of the motor neurons, upper motor neuron and lower motor neuron. The most common symptoms and signs are atrophy and muscle weakness, fasciculations, cramps, hypertonia and hyperreflexia. In more advanced stages, decreased respiratory muscle strength, progressive loss of body weight and changes in food intake are observed (Nelson et al., 2000). Several factors are inherent to the food intake in ALS, such as: lack of appetite, dysphagia, weakness, dyspnoea, and depression (Stanich et al., 2004; Nelson et al., 2000; Kasarskis et al., 1996; Welnetz, 1990; Slowie et al., 1983). ALS patients usually have rapid weight loss associated with reduced food intake, increased feeding time, fatigue, dehydration and depression (Wright et al., 2005). The combination of these factors may result in increased energy expenditure and therefore hypercatabolism.

Different studies confirm the correlation between the reduced Body Mass Index (BMI) and the decreased survival in subjects with ALS and the decreased food intake and decrease in tricipital skinfold (TSF) (Kasarskis et al., 1996; Desport et al., 2003; Desport et al., 1999; Desport et al., 2001; Heffernan et al., 2004; Slowie et al. 1983). They also show a high percentage of weight loss, greater than 15% (Mazzini et al. 1995), and prevalence of malnutrition.

Dysphagia, a common symptom with the disease progression, is a factor that makes difficult the maintenance of oral feeding, increasing the respiratory complications, with initiation of invasive ventilation, difficulty to move the patient for the outpatient care and depression (Mazzini et al., 1995).

In this context, taking the nutritional impairment experienced by ALS subjects into account, this chapter aims to discuss the key strategies of nutritional care of patients with ALS, with a tool for maximizing the nutritional status.

2. Amyotrophic lateral sclerosis and nutritional status

2.1 Food intake in ALS

Few studies on food intake in patients with ALS are available in the literature. Among these studies, Kasarskis et al. (1996) studies stand out, which found that 70% of the subjects experienced energy intake below the RDA and 84% of the patients experienced protein intake above the RDA. Slowie et al. (1983) found, as well as Kasarskis et al. (1996), 70% of inadequacy for energy, using the 24-hour recall in patients with ALS. Stanich et al. (2004), found values above the RDA for lipids in most ALS patients chosen in their study.

Silva et al. (2007a and 2007b) analyzed the nutritional profile of patients treated in Dysphagia and Neuromuscular Outpatient Clinics of the Hospital das Clínicas of Unicamp – HC/UNICAMP. Interdisciplinary assessments were performed, revealing a low caloric intake of approximately 1600 kcal for men. In women, a low caloric intake (approximately 1700 kcal/day) was also observed.

In another study conducted by Silva et al. (2008a) the food intake was quantitatively and qualitatively assessed in ALS patients regularly followed at the neuromuscular outpatient clinic of the HC-UNICAMP. The foods most consumed daily were oil, rice, beans, French bread and milk. The food was found to be inadequate regarding energy, fiber, calcium and vitamin E. A significant difference was observed between patients with ALS of bulbar and appendicular predominance, whereas, in patients with higher appendicular manifestation, a higher energy intake (p=0.02) of saturated fat (p=0.03), monounsaturated fat (p=0.04) and polyunsaturated fat (p=0.001), as well as cholesterol (p=0.001) and fibers (p=0.001) was observed when compared with the ALS of bulbar predominance. A higher swallowing impairment observed in patients with bulbar predominance may have influenced the qualitative and quantitative intake. While feeding is impacted by the disease features, the per capita income of patients seems to have influenced the low qualitative consumption of food. Based on the results obtained, the authors suggested that guidance regarding the consumption of foods and preparations with a higher content of high-biological proteins, fibers, calcium, and vitamin E is necessary.

In ALS, as in most neuromuscular diseases, changes can also be observed, which increase the muscle catabolism, directly impacting protein synthesis and mineral excretion. In the initial stages of the disease, according to the study conducted in 94 patients with ALS, it was observed no deficiency of vitamins E and C, but upon disease progression, clinical and biochemical manifestations of such deficiency were observed (Ludolph, 2006).

To estimate the dietary intake, some countries in Europe and Canada use as main practices the 24-hour recall, 3-day and 7-day food record. To estimate the energy requirements, professionals have used the equations of Schofield (1985) and Harris and Benedict (1919). To estimate the adequacy of macronutrients, the researchers used the standards of the Recommended Dietary Allowances (NCR, 1989), Department of Health (1991) and the Institute of Medicine (IOM, 2002; IOM, 2001; IOM 2000; IOM 1997).

To estimate the energy requirements, the most used equation was that of Harris and Benedict (1919) modified by Long; Schaffel; Geiger (1979).

According to Harris and Benedict:

$$\text{Men:} \quad \text{BMR*} = 66 + \left(13.7 \times \text{mass in kg}\right) + \left(5 \times \text{height in cm}\right) - \left(6.8 \times \text{age in years}\right)$$

$$\text{Women: BMR*} = 655 + \left(9.6 \times \text{mass in kg}\right) + \left(1.7 \times \text{height in cm}\right) - \left(4.7 \times \text{age in years}\right)$$

*BMR = basal metabolic rate
Modified by Long; Schaffel; Geiger (1979):
VET* = BMR x activity factor x injury factor
*TEV = total energy value

The activity factor is considered as 1.2 for patients unable to walk and 1.3 for patients able to walk. The injury factor is considered as 1.1 for chronic diseases (Long; Schaffel; Geiger, 1979). Considering a higher energy expenditure (10-20%) for individuals with ALS (Piquet, 2006), some professionals also employ 35 kcal/kg current body weight.

For water intake, the estimation according to Thomas (2001) should be 30-35mL/kg, taking the age into account.

2.2 Anthropometry and body composition

The nutritional status can be evaluated through objective methods, such as: anthropometry, body composition, biochemical parameters and dietary consumption; or subjective methods, such as: physical examination and subjective global assessment. Anthropometry involves obtaining measures of body size, their proportions and the relationship with standards that reflect the development of adult subjects. The most used measures are weight, height, circumferences and skinfolds (Almeida et al., 2010; Silva et al., 2008b; Silva et al., 2008c; Stanich et al., 2004; Kasarskis et al., 1996; Slowie et al., 1983).

2.2.1 Weight (W)

For patients unable to walk, in the absence of a metabolic scale, the weight is measured using a wheelchair. Prior to patient's weighing, the wheelchairs are weighted and their weight is deducted at the time of calibration of the scale. In patients able to walk, the body weight is measured standing on platform type or digital scales (Silva et al., 2008b; Stanich et al., 2004). The weight can also be measured in chair scales, available in the market.

2.2.2 Height (H)

The height for individuals unable to walk is measured with the subject seated closest to the edge of the chair with his/her left knee bent at 90 degrees. The length between the plantar surface and the knee is measured with the help of a measuring tape. The height is estimated according to the equations proposed by Chumlea; Roche; Steinbaugh (1985), where:

$$\text{Men's height} = \left[64.19 - (0.04 \times \text{age in years}) \right] + (2.02 \times \text{knee height in cm})$$

$$\text{Women's height} = [84.88 - (0.24 \times \text{age in years}) + (1.83 \times \text{knee height in cm})$$

2.2.3 Body mass index (BMI)

Usually, body mass-height ratio is used as an indicator of body mass index (BMI = body mass kg/height m^2).

The BMI classification is described below:

- BMI < 16 kg/m^2: severe malnutrition
- 16 - 16.9 kg/m^2: moderate malnutrition
- 17.0 - 18.49 kg/m^2: mild malnutrition
- 18.5 - 24.9 kg/m^2: eutrophic
- 25.0 - 29.9 kg/m^2: overweight
- 30.0 - 34.9 kg/m^2: grade I obesity
- 35.0 - 39.9 kg/m^2: grade II obesity
- >40 kg/m^2: grade III obesity (World Health Organization, 1985)

Kasarskis *et al.* (1996) confirm the correlation between reduced BMI and decreased life expectancy. In studies carried out by Mazzini *et al.* (1995), 53% of ALS patients showed BMI < 20Kg/m² and 55% had weight loss > 15% of usual weight.

2.2.4 Arm circumference (AC)

The arm circumference is measured at the non-dominant arm extended along the body, measured at the midpoint between the acromion and the olecranon process, using a flexible, non-elastic, plastic measuring tape (Lohman; Roche; Martorell, 1991). Desport; Maillot (2002) uses the AC to calculate the arm muscle circumference (AMC) and monitor the nutritional status of patients with ALS.

2.2.5 Skinfolds

Tricipital skinfold (TSF) is determined along the longitudinal axis of the arm, on its posterior face, whereas its exact point of repair is the average distance between the superior lateral edge of the acromion and the olecranon.

Bicipital skinfold (BSF) is determined towards the longitudinal axis of the arm, on its anterior face, in the mid-point of the humeral biceps.

Subscapular skinfold (SCSF) is obtained obliquely to the longitudinal axis following the direction of the ribs, and located 2 cm distant from the lower angle of the scapula.

Suprailiac skinfold (SISF) is measured by slightly placing the patient's right arm behind, trying not to influence the attainment of the measure. This fold is obliquely individualized 2 cm above the anterior superior iliac crest, at the anterior axillary line.

To evaluate the AC and skinfolds, the reference standard used is the work of Frisancho (1981).

2.3 Classification of nutritional status

According to the Percentile Distribution Table, the percentage of adequacy for the abovementioned parameters is calculated by considering the 50th percentile (P50) as standard.

$$\% \text{ adequacy} = \text{studied parameter value}/\text{P50 value} \times 100$$

Values in Table 1 are used for the classification of nutritional status.

Parameters	Obesity	Overweight	Eutrophy	mild PEM[1]	moderate PEM	severe PEM
AC[2]	≥ 120%	120-110%	110-90%	90-80%	80-70%	≤ 70%
TSF[3]	≥120%	120-110%	110-90%	90-80%	80-70%	≤ 70%

[1]PEM: Protein-energy malnutrition; [2]AC: arm circumference; [3]TSF: Tricipital skinfold.

Table 1. Classification of nutritional status according to the parameters proposed by Blackburn; Harvey (1982) and Blackburn; Thornton (1979).

For the determination of the nutritional status, the anthropometric parameters are analyzed together. The values obtained according to the percentage adequacy are classified by Protein-Energy Malnutrition (PEM) Score. The PEM Score is the sum of all parameters of nutritional assessment in percentage adequacy divided by the number of parameters assessed (Blackburn; Harvey, 1982).

$$\text{PEM Score} = \frac{\%\ \text{adq OW} + \%\ \text{adq TSF} + \%\ \text{adq AC} + \%\ \text{adq AMC} + \%\ \text{adq AMA}}{\text{Numbers of parameters}}$$

% adq OW = % adequacy from the optimal weight
% adq TSF = % adequacy of tricipital skinfold
% adq AC = % adequacy of arm circumference
% adq AMC = % adequacy of arm muscle circumference
% adq AMA = % adequacy of arm muscle area
The value obtained by PEM score allows for the classification of patients as:
Eutrophy: > 100%
Mild PEM: < 100% and > 80%
Moderate PEM: < 80% and > 60%
Severe PEM: < 60%

2.3.1 Percentage of weight loss (% WL)

The percentage change of usual weight or percentage of weight loss (% WL) is determined using the patient's usual and current weights, as per the following equation:

$$\%\ \text{WL} = \frac{\text{Usual Weight} - \text{Current Weight}}{\text{Usual Weight}} \times 100$$

The % WL highly reflects the extent of the disease. Patients with % WL values > 10% are classified as malnourished and above 10% severe malnutrition (Mahan; Escott-Stump, 2005).

2.4 Bioelectrical impedance analysis

Bioelectrical impedance analysis (BIA) is a non-invasive technique that can be used to estimate body composition. The method uses low amperage current (single or multiple frequencies) that passes between two electrodes placed on the skin under the assumption that the current resistance (impedance) ranges on an inversely proportional basis to the fluid contained in the tissues and the content of electrolytes. BIA has a good correlation with body composition made with the isotope dilution, under controlled conditions (O'Brien; Young; Sawka, 2002).
In ALS, due to the limitations and difficulties during nutritional assessment, BIA has been a good tool in nutritional diagnosis. It is an easy, non-invasive technique, where fat-free and fat mass are obtained, in addition to the estimation of the degree of hydration. In 2003, the equation for BIA was validated in patients with ALS through cross-sectional and longitudinal studies, which was optimized at 50 kHz (Desport et al., 2003).

2.5 Dual-emission X-ray absorptiometry (DEXA)

The dual-emission X-ray absorptiometry (DEXA) is an invasive method that has become a popular measure for the assessment of body composition in developed countries (Madsen; Jensen; Sorensen, 1997; Tothill et al., 1996; Snead; Birge; Kohrt, 1993). This method allows the structural assessment of body composition, dividing the body mass by three basic components: mineral- and fat-free soft tissue, bone mineral content and fat (Laskey, 1996).
Some studies show the use of such technique in ALS patients (Tadan et al., 1998; Nau et al., 1995; Kanda et al., 1994), however Desport et al. (2003) emphasizes the equipment is

very expensive, and the fact that the patient remains in a horizontal position with his/her arms extended along the body for more than 10 minutes can be a problem for subjects with ALS.

In a study conducted by Rio and Cawadias (2007), it was discussed the main techniques adopted by nutritionists of some centers for the treatment of ALS in Europe and Canada for nutritional assessment of ALS subjects. The researchers found only 22% of nutritionists had more than 4 years of experience in ALS. Amongst the most used nutritional assessment methods were weight, % WL, BMI and arm circumference, used by 100%, 96%, 83%, and 9% of the professionals, respectively. The bioelectrical impedance, validated by Desport et al. in 2003, as well as DEXA, were not reported by the professionals from the centers investigated by Rio and Cawadias.

Analyzing the measures adopted by the relevant literature, in ALS, as well as in other diseases, the use of parameters such as weight, % WL and BMI, as well as skinfolds, BIA, DEXA and indirect calorimetry can also be observed (Rio; Cawadias 2007; Desport et al., 2003; Desport et al., 2001; Silani; Kasarkis, Yanagisawa, 1998).

3. Dysphagia and ALS

With the clinical progression of ALS, manifestations such as dysarthria (speech impairment), dyspnoea (breathing alteration), dysphonia (voice alteration) and dysphagia (swallowing alteration) are common. These manifestations occur as a result of progressive respiratory muscle dysfunction, caused by motor neuron degeneration of corticobulbar tract (Chiappetta; Oda, 2004).

In 17 to 30% of ALS patients, bulbar muscles, especially the muscle groups of the velum and tongue are the first ones affected, resulting in progressive dysphagia, and therefore difficulty in swallowing food and liquids (Calia; Annes, 2003; Mitsumoto; Norris, 1994; Gubbay et al., 1985).

The oro-laryngo-pharyngeal weakness affects the survival of subjects with ALS, especially because of the continuous risk of aspiration pneumonia and sepsis, and the inadequate food intake, which can result in malnutrition (Karsarkis et al., 1996).

Malnutrition due to dysphagia, or other factors associated, such as muscle atrophy and diaphragm weakness, increases the relative risk of death almost eight times in ALS patients (Mitsumoto et al., 2003; Desport et al., 1999).

The involvement of the tongue muscles and lip orbicular muscles, upon ALS progression, triggers a decrease in pressure wave, pharyngeal peristalsis, and elevation and anteriorization of larynx, causing choking, even with saliva (Watts; Vanryckeghem, 2001; Strand et al., 1996).

In ALS, dysphagia for liquids is more common than for solids. The early escape, that is, when the food reaches the vallecula prior to initiation of pharyngeal swallowing, is more frequent with thin liquids and is the leading cause of tracheal aspiration. Pharyngeal residues are more commonly observed throughout the course of the disease. The pasty and solid consistencies may cause laryngeal penetration and tracheal aspiration after swallowing. Swallowing disorders occur due to the influence of oral transit, decreased movement of the tongue base, decreased elevation and anteriorization of the larynx and decreased pharyngeal contraction (Chiappetta; Oda, 2004; Logeman, 1998; Campbel; Enderby, 1984; apud Chiappetta, 2005).

In order to minimize respiratory and nutritional complications in the treatment of dysphagia, interdisciplinary assessment is extremely important, and the modification of the texture of foods is an alternative for the maintenance of the oral route.

3.1 Influence of viscosity

Food viscosity is one of the most important variables of swallowing. Thin liquids make difficult swallowing by patients with reduced laryngeal control, since they are quickly swallowed and do not maintain their shape inside the oral cavity, which can prematurely leak into the pharynx and, thus, penetrate the airways still open. To avoid such effect, the optimal viscosity must be determined so the swallowing may occur safety (Macedo & Furkim, 2000).

Viscosity influences many aspects of the assessment and management of dysphagia. It can be defined as the fluid resistance to the flow and is measured in Centipoise (ctps or cPs) (Silva et al, 2010).

There are different types of viscosity that can be easily achieved using commercial thickeners. These types can be classified in centipoise (cP) values (Table 1) as thin (1-50 cP), nectar (51-350 cP), honey (351-1750 cP) and pudding (> 1750 cP).

Classification	Viscosity (cP)
Thin	1-50
Nectar	51-350
Honey	351-1750
Pudding	> 1750

Source: ADA, 2002.

Table 2. Classification of viscosity, in centipoise (cP) values, according to the ADA (2002), for the nutritional care of subjects with dysphagia.

4. Nutritional therapy

Patients with symptoms of dysphagia limiting their intake of foods and liquids, hospitalized or at home, should be considered those at high risk of experiencing nutritional deficiencies and consequently should be treated.

Appropriate nutrition and hydration in patients with dysphagia are based on a complex balance between preparation, intake and absorption of foods and drinks (Steele & Lieshout, 2004).

When diagnosing the cause and severity of dysphagia, healthcare professionals can determine the texture of foods and the thickness of fluids for a safer swallowing by dysphagic patients, since the consistency of the diet should be individualized according to the type and extent of dysfunction. In case the recipe is not followed, the subject may face serious consequences for health (Silva et al, 2010; Macedo & Furquim, 2000).

Table 1 shows an example of a modified diet with restriction of "thin liquids" (1-50 cP) and solids for subjects with dysphagia and swallowing impairment.

Meal	Food	Ingredients (Servings)	Viscosity (cP)
Breakfast:	Dried milk porridge	Milk: 100 mL Dried Milk: 25 g	910
	Mashed banana	1 unit – 90 g	2.900
Snack:	Thickened papaya juice	Water: 30 mL Papaya: 170 g	870
Lunch:	Spaghetti and basil soup (liquefied)	Spaghetti (125 g), vegetable oil (2 tablespoons), onion (1 unit), mashed garlic cloves (2 units), nut (60 g), chicken bouillon (70 mL), fresh basil leaves (30 g), salt to taste, grated cheese (1 dessert spoon).	2.440
	Thickened orange juice	Orange juice: 200 mL Thickener: 10 g	320
Snack:	Juice of fruits (papaya, banana and apple)	Cold fluid milk (10º) (200 mL), papaya (100 g), banana (90 g), apple (50 g)	1.090
Dinner:	Vegetable broth	Water (2 L), turnips (2 units), carrots (2 units), garlic clove (1 unit), onion (1 unit), arracacha (1 unit), bunch of watercress (1 unit), basil (to taste), salt (to taste), and a drizzle of olive oil, raw large potato (1 unit) 100 g	4.680
	Lemon Mousse		8.000
Supper:	Maize porridge	Milk: 100 mL Maize bran: 25 g	840

* Adapted from Peres, Manzano and Silva (2007).

Table 3. Modified diet with restriction of "thin liquids" (1-50 cP) and "solids" for subjects with dysphagia and swallowing impairment. Features: Soft, wet and liquefied foods. Liquid foods are all thickened. The example menu contains approximately 2,000 kilocalories.

Changes in viscosity of foods and fluids can be achieved with the help of commercial thickeners. The choice of thickening agent is critical to achieve a homogeneous and lasting consistency. The thickeners should interfere as little as possible with the sensory properties of liquids (Silva et al, 2010)

Several agents can be used as food thickeners. Such thickeners are mostly composed of polysaccharides (carbohydrates), such as gums and starches, in addition to pectins and cellulose derivatives. Among them, the modified starch is one of the most used, since the starch physically or chemically treated improves the properties of thickening, cohesion, stability, gelatinization, luster and taste of the natural starch. In addition, they can also maximize the nutritional and water intake, facilitating a wide variety of textures (Silva & Ikeda, 2009). Therefore, these modified starch-containing thickeners can be used to prevent dehydration of subjects with dysphagia (Ada, 2002). However, the commercial thickeners are very expensive (approximately R$ 40.00 BRL/200 g), which limits the purchase and adjustment of the correct consistency.

It is known that the intake may be maximized by adjusting the consistency of foods through simple and low-cost techniques, without using commercial thickeners that are very expensive (Silva & Ikeda, 2009; Whelan, 2001). Thickening of foods by using the own foods in several preparations so as to adjust the correct consistency is still unknown by many patients, caregivers and healthcare professionals, limiting the food intake, resulting in high rates of malnutrition, dehydration and pulmonary aspiration, and increasing the risk of death[32]. These techniques are designed for this population, especially regarding the amount of food in household measures necessary to achieve optimal viscosity, according to the ADA standard (Silva et al., 2006a).

In 2006, researches were conducted in order to develop a guide with recent literature survey, standardized preparations for patients with dysphagia, viscosities adjusted according to the ADA, chemical composition and photographic record for healthcare professionals, caregivers and patients with dysphagia, for a safe dietary intake (Silva et al., 2006b). Studies like this are still scarce for this population.

The poor knowledge of the fundamental physical characteristics of the consistency of the preparations is considered a limiting factor to adjust the viscosity, which does not ensure a safe intake. Figure 1 shows a photographic representation of a preparation of heart of palm cream with the consistency of pudding. Its main characteristic is the formation of a heavy cake, in which there is low adherence on the spoon surface, forming no continuous filaments.

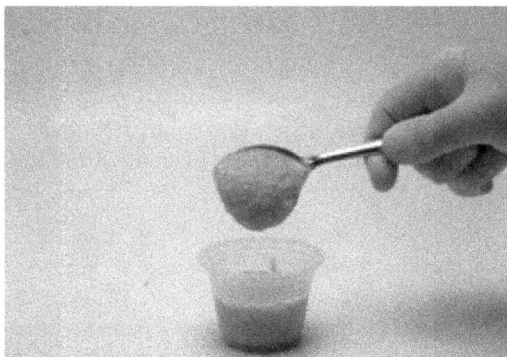

Fig. 1. Photographic representation of a preparation (heart of palm cream) with pudding consistency. pH = 3.73; viscosity = 2000 cP; amount of water for dilution = 0 mL

Figure 2 shows a photographic representation of the same preparation with the consistency of honey, in which there is a formation of continuous filament with the base of the spoon forming a characteristic "V".

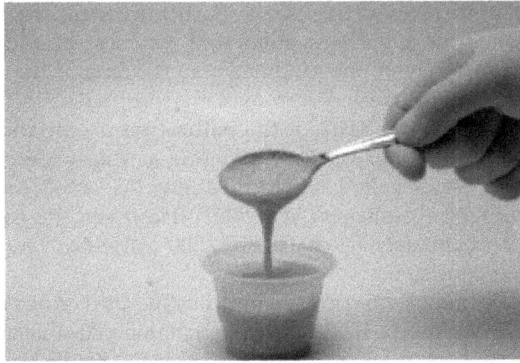

Fig. 2. Photographic representation of a preparation (heart of palm cream) with honey consistency. pH = 3.69; viscosity = 1080 cP; amount of water for dilution in 100 mL of the recipe with pudding viscosity = 14.23 mL

In the photographic representation of the nectar consistency (Figure 3), there is a formation of continuous filament thinner than the previous one, without a characteristic "V" at the base of the spoon.

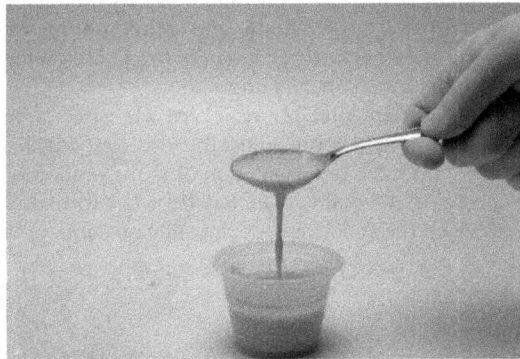

Fig. 3. Photographic representation of a preparation (heart of palm cream) with nectar consistency. pH = 3.71; viscosity = 240 cP; amount of water for dilution in 100 mL of the recipe with pudding viscosity = 42.88 mL

Figure 4 shows a photographic representation of the thin consistency of the same preparation; as the name implies, there is no formation of continuous filament, but only drops that fall from the spoon.

These alternatives are considered simple, low-cost and safe, and are extremely important to ensure a better quality of life for patients without dysphagia, without limiting the need for commercial thickeners, but guidelines concerning how to follow a correct preparation are still necessary. Currently, there are discussions on the improvement of the quality of life and reduction of potential complications, through education/health promotion programs, including specialized procedures and orientation programs for caregivers (Santoro, 2008)

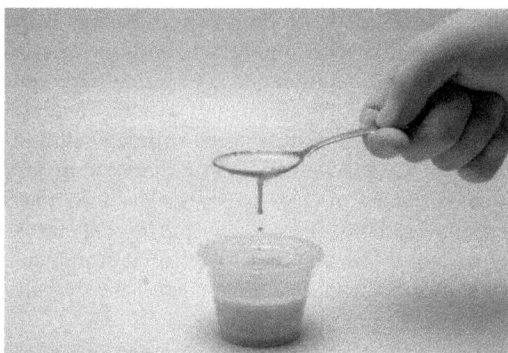

Fig. 4. Photographic representation of a preparation (heart of palm cream) with thin consistency. pH = 5.36; viscosity = 46 cP; amount of water for dilution in 100 mL of the recipe with pudding viscosity = 107.14 mL

Periodic and appropriate reassessments of the swallowing condition are critical aspects for the prevention/recovery from malnutrition. One study assessed the adequacy of the diet of elderlies admitted to nursing homes, where 91% of the patients had diets with a consistency below what they could tolerate safely. Both the nutritional status and the quality of life may be affected when patients are maintained on diets with inappropriate viscosity (Souza et al., 2003)

Patients with dysphagia may experience satiety quickly when they are given an extremely concentrated meal. Instead of providing three meals a day, these patients should receive smaller and more frequent portions (Silva et al., 2003). Of note, for patients with dysphagia, difficulty in performing the swallowing movements worsens when they are most tired. This is especially important for patients with diseases like Parkinson's, for which the medication effect can be reduced during the day, further reducing the patient's ability to swallow (Sachdev, 2005). The correct positioning of the patient may be of great help during meals, but it is important to follow the instructions of a speech therapist & audiologist.

If there is a high risk of aspiration or oral intake is insufficient to maintain the good nutritional status, the possibility of an alternative nutritional support must be considered. A soft and well tolerable tube can be inserted and radiologically guided. Percutaneous endoscopic gastrostomy is performed by inserting a gastrostomy tube into the stomach through a percutaneous abdominal route guided by the endoscopist and, if available, surgical gastrostomy is preferable (Ickenstein, 2003; Nguyen et al., 2006).

Therefore, the guidance on an individualized diet, precautions on the risk of aspiration, and appropriate choice regarding the route of access for feeding, help to prevent malnutrition in patients with dysphagia, where the care of a multidisciplinary team is required for the patient's welfare, as well as for a better quality of life. Nonetheless, the absence of detailed descriptions on the procedures for nutritional therapy makes unfeasible their efficient replication (Nguyen et al., 2006).

4.1 Nutritional support

Nutritional support may delay the weight loss and muscle atrophy. Researchers have shown the weight loss associated with bulbar changes (dysphagia and breathing) require early and specific nutritional support (Kasarskis et al., 1996; Slowie et al., 1983).

Constant muscle atrophy, characteristic of progressive diseases, may mask the increased metabolic demand. The increased baseline energy expenditure of patients with ALS occurs since the energies are focused on the maintenance of pulmonary ventilation (Stanich et al., 2004; Kasarskis et al., 1996; Nau et al., 1995; Shimizu; Hayashi; Tanabe, 1991).

In a study of ALS patients, under the oral nutritional supplementation program, there was a progressive decrease in body mass index (BMI) in patients with progressive bulbar palsy and preservation of such variables in ALS patients. The lean mass/fat mass ratio was maintained during the study for both groups. The nutritional status classification has not changed for 70% of the patients. The results showed that supplementation prevented the worsening of nutritional status, but was unable to correct the overall averages of adequacy (Stanich et al., 2004).

In clinical practice, the use of supplements of vitamins, especially vitamin E, is common. The supplementation of this vitamin, with quantity still not defined, is expected to improve the nutritional profile of subjects with ALS (Borasio; Voltz, 1997). Oral supplementation with creatine monohydrate at 3g/day showed no improvement of nutritional status in ALS. However, the energy and protein supplementation is used by many professionals, and has proven to be efficient in the nutritional status of subjects with ALS (Rio; Cawadias, 2007; Heffernan et al., 2004).

Silva et al., (2010) evaluated the efficacy of oral supplementation with milk whey proteins and modified starch (70%WPI:30%MS), on nutritional and functional parameters of patients with ALS. Sixteen patients were randomized to two groups, treatment (70%WPI:30%MS) and control (maltodextrin). They underwent prospective nutritional, respiratory and functional assessment for 4 months. Patients in the treatment group presented weight gain, increased BMI, increased arm muscle area and circumference, higher albumin, white blood cell and total lymphocyte counts, and reduced creatine-kinase, aspartate aminotransferase and alanine aminotransferase. In the control group, biochemical measures did not change, but weight and BMI declined. The results indicate that the agglomerate 70%WPI:30%MS may be useful in the nutritional therapy of patients with ALS.

4.2 Alternative feeding in ALS

Different authors report the need for alternative routes of nutrition from the following criteria: vital capacity of approximately 50% of the expected value, presence of moderate to severe dysphagia and 10% reduction in body weight over the past three months. (Stanich et al., 2004; Mitsumoto et al., 2003; Albert et al., 2001; Silani; Kasarskis; Yanagisawa, 1998; Lisbeth et al., 1994).

Percutaneous endoscopic gastrostomy (PEG) is an option for the symptomatic treatment of patients with ALS (Miller et al., 1999).

When comparing the use of enteral nutrition via nasogastric tube and percutaneous endoscopic gastrostomy (PEG) in patients with ALS, there is a significant difference in the body mass index (BMI) of patients with PEG compared to those with a nasogastric tube, as well as a better social acceptance and, consequently, quality of life of the patients studied, supporting the use of this technique when oral intake is not safe (Mazzini et al., 1995).

5. Conclusions

This chapter was conducted to support the hypothesis of the thesis and gathers scientific information listing the main practices for assessment, from the nutritional point of view, in patients with ALS. The relevant literature available for consultation is limited. Studies on food intake, specific techniques for assessment of nutritional status, and the use of supplements are scarce. However, the follow-up of nutritional status by monitoring the anthropometric evolution, body composition and clinical signs, such as dysphagia, may improve the quality of life of subjects with ALS.

6. References

ADA. (2002). National Dysphagia Diet Task Force. *National Dysphagia Diet: Standardization for Optimal Care*. The American Dietetics Association. pp 47

Albert, SM., Murphy, PL., Del Bene, M., Rowland, LP., Mitsumoto, H. (2001). Incidence and predictors of GEP placement in ALS/MND. *Journal of Neurological Sciences*, Vol.191, pp 115-119

Barros, PB., Manzano, FM., Silva, LBC. (2006). *Manual de Técnicas e Receitas para Espessamento de Alimentos: utilização de diferentes amidos espessantes*, São Paulo: Cescorf pp 10-68. *(In Portuguese)*

Blackburn, GL., Havey, KB. (1982). Nutritional assessment as a routine in clinical medicine. *Postgraduate Medicine*, Vol. 71, pp 46-63

Blackburn, GL., Thorrnton, PA. (1979). Nutrition assessment of the hospitalized patient. *Medicine Clinical Nutrition of American*, Vol 63, pp. 1103-1115

Borasio, GD., Voltz, R. (1997). Palliative care in amyotrophic lateral sclerosis. *Journal of Neurology*, Vol. 244, pp.S11-S7. Supl. 4.

Calia, LC., Annes, M. (2003). Afecções neurológicas periféricas. In: Levy, JA.; Oliveira, AS. *Reabilitação em doenças neurológicas – guia terapêutico prático*. São Paulo: Atheneu, pp. 31-64. *(In Portuguese)*

Campbell, MJ., Enderby, P. (1984). Management of motor neurone disease. *Journal of theNeurological Sciences*, Vol 64, pp. 65–71

Carvalho-Silva, LBC. (2011). Anthropometric wrist and arm circumference and their derivations: application to amyotrophic lateral sclerosis. In *Handbook of Anthropometry:Physical Measuresof Human Form in Health and Disease*. New York: Springer. DOI 10.1007/978-1-4419-1788-1_39.

Chiappetta, ALML. (2005). *Disfagia Orofaríngea em Pacientes com Doença do Neurônio Motor/Esclerose Lateral Amiotrófica*. São Paulo. 124. Tese (Doutor em Ciências) – Escola Paulista de Medicina, Universidade Federal de São Paulo.

Chiappetta, ALML., Oda, AL. (2004). Doenças neuromusculares. In: Ferreira, L. P., Benefilopes, D. M., Limongi, S. C. Ed. *Tratado de fonoaudiologia*. São Paulo: Roca, pp. 330-342

Chumlea, MAC., Roche, AF., Steinbaugh, ML. (1958). Estimating stature from knee height for persons 60 to 90 years of age. *Journal of American Geriatrics Society*, Vol. 33, pp. 116-120

Department of health. (1991). Report on health and social subjects. *Dietary reference values for food energy and nutrients for the UK*. No. 41

Desport, JC., Preux, PM., Bouteloup-Demange, C., Clavelou, P., Beaufrère, B., Bonnet, C., Couratier, P. P. (2003). Validation of bioelectrical impedance analysis in patients with amyotrophic lateral sclerosis. *American Journal of Clinical Nutrition*, Vol. 77, pp. 1179-1185

Desport, JC., Preux, PM., Magy, L., Boirie, Y., Vallat, JM., Beaufrère, B., Couratier, P. (2001). Factor correllted with hypermetabolism in patients with amyotrophic lateral sclerosis. *American of Journal Clinical Nutrition*, Vol. 74, pp. 328-3

Desport, JC., Preux, PM., Truong, TC., Vallat, JM., Sautereau, D., Couratier, P. (1999). Nutritional status is a prognostics factor for survival in ALS patients. *Neurology*, Vol. 53, pp. 1059-1063

Desport, JC., Maillot, F. Nutrition et Sclérose Latérale Amyotrophique (SLA). (2002). *Nutrition Clinique et Métabolisme*, Vol. 16, pp. 91-96

Frisancho, AR. (1981). New norms of upper limb fat and muscle areas for assessment of nutritional status. *American of Journal Clinical Nutrition*, Vol. 34, pp. 540-545

Gubbay, SS., Kahana, E., Zilber, N., Cooper, G., Pintov, S., Leibowitz, Y. (1985). Amyotrophic lateral sclerosis. A study of its presentation and prognosis. *Journal of Neurology*, Vol. 232, pp. 295-300

Harris, JA., Benedict, FG. (1919). A biometric study of basal metabolism in man. Washington, DC: Carnegie Istitute of Washington.

Heffernan, C., Jenkinson, C., Holmes, T., Feder, G., Kupfer, R., Leigh, R., McGowan, P. N., Rio, A., Sidhu, P. S. Nutritional management in MND/ALS patients: an evidence based review. *Amyotrophic Lateral Sclerosis and Other Motor Neuron Disorders*, Vol. 5, pp.72-83

Ickenstein GW., Kelly PJ., Furie K.L, Ambrosi D., Rallis N., Goldstein R et al. (2003). Predictors of feeding gastrostomy: tube removal in stroke patients with dysphagia. *Journal of Stroke and Cerebrovascular Diseases*, Vol.12(4), pp.169-74

Institute of medicine. (2002). Energy. In: Dietary Reference Intakes for energy, carbohydrate, fiber, fatty acids, cholesterol, protein, and amino acids. Washington, D.C.: The National Academy Press. <http://www.nap.edu> [2011 July 14].

Institute of medicine. (2001). In: Dietary Reference Intakes for vitamin A, vitamin K, arsenic, boron, chromium, copper, iodine, iron, manganese, molybdenum, nickel, silicon, vanadium, and zinc. Washington, D.C.: The National Academy Press, 2001. <http://www.nap.edu> [2011 July 14].

Institute of medicine. (2000). In: Dietary Reference Intakes for vitamin C, vitamin E, selenium, and carotenoids. Washington, D.C.: The National Academy Press. <http://www.nap.edu> [2011 July 14].

Institute of medicine. (1997). In: Dietary Reference Intakes for calcium, phosphorous, magnesium, vitamin D, and fluoride. Washington, D.C.: The National Academy Press. <http://www.nap.edu> [2007 Abril 14].

Kanda, F., Fujii, Y., Takahashi, L., Fujita, T. (1994). Dual-energy X-ray absorptiometry in neuromuscular diseases. *Muscle and Nerve*, Vol. 17, pp. 413-415

Kasarskis, E., Berryman, S., Vanderleest, JG., Schneider, AR., McClain, CJ. (1996). Nutritional status of patients with amyotrophic lateral sclerosis: relation to the proximity of death. *American Journal of Clinical Nutrition*, Vol. 63, pp.130-137

Lisbeth, MH., Mathus, V., Louwerse, LS., Merkus, MP., Tytgat, GNJ., Vianney, JMB. (1994). Percutaneous endoscopic gastrostomy in patients with amyotrophic lateral slerosis and impaired pulmonary function. *Gastrointestinal Endoscopy*, Vol. 40, pp. 463-469

Lohman, TG., Roche, AF., Martorell, R. (1991). *Anthropometric standardization reference manual*. Abrindged edition.

LONG, CL., Schaffel, N., Geiger, JW. (1979). Metabolic response to injury and illness: Estimation of energy and protein needs from indirect calorimetry and nitrogen balance. *Journal of Parenteral and Enteral Nutrition*, Vol. 3, pp. 452-456

Ludolph, AC. (2006). 135th ENMC International Workshop: Nutrition in amyotrophic lateral sclerosis 18-20 of March 2005, Naarden, The Netherlands. *Neuromuscular Disorders*, pp. 1-9

Macedo EDG, Furkim AM. (2000). *Manual de cuidados do paciente com disfagia*. São Paulo: Lovise. (In Portuguese)

Madsen, OR., Jensen, JEB., Sorensen, OH. (1997). Validation of a dual energy x- ray absortiometer: measurement of bone mass and soft tissue composition. European *Journal Applied Physiology*, Vol. 75, pp. 554-558

Mahan, K., Escott-Stump, S. (2005). Krause: alimentos, nutrição e dietoterapia. 11ª ed. São Paulo: Ed. Roca, 407 p. (In Portuguese)

Mazzini, L., Corrá, T., Zaccala, M., Mora, G., Del Piano, M., Galante, M. (1995). Percutaneous endoscopic gastrostomy and enteral nutrition in amyotrophic lateral sclerosis. *Journal of Neurology*, Vol. 242, pp. 695-698

Miller, R. G., Rosenberg, J. A., Gelinas, D. F., Mitsumoto, H., Newman, D., Sufit, R. (1999). Practice parameter: The care of the patient with amyotrophic lateral sclerosis (an evidence-based review). *Neurology*, Vol. 52, pp. 1311- 1323

Mitsumoto, H., Davidson, M., Moore, D., Gad, N., Brands, M., Ringel, S., Rosenfeld, J., Shefner, JM., Strong, MJ., Sufit, R., Anderson, FA. (2003). ALS CARE Study Group Percutaneous endoscopic gastrostomy (GEP) in patients with ALS and bulbar dysfunction. *ALS and other motor disorders*, Vol. 4, pp. 177-185

Mitsumoto, H., Norris, FH. (1994). *Amyotrophic Lateral A Comprehensive Guide to management*, pp. 342

National Research Council (US). (1989). *Recommended dietary allowances*. Washington: National Academic Press

Nau, KL. Individuals with amyotrofic lateral sclerosis are in caloric balance despite losses in mass. *Journal of the Neurological Sciences*, Vol. 192, pp.S47-S49

Nau, KL., Bromberg, MB., Forsshew, DA., Katch, VL. (1995). Individuals with amyotrophic lateral sclerosis are in caloric balance despite losses in mass. *Journal of the Neurological Sciences*, Vol. 129, pp. 47-49

Nelson, LM., Matkin, C., Longstreth, WT, McGuire, V. (2000). Population – based case – control study of amyotrophic lateral sclerosis in Western Washington State. II. Diet. *American Journal of Epidemiology*, Vol. 151, pp. 164-173

Nguyen NP, Moltz CC, Frank C, Vos P, Smith HJ, Nguyen PD, Nguyen LM, Dutta S, Lemanski C, Sallah S. (2006). Impact of swallowing therapy on aspiration rate following treatment for locally advanced head and neck cancer. *Oral Oncol.* Vol 43, pp.352-7

O'Brien, C., Young, AJ., Sawka, MN. (2002). *Bioelectrical impedance to estimate changes in hydration status. International Journal of Sports and Medicine, Vol. 23, pp. 361-366*

Piquet, MA. Nutritional Approach for patients with amyotrophic lateral sclerosis. *Revue Neurologique*, Vol. 2, pp. S177-4S187. (In French)

Rio, A., Cawadias, E. (2007). Nutritional advice and treatment by dietitians to patients with amyotrophic lateral sclerosis/motor neurone disease: a survey of current practice in England, Wales, Northern Ireland and Canada. *Journal of Human Nutrition and Dietetics*, Vol. 20, pp. 1-13

Sachdev PS. (2005). Neuroleptic-induced moviment disorders: an overview. *Psychiatr. Clin. N.Am*, Vol.28, pp.255-274

Santoro PP. (2008). Disfagia orofaríngea: panorama atual, epidemiologia, opções terapêuticas e perspectivas futuras. *Rev. CEFAC.* 10(2)

Schofield, WN. (1985). Predicting basal metabolic rate, new standards and a review of previous work. *Human Nutrition Clinical Nutrition*, Vol. 39, pp. 5-41

Shimizu, T., Hayashi, H., Tanabe, H. (1991). Energy metabolism of ALS patients Ander mechanical ventilation and tube feeding. *Clinical neurology and neurosurgery*, Vol. 31, pp. 255-259

Silani V., Kasarkis, E. J., Yanagisawa, N. (1998). Nutritional management in amyotrophic lateral sclerosis: a worldwide perspective. *Journal of Neurology*, Vol. 243, pp. S13-S19, 1998. Supl. 2.

Silva, LBC., Mourao, LF., Silva, AA., Lima, NMFV., Almeida, SRM., Franca Júnior, MC., Anamarli, N., Amaya-Farfán, J.. (2010). Effect of nutritional supplementation with milk whey proteins in amyotrophic lateral sclerosis patients. *Arquivos de Neuro-Psiquiatria*, Vol. 68, pp. 1

Silva, LBC., Ikeda, CM.. (2009). Cuidado nutricional na disfagia: uma alternativa para maximização do estado nutricional. *Revista Brasileira de Nutrição Clínica*, Vol. 27, pp. 1 *(in Portuguese)*

Silva, LBC., Mourao, LF., Silva, AA., Lima, NMFV., Franca Junior, M., Nucci, A., Amaya-Farfan, J. (2008a). Avaliação da ingestão alimentar de indivíduos com Esclerose Lateral Amiotrófica. *Revista Brasileira de Nutrição Clínica*, vol. 23, pp. 5-12 *(in Portuguese)*

Silva, LBC., Figueira, M.L., Silva, AA, Lima, NMFV., Almeida, SR., Franca Júnior, MC., Anamarli, N. Amaya-Farfán, J.. (2008b). Amyotrophic lateral sclerosis: combined nutritional, respiratory and functional assessment. *Arquivos de Neuro-Psiquiatria*, Vol. 66, pp. 354

Silva, LBC., Antunes, A., E., Botelho I., Paula A., Silva, A., A., Amaya-Farfan, J. (2008c). Nutrition and dysphagia: body mass index, food consistency and food intake. *Revista Brasileira de Nutrição Clínica.* Vol.6, pp. 23-91

Silva, LBC., Mourão, L., Lima, NMFV., Almeida, SRM., Franca, MJ., Nucci, A., Amaya-Farfan, J. (2007a). *Amyotrophic lateral sclerosis: nutritional status and functional conditions*, Annual Dysphagia Research Society Meeting, Vancouver, Canada, March 8-10

Silva, LBC., Mourão, L., Lima, NMFV., Almeida, SRM., Franca, MJ., Nucci, A., Amaya-Farfan, J. (2007b). *Amyotrophic Lateral Sclerosis (ALS): Nutritional profile and swallowing ability in patients with dysphagia*, Annual Dysphagia Research Society Meeting, Vancouver, Canada, March 8-10

Silva LBC., Mourão L., Lima NMFV., Aldeia SEM., Franca MJ., Nucci A. et al. (2007c). Amyotrophic lateral sclerosis (ALS): nutritional profile and swallowing ability in patients with dysphagia. *Annual Dysphagia Research Society Meeting*, Vancouver; Mar 8-10. Canada: 2007.

Silva LBC., Manzano FM., Moura RMX., Marques IL., Peres SPBA. (2006a). Viscosidade na terapia nutricional da disfagia: como espessar e alcançar a consistência desejada utilizando diferentes espessantes comerciais? 14° Congresso Latinoamericano de Nutrición; Nov 12-16. Florianópolis: 2006. *(In Portuguese)*

Silva LBC., De Paula A., Botelho I., Silva AA. (2006b). Perfil nutricional e de deglutição de pacientes atendidos no ambulatório de disfagia do HC-/Unicamp. 14° Congresso Latinoamericano de Nutrición; 2006 Nov 12-16. Florianópolis: 2006. *(In Portuguese)*

Souza BBA., Martins C., Campos DJ., Balsini ID., Meyer LR. (2003). *Nutrição e disfagia: guia para profissionais*, pp. 9-12.

Slowie, LA., Paige, MS., Antel, JP. (1983). Nutritional considerations in the management of patients with ALS amyotrophic lateral sclerosis. *Journal of the American Dietetic Association*, Vol. 83, pp. 44-47

Stanich, P., Pereira, AML., Chiappeta, ALML., Nunes, M., Oliveira, ASB., Gabbai, AA. (2004). Suplementação nutricional em pacientes com doença do neurônio motor/esclerose lateral amiotrófica.*Revista Brasileira de Nutrição Clínica*, Vol. 19, pp.70-78. *(in Portuguese)*

Steele CM., Van Lieshout PH. (2004). Influence of bolus consistency on lingual behaviors in sequential swallowing. *Dysphagia*, Vol.19, pp. 192-206

Strand, EA., Miller, RM., Yorkston, KM., Hillel, AD. (1996). Management of oral pharyngeal dysphagia symptoms in amyotrophic lateral sclerosis. *Dysphagia*, Vol. 11, pp. 129-139

Tadan, R., Krusinski, PB., Hiser, JR. (1998). *The validity and sensitivity of dual energy X-ray absorptiometry in estimulating lean body mass in amyotrophic lateral sclerosis*. In: Proceedings of the 9th International Symposium on ALS/MND, Munich, 16-18 November 1998. Munich: ALS Association, 1998. 48 p.

Thomas, B. (2001). *Manual of Dietetic Practice*. 3 rd edition. Oxford: Blackwell Science Ltd

Tothill, P., Han, TS., Avenell, A., McNeill, G., Reid, DM. (1996). Comparisons between fat measurements by dual-energy x-ray absorptiometry, underwater weighing and magnetic resonance imaging in healthy women. *European Journal of Clinical Nutrition*, Vol. 50, pp. 747-752

Watts, C. R., Vanryckeghem, M. (2001). Layngeal dysfunction in Amyotropic Lateral Sclerosis: a review and case report. *BMC Ear, Nose and Throat disorders*.

Welnetz, K. (1990). Maintaining adequate nutrition and hydration in the dysphagic ALS patient. *Journal of Continuing Education in Nursing*, Vol. 21, pp. 62-71

Whelan K. (2001). Inadequate fluid intakes in dysphagic acute stroke. *Clinical Nutrition*, Vol. 20, pp. 423-28

Wright, L., Cotter, D., Hickson, M., Frost, G. (2005). Comparison of energy and protein intakes of older people consuming a texture modified diet with a normal hospital diet. *Journal of Human Nutrition and Dietetics*, Vol. 18, pp. 213-219

12

How to Assess Disease's Severity and Monitor Patients with Amyotrophic Lateral Sclerosis: Lessons from Neurophysiology

Ferdinando Sartucci[1,2,3], Tommaso Bocci[1,4], Lucia Briscese[1],
Chiara Pecori[1,3], Chiara Rossi[1] and Fabio Giannini[4]
[1]*Department of Neuroscience, Unit of Neurology, Pisa University Medical School,*
[2]*Institute of Neuroscience, CNR, Pisa,*
[3]*Department of Neuroscience, Unit Outpatients Neurological Activity,*
Pisa University Medical School, Pisa,
[4]*Department of Neurological Neurosurgical and Behavioural Sciences,*
Siena University Medical School, Siena,
Italy

1. Introduction

Amyotrophic Lateral Sclerosis (ALS) is a fatal, neurodegenerative disorder affecting upper and lower motor neurons; it's the commonest of the motor unit diseases in Europe and North America, characterized by a broad spectrum of clinical presentations mimicking vertebral stenosis, motor polyradiculoneuropathies and myopathies (Juergens et al., 1980; Swash, 2001). Striking asymmetry and selective involvement of individual groups of muscles, especially of hand and forearm, are typical early features of the disease. On average, delay from onset of symptoms to diagnosis is about 14 months and expected survival commonly ranges from months to a few years (Andersen et al., 2007).

Clinical neurophysiology in ALS plays a fundamental role both in the diagnosis of suspected disease and in the assessment of its severity and progression, offering a promising perspective to quantify muscle involvement and evaluate response to therapy (Brooks et al., 2000; Olney and Lomen-Hoerth, 2000; Beghi et al., 2002). Neuroimaging using magnetic resonance imaging (MRI), magnetic resonance spectroscopy (1HMRS), positron emission tomography (PET) and functional MRI may prove valuable results (Pohl et al., 2001), although they are complex, expensive and not always available. On the other hand, blood tests are necessary: hypoglycaemia insulinoma-related and autoimmune hyperthyroidism can be mistaken for ALS as they cause generalized muscle weakness, sometimes accompanied by fasciculations without a significant sensory impairment. Spinal fluid analysis could be helpful to rule out rare conditions closely mimicking ALS, such as meningeal infiltration with lymphoma, multifocal motor neuropathy (MMN) or a motor variant of inflammatory demyelinating neuropathy (CIDP). EMG investigation, usually performed with concentric needle electrodes (Daube et al., 2000), plays an essential role in the diagnosis and monitoring of ALS (Bromberg et al., 1993; Eisen, 2001; de Carvalho et al.,

2005b). Amplitude, duration, area, shape, stability on repeated discharges of motor units (MU) and activity at full effort are parameters conventionally used to evaluate disease's stage. EMG may also assess the presence of activity of the denervation-reinnervation process and number of functioning motor units by evaluating recruitment-activation pattern (Brooks et al., 2000; Finsterer and Fuglsang-Frederiksen, 2001). However, these parameters represent only indirect indicators of the number of surviving muscle fibers.

A particular method to evaluate the full MU is the so-called macro-EMG (Stålberg, 1980; Stålberg and Fawcett, 1982; Stålberg, 1983; Dengler et al., 1990). This technique provides information from a larger area of the muscle than traditional needle EMG methods. The signal is recorded by most of the fibers inside the entire MU and is often employed to follow the degree of reinnervation. That represents a quantitative technique and can be applied to follow progression and effects of putative therapies (de Carvalho et al., 2005a; de Carvalho et al., 2005b) by evaluating size of individual MU (Stålberg, 1983; Guiloff et al., 1988).

Among quantitative electrodiagnostic (EDX) techniques, the methodology of Motor Unit Number Estimation (MUNE) has been previously employed in measuring loss of functioning MU in ALS patients (McComas et al., 1971; Daube, 1995; McComas, 1995; Wang and Delwaide, 1998; Gooch and Shefner, 2004; Daube, 2006; Sartucci et al., 2007).

2. Know your enemy. The useful association of MUNE and macro-EMG

MUNE is very sensitive in documenting disease progression in ALS. Some studies combining MUNE and standard electromyography showed a highly significant correlation between motor unit loss, clinical quantitative features and variations in compound motor action potential (CMAP) amplitude over time (Liu et al., 2009). That is not surprising considering their different targets; while MUNE assesses motor unit loss, changes in CMAP amplitude and duration also account for collateral reinnervation. A few longitudinal studies using MUNE in some ALS patients have been reported that MUNE decreases as the disease progresses and that MUNE is a very reliable and reproducible method in patients with ALS (Olney et al., 2000; Kwon and Lee, 2004; Boe et al., 2007; Hong et al., 2007; Sartucci et al., 2007; Sartucci et al., 2011). Its inter-individual and intra-individual reproducibility linearly increases as disease progresses, making this technique particularly useful in the symptomatic stage of the disease (Sartucci et al., 2007; Sartucci et al., 2011). However, results from MUNE might seem contradictory or not always conclusive in view of many studies were made on animals; in comparison with transgenic mice, it's worth remembering that the majority of cases of ALS are sporadic and the SOD-1 GD[93A] represents only about 20% of patients with hereditary ALS (Shefner et al., 2002; Zhou et al., 2007).

We routinely use the standard incremental technique, known as the McComas technique. Despite some limitations in comparison with statistical MUNE (alternation of motor unit, inability to recognize small motor units, small sample size), it is more reliable and less complex; in addiction, statistical MUNE cannot identify instable MUPs since it is based on the assumption that variability is due solely to the number of motor units responding in an intermittent manner (Shefner et al., 2007).

On the other hand, use of Macro-EMG is limited to muscles from which electrical activity can be elicited without any interference from other muscles (de Koning et al., 1988); moreover, it's difficult to perform it in the hands during the course of the disease due to the strong wasting of the intrinsic hand muscles. Because of these limitations, our twenty-years experience led us to combine the two techniques in order to improve diagnostic accuracy.

3. Methodological and technical considerations

The most used MUNE technique relays on manual incremental stimulation of the motor nerve, known as the McComas technique (McComas, 1995), modified by Ballantyne and Stålberg. The following test settings were used: sweep duration 50 ms, gain 2 mV/Div for M wave, 0.5 mV/Div for each step; filters 20 – 10 KHz (Keypoint Clinical Manual, 1999). The use of specific software for MUNE detects "alternation", eliminates subjectivity and the sampling of artifactually small motor units in ALS patients (McComas, 1995; Hong et al., 2007); ten incremental steps are commonly recorded (Sartucci et al., 2007).

Percutaneous stimuli were delivered over musculocutaneous nerve immediately below axilla, recording from BB muscles, and ulnar nerve at the wrist by recording from the ADM muscle of the same upper limb (Sartucci et al., 2007; Sartucci et al., 2011). Signals are detected with common surface electrodes, Ag/AgCl type, tapered on the cutis over the target muscles with a common muscle-belly tendon montage. In those patients who underwent follow-up after several months, each test was performed exactly on the same side with the same electrode position (spatial coordinates have been annotated in patients schedule).

At least two consecutive MUNE measures are usually performed on each patient to verify the consistency of our results; when required, further estimation was made until the MUNE was clearly stable. The mean of the two or more tests was calculated (Henderson et al., 2007). The results showed an excellent reproducibility with test-retest correlation coefficients ranging from 0.75 to 0.86 (Sartucci et al., 2007).

The standard macro-EMG method is routinely applied in our patients (Stålberg, 1983). We employ a recording electrode, consisting of a modified single fibre EMG (SFEMG) electrode with the cannula Teflon insulated except for the distal 15 mm. The SFEMG recording surface is exposed 7.5 mm from the tip and the recording is made using two channels: the first one in whom the SFEMG activity is displayed (using the cannula as reference) and used to identify the MU and trigger the averaging procedure (band-pass filter for this channel: 500-10 kHz); fiber density (FD) of the triggering single fibre electrode is recorded. The second channel averaged the activity from the cannula until a smooth baseline and a constant macro MUP was obtained (Filter pass-band: 5-10 kHz).

Total area between the curve and the baseline, the maximal peak-to-peak amplitude (macro-MUP) during the total sweep time of 70 ms are measured (Bauermeister and Jabre, 1992). Results are expressed as individual area values from at least 20 recordings. The relative macro amplitude is expressed as the obtained mean value (Stålberg, 1983). Fibre density is expressed as number of time locked spikes obtained on the SFEMG channel (Sanders and Stålberg, 1996).

4. Our experience

Compared with previous studies (Bromberg et al., 1993; de Carvalho et al., 2005b), our idea was taking into consideration simultaneously Macro-EMG and MUNE changes, both in proximal and distal muscles, in the same sample of patients with a one-year follow-up. Sixty-one ALS patients (34 male: mean age ± SD 60.0 ± 15.5, range 20-82 yrs; 27 female: mean age ± SD 62.0 ± 9.2 yrs, range 30-82 years), were enrolled in the study and examined basally (T0) and every 4 months (T1, T2 and T3). Macro Motor Unit Potentials (macro MUPs) were derived from Biceps Brachialis (BB) muscle; MUNE was performed both in BB and Abductor Digiti Minimi (ADM) muscles of the same side. Thirty-three healthy volunteers (13 women and 20 men, mean age: 57.7 ± 13.8 years, range 28 - 77 years) served as controls.

All patients had probable or definite ALS, according to the criteria of the World Federation of Neurology (Brooks et al., 2000).

The sample group of patients included cases with a disease duration from clinical onset of symptoms to the time of the first examination less than 48 months (mean ± 1SD: 12.2 ± 11.0 months); only few cases had a disease duration behind this limit (11 patients; about 14.3 %). Twenty-two patients presented a bulbar onset and the remaining a spinal one (Brooks et al., 2000). Muscle strength over time was evaluated by MRC score for all muscles (0-5 grading system). Forty patients were in treatment with riluzole (Rilutek® 50 mg), at a mean daily dosage of 100 mg (50 mg BID) throughout the entire period of EDX follow-up.

In twenty-nine patients (subgroup 1, SG1: 19 males and 10 females; mean age ± 1SD: 60,0 ± 11,8 years; range 30-78 years; spinal/bulbar onset: 22/7; mean disease duration 29,7 months) macro EMG was repeated after 4 months (T1). Among the second subgroup, eleven patients (subgroup 2, SG2: 8 males and 3 females; mean age ± SD: 57,0 ± 12,8 years; range 30-72 years; spinal/bulbar onset: 10/1; mean disease duration 31 months) were re-tested after 8 months (T2) and in 8 (Subgroup 3, SGP3; 7 males and 1 female; mean age ± SD: 58,0 ± 13,6 years; range 31-82 years; spinal/bulbar onset: 7/1; mean disease duration 37 months) after 12 months from the first examination.

Both patients and controls gave their written informed consent prior to participation in the study that had been approved by the local ethical Committee and followed the tenets of Helsinki.

5. Results

Macro-EMG in control subjects showed a mean area 1139.9 ± 182.8 µVms, a mean amplitude of 168.0 ± 63.7 µV, and a FD 1.24 ± 0.13 (a summary of results is given in *Figures 1* and *2*).

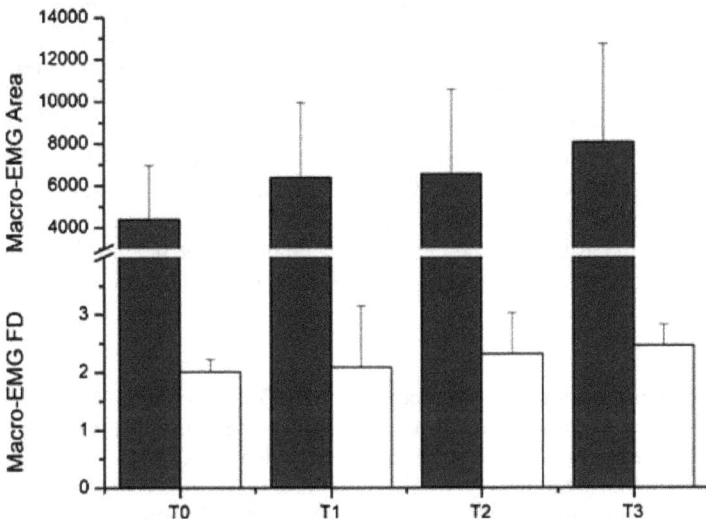

Fig. 1. Time evolution of macro-EMG FD (white columns) and of macro EMG area (gray columns; note the break and the different scale in ordinate) in ALS pt. The macro EMG area increase continuously with the time, paralleled by FD value, up to T2 (modified from Sartucci et al., 2011).

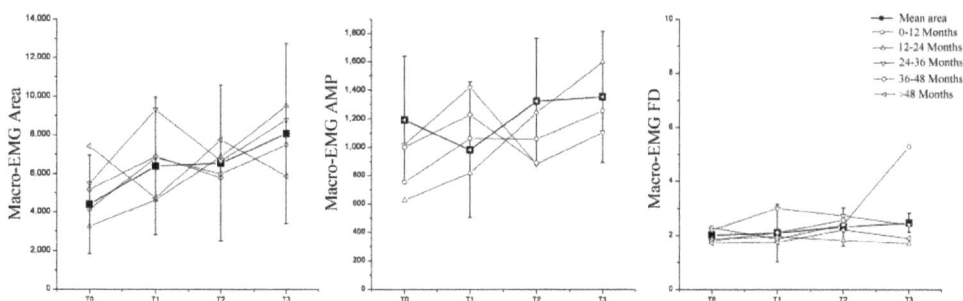

Fig. 2. Time evolution of each macro EMG parameters (area, amplitude and FD) with the
time, keeping in the consideration disease duration at the beginning of the observation.
Sample with a disease duration of 12-24 months exhibited a more steep slope (modified
from Sartucci et al., 2011).

In ALS patients at T0, both Macro-MUP area and FD were above upper normal limits:
macro-MUP area was 4397.6 ± 2554.9 µVms (+ 285.8%; p < 0.001), mean FD 2.01 ± 0.2
(+62.1%; p < 0.005).
The macro EMG MUP area was abnormal in 57 (93.4%). and normal in 4 (6.6%) patients, the
FD resulted increased in 55 pt. (90%) and normal in 6 (10%). Macro EMG MUP area and
peak-to-peak amplitude exhibited a good correlation (Spearmann coeff. of correlation =
0.888) at every time of testing (Gan and Jabre, 1992).
Macro MUPs area (*Figure* 2) resulted progressively increased at every time, especially at T3
compared with T0: Area: + 45.3% (T1); + 49.0% (T2); + 83.6% (T3); FD showed a trend to
increase up to T3: +3.5% (T1); +15.4% (T2); +22.4% (T3) (Fig 2).
FD resulted increased in cases with longer disease duration (*Figure* 2). Anyway, the FD
was generally increased when macro EMG amplitude was also increased in the first stage
of disease; after less than one year (about 8 months) they showed a large dispersion of
value.
MUNE (*Figure 3*) in controls resulted in BB muscle 91.9 ± 18.9, with a mean step area of 2.09
± 0.7 µV/ms and a Mean Maximal M wave of 131.9 ± 36.0 mV; for the ADM muscle 87.7 ±
14.6, with a mean step area of 1.05 ± 0.4 mV/ms and Mean Maximal M wave of 61.3 ± 21.2
mV. In ALS patients, values were behind normal limits in 56 (91.8%) and within normal
limits in 5 (8.2%) in BB muscle; in 60 (98.4%) and in 1 (1.6%) in ADM muscle. Functioning
MUs number progressively decreased in both muscles throughout the entire follow-up
period. The Pearson's correlation coefficient was 0,61, suggesting the rate and amount of
MU decrease was approximately similar in both muscles (Cuturic et al., 2005). In ALS
MUNE exhibited a parallel trends in proximal and distal muscles (BB and ADM),
independently of disease duration (see *Figures 3 and 4*); mean step area, instead, increased
more in BB, especially in patients with longer disease duration. MUP amplitude at T0 did
not show any significant difference between females and males, even if a bit higher in males
(p>0.05, Figure 5).

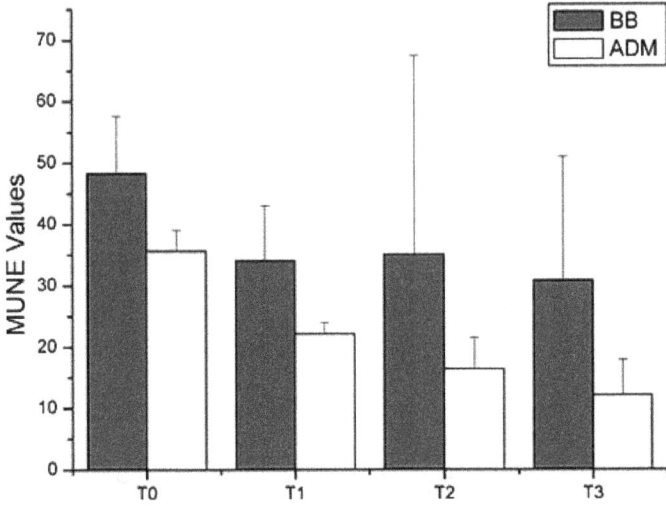

Fig. 3. Histogram showing MUNE values in both BB (gray columns) and ADM (white columns) muscles at every time of measurement. The trends is similar even if more evident in ADM (modified from Sartucci et al., 2011).

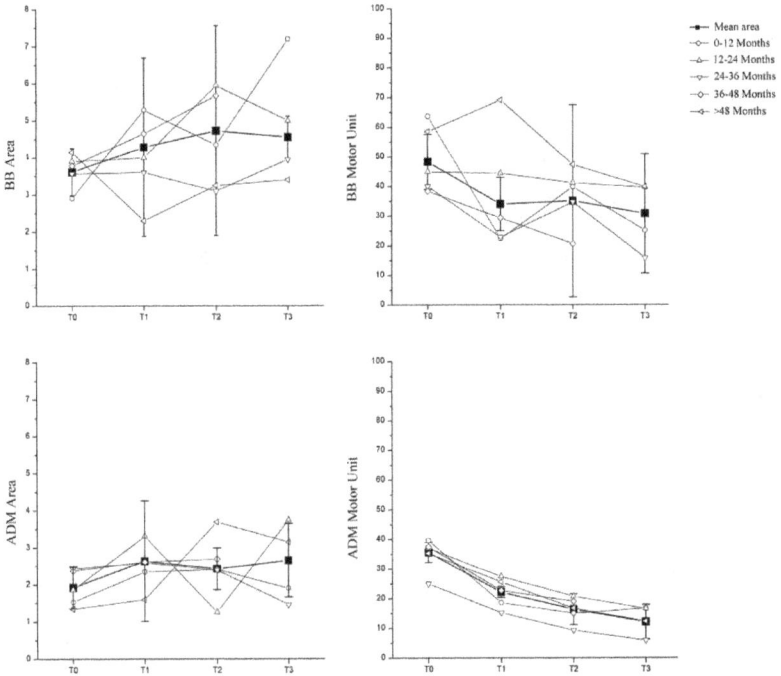

Fig. 4. MUNE values in both BB and ADM muscles at every time of evaluation in pt. with different disease duration and their mean value (filled circles) (modified from Sartucci et al., 2011).

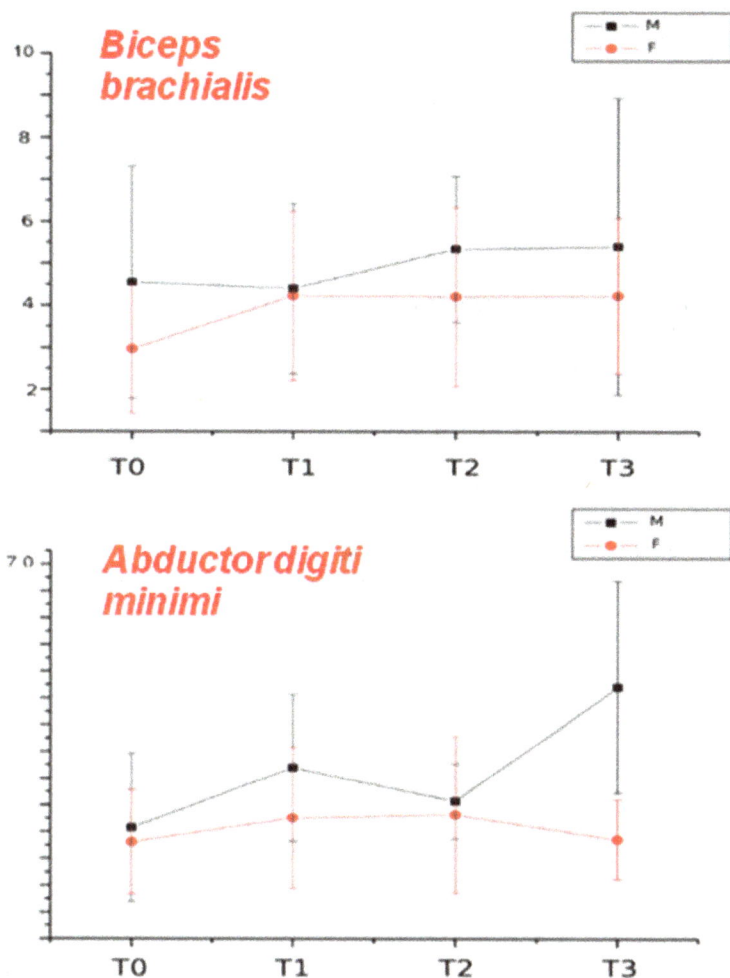

Fig. 5. MUP amplitude at T0 did not show any significant difference between females and males, both in spinal and bulbar form, even if a bit higher in males (p>0.05; Sartucci et al., personal data).

5.1 Correlation between macro-MUP and MUNE

All main macro-EMG parameters (area, amplitude and FD), as well as MUNE features (number of MUPs and mean step area either in the BB and ADM), did not disclose any significant difference between patients intaking the drug for both disease type (spinal or bulbar) at any time during the follow-up period (*Figure* 6). As concerns as Macro-EMG area, the difference in the mean values among the different levels of treatment is not great enough to exclude the possibility that the difference is just due to random sampling variability. There is not a statistically significant difference between riluzole vs. control (p = 0.321), as confirmed by FD measures over time (p = 0.588).

6. Conclusions and unanswered questions

Our study design was a prospective study to evaluate ongoing denervation/reinnervation process. Main aim was to objectively measure the extent of MU loss and the accompanying changes in innervation pattern during the time in ALS patients (Stålberg, 1983; Jabre, 1991), and therefore is often impossible to perform it in a hand muscle in the course of ALS due to the strong wasting of the intrinsic hand muscles; consequently to evaluate distal time disease evolution and its behaviour compared with proximal district we had to use only MUNE.

Area and amplitude of the Macro-MUP reflect number and size of muscle fibers in the motor unit (Schwartz et al., 1976; Stålberg et al., 1976). MUNE instead is the ideal tool for the assessment of disease in which primary defect is MU loss (Strong et al., 1988; Gooch and Shefner, 2004; Daube, 2006; Sartucci et al., 2007).

ALS is featured by repetitive cycles of denervation/reinnervation and the mechanism lead to a variation of fibre density within a given motor unit (Stålberg, 1983; de Carvalho et al., 2005a; de Carvalho et al., 2005b). If this rearrangement is interrupted by new processes of denervation, following further motor neuron loss, this will lead to areas of grouped atrophy and loss of muscle fibers. Reinnervation process are strictly interwoven with lower motor neuron loss; quantization and tracking of MU loss with simultaneously gauging countervailing collateral dynamic innervation may be assessed by combining MUNE and macro-EMG (Gooch and Shefner, 2004; Pouget, 2006). The macro-EMG gives a global view of the MU. First, the physical length of the electrode (15 mm), cover the entire diameter of an average sized MU; the large electrode surface suppresses the contribution of the closest action potentials and favours the relative influence of slow components so including distant fibers (Sanders and Stålberg, 1996).

Macro-EMG parameters in controls were in agreement with data of others authors (Stålberg and Fawcett, 1982; Stålberg, 1983; Jabre, 1991). Both macro-MUP area, amplitude and FD were beyond upper normal limits, as expected, in ALS (Bauermeister and Jabre, 1992; Gan and Jabre, 1992). Macro-EMG parameters progressively increased, at least in the first eight months compared with baseline as proved by coefficient of correlation at each time displaying a progressive increment of correlation up to 8 months, suggesting the process of MU rearrangement begins to fail after 8 months of disease course. Also when macro EMG area and amplitude were increased, FD was parallely increased.

The time elapsed from disease onset plays a fundamental role, since patients included with a diseases duration between 12 and 24 months showed largest changes in Macro EMG features, suggesting a higher efficiency of compensatory mechanisms at least in early stages of disease. Evidence of some MU loss at baseline compared with controls and its trend over time, together with a broader mean step area, yields novel insights into the pathophysiology of MU loss and its relationship to motor function in patients with ALS (Daube et al., 2000; Sartucci et al., 2007). Fluctuation of MU estimates between separate time could suggest reversible motoneurons dysfunction (Gooch and Shefner, 2004). The coefficient of correlation for MUNE – macro EMG mean area regression line was not significant (= - 0.17) in BB muscle, suggesting that both processes go on in some way independently. In more advanced stages, a decline of the strength of the surviving MUs, especially those with higher thresholds, seems to contribute to the progressive muscle weakness, in addition to both corticospinal degeneration and reduction in motoneurons number (Dengler et al., 1990). Our study also showed a significant correlation between MRC scores and EDX measurements throughout the whole course of the disease only for ADM muscle. The absence of a significant correlation between MUNE and MRC values (p > 0.05) for BB could confirm the specificity of EDX investigations to track over time changes in muscle MU features and number. Muscle strength seems to decline more linearly than MUNE values: that could be explained, as recently suggested by Liu et al. (2009) with the persistence of a small proportion of lower motor neurons long-term surviving.

6.1 Gender and amyotrophic lateral sclerosis. Lessons from motor unit estimation

Another interesting result is about gender differences (*Figure 5*); in fact, some studies have reported a significant male predominance until the sixth decade of life and an older average age at onset for females, sometimes explained with a possible protective effect of estrogen. In our experience, MUP amplitude at T0 did not show any significant difference between females and males, even if a bit higher in males: MUP amplitudes were 86.9 ± 21.2 µV and 84.1 ± 17.5 µV for the biceps brachii and abductor digiti minimi muscle, respectively, in females, 90.7 ± 17.3 µV and 88.2 ± 16.8 µV in males (p>0.05). This is only a trend, as gender don't influence motor unit loss neither corresponding decline in MRC values over time. The lack of significant differences between females and males in both spinal and bulbar form, as emerged from our sample, is consistent with results reported by Hegedus (Hegedus et al., 2009): the antioxidant effects of estrogens and their proved role in preventing glutamate-related toxicity *in vitro* (Kruman et al., 1999; Nakamizo et al., 2000) could not delay both the early retraction of nerve terminals from neuromuscular end-plates and the dying-back of the axons during asymptomatic phase *in vivo*, as well as the denervation/reinnervation process in later stages. However, there is a substantial lack of studies describing the contribution of gender in progression of ALS; that's likely due to the discrepancy between humans patients and animal models, in terms of disease and presymptomatic phase duration, absence of sensitive biological markers and different pathogenesis (sporadic vs. SOD1-related; Zhou et al., 2007).

6.2 MUNE and Macro-EMG in evaluating response to treatment

Our investigation was aimed to evaluate also the EDX effects of one of the most common drug employed in the ALS, riluzole (Leigh et al., 2003), on the fundamentals process of ALS: the primary process of motorneurons loss and denervation, and the secondary process of reinnervation. Riluzole is a benzothiazole derivative with a wide range of effects on glutamate pathways including inhibition of presynaptic glutamate release; it is relatively safe and well tolerated. Prescription of riluzole is restricted to patients with probable or definite ALS. At the moment, there is no convincing evidence that treatment at 100 mg daily is associated with a significant increase in survival (Miller et al., 2007); its effects on quality of life and survival are weak especially in older patients (over 75 years), in those with bulbar onset and at more advanced stages (Miller et al., 2003). We did not detect any significant electrophysiological difference between patient intaking the drug and those who didn't (see *Figure 6*), but considering the high attrition rate it's quite difficult to draw any conclusion about the effect of pharmacological treatments on neurophysiological parameters. Future studies are then required to solve this dilemma.

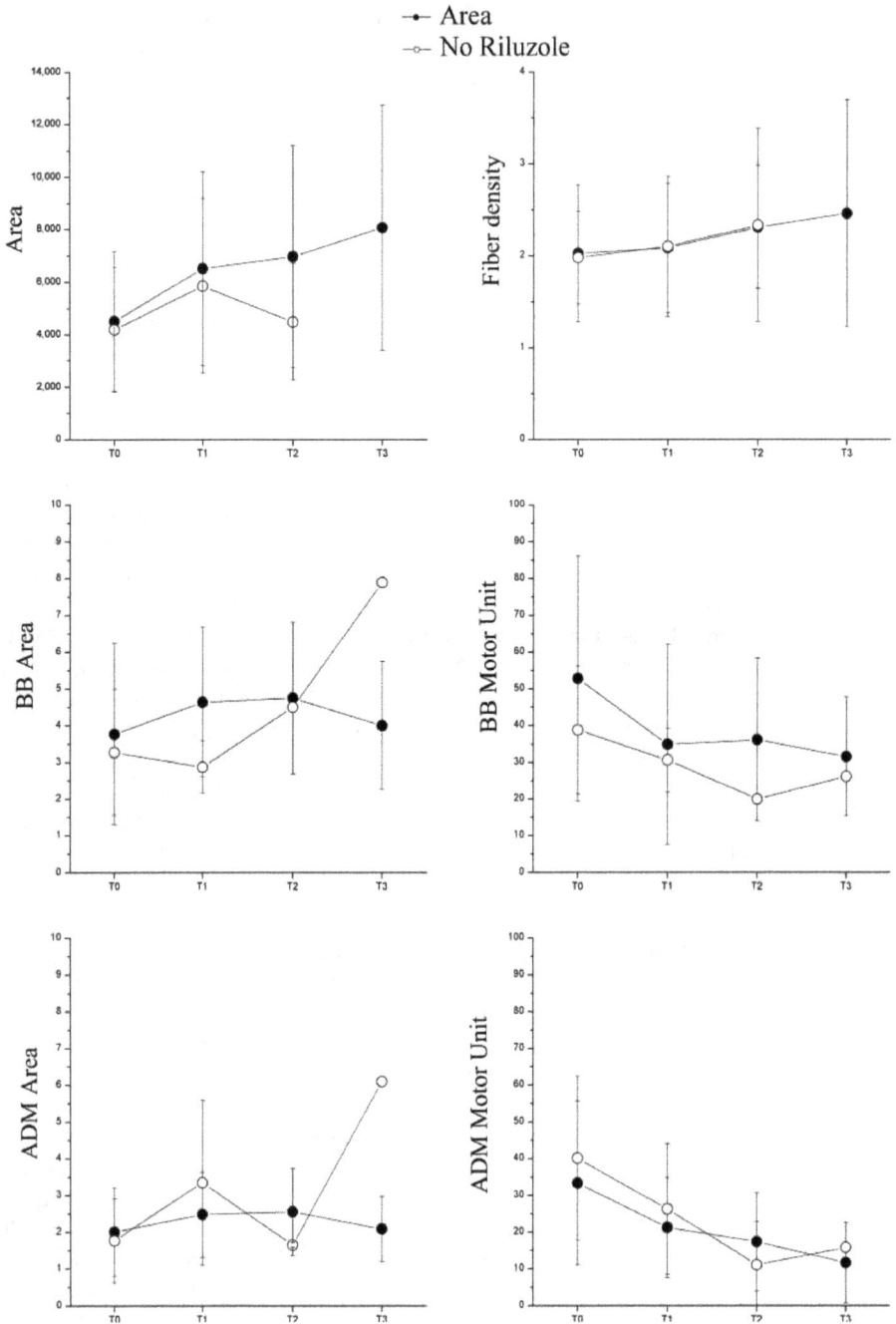

Fig. 6. Effects of Riluzole on the macro EMG and MUNE parameters with the time, in patients intaking (filled circle) or not (empty circle) the drug (modified from Sartucci et al., 2011).

7. References

Andersen PM, Borasio GD, Dengler R, Hardiman O, Kollewe K, Leigh PN, Pradat PF, Silani V, Tomik B (2007), Good practice in the management of amyotrophic lateral sclerosis: clinical guidelines. An evidence-based review with good practice points. EALSC Working Group. Amyotroph Lateral Scler 8:195-213.

Bauermeister W, Jabre JF (1992), The spectrum of concentric macro EMG correlations. Part I. Normal subjects. Muscle Nerve 15:1081-1084.

Beghi E, Balzarini C, Bogliun G, Logroscino G, Manfredi L, Mazzini L, Micheli A, Millul A, Poloni M, Riva R, Salmoiraghi F, Tonini C, Vitelli E (2002), Reliability of the El Escorial diagnostic criteria for amyotrophic lateral sclerosis. Neuroepidemiology 21:265-270.

Boe SG, Stashuk DW, Doherty TJ (2007), Motor unit number estimates and quantitative motor unit analysis in healthy subjects and patients with amyotrophic lateral sclerosis. Muscle Nerve 36:62-70.

Bromberg MB, Forshew DA, Nau KL, Bromberg J, Simmons Z, Fries TJ (1993), Motor unit number estimation, isometric strength, and electromyographic measures in amyotrophic lateral sclerosis. Muscle Nerve 16:1213-1219.

Brooks BR, Miller RG, Swash M, Munsat TL (2000), El Escorial revisited: revised criteria for the diagnosis of amyotrophic lateral sclerosis. Amyotroph Lateral Scler Other Motor Neuron Disord 1:293-299.

Cuturic M, Shamsnia M, Palliyath S (2005), Lateral asymmetry of motor unit number estimate (MUNE). Electromyogr Clin Neurophysiol 45:233-239.

Daube JR (1995), Estimating the number of motor units in a muscle. J Clin Neurophysiol 12:585-594.

Daube JR (2006), Motor unit number estimates--from A to Z. J Neurol Sci 242:23-35.

Daube JR, Gooch C, Shefner J, Olney R, Felice K, Bromberg M (2000), Motor unit number estimation (MUNE) with nerve conduction studies. Suppl Clin Neurophysiol 53:112-115.

de Carvalho M, Chio A, Dengler R, Hecht M, Weber M, Swash M (2005a), Neurophysiological measures in amyotrophic lateral sclerosis: markers of progression in clinical trials. Amyotroph Lateral Scler Other Motor Neuron Disord 6:17-28.

de Carvalho M, Costa J, Swash M (2005b), Clinical trials in ALS: a review of the role of clinical and neurophysiological measurements. Amyotroph Lateral Scler Other Motor Neuron Disord 6:202-212.

de Koning P, Wieneke GH, van der Most van Spijk D, van Huffelen AC, Gispen WH, Jennekens FG (1988), Estimation of the number of motor units based on macro-EMG. J Neurol Neurosurg Psychiatry 51:403-411.

Dengler R, Konstanzer A, Kuther G, Hesse S, Wolf W, Struppler A (1990), Amyotrophic lateral sclerosis: macro-EMG and twitch forces of single motor units. Muscle Nerve 13:545-550.

Eisen A (2001), Clinical electrophysiology of the upper and lower motor neuron in amyotrophic lateral sclerosis. Semin Neurol 21:141-154.

Finsterer J, Fuglsang-Frederiksen A (2001), Concentric-needle versus macro EMG. II. Detection of neuromuscular disorders. Clin Neurophysiol 112:853-860.

Gan R, Jabre JF (1992), The spectrum of concentric macro EMG correlations. Part II. Patients with diseases of muscle and nerve. Muscle Nerve 15:1085-1088.

Gooch CL, Shefner JM (2004), ALS surrogate markers. MUNE. Amyotroph Lateral Scler Other Motor Neuron Disord 5 Suppl 1:104-107.

Guiloff RJ, Modarres-Sadeghi H, Stålberg E, Rogers H (1988), Short-term stability of single motor unit recordings in motor neuron disease: a macro EMG study. J Neurol Neurosurg Psychiatry 51:671-676.

Hegedus J, Putman CT, Gordon T (2009), Progressive motor unit loss in the G93A mouse model of amyotrophic lateral sclerosis is unaffected by gender. Muscle Nerve 39:318-327.

Henderson RD, Ridall PG, Hutchinson NM, Pettitt AN, McCombe PA (2007), Bayesian statistical MUNE method. Muscle Nerve 36:206-213.

Hong YH, Sung JJ, Park KS, Kwon O, Min JH, Lee KW (2007), Statistical MUNE: a comparison of two methods of setting recording windows in healthy subjects and ALS patients. Clin Neurophysiol 118:2605-2611.

Jabre JF (1991), Concentric macro electromyography. Muscle Nerve 14:820-825.

Juergens SM, Kurland LT, Okazaki H, Mulder DW (1980), ALS in Rochester, Minnesota, 1925-1977. Neurology 30:463-470.

Kruman, II, Pedersen WA, Springer JE, Mattson MP (1999), ALS-linked Cu/Zn-SOD mutation increases vulnerability of motor neurons to excitotoxicity by a mechanism involving increased oxidative stress and perturbed calcium homeostasis. Exp Neurol 160:28-39.

Kwon O, Lee KW (2004), Reproducibility of statistical motor unit number estimates in amyotrophic lateral sclerosis: comparisons between size- and number-weighted modifications. Muscle Nerve 29:211-217.

Leigh PN, Abrahams S, Al-Chalabi A, Ampong MA, Goldstein LH, Johnson J, Lyall R, Moxham J, Mustfa N, Rio A, Shaw C, Willey E (2003), The management of motor neurone disease. J Neurol Neurosurg Psychiatry 74 Suppl 4:iv32-iv47.

Liu XX, Zhang J, Zheng JY, Zhang S, Xu YS, Kang DX, Fan DS (2009), Stratifying disease stages with different progression rates determined by electrophysiological tests in patients with amyotrophic lateral sclerosis. Muscle Nerve 39:304-309.

McComas AJ (1995), Motor unit estimation: anxieties and achievements. Muscle Nerve 18:369-379.

McComas AJ, Fawcett PR, Campbell MJ, Sica RE (1971), Electrophysiological estimation of the number of motor units within a human muscle. J Neurol Neurosurg Psychiatry 34:121-131.

Miller RG, Mitchell JD, Lyon M, Moore DH (2003), Riluzole for amyotrophic lateral sclerosis (ALS)/motor neuron disease (MND). Amyotroph Lateral Scler Other Motor Neuron Disord 4:191-206.

Miller RG, Mitchell JD, Lyon M, Moore DH (2007), Riluzole for amyotrophic lateral sclerosis (ALS)/motor neuron disease (MND). Cochrane Database Syst Rev CD001447.

Nakamizo T, Urushitani M, Inoue R, Shinohara A, Sawada H, Honda K, Kihara T, Akaike A, Shimohama S (2000), Protection of cultured spinal motor neurons by estradiol. Neuroreport 11:3493-3497.

Olney RK, Lomen-Hoerth C (2000), Motor unit number estimation (MUNE): how may it contribute to the diagnosis of ALS? Amyotroph Lateral Scler Other Motor Neuron Disord 1 Suppl 2:S41-44.

Olney RK, Yuen EC, Engstrom JW (2000), Statistical motor unit number estimation: reproducibility and sources of error in patients with amyotrophic lateral sclerosis. Muscle Nerve 23:193-197.

Pohl C, Block W, Traber F, Schmidt S, Pels H, Grothe C, Schild HH, Klockgether T (2001), Proton magnetic resonance spectroscopy and transcranial magnetic stimulation for the detection of upper motor neuron degeneration in ALS patients. J Neurol Sci 190:21-27.

Pouget J (2006), [Electroneuromyographic criteria of amyotrophic lateral sclerosis]. Rev Neurol (Paris) 162 Spec No 2:4S34-34S42.

Sanders DB, Stålberg EV (1996), AAEM minimonograph #25: single-fiber electromyography. Muscle Nerve 19:1069-1083.

Sartucci F, Maritato P, Moscato G, Orlandi G, Calabrese R, Domenici GL, Murri L (2007), Motor unit number estimation (mune) as a quantitative measure of disease progression and motor unit reorganization in amyotrophic lateral sclerosis. Int J Neurosci 117:1229-1236.

Sartucci F, Moscato G, Rossi C, Caleo M, Bocci T, Murri L, Giannini F, Rossi A (2011), Macro-EMG and MUNE Changes in Patients with Amyotrophic Lateral Sclerosis: One-Year Follow Up. Int J Neurosci 121(5):257-66.

Schwartz MS, Stålberg E, Schiller HH, Thiele B (1976), The reinnervated motor unit in man. A single fibre EMG multielectrode investigation. J Neurol Sci 27:303-312.

Shefner JM, Cudkowicz ME, Brown RH, Jr. (2002), Comparison of incremental with multipoint MUNE methods in transgenic ALS mice. Muscle Nerve 25:39-42.

Shefner JM, Cudkowicz ME, Zhang H, Schoenfeld D, Jillapalli D (2007), Revised statistical motor unit number estimation in the Celecoxib/ALS trial. Muscle Nerve 35:228-234.

Stålberg E (1983), Macro EMG. Muscle Nerve 6:619-630.

Stålberg E (1980), Macro EMG, a new recording technique. J Neurol Neurosurg Psychiatry 43:475-482.

Stålberg E (1983), Macro EMG. Muscle Nerve 6:619-630.

Stålberg E, Fawcett PR (1982), Macro EMG in healthy subjects of different ages. J Neurol Neurosurg Psychiatry 45:870-878.

Stålberg E, Schwartz MS, Thiele B, Schiller HH (1976), The normal motor unit in man. A single fibre EMG multielectrode investigation. J Neurol Sci 27:291-301.

Strong MJ, Brown WF, Hudson AJ, Snow R (1988), Motor unit estimates in the biceps-brachialis in amyotrophic lateral sclerosis. Muscle Nerve 11:415-422.

Swash M (2001), ALS and motor neuron disorders today and tomorrow. Amyotroph Lateral Scler Other Motor Neuron Disord 2:171-172.

Wang FC, Delwaide PJ (1998), Number and relative size of thenar motor units in ALS patients: application of the adapted multiple point stimulation method. Electroencephalogr Clin Neurophysiol 109:36-43.

Zhou C, Zhao CP, Zhang C, Wu GY, Xiong F, Zhang C (2007), A method comparison in monitoring disease progression of G93A mouse model of ALS. Amyotroph Lateral Scler 8:366-372.

13

Protection of Motor Neurons in Pre-Symptomatic Individuals Carrying SOD 1 Mutations: Results of Motor Unit Number Estimation (MUNE) Electrophysiology

Arun Aggarwal
University of Sydney
Australia

1. Introduction

Amyotrophic lateral sclerosis (ALS) is a progressive degenerative disease of motor neurones. There is a family history in approximately 10% percent of cases. Only 20% of such families have point mutations in the Cu, Zn superoxide dimutase 1 (SOD1) gene. Pre-symptomatic loss of motor neurons has been identified prior to the onset of symptoms in SOD1 mice. This loss was biphasic with initial loss in the pre-symptomatic phase followed by a period of stabilisation and then gradual loss at time of weakness to death. (Kong & Xu, 1998).

In order to determine the time course of motor neurone loss prior to symptomatic onset of disease, a longitudinal study of at-risk asymptomatic individuals (i.e. SOD1 mutation carriers with no neurological symptoms or signs as determined by a neurologist) was performed.

There was no detectable difference in the number of motor units in SOD1 mutation carriers compared to their SOD1 negative family controls. (Aggarwal & Nicholson, 2001). This may indicate that mutation carriers have undetectable loss of motor neurones until rapid and widespread cell death of motor neurones occurs, coinciding with the onset of symptomatic features. This implies that the disease is not the end result of the slow attrition of motor neurones. (Aggarwal, 2009).

The longitudinal study was extended on 20 asymptomatic carriers of the Cu, Zn superoxide dimutase 1 (SOD1) point mutation. In 2 of the 20 mutation carriers, there was a sudden reduction in MUNE, several months prior to the onset of weakness. (Aggarwal & Nicholson 2002), which also occurred in another 3 mutation carriers over the course of the study. (Aggarwal, 2009).

This suggests that gradual pre-clinical loss of motor neurones does not occur in asymptomatic SOD1 mutation carriers and supports the observation that sudden, catastrophic loss of motor neurones occurs immediately prior to the onset of symptoms and the development of the disease, rather than a gradual attrition of motor neurones over time. These results suggest that there may be a biological trigger initiating rapid cell loss, just prior to the onset of symptoms. This observation is an important contribution to the current understanding of the pathogenesis of MND.

Regular follow-up of SOD1 carriers with MUNE may lead to early diagnosis, creating an opportunity for future approaches and therapies aimed at preserving motor neurones rather than replacing lost motor neurones. Detecting the onset of motor neurone loss in asymptomatic individuals will identify those who may benefit from early institution of an active management program to improve their quality of life, until more effective treatment modalities are available for this devastating condition.

2. Background

Amyotrophic lateral sclerosis (ALS) is a group of fatal, neurodegenerative disorders, which is characterised pathologically by progressive degeneration and loss of motor neurones in the anterior horn cells of the spinal cord, motor nuclei of the brainstem and the descending pathways within the corticospinal tracts. The term amyotrophic lateral sclerosis (ALS) is used synonymously with motor neurone disease (MND) in the USA, but in the UK and Australia is used only to refer to patients who have a combination of upper and lower motor neurone dysfunction. (Talbot, 2002).

It is primarily a condition of middle to late life, with onset of symptoms between the ages of 50 and 70 and a mean age of onset of 57.4 years. (Ringel et al., 1993). Occasionally, it arises as early as the 2nd decade or as late as the 9th decade. In a natural history study, the overall median survival is 4.0 years from the onset of symptoms, but only 2.1 years from the time of diagnosis. (Ringel et al., 1993). In a study performed at the Mayo clinic, approximately 50% of patients died within 3 years of referral, but 20% were still alive at 5 years and 10% were still alive at 10 years. (Mulder & Howard, 1976).

Aging, motor neurone diseases and many peripheral neuropathies are all associated with loss of motor neurones or axons. When the disorders are recent or rapidly progressive, the extent of the loss may be indicated by weakness and wasting. In slowly progressive denervating conditions, like MND, loss of more than 50-80% of motor units may occur with little or no clinically apparent weakness.

It has been showed that patients with substantial chronic denervation could maintain normal muscle twitch tension until loss of about 70-80% of motor units occurred. (McComas, 1971). The surviving motor neurones enlarge their territories, through collateral sprouting (reinnervation) to keep pace with cell loss, to maintain the muscle maximum compound muscle action potential (CMAP), until late in the disease. At this point, collateral reinnervation is no longer able to provide full functional compensation. (Campbell et al., 1973).

In MND, needle electromyography often reveals evidence of chronic reinnervation (increased motor unit action potential amplitudes and duration with reduced recruitment), but provides little direct evidence to the extent of motor neurone and axonal loss. The supramaximal CMAP amplitude also provides little direct evidence of the extent of motor neurone loss. Normal CMAP amplitudes might mistakenly suggest that motor neurone loss has not occurred yet. (Shefner, 2001).

Motor unit number estimation (MUNE) is a more reliable method for following changes in neurogenic disorders than the CMAP amplitude. It estimates the number of functioning lower motor neurones innervating a muscle or a group of muscles i.e. the number of motor units, which can be excited by electrical stimulation. It is therefore an indirect measure of motor neurone loss, rather than a measure of primary pathology. It can identify that the number of motor units may be well below normal, in the presence of normal CMAP amplitudes. (Brown, 1976).

Pre-symptomatic loss of motor neurones has been identified in an animal model of the disease (transgenic mice expressing mutant human SOD1-G93A). The initial loss in the pre-symptomatic phase related to severe motor axonal degeneration due to vacuolar changes in motor neurones and a slow decrease in CMAP amplitudes. After a period of stabilisation, there was a gradual loss of motor neurones and a rapid decrease in CMAP amplitude, at the onset of weakness due to myelin alteration. At this point, there was a striking loss of motor units. There was also decrease in evoked motor potentials (an indirect measure of the number of motor units), prior to the onset of symptoms. The onset of disease in transgenic G93A mice involves a sharp decline of muscle strength and a transient explosive increase in vacuoles derived from degenerating mitochondria, but little motor neurone death. These did not die until the terminal stage. (Kong & Xu, 1998). The decline exhibited kinetics consistent with both a constant and exponentially decreasing risk of neuronal death. An escalating risk forced by cumulative damage was not responsible for cell death. (Azzouz et al., 1997).

It is possible that the high metabolic activity in motor neurones, combined with the toxic oxidative properties of the mutant SOD1, causes massive mitochondrial vacuolation in motor neurones, resulting in degeneration, earlier than other neurones, triggering the onset of weakness. The involvement of mitochondrial degeneration in the early stages is consistent with a direct effect of toxicity, mediated by properties gained by the mutant enzyme in catalysing redox reactions. (Beckman et al., 1993).

Until recently, it has not been possible to address this in humans, as pre-symptomatic diagnosis was not possible. Now, with the ability to identify Cu, Zn superoxide dismutase 1, (SOD1) mutation carriers, a group of human pre-symptomatic subjects can be studied to determine whether there was gradual lifelong pre-symptomatic loss of motor neurones or whether sudden catastrophic loss of motor neurones occurs just prior to the onset of clinical symptoms.

3. Familial ALS

The only forms of MND in which a clear cause has been established are the genetic variants. 20% of all familial cases are the dominantly inherited adult onset form of MND, which is clinically indistinguishable from the sporadic form of MND. These are due to a point mutation in the cytosolic Cu, Zn superoxide dismutase 1, (SOD1) gene on long arm of chromosome 21 (21q22.1). (Siddique & Deng, 1996). Mutations in other genes, alsin and the heavy subunit of neurofilament (NEFH) can also result in motor neurone degeneration in humans. Two other genes that have been investigated are the other isoforms of SOD. MnSOD (SOD2) maps to chromosome 6q25 and is primarily located in mitochondria and extracellular SOD (SOD3) maps to chromosome 4p15.2. Neither of these genes have yet to be linked to FALS. (Hand & Rouleau, 2002). There is however genetic heterogeneous and other causal genes remain to be found to explain the vast majority of FALS cases. (Siddique et al., 1989).

The initial study to establish a causal link between the SOD1 gene and familial MND (FALS) identified a total of 11 missense mutations in two exons studied in 13 autosomal dominant MND families. (Rosen et al., 1993). This led to an explosion of SOD1 gene screening in MND pedigrees. To date 112 different mutations in the SOD1 have been found which can lead to changes throughout the protein. There have been 99 substitutions, 5 polymorphisms, 3 insertions, 4 deletions and 1 compound mutation types identified. Mutations have been identified in all five exons of the gene. These include 20 on exon 1, 13 on exon 2, 8 on exon 3,

39 on exon 4 and 29 on exon 5 (Figure 1). There have also been 2 non-exon mutations identified on intron 4 and intron 1 and 14 'apparently' sporadic cases described with 6 different SOD1 mutations. (Shaw et al., 1998).

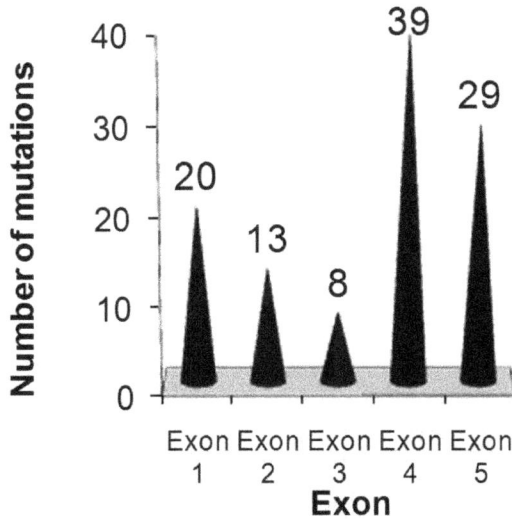

Fig. 1. Number of SOD1 mutations identified for each exon

Most are autosomal dominant in inheritance, but there is one confirmed autosomal recessive mutation, the D90A mutation in exon 4. This is unique in that it exists in dominant families in a heterozygous state, but in a number of pedigrees, specifically those of Scandinavian ancestry, homozygous mutations are required for disease. (Anderson et al., 1997).

Mutations in the heavy polypeptide 200kDa subunit of neurofilaments (NEFH) have been identified in sporadic MND cases, (Figlewicz et al., 1994) and in one FALS case. (Al-Chalabi et al., 1999). Accumulation of neurofilaments in cell bodies and axons of motor neurons is a pathological hallmark of early stages of many neurodegenerative diseases. These mutations lie in the region of the protein involved in cross-linking and thus may disrupt normal aggregation of filaments. Thus far, 1 insertion and 5 deletion mutations have been identified on exon 4. Analysis of the NEFH locus on chromosome 22 however has failed to detect linkage in MND families. (Vechio et al., 1996). Genome search on a large pedigree with autosomal dominant juvenile onset MND found strong evidence for linkage to chromosome 9q34 (ALS4). The average age of onset is 17 years, with slow progression of disease. (Chance et al., 1996). There is also an autosomal recessive, juvenile onset MND, with linkage to a locus on chromosome 15 (ALS5). (Hentati et al., 1998).

The other 90% of all MND patients have the sporadic form. There is no recognisable phenotypic difference between FALS and sporadic MND. The male: female ratio is 1:1 in FALS and 1.7:1 in sporadic MND. (De Belleroche et al., 1995). This decreases with increasing age of onset and approaches 1:1 after the age of 70. (Haverkamp et al., 1995). The site of onset is variable. Survival does not seem to be affected by age or gender, but rather the site of symptom onset. Generally, bulbar onset disease has a worse prognosis, and upper limb onset is more favourable. (Mulder et al., 1986).

It has be postulated that sporadic MND may be the final development of a chain of events that may be set in motion at one or more places in the central nervous system by endogenous and exogenous causes, or both. The aetiology of MND however remains unknown and is probably multifactorial. (Eisen 1995). There is no evidence to support the cause of sporadic MND being due to accumulation of heavy metals in the environment, (Needleman, 1997), deficiencies or excess of essential trace metals, (Mena et al., 1967) or exposure to environmental poisons and industrial solvents. (Leigh, 1997). There is also no evidence to support the cause of sporadic MND being due excessive physical activity or antecedent trauma.

4. Possible patterns of motor neurone loss

In normal healthy individuals, it has been shown that there is little loss of functioning motor neurones before the age of 60. The normal aging process then accounts for loss of approximately 3.9% of the original motor neurone pool per annum after the age of 60. (Brown, 1972). In this situation, the number of motor neurones remain fairly constant up to the age of 60, after which there is a gradual steady decline with age.

MND may be due to a slow attrition of motor neurones over time (Pattern 1 in Figure 2). If this were the case, pre-symptomatic motor neurone loss may be identifiable in SOD1 mutation carriers, as eventually there may be a gradual decline over time (Figure 2).

Another possible course of MND is that normal numbers of motor neurones are maintained until sudden, rapid multi-focal cell death of motor neurones occurs, corresponding with the development of symptoms (Pattern 2 in Figure 2). If this situation, it would be expected that SOD1 mutation carriers have a normal number of motor neurones during the pre-symptomatic phase. In this case, cell death occurs as neurones gradually accumulate damage, secondary to the mutation, which ultimately overwhelms cellular homeostasis. This is the cumulative damage hypothesis. (Clarke et al., 2000).

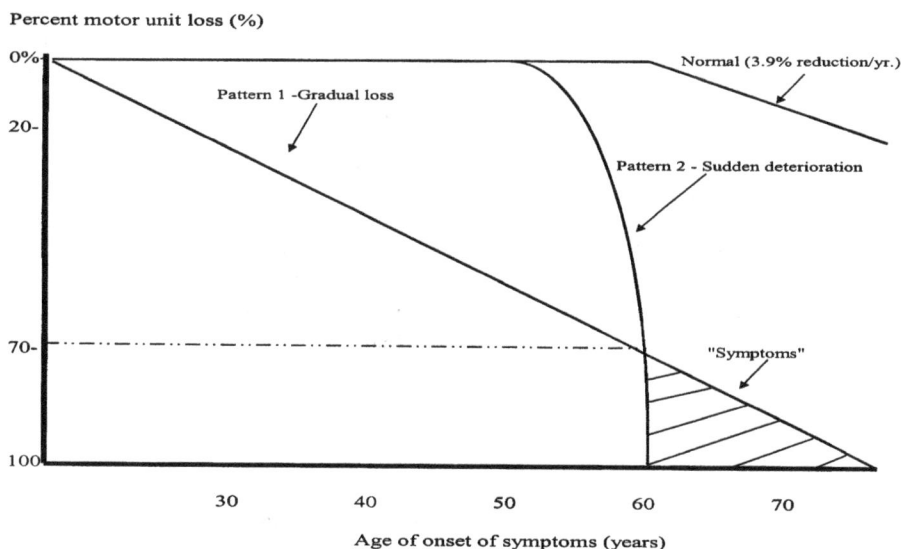

Fig. 2. Diagrammatic representation of possible patterns for motor neurone loss in an individual.

One of the mechanisms most frequently proposed to underlie cumulative damage is oxidative stress, in which an imbalance between the production of reactive oxygen species and cellular antioxidant mechanisms results in chemical modifications of macromolecules, thereby disrupting cellular structure and function. (Robberecht, 2000). A key prediction of the cumulative damage hypothesis is that the probability that any individual neurone will become committed to apoptosis increases as damage accrues within it. A mutant neurone in an older patient will have accumulated a greater amount of damage and is therefore be more likely to die than in a younger patient. Consequently, early in the course of disease, the chance of a cell containing a sufficient amount of damage to initiate apoptosis is small, and the rate of cell loss is correspondingly low. However, as the amount of intracellular damage increases, the chance that a cell will die also increases

It has been shown that the kinetics of neuronal death in a number of inherited neurodegenerative diseases was best explained by models in which the risk of cell death remains constant throughout life of the neurone and that cell death occurred randomly in time and was independent of any other neurone. This implies a "one-hit" biochemical phenomenon in which the mutant imposes an abnormal mutant steady state on the neurone and a single catastrophic event randomly initiates cell death and apoptosis. The principal features of the mutant steady state are that the living mutant neurones function very well for years or even decades and that the predominant feature of the mutant neurones is that they are all at a risk of death. This argues against the multiple environmental factors hypothesis as a cause of MND, as a random process is probably responsible for the initiation of disease. (Clarke et al., 2001).

5. Cu/Zn superoxide dismutase (SOD1) mutations

Linkage studies for familial MND (FALS) on chromosome 21q22.1 led to the identification of point mutations in the gene for Cu/Zn superoxide dismutase (SOD1) as a cause of MND. (Siddique 1991). Superoxide (O2-) is an unstable and highly active molecule, which causes oxidation of cell constituents either directly or through toxic and stable derivatives. The major superoxide dismutase activity in cytoplasm is from SOD1, which consists of 5 small exons that encode 153 highly conserved amino acids with a molecular weight of 16Kda. SOD1 is a homodimer. Within each monomer, there is an active site containing one atom each of copper and zinc. (Radunovic & Leigh, 1996).

The most common SOD1 gene mutation seen in FALS is an alanine to valine shift at codon 4 (Ala4Val). This accounts for 50% of all mutations in the USA. (Rosen, 1993). Of all the clinical variables, only bulbar onset and three specific mutations seem to influence age of onset of MND. Bulbar patients are older when their illness begins, whereas the Gly37Arg and Leu38Val mutations predict an earlier age of onset.). Leu38Val is associated with the earliest onset (mean 35.5 years) and Ile113Thr with the latest onset (mean 58.9 years).

In terms of survival, Ala4Val correlated with the shortest survival of 1.5 years. Whereas, Gly37Arg, Gly41Asp, and Gly93Ala mutation predicted longer survival. The mutations that predict earlier onset are not the same as those that correlate with shortest duration of disease. (Cudkowicz et al., 1997). This suggests that the factors that influence onset of disease differ from those that influence the rate of progression of the disease.

Determining the mechanism by which mutations in the Cu/Zn superoxide dismutase (SOD1) gene triggers the destruction of motor neurones causing MND remains a challenging and complex problem. Five primary hypotheses have been postulated for the

pathogenesis of FALS (Figure 3). (Hand & Rouleau, 2002). At present the favoured
hypotheses is that the mutation causes disease as a result of a toxic gain of function by the
mutant SOD1 provoking selective neurotoxicity, probably disrupting the intracellular
homeostasis of copper and/or protein aggregation. (Clevland, 1999).

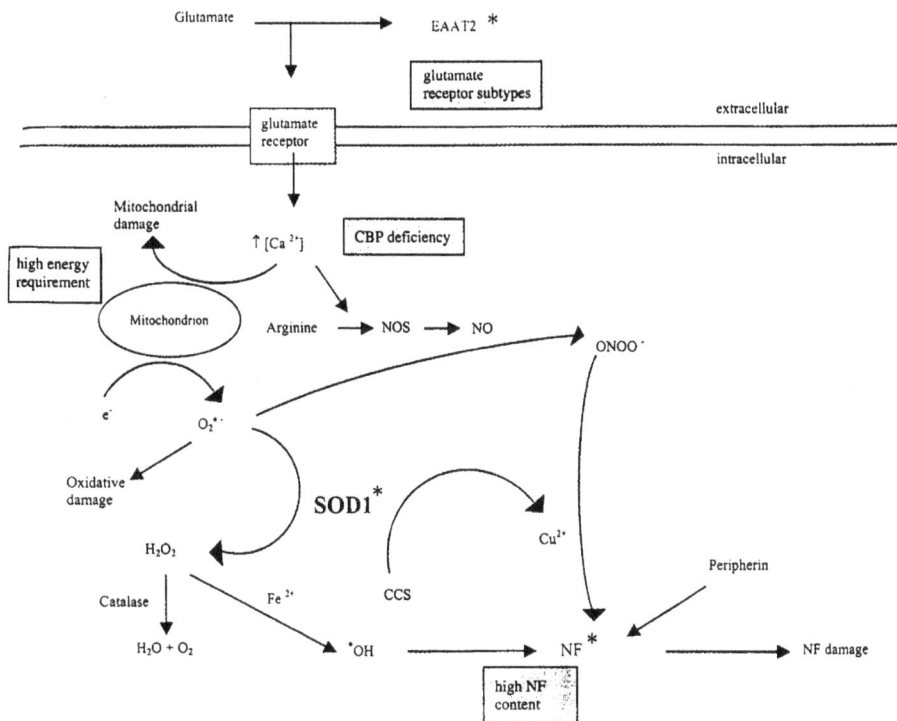

Fig. 3. Pathways that have been implicated in motor neurone cell death in amyotrophic
lateral sclerosis (Reproduced from Hand CK. Familial Amyotrophic Lateral Sclerosis.
Muscle Nerve 2002; 25:137).

The mutant SOD1 enzyme has altered reactivity with certain substrates, (Noor et al., 2003), in
addition to the major superoxide dismutase activity. The SOD1 enzyme catalyses the reduction
of hydrogen peroxide (H_2O_2), therefore acting as a peroxidase. This leads to the formation of
hydoxyl radicals that can also alter the neurofilament network. Motor neurones have high-
energy requirements and thus contain many mitochondria that generate superoxide radials
(O_2-) through normal metabolism. SOD1 is an anti-oxidant defence which catalyses conversion
of superoxide free radical anion (O2-) to hydrogen peroxide (H_2O_2), which is reduced to H_2O
and O_2 by catalse. Mutations at SOD1 binding sites, alter the redox behaviour of the enzyme
and destabilise the SOD1 ligand, leading to increased oxidative damage as hydrogen peroxide
and its derivatives are toxic to the cell. (Yim et al., 1990).

This supports the hypothesis that the pathogenesis of SOD1 related FALS may be due to
increased peroxidase activity of mutant SOD1 resulting in oxidative damage mainly to
lipids of the cell membrane.

Mapping of the mutation sites predicted that these mutations destabilise the protein structure, leading to a less active enzyme i.e. "loss of function". This is however not supported by the fact that transgenic mice over expressing SOD1 gene developed disease similar to MND in humans, while those over-expressing normal SOD1 remained unaffected. This suggests that the mutant mice develop the disease independent of the level of SOD1 activity and suggests that the mutant protein itself is selectively toxic to motor neurones and that there is a "gain of toxic function" rather than a "loss of function". (Gurney et al., 1993). Also, although most mutations in SOD1 gene cause decrease in steady state of cytosolic SOD1 activity, Gly37Arg and Asp90Ala, have no significant decrease in SOD1 activity. (Shaw et al., 1998).

As most SOD1 mutations destabilise SOD1 protein (except Asp90Ala), it is possible that the mutant protein, with altered conformation may become unstable and precipitate to form aggregates or inclusions in motor neurons. These aggregates may then disturb normal cell function and lead to cell death. They are easily formed when SOD1 protein stability is decreased because this protein exists in large amounts accounting for 0.5-1% of total cytosolic protein in neurons. Alternations in the length of the coding sequence, folding, solubility or degradation results in the formation of aggregates. (Yim et al., 1990). Structural changes of mutant SOD1 may distort the rim of the electrostatic guidance channel and allow the catalytic site to become exposed and shallow. Molecules that are normally excluded may gain access to the catalytic reactive site. This results in less buffering of copper and zinc, which then become neurotoxic. (Radunovic & Leigh, 1996).

The nitric oxide (NO) produced by nitric oxide synthase (NOS) reacts spontaneously with O_2- to generate peroxynitrite (ONOO-), which nitrosylates proteins leading to damage. Excess NO may also cause an increase in O_2- production by inhibition of mitochondrial electron flow, resulting in further generation of peroxynitrite. This facilitates nitrosylation of tyrosine residues of critical cytosolic proteins thus injuring cells. This reaction is copper dependent. The source of free copper may be mutant SOD1, which cannot accept the ion from the copper chaperone (CCS) protein. Mutant SOD1 possibly exhibit metal mediated cytotoxicities by disrupting the intracellular homeostasis of Cu and Zn, which are potential neurotoxins. (Gurney & Tomasselli, 2000).

The target proteins for nitrosylation include the neurofilament (NF) subunits, which may result in abnormal NF accumulation and subsequent disruption of the NF network and axonal transport, as there is a high neurofilament content in motor neurones. It has also been demonstrated that transgenes encoding mutant NF subunits can directly cause selective degeneration and death of motor neuones. (Cleveland, 1999). Conformational changes have been described in the mutations, Ala4Val, Gly37Arg and His6Arg that may affect the rim of the electrostatic guidance channel coded by exon 3. (Sjalander et al., 1995).

Glutamate is released from the presynaptic terminal activates the glutamate receptor on the postsynaptic cell membrane. It is then cleared from the synaptic cleft by specific glutamate transporters such as EAAT2. (Trotti et al., 1999). Astrocyte (glial cell) dysfunction may result in selective loss of EAAT2, interfering with the normal clearance of glutamate and allowing it to accumulate in the cell membrane and continue to activate the receptor. (Bruijin et al., 1997). Once activated, the glutamate receptor causes a calcium influx and a cascade of toxicity. The neurone does not have the capacity to buffer this efficiently due to a deficiency in calcium binding proteins (CBP's). This results in disturbances in mitochondrial metabolism and as a consequence, motor neurone cell death. (Beal, 1996).

To date, the only effective approved treatment for amyotrophic lateral sclerosis is Riluzole, (Cheah et al., 2010), which has a neuroprotective role, possibly due to pre-synaptic inhibition of glutamate release. (Doble, 1996). Treatment of human ALS patients or transgenic Cu, Zn superoxide dimutase 1 (SOD 1) mice, most commonly produce a modest but significant increase in survival. (Bensimon et al., 1994). It has also been shown to have a small beneficial effect on bulbar function, but not muscle strength. (Miller et al., 2007).

Apoptosis is characterised by a series of cellular changes leading to non-inflammatory cell death. Mitochondrial involvement in the apoptotic pathway also leads to the release of cytochrome c, an activator of the initiator caspase-9, which in turn activates caspase-3, which are executioners in the breakdown of essential cellular proteins. There is evidence that the mutant SOD1 transgene causes motor neurone death in mice through caspase-mediated programmed cell death. (Li et al., 2000). This may then be a target for inhibiting the apoptotic cascade, as it has been shown in a SOD1 transgenic mouse model that a small peptide caspase inhibitor (*zVAD-fmk*), prolonged survival after onset of disease by nearly 70%. (Kosti et al., 1997). It has also been reported that there are elevated levels of *bax* protein in MND spinal motor neurones, which promotes apoptosis. (Mu et al., 1996).

6. Methods

The Department of Molecular Medicine at Concord hospital had a large database of family members with a known family history of MND, who had blood samples collected for DNA, as part of a previous linkage study. From this database, family members were contacted by telephone by the department's genetic counsellor and informed about the study.

The regional committees for Ethics in Medical Research from Central Sydney Area Health Service, Royal North Shore Hospital and Prince Charles Hospital, approved this study.

All individuals participated without knowledge of their mutation status and on the understanding that this would not be revealed to them. Subjects were also aware that the results obtained from the study would not be available to them and that the information would only be used for research purposes. New consents were obtained from all individuals who participated in the study. The neurologist performing the MUNE studies also had no knowledge of their mutation status. The mutation status was only used in the final analysis of results. Subsequently, they were divided into "SOD1 negative family controls" and "asymptomatic SOD1 mutation carriers".

In addition, studies were also carried out on normal individuals, such as department technicians, spouses of SOD1 family members and individuals from the general population who attended MND support meeting and had an interest in helping to advance research into MND. This group was used as "population controls", to test the validity and reproducibility of the MUNE technique used.

Sporadic MND subjects were also initially studied once the MUNE technique had been validated to demonstrate that the MUNE technique used was able to detect a loss of motor neurones, when present. These were used as "positive controls".

6.1 Motor unit number estimation

Motor unit number estimation (MUNE) estimates the number of functioning lower motor neurones innervating a muscle or a group of muscles and is a measure of the primary pathologic process of motor neurone loss. The concept of motor unit number estimation

(MUNE) originated in 1967. At the time there was no satisfactory method of assessing the extent of denervation in muscles during life. Analysis of the density of the electromyographic interference pattern during maximal effort was not quantitative, and required the full co-operation of the patient.

The principle of MUNE is that if one can measure the mean single motor unit amplitude (SMUP), it is possible to obtain an estimate of the total number of motor units in the muscle. The results achieved were comparable with estimates of alpha motor fibres obtained by counting axons in specimens of motor nerves. (McComas, 1971).

MUNE has been performed in a number of different ways, each with their advantages and limitations. (Stein & Yang, 1990). The choice of technique depends on the speed and simplicity of the technique, as well as its accuracy and reproducibility. Some methods sample a very small proportion of the number of motor units innervating a muscle (typically 10-20). The coefficient of variation associated with different methods range from 10-45%. (McComas, 1991). If the variability is too large, then the technique cannot be used to follow motor unit loss reliably over time.

The way the average single motor unit potential (SMUP) size is obtained distinguishes the several techniques available. Most employ electrical stimulation of the motor nerve to determine the sizes of the SMUP, but a few use needle EMG.

Each method measures both the average size of the potentials generated by single motor units - single motor unit potentials (SMUP) and the size of the compound muscle action potential (CMAP) obtained with maximal stimulation of a motor nerve.

The motor unit number estimate is calculated by:

$$MUNE = \frac{\text{Maximum CMAP amplitude (or area)}}{\text{Average single motor unit potential (SMUP) amplitude or area.}}$$

Whereas the methods of measuring the average SMUP differ, they have common assumptions about the measurement of the supramaximal CMAP and the measurement of the average SMUP.

i.   Maximal stimulation of any peripheral motor nerve activates all the muscles innervated by that nerve distal to the point of stimulation. Therefore, measurements of the CMAP are the summation of activity from multiple muscles and the MUNE is more accurately an estimate of the number of motor units in a group of muscles rather than in a single muscle.

For example, the median CMAP recorded at abductor pollicis brevis (APB) is more correctly a "thenar MUNE", as it is a summation of the activity of APB, opponens pollicis, flexor pollicis brevis, and to a lesser extent, the lateral lumbricals.

Extensor digitorum brevis (EDB) on the other hand, is a muscle innervated by the deep peroneal nerve. The only source of interfering muscle action potential is from extensor hallucis longus, which can be reduced by correct position of the stimulating electrodes. The muscle belly is flat in profile, eliminating deeper motor units as a cause of small potentials. The recording electrode is placed transversely across the innervation zone, resulting in a simple biphasic negative-positive M wave.

ii. The motor unit potentials used in the calculation of the average SMUP are representative of those generated by the total population of units. All methods, select a subset of the total population of motor units, measure their sizes and calculate an average SMUP for that subgroup.

iii. Finally, there is a phenomenon caused "alternation". This refers to fluctuations in the
      CMAP amplitude of the same motor unit with similar stimulation intensities. The
      thresholds of the first few motor axons excited are not sufficiently separate from one
      another, so that when graded increases in the stimulus intensity occur, the motor axons
      excited often overlap and add more than one SMUP to the CMAP being recorded. This
      can result in an underestimation of the mean SMUP size, as it may appear that there are 7
      or 8 motor units when there are only 2 or 3 present, which in turn results in an over-
      estimation of the MUNE.

6.2 Statistical MUNE method

We used the statistical electrophysiological technique of motor unit number estimation
(MUNE), (Daube, 1998), was used to estimate the number of motor units in thenar and
extensor digitorum brevis muscles. The statistical method estimates the average size of
SMUP's and the number of motor units in a group of muscles innervated by the nerve being
stimulated, based on the normal variation of the submaximal CMAP evoked with constant
stimuli. No attempt is made to identify individual motor unit potentials. The method relies
on the known relation between the variance of multiple measures of step functions and the
size of the individual steps when the steps have a Poisson distribution. S.D. Poisson was a
French mathematician (1781-1840).

Poisson statistics are useful when the distribution arising for events occur randomly in time
or when small particles are distributed randomly in space. They have been used to calculate
the number of quanta released from a nerve terminal at the neuromuscular junction when
the individual quanta are too small to be distinguished, as in myasthenia gravis. (Lomen-
Hoerth & Slawnych, 2003).

In pure Poisson statistics, the size of a series of measurements is multiples of the size of a
single component. In a Poisson distribution there is a discrete asymmetrical distribution in
which responses are found at some levels and others where there are no responses (Figure 4).
(McNeil, 1996).

A pure Poisson distribution has decreasing numbers at higher values. In Poisson
distribution, the variance of these 30 measurements is equal to the size of the individual
components making up each measurement. The variance can thus provide an estimate of
the average size of the SMUP's.

The statistical method looks only at variance of the CMAP and does not require
identification of individual components. It can be used when the sizes of SMUP's are too
small to be isolated. The statistical method assumes that each motor unit has a similar size
and that it is the same size each time it is activated.

Sequences of 30 submaximal stimuli are given. The inherent variability of the threshold of
individual axons causes variations in the size of the CMAP. The average change in the
submaximal CMAP amplitude caused by alternation (addition and subtraction of motor
axons) is derived by Poisson statistics.

The occurrence of alternation with changing units that are activated does not modify the
accuracy of the statistical method, because the method is a statistical measurement, a
different result is found with each series of 30 stimuli. Therefore, multiple trials are needed
to obtain the most accurate measurement. (Olney et al., 2000).

Experimental testing with trials of >300 stimuli has shown that repeated measurement of
groups of 30 until the standard deviation of the repeated trials is <10% provides a close

estimate of the number obtained with many more stimuli.[86] Estimates of the SMUP size and of the number of motor units are also most reliable if made at multiple different stimulus intensities to test axons with different thresholds.

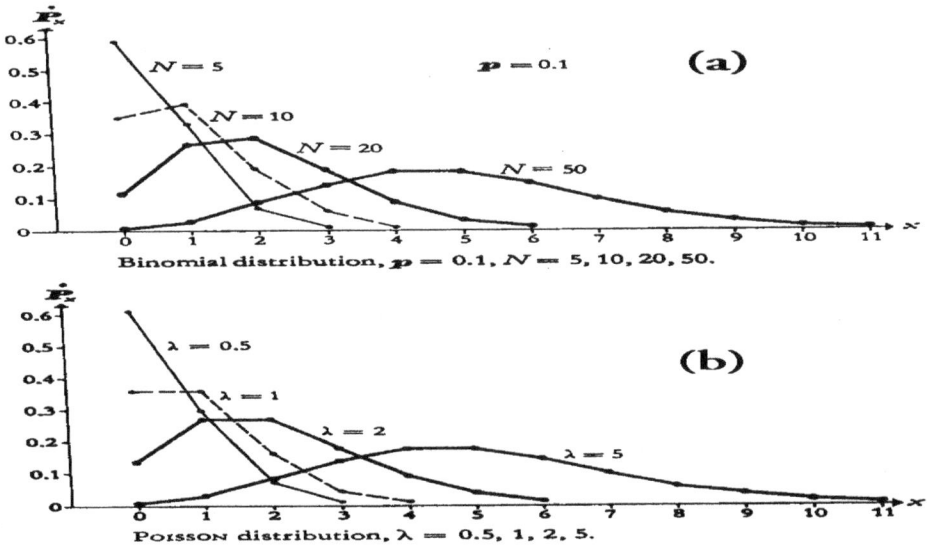

Fig. 4. Graphs illustrating Binomial and Poisson distribution (Reproduced from McNeil D. Statistical Methods. 1996; 184). The top graph (a) illustrates that binomial distribution resembles normal distribution with increasing sample size (n=50). The lower graph (b) illustrates that smaller values (λ=5) result in a normal distribution - Poisson distribution.

MUNE is calculated with the number weighted statistical method, where the mean SMUP amplitude at each level is multiplied by the number of motor units estimated at each level.

The steps in statistical MUNE are as follows:

1. Recording surface electrodes are applied as for standard nerve conduction studies.
2. An initial scan of the CMAP is performed using a series of 30 submaximal stimuli at 1 Hz, increasing in equal increments to identify unusually large steps at which further information is required.
3. On the basis of the scan, three or four 10% stimulus ranges are identified, according to an internal algorithm. Usually, one range includes the smallest step and the other ranges where the steps are >15% (Figure 5).
4. At each intensity, groups of 30 responses are captured at a rate of 3Hz. Estimates are most reliable if 10 groups of 30 responses are recorded. To minimise patient discomfort, however, repetition is repeated until the standard error of the MUNE SMUP size is less than 10%.
5. Statistical MUNE estimates the average size of SMUP's and the number of motor units in a group of muscles innervated by the nerve being stimulated, based on the normal variation of the sub-maximal CMAP evoked with constant stimuli (Figure 6).

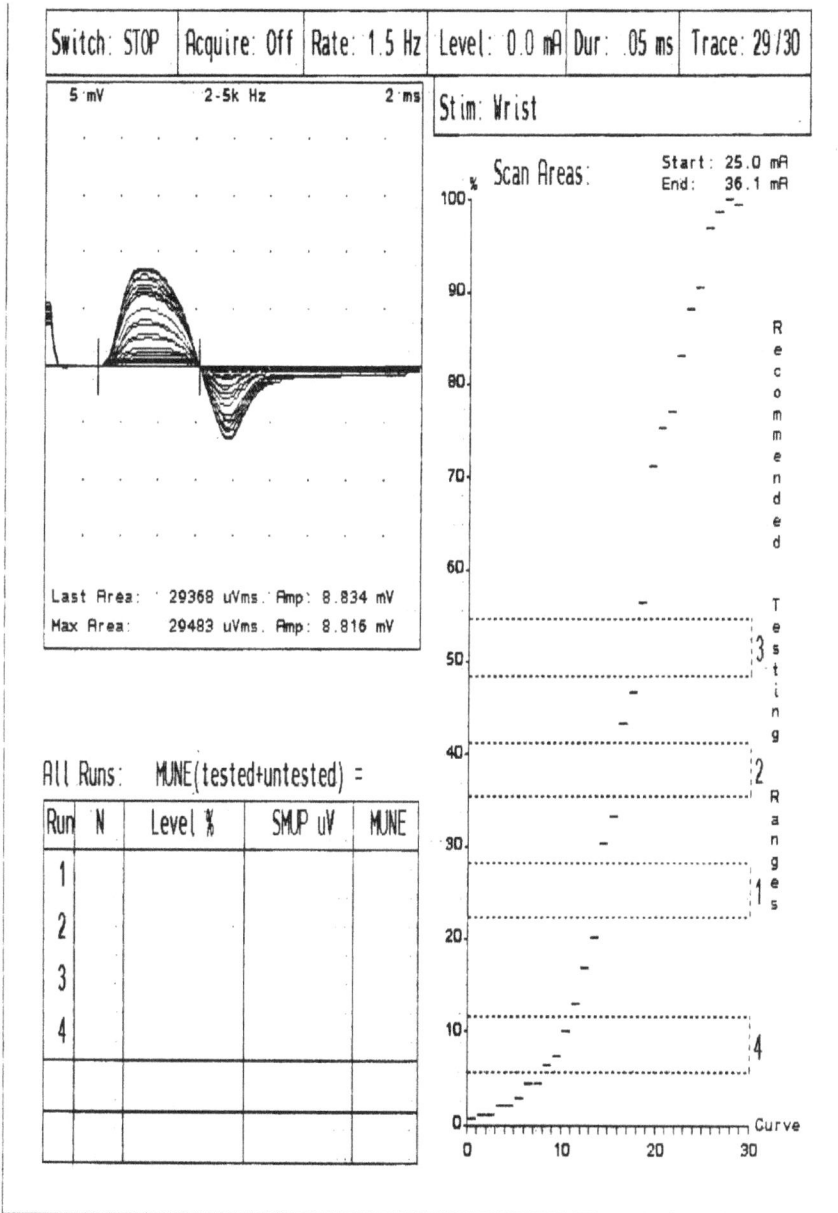

Fig. 5. An initial scan of the CMAP (right) recorded from APB muscles in response to 30 sub-maximal stimuli (x-axis) with equal increments between threshold and maximum stimulation. On the basis of the scan, 10% stimulus ranges are identified, according to an internal algorithm. The CMAP increments are shown at the top left and the eventual table of results in the bottom left corner.

| Switch: STOP | Acquire: Off | Rate: 3 Hz | Level: 0.0 mA | Dur: .05 ms | Trace: 30/30 |

5 mV   2-5k Hz   2 ms

Stim: Wrist

Run 4 areas

Last Area: 2696 uVms. Amp: 0.734 mV
Max Area: 29483 uVms. Amp: 8.816 mV

Run 4:   Area Test Range: 6 - 12 %

Group	Amp mV	SMUP uV	MUNE
1	0.8	76	116
2	0.7	91	97
3			
4			
5			
6			
7			
8			
9			
10			
Avg:	0.8	83± 7	106

All Runs: MUNE(tested+untested) = 116

Run	N	Level %	SMUP uV	MUNE
1	180	22- 28	100±13	5
2	60	36- 41	73± 0	7
3	60	49- 55	84± 5	6
4	60	6- 12	83± 7	6
	360	24% tested	85± 5	24
NONE	76% untested	73	92

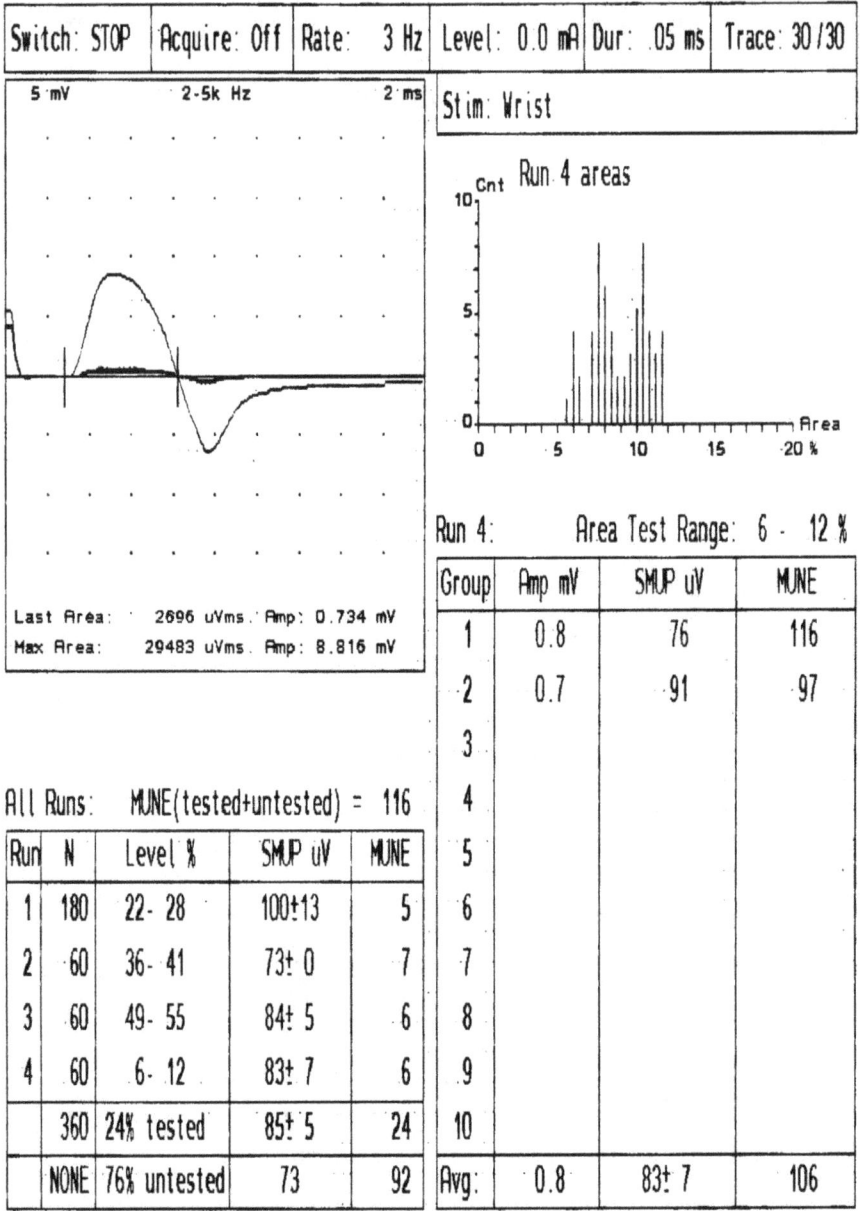

Fig. 6. At each intensity level (runs 1-4), groups of 30 responses are captured at a rate of 3Hz. The CMAP amplitudes are shown at the top left, with the histogram of results at the top right. The thenar MUNE results from repeated trials are shown in the bottom left table.

The statistical technique of estimating the size of the SMUP was performed using proprietary software on a Nicolet Viking IV electromyography machine. This technique uses direct stimulation of the motor nerve. The low frequency filter was set at 2 Hz and the high frequency filter at 5 kHz. The gain for extensor digitorum brevis was set at 2 mV/div and for abductor pollicis brevis studies at 5 mV/div. The sweep speed was 2 ms/div. This method had excellent test-retest reproducibility (+/-2.8%). The method was quick to use and well tolerated.

This technique has been greatly modified since its original description, but numerous studies have shown that MUNE can change systematically in ALS patients when used by experienced technicians, even though evaluator bias needs to be taken into account. (Shefner et al., 2004). The statistical MUNE method has also been shown to be unreliable in the presence of clinical weakness due to motor unit instability. (Shefner, 2009). Our study however was performed on asymptomatic patients, without clinical weakness.

6.3 MUNE technique

Motor unit numbers were estimated in abductor pollicis brevis (resulting in a thenar MUNE) and the extensor digitorum brevis (EDB) muscle. These muscles were used, as both are easily accessible distal muscles. The electrical activity can be recorded without interference, and in the case of EDB, the muscle belly is flat.

Self-adhesive surface recording electrodes (G1) were placed transversely across the innervation zone of each muscle, resulting in a simple biphasic negative-positive M wave, with G2 placed over a bony prominence. The deep peroneal nerve was stimulated just above the ankle and the median nerve at the wrist with a surface stimulator. This was performed by strapping the stimulating electrode onto the surface of the skin, at the point where the threshold of the nerve to electrical stimulation was at its' lowest. A hand-held stimulator was not used, as reproducibility is enhanced when the stimulating electrodes are fixed to the surface of the skin.

Initially, bilateral thenar and EDB MUNE's were obtained from all subjects. After the reproducibility phase of the study, generally only right-sided studies were performed. Once a reduction in MUNE was identified, bilateral studies were once again performed on selected subjects. The protocol was also modified depending on the subjects' tolerance to the procedure. Median nerve stimulation at the wrist for thenar MUNE was generally well tolerated by most subjects, as the stimulation intensity required to obtain an adequate response was generally less than 20mA with duration of 0.05-0.1ms.

Peroneal nerve stimulation required for EDB MUNE resulted in slightly more discomfort, as the nerve is located further away from the surface of the skin. The stimulus intensity required, in some cases was up to 50-80mA with duration of between 0.1-0.3ms. Some subjects indicated that they were unwilling to continue to participate in the study due to the discomfort caused by performing EDB MUNE. In these subjects, only thenar MUNE's were performed.

To assess the test-retest reproducibility of the technique, SOD1 family members and population controls were followed over a 1-year period, with thenar and EDB MUNE tests repeated every 3 to 6 months. The difference between MUNE results from the first and second study, and if possible, first and third studies were divided by the MUNE of the first study, and expressed as a percentage change. The results were analysed using Pearson and Spearman correlation coefficients.

All results were entered into a database and analysed using a standard statistical software package (SPSS 9.05 for Windows). For the initial part of the study, the MUNE results from asymptomatic SOD1 mutation carriers were grouped together. Although different mutations in SOD1 have different effects on the progression of the disease once symptoms occur, these different mutations do not influence on the age of onset of symptoms.[67]

Motor unit estimates in carriers were compared to age and sex matched family controls without the SOD1 mutation, and sporadic (non-SOD1) MND patients. To determine whether groups had different numbers of motor units, an unpaired t-test was used. Although there were some outlying results, the distributions were not sufficiently skewed to contradict the use of the t-test. Statistical significance was accepted at a p-value of <0.05.

The group of asymptomatic SOD1 mutation carriers were followed over the next 2 to 5 years, depending on the volunteers' motivation, both clinically and by MUNE. Results were compared to their initial baseline MUNE and the date of the study when this reduction was first detected, was used as the date when motor neurone loss commenced.

6.4 Maximal voluntary isometric contraction testing

It has been suggested that the traditional neurological examination is inadequate for documenting motor performance impairment with reliability. (Hanten et al., 1999). Generally, manual motor testing used in a standard neurological motor examination does not allow objective documentation of change in performance, as it may be influenced by the patient's history and progress. Major changes are apparent, but subtle changes are difficult to determine with accuracy.

There are a number of methods that have been developed to quantify maximal voluntary isometric contraction (MVIC). It has been proposed that this is a clinically useful, reliable, reproducible, time efficient and quantitative measure for monitoring disease progression in MND. (Hoagland et al., 1997). This would be surprising, given that in a slowly progressive denervating process, patients with substantial chronic denervation could maintain normal muscle twitch tension until loss of about 70-80% of motor units occurs. (McComas, 1971).

The methods used to quantify maximal voluntary isometric contraction have included an electronic strain-gauge tensiometer and a hand-held Jamar hydraulic dynamometer. In this study, maximum bilateral isometric grip strength was obtained using the Jamar hydraulic dynamometer to determine whether this correlated with the number of functional motor neurones in the thenar group of muscles, as measured by MUNE. Standardised (middle handle) positioning and instructions were given to all subjects. Handgrip force was measured with subjects in the sitting position and with the arm flexed at 90 degrees. Two trials were performed on each hand, and the best result used for analysis. This method was used as previous studies of grip strength reliability showed that there was no significant difference in reliability between one attempt, the mean score of two or three attempts, or the highest score of three attempts. (Hamilton et al., 1994).

Clinical neurological examination was performed, with power of thumb abduction, finger flexion and finger abduction measured according to the Medical Research Council (MRC) grading system and compared to thenar (APB) MUNE.

Felice showed that in twenty one MND patients, changes in thenar MUNE was the most sensitive outcome measure for following disease progression, when compared to other quantitative tests, such as CMAP, isometric grip strength, forced vital capacity and Medical Research Council manual muscle testing. (Felice, 1997).

7. Results

7.1 Demographics
A total of eighty-eight (88) subjects (45 males and 43 females) gave informed consent. The subjects were divided into four test groups.
1.   24 population controls;
2.   32 SOD1 negative (normal) family controls;
3.   20 asymptomatic (pre-clinical) SOD1 mutation carriers (test group),
   a.   5 subjects with point mutation in exon 4, codon 100, GAA to GGA, Glu to Gly) – glu100gly;
   b.   5 subjects with point mutation in exon 4, codon 113, ATT to ACT, Ile to Thr) – ile113thr;
   c.   5 subjects with point mutation in exon 5; codon 148, GTA to GGA, Val to Gly) – val148gly;
   d.   5 subjects with point mutation in exon 5, codon 148, GTA to GGA, Val to Ile) val148ile.
4.   12 sporadic symptomatic MND patients (positive controls).
There was no statistically significant difference in age distribution between these groups, with a range of 16 to 73 years of age.

7.2 Motor units in asymptomatic FALS (SOD1) carriers
For the initial part of the study, the baseline MUNE results were grouped together and the means of the groups were compared. The initial aim of the study was to determine if MND was due to a slow gradual attrition of motor neurones over time. If this were the case, the group of asymptomatic SOD1 mutation carriers, would be expected to have a reduced number of motor units, indicating the presence of pre-clinical motor neurone loss. Motor unit estimates in the group of asymptomatic SOD1 mutation carriers were compared to age and sex matched family controls without the SOD1 mutation, and sporadic (non-SOD1) MND patients. To determine whether groups had different numbers of motor units, an unpaired t-test was used. Statistical significance was accepted at a p-value of <0.05.
The numbers of motor units in the groups of population controls, SOD1 negative family controls and asymptomatic SOD1 mutation carriers were similar. In population controls the mean thenar MUNE was 148 with a range of 115 - 254, in SOD1 negative family controls was 138 with a range of 106 - 198 and in asymptomatic SOD1 mutation carriers, 144 with a range of 109 - 199. There was no detectable difference in the mean number of thenar motor units in the group of asymptomatic SOD1 mutation carriers compared to the group of SOD1 negative family controls (thenar p>0.46), or population controls (thenar p>0.70) (Table 1 and Figure 7).

| | Thenar (APB) muscle | |
	Cases	MUNE (Range)
Population Controls	24	148 (115-254)
SOD1 Negative Family Controls	32	138 (106-198)
SOD1 Mutation Carriers	20	144 (109–199)
Sporadic MND patients	12	45 (5–84)

Table 1. Thenar (APB) motor unit number estimates (MUNE number represents mean MUNE).

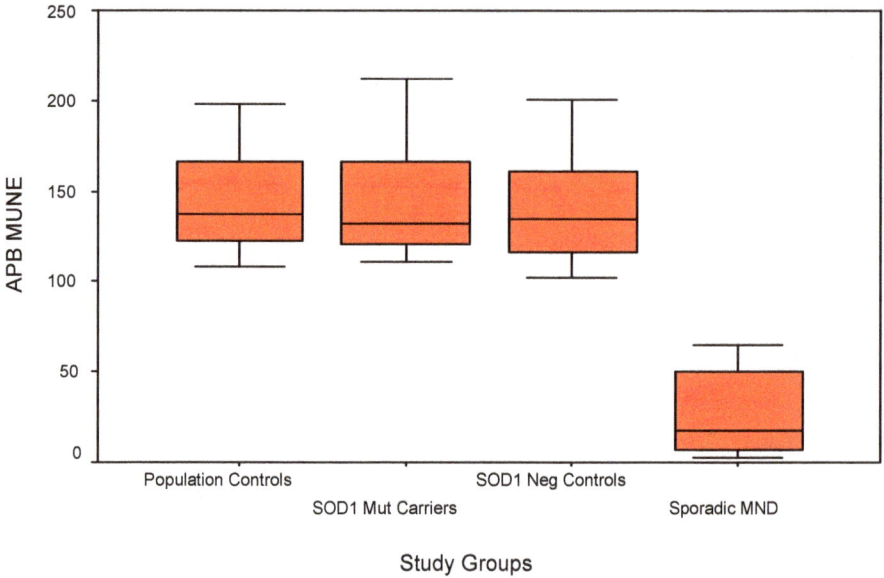

Study Groups

Fig. 7. Baseline thenar (APB) MUNE subdivided into study groups (The lower boundary of the box is the 25th percentile, and the upper border is the 75th percentile of MUNE. The horizontal line inside the box represents the median MUNE. The whispers represent the largest and smallest observed values, i.e. the range). Data is shown in Table 1.

In population controls the mean EDB MUNE was 138 with a range of 119 - 169, in SOD1 negative family controls was 134 with a range of 107 - 180 and in asymptomatic SOD1 mutation carriers, 136 with a range of 111 - 187.

Once again, there was no detectable difference in the mean number of EBD motor units in the group of asymptomatic SOD1 mutation carriers compared to the group of SOD1 negative family controls (EDB $p > 0.95$), or population controls (EDB $p > 0.50$) (Table 2 and Figure 8).

	Extensor Digitorum Brevis	
	Cases	MUNE (Range)
Population Controls	13	138 (119-169)
SOD1 Negative Family Controls	30	134 (107-180)
SOD1 Mutation Carriers	14	136 (111-187)
Sporadic MND patients	9	70 (8-82)

Table 2. EDB motor unit number estimates (MUNE number represents mean MUNE).

Symptomatic sporadic MND subjects showed a definite loss of motor units with fewer motor units compared to all other groups ($p < 0001$) with a mean thenar MUNE of 45 with a range of 5 - 84 and a mean EDB MUNE of 70 with a range of 8 - 82 (Tables 1 and 2).

There was no cross over between thenar and EDB MUNE results in symptomatic and asymptomatic subjects.

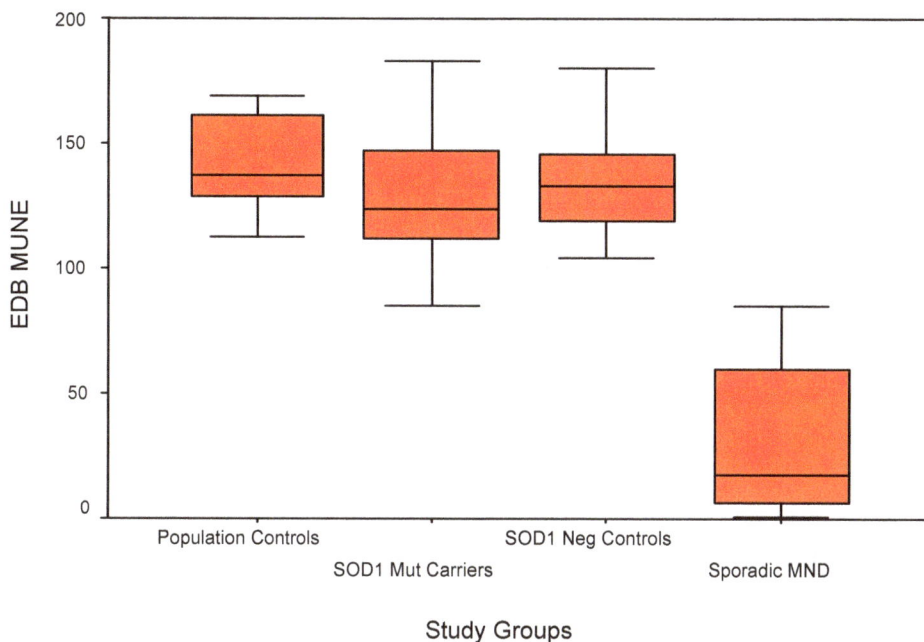

Study Groups

Fig. 8. Baseline EDB MUNE subdivided into study groups (The lower boundary of the box is
the 25th percentile, and the upper border is the 75th percentile of MUNE. The horizontal line
inside the box represents the median MUNE. The whispers represent the largest and
smallest observed values, i.e. the range). Data is shown in Table 2.

7.3 Reproducibility of MUNE technique

To assess the test-retest reproducibility of the technique, 69 of the 88 SOD1 family members
and population controls were followed over a 1-year period, with thenar and extensor
digitorum brevis (EDB) MUNE tests repeated every 3-6 months, depending on patient
availability. The difference between MUNE results from the first and second study, and if
possible, first and third studies were divided by the MUNE of the first study, and expressed
as a percentage change. The results were analysed using Pearson and Spearman correlation
coefficients.

The test-retest correlation of thenar MUNE in asymptomatic subjects was high with a
Pearson correlation coefficient of 0.93. The mean difference between MUNE results on
separate occasions on the same individual was +/- 3.6%, with a range of 0-11.7% (Table 3).

	Number of Cases	Mean MUNE
Thenar 1	88	145.7
Thenar 2	69	140.1
Thenar 3	33	140.0
Thenar Change	**Range (0 - 11.7%)**	**3.6%**

Table 3. Reproducibility of mean thenar (APB) motor unit number estimates in
asymptomatic subjects on separate reviews over a one-year period.

For EDB MUNE, the Pearson correlation coefficient was also high, 0.88, with a mean difference between MUNE results on separate occasions on the same individual of +/- 4.6%, with a range of 0-15.7%. The test-retest correlation was high with a Pearson correlation coefficient of 0.91, when groups were broken down into the different study groups.

7.4 Maximal voluntary isometric contraction

Maximal voluntary isometric contraction (MVIC), using the Jamar hand dynamometer was used to measure isometric grip strength to determine whether this correlated with the number of functional motor neurones in the thenar group of muscles as measured by MUNE. Isometric grip strength tests, thenar MUNE and MRC power were performed on 69 asymptomatic subjects twice within a 3-6 month period to assess the test-retest reproducibility of this technique. Pearson correlation coefficients between study 1 and study 2 of right hand grip strength was 0.941, left hand grip strength 0.910 and thenar MUNE results 0.937. These results indicate that the reproducibility of these techniques was high.

Right hand grip strength correlated with left hand grip strength, with Pearson correlation coefficients of 0.959 and Spearman correlation coefficients of 0.956 Two-way analyses of variance showed a no significant difference between the right and left hands (Figure 9). There was no correlation between right grip strength and right thenar motor unit number, with Pearson correlation coefficients of 0.483 and Spearman correlation coefficient of 0.34 (Figure 10).

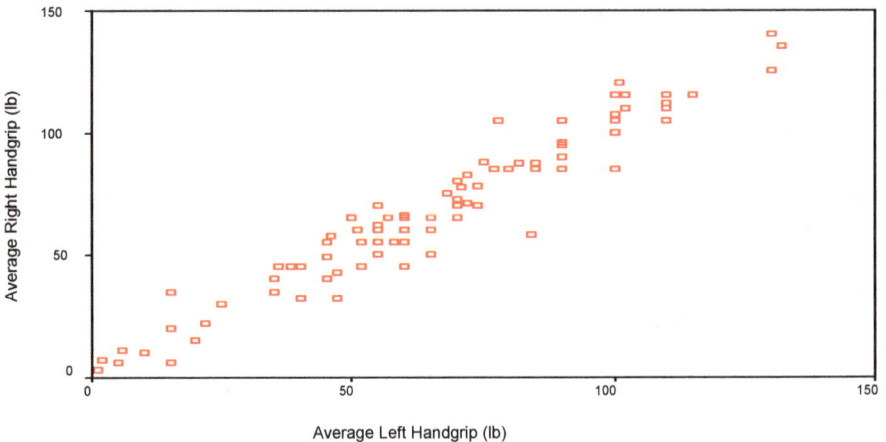

Fig. 9. Graph showing the correlation between right and left handgrip

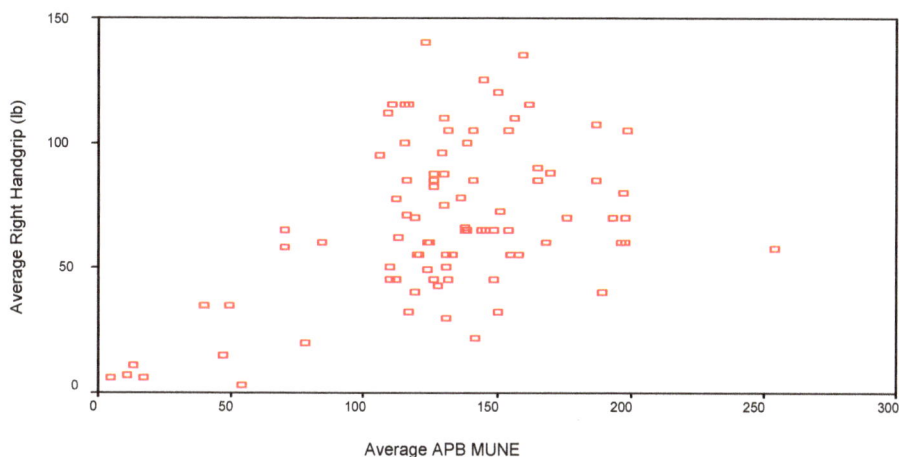

Fig. 10. Scatter graph showing the lack of correlation between right handgrip and right thenar (APB) MUNE

7.5 Detection of pre-symptomatic motor neurone loss in SOD1 mutation carriers

The MUNE results, after validating their reproducibility, were used as a baseline to follow the number of motor units over time in individual pre-symptomatic SOD1 mutation carriers over the next 2-5 years, to determine whether pattern of motor neurone loss is either a slow attrition of motor neurones over time or whether normal numbers of motor neurones are maintained until sudden, rapid multi-focal cell death of motor neurones occurs, corresponding with the development of symptoms.

During the course of the study, 5 of the SOD1 mutation carriers developed leg weakness. A significant fall in motor unit number was detected in these 5 SOD1 mutation carriers, were there was a detectable reduction of motor units, 4-10 months prior to the onset of weakness and the diagnosis of familial ALS being made. There was no detectable loss of motor units in the other 15 SOD1 mutation carriers or in the group of SOD1 mutation negative relatives, during the study period.

In individual cases, there was:

51% loss of motor units, 4 months prior to onset of weakness in Case 1

37% loss of motor units, 10 months prior to onset of weakness in Case 2

28% loss of motor units, 6 months prior to onset of weakness in Case 3

46% loss of motor units, 6 months prior to onset of weakness in Case 4

68% loss of motor units, 8 months prior to onset of weakness in Case 5

There was further motor unit loss as weakness progressed, at which point the diagnosis of MND was confirmed.

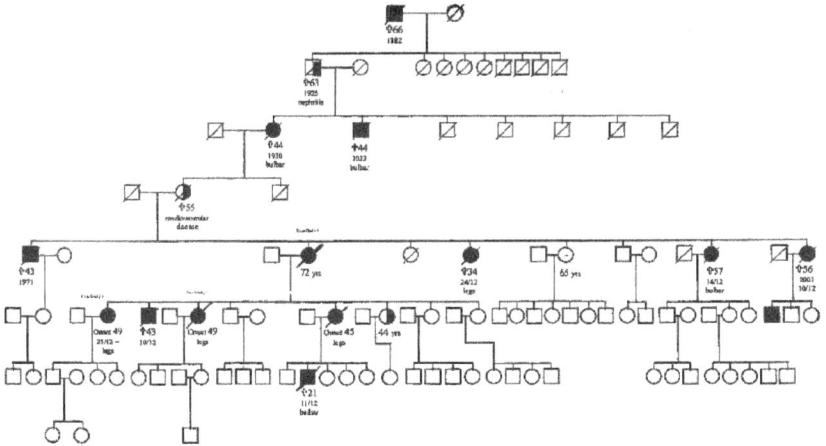

Fig. 11. Pedigree of cases 1, 2 and 3

7.5.1 Case study 1

A 48-year-old lady from a family with a strong history of familial ALS. Pedigree is shown in Figure 11. This family has a point mutation in the SOD1 gene at val148gly. At the time of recruitment, October 1998, the subject was asymptomatic, with a normal neurological examination and no evidence of wasting, weakness or fasciculations. Progress MUNE results are shown in Table 4 and Figure 12.

Months before and after weakness	-26	-24	-21	-13	-7	-4	0	+3	+5	+8	+17
Date of study	Oct-98	Dec-98	Mar-99	Nov-99	Jul-00	Nov-00	Mar-01	Jun-01	Aug-01	Nov-01	Aug-02
R Handgrip	60	65	68	60	60	65	65	62	60	45	Died
R Thenar MUNE	130	131	126	131	115	113	115	110	83	49	
L Handgrip	60	60	60	60	60	60	55	45	37	18	
L Thenar MUNE	122		114	110		122	83	52	40	0	
R EDB power	5/5	5/5	5/5	5/5	5/5	5/5	5/5	3/5	0/5	0/5	
R EDB MUNE	124	120	132	116	116	114	114	72	53	0	
L EDB power	5/5	5/5	5/5	5/5	5/5	5/5	0/5	0/5	0/5	0/5	
L EDB MUNE	130		125		64	0	0	0	0		

Table 4. Case 1 progressive handgrip, dorsiflexion power and thenar and EDB MUNE results

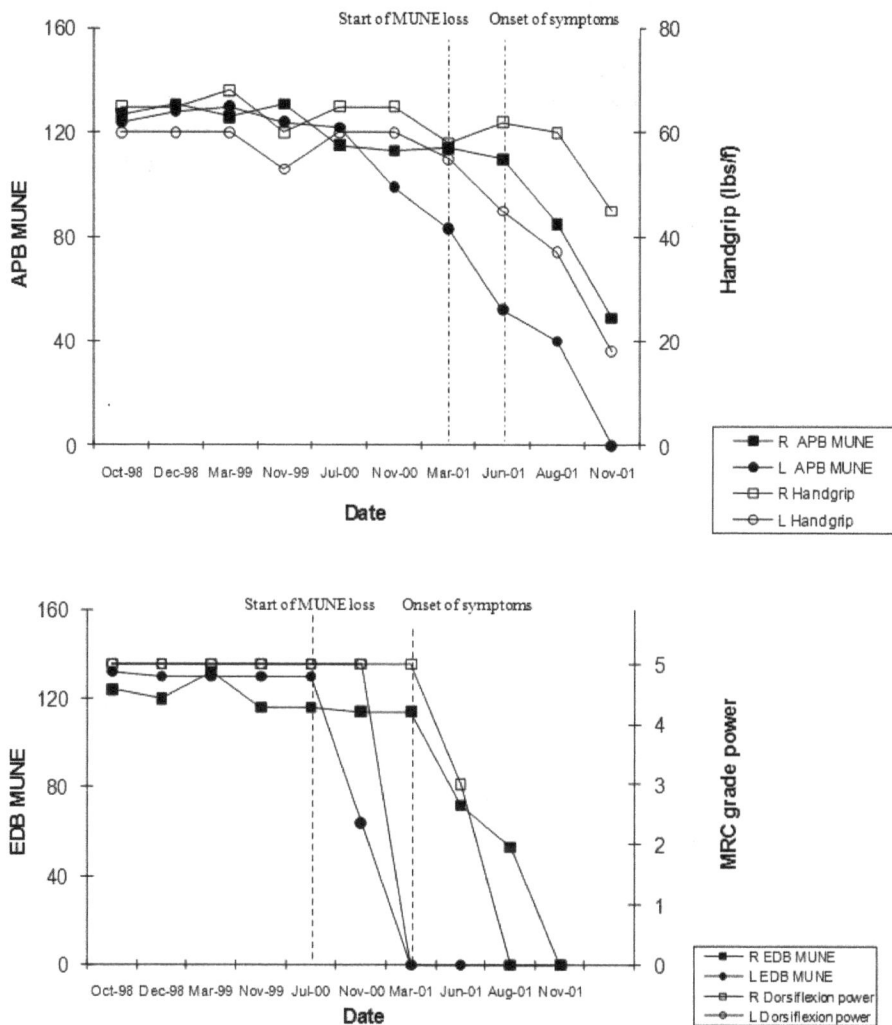

Fig. 12. Progressive results of case 1 showing the change in APB and EDB motor unit estimates over time in relation to handgrip strength and power. There is a reduction of APB and EDB MUNE prior to the onset of weakness.

The MUNE results remained stable over the first 2 years of the study. By November 2000, her left EDB MUNE had dropped to 64 (total reduction of 51%), but she only developed wasting and weakness of the anterior compartment muscles of her left leg, 4 months later, when she had MRC grade 2/5 of dorsiflexion and eversion, 3/5 plantarflexion and inversion 3/5. Proximal muscles, upper limb and right leg muscles were normal. Deep tendon reflexes were brisk in the upper and lower limbs. Over the next 6 months, her right thenar MUNE from 130 to 115 (12%) She had no detectable right arm weakness at the time and her handgrip strength remained at around 65 pounds.

An independent neurologist performed needle EMG, which showed extensive denervation in left leg muscles with fibrillation potentials in the left tibialis posterior, gastrocnemius, vastus medialis and L5/S1 paraspinal muscles. There were no changes in the right vastus medialis, biceps brachialis, triceps, left deltoid and the tongue. It was felt that these changes were not enough to make a diagnosis of ALS. She went on to have a MRI scan of her lumbar spine showed degenerative disc disease of L4/5 and L5/S1, with no evidence of neural compression.

Over the next 6 months, her right EDB MUNE continued to drop from 114 to 72 and subsequently to 53, a 54% reduction. Her left thenar MUNE also dropped from 122 to 83 motor units, a 36% reduction. Her right foot power remained normal until August 2001, 7 months after the reduction was noted. At that time, she developed upper limb weakness, with a reduction of left handgrip strength to 45 pounds.

Repeat needle EMG examination showed severe denervation in the left tibialis anterior and gastrocnemius, but still no changes in proximal right lower limb or upper limb muscles. Once again, this was considered not to be diagnostic for ALS. Her EDB and thenar MUNE however continued to drop and she developed upper and lower limb weakness and became wheelchair bound. She subsequently died with respiratory failure in August 2002.

7.5.2 Case study 2

A 43-year-old sister of case 1. She had the same strong family history of ALS, with a point mutation in SOD1 gene at val148gly. Her pedigree is shown in Figure 11. She was asymptomatic at the time of recruitment with a normal neurological examination, and no evidence of wasting, weakness or fasciculation. Her right and left thenar MUNE's remained stable for the first 2½ years of the study at around 115-120 motor units. Progress MUNE results are shown in Table 5 and Figures 14.

Months pre and post weakness 1st detected	-42	-40	-37	-29	-20	-10	0	+11	+21	+27
Date of study	Oct-98	Dec-98	Mar-99	Nov-99	Jul-00	Jan-01	Nov-01	Oct-02	Aug-03	Feb-04
R Handgrip	60	60	65	65	60	70	65	65	65	65
R Thenar MUNE	111	111	117	119	120	114	96	97	86	85
L Handgrip	60	55	60	65	63	65	65	60	60	60
L Thenar MUNE	117				119	111	89	86	79	81
R EDB power	5/5	5/5	5/5	5/5	5/5	5/5	4+/5	4+/5	4+/5	4+/5
R EDB MUNE	104	111	119	108	104	92	71	75	75	65
L EDB power	5/5	5/5	5/5	5/5	5/5	5/5	5/5	5/5	5/5	5/5
L EDB MUNE	112						89	80	80	81

Table 5. Case 2 progressive handgrip, dorsiflexion power and thenar and EDB MUNE results

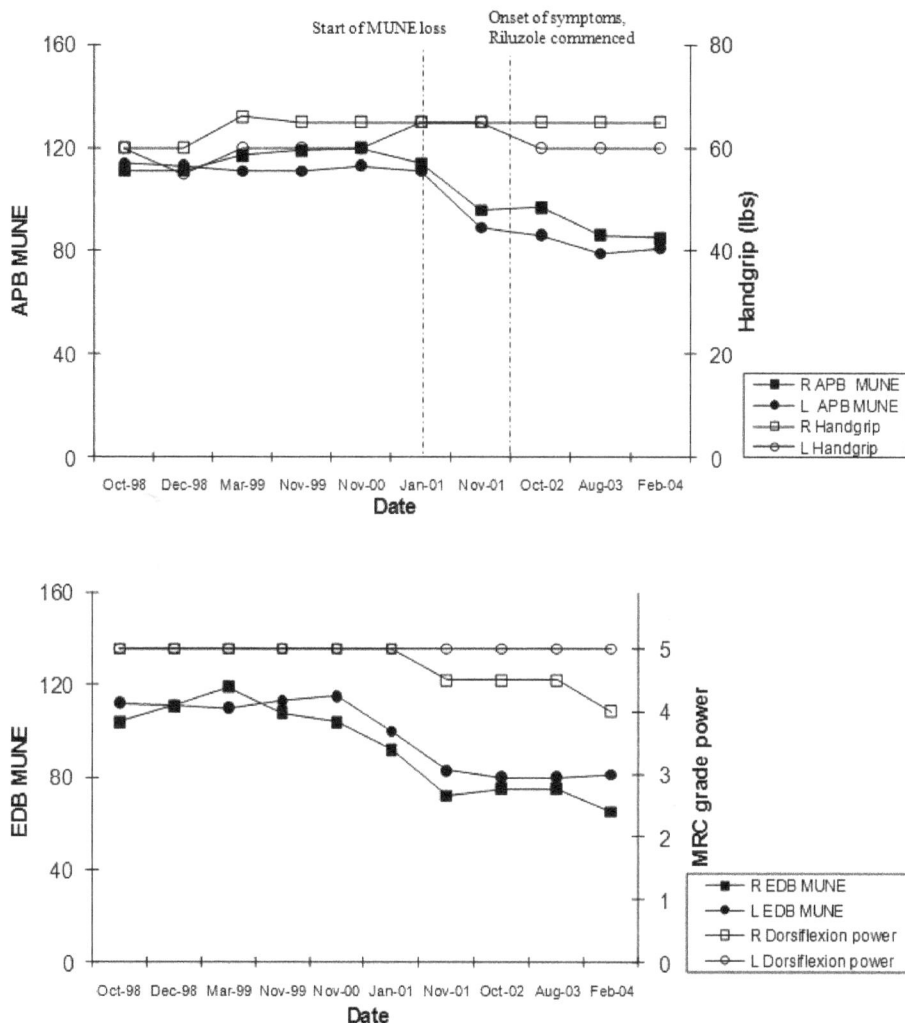

Fig. 14. Progressive results of case 2 showing the change in APB and EDB motor unit
estimates over time in relation to handgrip strength and power. There is a reduction of APB
and EDB MUNE even though strength has remained stable.

Over the next 6 months, there was a reduction in her right thenar MUNE to 96 (20%) and her
left thenar MUNE to 89 (19%), with no detectable weakness. Her right EDB MUNE also
dropped from 111 to 92 (17%), but she only had detectable weakness 10 months later of
MRC grade 4+/5 in right dorsiflexors, at which time her right EDB MUNE had dropped
further to 71 motor units (35%). The left EDB MUNE also dropped from a baseline of 112 (2
years previously) to 89 (20%), but with no detectable weakness.

An independent neurologist performed needle EMG examination, which showed high
amplitude motor units with reduced recruitment in vastus medialis, tibialis anterior and

extensor carpi radialis longus, bilaterally but no fibrillation potentials were seen. It was felt that these changes were not enough to make the diagnosis of ALS.

In view of her strong family history, a presumed diagnosis of familial ALS was made and she was commenced on Riluzole in February 2002.

Over the next 3 years, her EDB MUNE results have stabilised. Her weakness has not progressed significantly. In February 2004, she still had MRC grade 4+/5 power of her right dorsiflexors and no symptomatically apparent weakness in her left dorsiflexors or upper limbs.

7.5.3 Case study 3

A 68 year-old mother of case 1 and 2. She had the same family history of ALS, with a point mutation in SOD1 gene at val148gly. Her pedigree is shown in Figure 12. She was also asymptomatic at the time of recruitment. Her right and left thenar MUNE's remained stable at around 130 motor units. Due to her age, she was not followed as regularly as her daughters.

On her review in November 2001, there had been a reduction of her right thenar MUNE to 98 (23%) and her left thenar MUNE to 98 (25%), with no detectable weakness. Her right EDB MUNE also dropped from 147 to 106 (28%), but she did not have any detectable weakness. She subsequently developed voice change 6 months later in May 2002, and died of respiratory failure in August 2002. Progress MUNE and handgrip results are shown in Table 6.

Months pre and post weakness 1st detected	-43	-41	-38	-6	0	+3
Date of study	Oct-98	Dec-98	Mar-99	Nov-01	May-02	Aug-02
R Handgrip	55	55	55	55	Voice	Died
R Thenar MUNE	127	135	130	98	Change	
L Handgrip	60	50	50	45		
L Thenar MUNE	130			125		
R EDB power	5/5	5/5	5/5	5/5		
R EDB MUNE	147	153	150	106		

Table 6. Case 3 progressive handgrip, dorsiflexion power and thenar and EDB MUNE results

7.5.4 Case study 4

A 48-year-old lady with a strong family history of ALS. This family had a point mutation in SOD1 gene at glu100gly. At the time of recruitment, the subject was asymptomatic, with a normal neurological examination and no evidence of wasting, weakness or fasciculations. Progress MUNE results are shown in Table 7.

The MUNE results remained stable over the first 2½ years of the study. Her right EDB MUNE results remained stable at around 120 motor units. It was then noted that her left EDB MUNE had dropped from 118 to 64 (46% reduction) and her right thenar MUNE had also dropped from 153 to 123 (20% reduction). She did not have any detectable weakness of her upper or lower limbs. Needle EMG showed neurogenic changes, but not sufficient to fulfil the criteria for ALS.

She subsequently developed left lower leg weakness with inversion and eversion of MRC
grade 3/5 and dorsiflexion and plantarflexion 4/5, 6 months later. Her disease progressed
rapidly and died within the 4 months of diagnosis, in March 2002 of respiratory failure.

Months pre and post weakness 1st detected	-33	-30	-25	-14	-6	0	+4
Date of study	Apr-98	Jul-98	Dec-98	Nov-99	Apr-01	Oct-01	Mar-02
R Handgrip	60	66	70	80	60	70	Died
R Thenar MUNE	149	144	142	151	153	123	
L Handgrip	50	60	65	60	55	58	
L Thenar MUNE	128						
R EDB power	5/5	5/5	5/5	5/5	5/5	5/5	
R EDB MUNE	126	132	137	119	118	118	
L EDB power	5/5	5/5	5/5	5/5	5/5	3/5	
L EDB MUNE	123			118	64	42	

Table 7. Case 4 progressive handgrip, dorsiflexion power and thenar and EDB MUNE results

7.5.5 Case study 5

A 44-year-old man with a strong family history of ALS and a 2nd cousin once removed of
case 4. His family also had a point mutation in SOD1 gene at glu100gly. At the time of
recruitment, the subject was asymptomatic, with a normal neurological examination and no
wasting, weakness or fasciculations. Progress MUNE results are shown in Table 8.

Months pre and post weakness 1st detected	-50	-48	-44	-35	-22	-8	0
Date of study	May-98	Jul-98	Nov-98	Aug-99	Sep-00	Nov-01	Jul-02
R Handgrip	115	110	120	115	110	115	120
R Thenar MUNE	127	117	107	116	138	116	121
L Handgrip	100	100	105	105	105	100	100
L Thenar MUNE	135					122	120
R EDB power	5/5	5/5	5/5	5/5	5/5	0/5	0/5
R EDB MUNE	125	114	129	106	115	0	0
L EDB power	5/5	5/5	5/5	5/5	5/5	5/5	4/5
L EDB MUNE	127				114	36	0

Table 8. Case 5 progressive handgrip, dorsiflexion power and thenar and EDB MUNE results

The MUNE results remained stable over the first 3 years of the study. The right EDB MUNE
dropped from 115 down to being not recordable. Thenar MUNE remained stable at about
130 motor units. He had occasional fasciculations in the right quadriceps region, weakness
of the right quadriceps and MRC grade 0/5 weakness of right dorsiflexion. He was unsure

as to when weakness developed. Needle EMG showed changes of active and chronic denervation limited to the right quadriceps muscle, which was not considered diagnostic for ALS.

Over the next 6 months, there was a reduction of the left EDB MUNE as well from 114 to 36 (68% reduction), but with no detectable weakness. In July 2002, 8 months later, he was reviewed by his neurologist and was found to have only slightly reduced left ankle power with MRC grade 4/5 and weakness of knee flexion bilaterally. He progressed rapidly after that and by October 2002 had bilateral lower limb weakness to a point were he was unable to stand without assistance and became wheelchair bound. He commenced Riluzole, in May 2003, but over the next year there was progression of upper limb weakness. Currently, his forced lung capacity is around 30% and he is using BiPAP ventilation at night and receives PEG feeding.

8. Conclusion

Motor neurone disease (MND) is a group of fatal, progressive neurodegenerative disorders, with an overall median survival is approximately 4.0 years from the onset of symptoms. By the time most patients with MND are aware of clinical weakness and seek review by their primary physician or neurologist, a significant proportion of motor units have already been lost. Early detection of motor neurone loss in clinically apparently unaffected muscles is therefore important to establish an early diagnosis of the condition.

Motor unit number estimates in the group of asymptomatic SOD1 mutation carriers were compared to age and sex matched family controls without the SOD1 mutation, and sporadic (non-SOD1) MND patients. There was no detectable difference in the number of thenar motor units in the group of asymptomatic SOD1 mutation carriers compared to the group of SOD1 negative family controls (thenar $p>0.46$), or population controls (thenar $p>0.70$).. In addition, there was no detectable difference in the number of EBD motor units in the group of asymptomatic SOD1 mutation carriers compared to the group of SOD1 negative family controls (EDB $p>0.95$), or population controls (EDB $p>0.50$). Symptomatic sporadic MND subjects showed a definite loss of motor units with fewer motor units compared to all other groups ($p<0.001$). There was no overlap between MUNE results in symptomatic and asymptomatic subjects.

These results indicate that the group of asymptomatic carriers of the SOD1 mutation have no significant difference in the number of motor neurones, when compared to age and sex matched controls. All carriers had a full complement of motor neurones during the asymptomatic phase, indicating that mutation carriers have normal survival of motor neurones and that symptomatic MND is not the end result of a slow attrition of motor neurones. This implies that gradual pre-symptomatic loss of motor neurones does not occur in asymptomatic SOD1 mutation carriers. This supports the observation that sudden, catastrophic loss of motor neurones occurs immediately prior to the onset of symptoms and the development of the disease, rather than a gradual attrition of motor neurones over time. These results suggest that there may be a biological trigger initiating rapid cell loss, just prior to the onset of symptoms. This observation is an important contribution to the current understanding of the pathogenesis of MND. (Aggarwal & Nicholson, 2001).

The statistical MUNE technique was used for the study. This technique has been greatly modified since its original description, but numerous studies have shown that MUNE can change systematically in ALS patients when used by experienced technicians, even though evaluator bias needs to be taken into account. Shefner demonstrated that the statistical MUNE was unreliable in the presence of clinical weakness due to motor unit instability. The difference is that our study was performed on asymptomatic patients, without clinical weakness.

It also showed that MUNE may be used as a reliable method of pre-symptomatic detection of motor unit loss in SOD1 mutation carriers. Following 69 SOD1 family members and population controls over a 1-year period, with thenar and EDB MUNE tests repeated every 3 to 6 months, assessed the test-retest reproducibility of the technique. The mean difference between thenar MUNE results on separate occasions in asymptomatic subjects was +/- 3.6%, with a range of 0-11.7%, and +/- 4.6%, with a range of 0-15.7% in EDB MUNE. These results indicate that the reproducibility of this technique and the results achieved was high, so that individual results could be used as a baseline for serial MUNE studies. (Aggarwal, 2009).

During the course of the study, however, a significant fall in motor unit number was detected in 5 of the SOD1 mutation carriers, several months before the onset of weakness and the diagnosis of motor neurone disease (MND) being made. There was no detectable loss of motor units in the other 15 SOD1 mutation carriers or in the group of SOD1 mutation negative relatives. From the study, a threshold MUNE of less than 100 was considered to imply that symptoms were imminent.

In individual cases, there was a reduction of 68% 8 months prior, 51% 4 months prior, 46% 6 months prior, 35% 10 months prior and 28% 6 months prior to the onset of weakness. Further motor unit loss occurred as weakness progressed and the diagnosis of MND being made.

Case 1 was a 48-year-old lady from a family with a strong history of familial MND, with a point mutation in the SOD1 gene at val148gly. At the time of recruitment in October 1998, she was asymptomatic. Her MUNE results remained stable over the first 2½ years, after which her left EDB MUNE dropped by 51%, and she only had detectable weakness of her left foot 4 months later with wasting and weakness of the anterior compartment muscles of her left leg of MRC grade 2-3/5. Over the next 6 months, her right EDB MUNE dropped by 56%, but she only developed right foot weakness 3 months later in June2001.

Her 43-year-old sister also showed a reduction in MUNE prior to the onset of symptoms. About 3 years into the study, there was a reduction in her right thenar MUNE to 96 (20%) and her left thenar MUNE to 89 (19%), with no detectable weakness. Her right EDB MUNE also dropped by 17%, but she only had detectable weakness 10 months later of MRC grade 4+/5 in right dorsiflexors, at which time her right EDB MUNE had dropped by a total of 35%. In view of her strong family history, a presumed diagnosis of MND was made and she was commenced on Riluzole in February 2002. Over the last 2 years, her EDB MUNE have not shown any decline. Her weakness has not progressed significantly, as on her last review in February 2004, she still had MRC grade 4/5 power of her right dorsiflexors and no clinically apparent weakness in her left dorsiflexors or upper limbs. It is possible that since "treatment" was commenced prior to the loss of a significant number of motor neurones, this may have slowed down the progression of the disease in this individual case. (Aggarwal & Nicholson, 2002).

Her mother also had a detectable reduction right thenar MUNE of 23% and left thenar MUNE of 25%, with no clinically apparent weakness. Her right EDB MUNE also dropped by 28%, with no detectable weakness. She subsequently developed bulbar symptoms 6 months and died of respiratory failure.

Case 4 was a 48-year-old lady with a strong family history of MND and a point mutation in SOD1 gene at glu100gly. At the time of recruitment, she was asymptomatic and her MUNE results remained stable over the first 3 years of the study. It was then noted that her reduction of her left EDB MUNE of 46% reduction, but with no detectable weakness. She subsequently developed left lower leg weakness of MRC grade 3/5 about 6months later.

Finally, her 2nd cousin, once removed, is a 44-year-old man who also had a point mutation in SOD1 gene at glu100gly. His MUNE results also remained stable over the first 3 years of the study. The right EDB MUNE dropped from 115 down to being not recordable over a 12-month period. At that time, he had occasional fasciculations in the right quadriceps region and MRC grade 0/5 weakness of right dorsiflexion. He was unsure as to when the weakness had developed. Over time, his left EDB MUNE has reduced by 68%, but his left ankle power remained normal until 8 months later, when it reduced slightly to MRC grade 4/5.

This study also shows that there can be substantial loss in MUNE and still have an essentially normal EMG with minimal signs of acute denervation or motor unit potential remodelling, as one would expected that at a minimum, the muscles with transiently reduced MUNE numbers should have reduced recruitment during EMG studies.

Four of the five SOD 1 mutation carriers who had a pre-symptomatic loss of motor neurones had needle EMG studies performed by an independent neurologist, which showed neurogenic changes but not sufficient to fulfil the criteria to make the diagnosis of MND. All had a reduction in MUNE at the time of the EMG study of which the independent neurologist was not aware. This implies that MUNE may be a more reliable and sensitive method for diagnosing MND than needle EMG. MUNE can be used as a non-invasive method of predicting impending decline in motor neurones and estimating the rate of neuronal death in asymptomatic subjects. This indicates that loss of motor neurones is detectable in the pre-symptomatic phase and this loss was detectable before significant needle EMG changes of pathology occur. McComas showed that patients with substantial chronic denervation could maintain normal muscle twitch tension until loss of about 70-80% of motor units, before collateral reinnervation was unable to provide functional compensation, and this is the probable explanation of this finding.

As MUNE is a measure of the primary pathologic process of motor neurone loss and can identify that the number of motor units are reduced, even in the presence of a non-diagnostic needle EMG. Needle electromyography may reveal evidence of chronic reinnervation, but provides little direct evidence to the extent of motor neurone and axonal loss.

This lack of corroboration with needle EMG in the pre-symptomatic stage requires a paradigm shift in the traditional concept that needle EMG is the "gold" standard for the diagnosis of ALS. We are aware that traditional neurologists and neurophysiologists will find this difficult to accept, as it would be expected that at a minimum, the muscles with transiently reduced MUNE numbers should have reduced recruitment during EMG studies. It is hard to understand physiologically how there can be substantial loss in MUNE and still have normal EMG with no signs of acute denervation or motor unit potential remodelling. These cases clearly indicate that loss of motor neurones is detectable in the pre-symptomatic phase and this loss was detectable before significant needle EMG changes of pathology occur. Even though some may argue that a reduction in MUNE cannot be used to support or diagnosis FALS, once changes occur on conventional EMG studies, the window of opportunity to influence the progression of this condition has been missed.

Maximum isometric grip strength using the Jamar hydraulic dynamometer also does not correlate with the number of functional motor neurones in thenar group of muscles as measured using the statistical method of MUNE, indicating that MUNE is a more sensitive test than MVIC for monitoring disease progression in MND. It has also been shown that MUNE is able to identify deterioration in functional motor units before handgrip maximal voluntary isometric contraction (MVIC).

This confirms McComas' observation that patients with substantial chronic denervation could maintain normal muscle twitch tension until loss of about 70-80% of motor units occurs. This suggests that handgrip MVIC is not as sensitive as thenar MUNE for monitoring disease progression, as it is unable to detect early motor neurone loss due to the presence of compensatory mechanisms. The surviving motor neurones enlarge their territories, through collateral sprouting (reinnervation) until late in the disease, when collateral reinnervation is no longer able to provide full functional compensation. Thenar MUNE however does examine all of the motor units that are involved in handgrip MVIC, as forearm flexors and ulnar-innervated muscles are involved in the generation of handgrip MVIC. It also confirms Felice's study which showed that in patients with MND, changes in thenar MUNE was the most sensitive outcome measure for following disease progression, when compared to other quantitative tests, such as CMAP, isometric grip strength, forced vital capacity and Medical Research Council manual muscle testing.

As motor neurone loss once it occurs is rapid and precipitous, any potential treatment will need to be given early to SOD1 mutation carriers. Once the disease progresses, resulting in functional impairment and disability, restorative treatments to replace lost motor neurones becomes less feasible. To date there have been a number of drugs which have undergone clinical trials in MND, for which there is no evidence of benefit. These include creatinine, high dose vitamin E, Gabapentin and nerve growth factors such as brain derived neurotrophic factor and insulin-like growth factor-1. If effective treatment for MND were to be developed to arrest the process of degeneration, therapies aimed at preserving functional motor neurones would be more feasible. This requires the ability to be able to identify individuals at risk of developing the disease, which currently are SOD1 mutation carriers.

Currently, the only effective approved treatment for MND is Riluzole, which has a neuroprotective role, possibly due to pre-synaptic inhibition of glutamate release. Riluzole is an anti-glutamate agent that has been approved for the treatment of patients with amyotrophic lateral sclerosis in most countries. There have been a least three large randomised trials involving hundreds of patients that have been unable to show that Riluzole is a disease altering agent nor does it have any restorative reports.

In one of the cases in the study, Riluzole was commenced once she developed mild weakness. At the time, there was a slight reduction in MUNE, but conventional needle EMG examination did not fulfil the criteria to make the diagnosis of MND. In view of her strong family history and positive genetic testing, a presumed diagnosis of MND was made. Since commencing Riluzole there has been no significant reduction in her EDB MUNE over the last 2 years, and her weakness of right dorsiflexors has only progressed marginally from MRC grade 4+/5 to 4/5 power. It is possible that since "treatment" was commenced prior to the loss of a significant number of motor neurones, this may have slowed down the progression of the disease in this individual case. Early in the course of ALS, the rate of cell death is low as the amount of neuronal damage caused by the mutation is small. As the amount of intracellular damage increases, a critical threshold is reached, which overwhelms cellular homeostasis, resulting in rapid apoptosis and cell death. The increase in MUNE numbers may be either due to reinnervation of the damaged muscle or repair of poorly functioning synapses, at the early stage of the disease, without resulting in a change in CMAP.

We would argue that previous trials have all be performed in the symptomatic phase of the disease when 70-80% of motor units have already been lost, rather than in the pre-symptomatic phase of the disease, when the therapeutic benefit might change, as "treatment" is commenced prior to significant motor neurone loss occurring and therefore, the progression of disease can be slowed down. MUNE numbers are believed to reduce because of remodelling of the motor unit and in our study, the compound muscle action potential amplitudes (CMAP) were retained as early in the course of the disease, the rate of cell death is low. The increase in MUNE numbers may be either due to reinnervation of the damaged muscle or repair of poorly functioning synapses, at the early stage of the disease, without resulting in a change in CMAP.

This longitudinal study showed that it was possible to detect loss of motor neurones in the pre-symptomatic stage of MND in humans. This study provided further evidence that considerable motor neurone loss occurred just before the onset of symptoms or weakness. (Aggarwal, 2009).

This study indicates that SOD1 mutation carriers have normal survival of motor neurones, with as carriers had a full complement of motor neurones during the asymptomatic phase. Significant pre-symptomatic loss of motor neurones did not occur in asymptomatic SOD1 mutation carriers. Sudden and widespread motor neurone death occurs at the time development of the symptomatic symptoms, rather than life-long motor neurone loss. Sudden, catastrophic and multifocal loss of motor neurons occurs immediately prior to the onset of symptoms and the development of MND. This suggests that there may be a biological trigger initiating rapid cell loss, just prior to the onset of symptoms, rather than life-long motor neurone loss. Also, if the trigger initiating motor neurone loss can be identified, it may be possible to prevent motor neurone loss in familial ALS and develop treatments for sporadic MND. The mutant SOD1 protein itself cannot be the trigger, as it is constantly expressed. There may however be a gradual accumulation of a toxic product, possibly SOD1, which has changed into a new toxic conformation or aggregate, resulting in neuronal damage. The possibility of an individual neuron undergoing apoptosis increases as damage accumulates . This cumulative damage may be due to oxidative stress, resulting in disruption of the cellular structure and function.

Neurofilament heavy polypeptide (NF-H) is an abundant stable cytoplasmic protein located in neuronal cells in large axons and may be used as a cell type marker. Abnormal accumulation of NF-H in motor neurones is associated with ALS, but it is unclear to what extent these contribute to human disease. Analysis of blood serum markers looking for increased levels of NF-H was not performed in this study, but would be interesting to be done in the future to the compare levels of NF-H in the carriers.

The results of this study indicate that the risk of cell death probably remains constant throughout life of the neurone and that cell death occurs randomly in time and is independent of that of any other neurone. This suggests a "one-hit" biochemical phenomenon in which the mutation imposes an abnormal mutant steady state on the neurone and a single catastrophic event randomly initiates cell death and apoptosis. Early in the course of MND, the rate of cell death is low as the amount of neuronal damage caused by the mutation is small. The delay in clinical onset was thought to reflect the gradual accumulation of damage within the neurones, as a result of the mutation, which ultimately overwhelms cellular homeostasis leading to cell death. The living mutant neurons function very well for years or decades but the probability that an individual neurone undergoes apoptosis increases as damage accumulates within it. A mutant neurone in an older patient will have accumulated a greater amount of damage and will therefore be more likely to die than in a younger patient. Consequently, early in the course of disease, the chance of a cell containing a sufficient amount of damage to initiate apoptosis is small, and the rate of cell loss is correspondingly low. The mutant neurones appear to function normally for decades, with weakness only occurring once apoptosis and cell death occurs due to a gradual accumulation of damage within the cell. Therapies aimed at preserving motor neurones may be more feasible than trying to replace lost motor neurones. A number of treatment or preventative strategies arise, such as measures to diminish SOD1 aggregation or interactions to specifically reduced apoptosis in motor neurones. As motor neurone loss at this stage is rapid and precipitous, any potential treatment will need to be given much earlier in SOD1 mutation carriers.

Determining the mechanism by which mutations in the Cu/Zn superoxide dismutase (SOD1) gene triggers the destruction of motor neurones causing MND remains unknown. At present, the favoured hypothesis is that the mutation causes disease as a result of a toxic gain of function by the mutant SOD1 provoking selective neurotoxicity, probably disrupting the intracellular homeostasis of copper and/or protein aggregation. However, as the amount of intracellular damage increases, the chance that a cell will die also increases. This cumulative damage may be due to oxidative stress, in which an imbalance between the production of reactive oxygen species and cellular antioxidant mechanisms results in chemical modifications of macromolecules, thereby disrupting cellular structure and function. It is possible that the high metabolic activity in motor neurones, combined with the toxic oxidative properties of the mutant SOD1, causes massive mitochondrial vacuolation in motor neurones, resulting in degeneration, earlier than other neurones, triggering the onset of weakness. Prominent cytoplasmic intracellular inclusions in motor neurones and within astrocytes surrounding them developed by the onset of clinical disease and in some cases represented the first pathological sign of disease. These aggregates increased in number as the disease progressed. This indicates that the mutant SOD1 toxicity is mediated by damage to mitochondria in motor neurones and this damage triggers the functional decline of motor neurones and the clinical onset of symptoms. The absence of motor neurone death in the early stages of the disease indicates that the majority of motor neurones could be rescued after early clinical diagnosis.

Regular follow-up of SOD1 carriers with MUNE may lead to early diagnosis, creating an opportunity for future novel approaches and therapies aimed at preserving motor neurones rather than replacing lost motor neurones. If the trigger initiating motor neurone loss can be identified, it may be possible to prevent motor neurone loss in familial ALS. At this stage, detecting the onset of motor neurone loss in asymptomatic individuals will identify those who may benefit from early institution of an active management program to improve their quality of life, until more effective treatment modalities become available for this devastating condition This observation is an important contribution to the current understanding of the pathogenesis of MND, as it shows that motor neurone disease does not seem to be the end result of slow attrition of motor neurones. MUNE may be able to be used as a method of pre-symptomatic testing of individuals who on genetic testing are SOD1 mutation carriers. Regular follow-up of SOD1 carriers with MUNE may lead to early diagnosis, creating an opportunity for future novel approaches and therapies aimed at preserving motor neurones rather than replacing lost motor neurones.

9. Acknowledgments

Prof. Garth Nicholson who introduced me to research into motor neurone disease and his continuing support. Prof. David Burke and Assoc. Prof. Alastair Corbett for their professional guidance and Prof. Jasper Daube for his technical assistance regarding the technique used in this research. The research was supported by the Motor Neurone Disease Association of NSW (Northern Region), ANZAC Health and Medical Research Foundation, Motor Neurone Disease Research Institute of Australia Inc. and the Nerve Research Foundation.

10. References

Aggarwal, A. (2009). Motor unit number estimation in asymptomatic familial amyotrophic lateral sclerosis. *Supplements to Clinical Neurophysiology.* 60:163-169.

Aggarwal, A. (2009). Detection of pre-clinical motor unit loss in familial amyotrophic lateral sclerosis. *Supplements to Clinical Neurophysiology.* 60:171-179.

Aggarwal, A. & Nicholson, GA. (2001). Normal complement of motor units in asymptomatic familial (SOD1 mutation) amyotrophic lateral sclerosis. J. *Neurology, Neurosurgery and Psychiatry.* 17 (4), 472-48.

Aggarwal, A. & G, Nicholson. (2002). Detection Of pre-clinical motor neurone loss in SOD1 mutation carriers using motor unit number estimation. *J of Neurology, Neurosurgery & Psychiatry.* 73(2):199-201.

Al-Chalabi, A., Andersen, P.M., Nilsson, P., Chioza, B., Andersson, J.L., Russ, C., Shaw, C.E., Powell, J., Leigh, P.N. (1999). Deletions of the heavy neurofilament subunit tail in amyotrophic lateral sclerosis. *Hum Mol Genet.*8: 157-164.

Andersen, P.M., Nilsson, P., Keranen, M.L., Forsgren, L., Hagglund, J., Karlsborg, M., Ronnevi, L.O., Gredal, O., Marklund, S.L. (1997). Phenotypic heterogenicity in motor neurone disease patients with CuZn superoxide dismutase mutations in Scandinavia. *Brain.* 120:1723-1737.

Azzouz, M., Leclerc, N., Gurney, M., Warter, J,M., Poindron, P. & Borg, J. (1997). Progressive motor neuron impairment in an animal model of familial amyotrophic lateral sclerosis. *Muscle Nerve.*20: 45-51.

Beal, M.F. (1996). Mitochondria, free radicals and neurodegeneration. *Curr Opin Neurobiol.* 6: 661-666.

Beckman, J.S., Carson, M., Smith, C.D. & Koppenol, W.H. (1993). ALS, SOD and peroxinitrate. *Nature.*364: 584.

Bensimon, G., Lacomblez, L. & Meiniger, V. (1994). A controlled trial of Riluzole in amyotrophic lateral sclerosis. ALS/Riluzole study group. *N Engl J Med.* 330 (9): 585-591.

Brown, W.F. (1972). A method for estimating the number of motor units in thenar muscles and the changes in motor unit counting with aging. *J Neurol Neurosurg Psychiatry.*35: 845-852.

Bruijn, L.I., Becher, M.W., Lee, M.K., Anderson, K.L., Jenkins, N.A., Copeland, N.G., Sisodia, S.S., Rothstein, J.D., Borchelt, D.R., Price, D.L.& Cleveland, D.W. (1997). ALS-linked SOD1 mutant G85R mediates damage to astrocytes and promotes rapidly progressive disease with SOD1-containing inclusions. *Neuron*. 18: 327-338.

Campbell, M.J., McComas, A.J. & Petito, F. (1973). Physiological changes in ageing muscles. *J Neurol Neurosurg Psychiatry*. 36: 174-182.

Chance, P.F., Rabin, B.A., Ryan, S.G., Ding, Y., Scavina, M., Crain, B., Griffith, J.W., Cornblath, D.R. (1998). Linkage of the gene for an autosomal dominant form of juvenile amyotrophic lateral sclerosis to chromosome 9q34. *Am J Hum Genet*. 62: 633-640.

Cheah, B.C., Vucic, S., Krishnan, A.V., Kiernan, M.C. (2010). Riluzole, neuroprotection and amyotrophic lateral sclerosis. *Curr Med Chem* 17(18): 1942-49.

Clarke, G., Collins, R.A., Leavitt, B.R., Andrews, D.F., Hayden, M.R., Lumsden, C.J. & McInnes, R,R. (2000). A one hit model of cell death in inherited neuronal degenerations. *Nature*. 406: 195-199.

Clarke, G., Lumsden, C.J. & McInnes, R.R. (2001). Inherited neurodegenerative disease: the one hit model of neurodegeneration. *Human Molecular Genetics*. 10: 2269-2275.

Cleveland, D.W. (1999). From Charcot to SOD1: Mechanisms of selective motor neuron death in ALS. *Neuron*. 24: 515-520.

Cudkowicz, M.E., McKenna-Yasek, D., Sapp, P.E., Chin, W., Geller, B., Hayden, D.L., Schoenfeld, D.A., Hosler, B.A., Horvitz, H.R., Brown, R.H. Jr. (1997). Epidemiology of mutations in superoxide dismutase in amyotrophic lateral sclerosis. *Ann Neurol*. 41: 210-221.

Daube, J.R. (1995). Estimating the number of motor units in a muscle. *J Clin Neurophysiol*. 12(6): 585-594.

de Belleroche, J., Orrell, R., King, A. J. (1995). Medical Genetics. Familial amyotrophic lateral sclerosis/motor neurone disease (FALS): a review of current developments. *J Med Genet*. 32: 841-847.

Doble, A. (1996). The pharmacology and mechanism of action of riluzole. *Neurology*. 47: S233-241.

Eisen, A. (1995). Amyotrophic lateral sclerosis is a multifactorial disease. *Muscle Nerve*. 18:741-752.

Felice, K.J. (1997). A longitudinal study comparing thenar motor unit number estimation to other quantitative tests in patients with amyotrophic lateral sclerosis. *Muscle Nerve*. 20: 179-185.

Figlewicz, D.A., Krizus, A., Martinoli, M.G., Meininger, V., Dib, M., Rouleau, G.A., Julein, J.P. (1994). Variants of the heavy neurofilament subunit are associated with the development of amyotrophic lateral sclerosis. *Hum Mol Genet* 3: 1757-1761.

Gurney, M.E., Pu, H., Chiu, A.Y., Dal Canto, M.C., Polchow, C.Y., Alexander, D.D., Caliendo, J., Hentati, A., Kwon, Y.W., Deng, H.X., Chen, W., Zhai, P., Sufit, R.L. & Siddique, T. (1994). Motor neuro degeneration in mice that express a human Cu/Zn superoxide dismutase mutation. *Science*. 264: 1772-1775.

Gurney, M.E., Tomasselli, A.G., Heinrikson, R.L. (1994). Stay the Executioner's hand. *Science* 2000; 288: 283-284.

Hamilton, A., Balnave, R. & Adam, R. Grip strength reliability. *J Hand Therapy*. 7(3): 163-170.

Hand, C.K. & Rouleau, G.A. (2002). Familial Amyotrophic Lateral Sclerosis. *Muscle Nerve*. 25: 135-159.

Hanten, W.P., Chen, W.Y., Austin, A.A., Brooks, R.E., Carter, H.C., Law, C.A., Morgan, M.K., Sanders, D.J., Swan, C.A. & Vanderslice, A.L. (1993). Maximum grip strength in normal subjects from 20 to 64 years of age. *J. Hand Therapy*. 12(3): 193-200.

Haverkamp, L.J., Appel, V., Appel, S.H. (1995). Natural history of amyotrophic lateral sclerosis in a database population. Validation of a scoring system and a model for survival prediction. *Brain*. 118: 707-719.

Hentati, A., Pericak-Vance, M.A., Nijhawan, D., Ahmed, A., Yang, Y., Rimmler, J., Hung, W-Y., Schlotter, B., Ahmed, A., Ben Hamida, M., Hentati, F., Siddique, T. (1998). Linkage of a commoner form of recessive amyotrophic lateral sclerosis to chromosome 15q15-q22 markers. *Neurogenetics*. 2: 55-60.

Hoagland, R.J., Mendoza, M., Armon, C., Barohn, R.J., Byran, W.W., Goodpasture, J.C., Miller, R.G., Parry, G.J., Petjan, J.H., Ross, M.A. & the Syntex / Synergen Neuroscience Joint Venture rhCNTF ALS Study Group. (1997). Reliability of maximal isometric contraction testing in multicenter study of patients with amyotrophic lateral sclerosis. *Muscle Nerve*. 20: 691-695.

Kong, J. & Xu,Z. (1998). Massive mitochondria degeneration in motor neurons triggers the onset of amyotrophic lateral sclerosis in mice expressing a mutant SOD1. *J Neurosci*. 18: 3241-3250.

Kosti, V., Jackson-Lewis, V. & Bilbao, F.D. (1997). Bcl-2: prolonging life in a transgenic mouse model of familial amyotrophic lateral sclerosis. *Science*. 227: 577.

Leigh, P.N. Amyotrophic lateral sclerosis and other motor neurone diseases. (1997). *Current Opinion Neuro Neurosurg*. 3: 567.

Li, M., Ona, V.O., Gueng, C., Chen, M., Jackson-Lewis, V., Andrews, L.J., Olszewski, A.J., Steig, P.E., Przedborski, S. & Friendlander, R.M. (2000). Functional role of caspase-1 and caspase-3 in an ALS transgenic mouse model. *Science*. 288: 335-339.

Lomen-Hoerth, C. & Slawnych, M.P. (2003). Statistical motor unit number estimation: From theory to practice. *Muscle Nerve*. 28: 263-272.

McComas, A.J., Fawcett, P.R.W., Campbell, M.J. & Sica, R.E.P. (1971). Electrophysiological estimation of the number of motor units within a human muscle. *J. Neurology, Neurosurgery and Psychiatry*. 34: 121-131.

McComas, A.J. (1971). Functional compensation in partially denervated muscles. *J Neurol Neurosurg Psychiatry* 34:453-460.

McComas, A.J. (1991). Motor unit estimation: Methods, results and present status. *Muscle Nerve*. 14: 585-597.

McComas, AJ. (1995). Motor unit estimation: The beginning. *J Clin Neurophysiol*. 12(6): 560-564.

McNeil, D. (1996). Statistical Methods.1st Edition. New York. *Wiley & Sons*; 184.

Mena, I., Marin, O., Fuenzalida, S., Cotzias, G.C. (1967). Chronic manganese poisoning. Clinical picture and manganese turnover. *Neurology*. 17: 128-136.

Miller, R.G., Mitchell, J.D., Lyon, M., Moore, D.H. (2007). Riluzole for amyotrophic lateral sclerosis (ALS / motor neuron disease (MND). *Cochrane Database Syst Rev*. 1: CD001447.

Mu, X., He, J, Anderson, M. (1996). Altered expression of bcl-2 and bax mRNA in amyotrophic lateral sclerosis spinal cord motor neurones. *Ann Neurol*. 40: 379.

Mulder, D.W., Howard, F.M. Jr. (1976). Patient resistance and prognosis in amyotrophic lateral sclerosis. *Mayo Clin Proc.*51: 537-541.

Mulder, D.W., Kurland, L.T, Offord, K.P., Beard, C.M. (1986). Familial adult motor neurone disease: amyotrophic lateral sclerosis. *Neurology.* 38: 511-517.

Needleman, H.L. (1997). Exposure to lead: Sources and effects. *N Engl J Med.* 297: 943-945.

Noor, R., Mittal, S., & Iqbal E. (2003). Superoxide dismutase – applications and relevance to human diseases. *Med Sci Monit.* 8(9): 210-215.

Olney, R.K., Yuen, E.C. & Engstrom, J.W. (2000). Statistical motor unit number estimation: Reproducibility and sources of error in patients with amyotrophic lateral sclerosis. *Muscle Nerve.* 23: 193-197.

Radunovic, A., Leigh, P.N. (1996). Cu/Zn superoxide dismutase gene mutations in amyotrophic lateral sclerosis: correlation between genotype and clinical features. *J. Neurology, Neurosurgery and Psychiatry.* 61: 565-572.

Ringel, S.P., Murphy, J.R., Alderson, M.K., Byran, W., England, J.D., Miller, R.G., Petajan, J.H., Smith, S.A., Roelofs, R.I., Ziter, F., Lee, M.Y., Brinkmann, J.R., Almada, A., Gappmaier, E., Graves, J., Herbelin, L., Mendoza, M., Mylar, D., Smith, P. & Yu, P.(1993). The natural history of amyotrophic lateral sclerosis. *Neurology.* 43: 1316-1322.

Robberecht,W. (2000). Oxidative stress in amyotrophic lateral sclerosis. *J. Neuro.* 247 (Suppl. 1): 111-116.

Rosen, D.R., Siddique, T., Patterson, D., Figlewicz, D.A., Sapp, P., Hentati, D., Donaldson, D., Goto, J., O'Regan, J.P., Deng, H.X., Rahmani, Z., Krizus, A., McKenna-Yasek, D., Cayabyab, A., Gaston, S., Berger, M., Tanzi, R.E., Halperin, .J.J, Herzfeldt, B., Van den Bergh, R., Hung, W.Y., Bird, T., Deng, G., Mulder, D.W., Smyth, C., Laing, N.G., Soriano, E., Pericak-Vance, M.A., Haines, J., Rouleau, G.A., Gusella, J.S., Horvitz, H.R. & Brown R.H., Jr. (1993). Mutations in Cu, Zn superoxide dismutase gene are associated with familial amyotrophic lateral sclerosis. *Nature.*362: 59-62.

Shaw, C.E., Enayat, Z.E., Powell, J.F., Anderson, V.E., Radunovic, A., Powell, J.F., Leigh, P.N. (1998). Mutations in all five exons of SOD1 may cause ALS. *Ann Neurol.* 43: 390-394.

Shefner, J.M. (2001). Motor unit number estimation in human neurological diseases and animal models. *Clin Neurophysiolo.* 112: 955-964.

Shefner, JM. (2009). Statistical motor unit number estimation and ALS trials: the effect of motor unit instability. *Suppl Clin Neurophysiol .*60: 135-41

Shefner, J.M., Cudkowicz, M.E., Zhang, H., Schoenfiekd, D. & Jillapalli, D. (2004). Northeast ALS Consortium. The use of statistical MUNE in multicentre clinical trials. *Muscle Nerve.* 30: 463-9.

Sica, R.E.P., McComas, A.J., Upton, A.R.M. & Longmire, D. (1974). Motor unit estimations in small muscles of the hand. *J Neurol Neurosurg Psychiatry.*37: 55-67.

Siddique, T. & Deng, H.X. (1996). Genetics of amyotrophic lateral sclerosis. *Human Mol Gen.* 5: 1465-1470.

Siddique, T., Figlewicz, D.A., Pericak-Vance, M.A., Haines, J.L., Rouleau, G.A., Jeffers, A.J., Sapp, P., Hung, W.Y., Bebout, J., McKenna-Yasek, D., Deng, G., Horvitz, H.R., Gusella, J.S., Brown, R.H., Jr., Roses, A.D. and Collaborators.(1991). Linage of a gene causing familial amyotrophic lateral sclerosis to chromosome 21 and evidence of genetic locus heterogenicity. *N Engl J Med.* 324: 1381-1384.

Siddique, T., Pericak-Vance, M.A. & Brooks, B.R. (1989). Linkage analysis in familial amyotrophic lateral sclerosis. *Neurology.* 39: 919-925.

Sjalander, A., Beckman ,G., Deng, H.Z. (1995). The D90A mutation results in a polymorphism of Cu/Zn superoxide dismutase that is prevalent in northern Sweden and Finland. Hum Mol Genet 1995; 4: 1105-1108.

Stein, R.B. & Yang, J.F. (1990). Methods of estimating the number of motor units in human muscles. *Ann Neurol.* 28: 487-495.

Talbot, K. (2002). Motor neurone disease. *Muscle Nerve.* 25: 513-519.

Trotti, D., Rolfs, A., Danbolt, N.C., Brown, R.H. Jr, Hediger, M.A. (1999). SOD1 mutations linked to amyotrophic lateral sclerosis selectively activates a glial glutamate transporter. *Na Neurosci.* 19: 427-433.

Vechio, J.D., Bruijn, L.I., Xu, Z., Brown, R.H. Jr, (1996). Cleveland ,D.W. Sequence variants in the human neurofilament proteins: absence of linkage to familial amyotrophic lateral sclerosis. Ann Neurol 1996; 40: 603-610.

Yim, M.B., Chock, P.B. & Stadtman, E.R. (1990). Copper, zinc superoxide dismutase catalyses hydroxyl radial production from hydrogen peroxide. *Proc Natl Acad Sci.* 87:5006-5010.

14

Overview of Cognitive Function in ALS, with Special Attention to the Temporal Lobe: Semantic Fluency and Rating the Approachability of Faces

Heike Schmolck[1,3], Paul Schulz[1,2,4] and Michele York[1,2]

[1]*Baylor*
[2]*Veterans Hospital*
[3]*Ruan Neuroscience Center*
[4]*University of Texas*
USA

1. Introduction

Amyotrophic lateral sclerosis (ALS) is a progressive neurodegenerative disorder that affects upper and lower motor neurons and is more recently known to be associated with declines in cognitive and behavioral functions for a subset of patients (Strong, et al., 1996; Strong et al., 2009). The cognitive changes associated with ALS can vary from mild impairments that may or may not affect the individual's daily functioning to more severe cognitive and behavioral changes that meet criteria for a diagnosis of frontotemporal dementia (ALS-FTD). There are at least mild cognitive changes in 40 to 60% of sporadic and familial ALS patients (Massman et al., 1996; Phukan et al., 1996; Ringholz et al., 2005; Wheaton et al., 2007). The cognitive and behavioral changes associated with ALS follow a pattern consistent with involvement of the frontal and temporal lobes (Strong et al., 2009, Hodges et al., 2004), presenting as difficulties with attention, working memory, verbal fluency, and semantic abilities (Abe et al., 1997; Ringholz et al., 2005; Rippon et al., 2006, Schmolck et al., 2007; Strong et al, 1999; Strong et al., 2009). Furthermore, 15% of ALS patients demonstrate more severe cognitive and behavioral changes consistent with ALS-FTD (Lomen-Hoeth et al., 2002; Ringholz et al., 2005; Wheaton et al., 2007), presenting as declines in judgment, problem solving, and reasoning, which are more frontally mediated cognitive functions. In addition to cognitive changes, up to 25% of patients with ALS may also experience significant changes in their behavior, mood, and personality characteristics (Hodges et al., 2004; Kertesz et al., 2005), including a loss of empathy, problems with organization and planning, changes in social behavior and personality, difficulties with impulse control, and apathy.

The temporal lobes are purported to be involved in auditory perception, language comprehension, naming, processing of semantic knowledge and long-term memory storage, high-level visual processing of complex stimuli such as faces and scenes, and episodic memory (Lezak, 1995). In addition, they contain the amygdala and associated limbic areas, which are key structures for processing emotional stimuli and detecting threat from the environment, and are of particular interest for ALS patients. ALS patients show a lack of memory enhancement for highly emotional stimuli (Abrahams et al., 2005). Furthermore, social judgment was found to be decreased in individuals with ALS as compared to healthy controls (Flaherty-Craig et al., 2011). Behavioral dysfunction has been linked to decreased performance on cognitive measures; however it is unclear if these changes present and/or progress independently (Wooley et al., 2009). The relationship between the fontal and temporal cognitive and behavioral changes in ALS is not well understood. Here, we report on two studies examining temporal cognitive changes in ALS.

Indentifying and acknowledging that ALS patients may also be dealing with cognitive and/or behavioral changes in addition to their debilitating motor declines may help their physicians and caregivers to better care for the individual with ALS and anticipate problems that they may experience throughout the disease progression (Hecht et al., 2003). These cognitive changes can affect the everyday social interactions of ALS patients, and they are vital for the execution of more complex tasks such as decision-making, problem solving, and management of occupational demands (e.g., multi-tasking). Patients with these types of impairments have significantly shorter survival than other ALS patients and are twice as likely to be noncompliant with interventions (Woolley et al., 2008). Safety, financial planning, driving, and occupational performance can be of concern in patients who demonstrate impairments in these cognitive domains. Consequently, the predictive value of these cognitive abilities may aid in the clinical management of ALS patients, aiding physicians in making decisions concerning the overall safety of their patients and their patients' ability to work, drive, and manage their medication regimen. Educating the patients and family members to better understand these cognitive and behavioral changes as part of the disease process can help improve the patient's quality of life and reduce the feelings of caregiver burden (Murphy et al., 2009).

2. Rating the approachability of faces in ALS – Too much or not enough fear?

We hypothesize that alterations in emotional cognition indicative of amygdala dysfunction occur in ALS, but are often unrecognized. Changes in the emotional expression of ALS patients are reported by clinicians, and often by patients themselves. Pseudobulbar affect is a common problem. ALS patients also have a lower incidence of depression than patients afflicted with similarly debilitating diseases (Rabkin et al., 2005), and many have a stunning lack of concern regarding their grave illness. They often have a very pleasant personality, which has lead clinicians to call ALS the "nice guy's disease". Emotional lability and mild disinhibition are commonly found.

None of the above observations can be explained satisfactorily by behavioral changes commonly seen with frontal dysfunction alone. Thus, while examining frontal contributions to social and emotional cognitive changes in ALS has been fruitful, other areas that have been implicated in social cognition have not been studied much. In one study, ALS patients have been found to show a lack of memory enhancement for highly emotional stimuli, which is consistent with amygdala dysfunction (Abrahams et al., 2005). We have previously shown in a small group of patients that ALS patients have a tendency to rate faces inappropriately approachable compared to normal controls (Schmolck et al., 2007); this behavior is also consistent with amygdala dysfunction. Lastly, a study by Zimmerman and colleagues (2007) found that over 62% of patients with bulbar ALS had deficits in their ability to properly recognize the emotions of others (emotional perceptual deficits).

Few neuropathologic studies have examined non-frontal areas in ALS brains. In the ALS-Parkinson-dementia complex of Guam, tau and alpha-synuclein aggregates are a common finding in the amygdala (for example, Yamazaki et al., 2000). Case series of sporadic ALS patients with and without dementia have demonstrated ubiquitinated intraneuronal inclusions and spongiform changes in the amygdala and other limbic structures (Kawashima et al., 2001; Kato et al., 1994; also Tsuchiya 2002).

The amygdala is a key structure for processing emotional stimuli and detecting threat from the environment (e.g., Adolphs 2003a; Adolphs 2003b). Patients with bilateral amygdala damage are impaired at recognizing negative basic emotions in facial expressions, most notably fear (e.g., Adolphs et al., 1994; Broks et al., 1998;, Schmolck & Squire 2001) . In a much broader sense, they also have difficulties making social judgments, and interpreting social signals about intentions and internal states (e.g. Adolphs 2003b); for example, patients are differentially impaired at recognizing complex social emotions relative to complex non-social emotions (Adolphs et al., 2002), and assigning emotional states to people (e.g. Fine et al., 2001) and objects (anthropomorphizing; Heberlein & Adolphs, 2004). This is also seen clinically when patients get themselves into unfavorable situations because they are unable to correctly read and act on threatening environmental and social stimuli. Adolphs et al. (1998) replicated this observation most closely in a laboratory experiment, showing that patients indiscriminately rated unfamiliar faces as approachable and trustworthy while controls did not.

We administered the same task to ALS patients hypothesizing that their "nice" personalities and strikingly good morale in facing a debilitating disease might be due, at least in part, to amygdala dysfunction as part of a broader multi-system disorder.

2.1 Participants

91 ALS patients were recruited from the MDA-ALS clinic and the ALSA clinic at Baylor College of Medicine. 78 age and gender matched controls were recruited from 2 groups – family members and friends of ALS patients, as well as patients from the Baylor Cardiology CHF clinic (n = 24). The latter group was chosen to control for the effects of living with a serious life threatening chronic illness. Data from both control groups were combined in the final analysis, as there were no significant differences between groups. Please see Table 1 for demographic characteristics for both groups.

	ALS	CON
Gender		
Male	54.9%	54.3%
Female	45.1%	45.7%
Age		
Mean	50.4	58
Range	22-78	30-84
Disease Type		
Limb onset	61.5%	
Bulbar onset	27.5%	
No information	10.9%	
Disease Duration		
Mean	2.5 years	
Range	0.5 – 14 years	

Table 1. Demographic Characteristics of Participants

2.2 Methods

Participants viewed 60 images of faces (Adolphs et al., 1998) in a pseudo-random order on a computer screen. 40 faces were excluded to reduce testing time. We chose the 20 most approachable, the 20 least approachable, and the 20 intermediate faces. Faces expressed a mix of neutral or emotional expressions. Before viewing, participants were given the following case scenario:

"Imagine you are in a city you do not know well, you are by yourself, it is getting dark and you have lost directions. You see many people on the street. You need to decide who you would like to approach to ask for directions.

We will show you 60 faces. For each face, we would like you to decide how approachable that person is in the particular situation that you are in."

Participants were then instructed to respond with an answer between –3 and 3, and were given examples of what each rating would mean. There was no time limitation. Answers were recorded by the examiner. To minimize gender effects, all faces that had received different ratings ($p < .10$) from male and female controls were eliminated from further analysis; 51 faces remained.

As part of their initial ALS evaluation in the MDA-ALS or ALSA Clinic, several patients (n = 49) were given a comprehensive neuropsychological interview and testing battery and received a cognitive diagnosis: cognitively intact, subtle deficits, mild-to-moderate or severe (FTD) deficits (see Table 2).

2.3 Results

For each participant, three means were calculated – overall mean rating, mean rating for the 10 most approachable faces, and mean rating for the 10 least approachable faces. We then divided participants into Trusters, Suspicious Responders (SR) and Conventional Responders (CR). Participants were labeled Trusters if their average rating for the 10 least approachable faces was above zero; i.e. they regarded even those faces as approachable that controls would not have approached. They were labeled Suspicious Responders if their average rating for the 10 most approachable faces was lower than 1, indicating that they felt faces difficult to approach that controls found very approachable.

While 65.4% of participants in the control group were CR, 62.6% in the ALS group were either Trusters or Suspicious Responders (Figure 1 "minority responders"; Chi square test $p < .001$).

Thirty-one ALS patients were Trusters, 26 were SR, and 34 were CR (34.1%, 28.6% and 37.4%, respectively). In the control group, 16 were Trusters, 11 SR and 51 CR (20.5%, 14.1% and 65.4%, respectively). Both Trusters (34.1% vs. 20.5%) and Suspicious Responders (28.6% vs. 14.1%) were significantly more common in the ALS group (Chi Square tests; both ps < .01) than in the control group.

We previously reported results on 26 patients (Schmolck et al., 2007); only Trusters were identified in that subgroup (n = 14) since that was a common response pattern. In retrospect, the SR pattern was present in 3 patients but not recognized at the time. Our finding in a large group of ALS patients thus not only confirms our earlier results, but also expands them to describe a new common response pattern in the ALS group.

In the subgroup of 49 patients with neuropsychological testing, there was no clear correlation between cognitive diagnosis and performance on the faces task (Table 2). In the small number of patients with FTD (n = 8), half of patients were CR and half of patients were Trusters (Table 2).

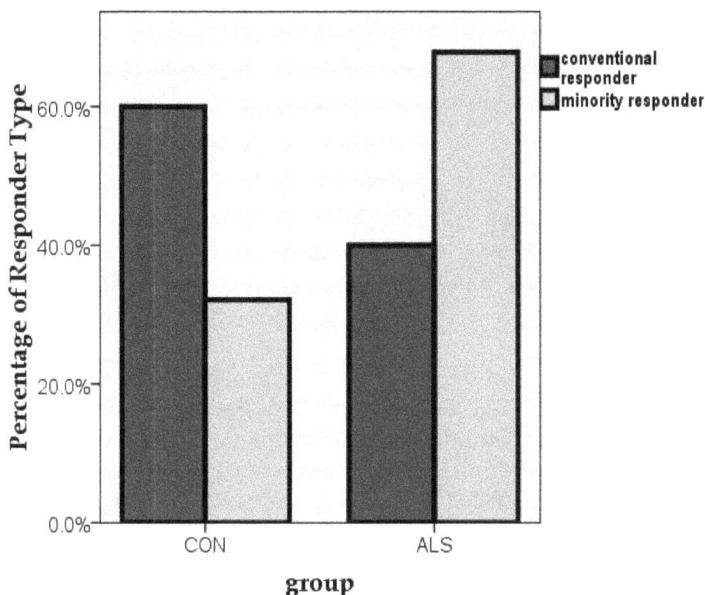

Fig. 1. Significantly more ALS patients were minority responders (Trusters and Suspicious
Responders combined)

	Cognitive Diagnosis				
	Intact	Subtle	MiMo	FTD	Total
Conventional Responder	10	3	3	4	20
Truster	10	1	1	4	16
Suspicious Responder	5	2	6	0	13
Total	25	6	10	8	49

Table 2. Cognitive Performance and Responder Type in the subgroup of patients with
neuropsychological testing results. MiMo – Mild to moderate impairment

2.4 Discussion

We have shown that more than half of our patients with ALS have an abnormal response
pattern. One response pattern (Trusters) shows similar behavioral characteristics to patients
with bilateral amygdala damage on a paradigm asking participants to judge the
approachability of unfamiliar faces. This difficulty can be generalized as an inability to
correctly recognize threat in a given social context. A person with this behavioral pattern
would be expected to be trusting, friendly and open to cooperation, and show very little
hostility or suspicion. Many clinicians caring for ALS patients have noted this type of
personality in ALS patients. The second response pattern is that of overly suspicious
behavior (SR). These patients will be overly reluctant to approach unfamiliar faces, also
showing poor discrimination between approachable and less approachable faces. These

patients show a response pattern that might be seen in autism (e.g. Baron-Cohen et al., 2001), or patients with anxiety disorder or social phobia, which have both been linked to hyperactivity of the amygdala (e.g. Freitas-Ferrari et al., 2010; Blair et al., 2011). Clinically, this patient population might not be easily recognized if not specifically probed by the examiner during history taking.

There are some clues regarding the basic mechanism by which amygdala damage leads to impairments making social judgments from faces. Complex mental states are recognized disproportionately from the eye region of the face, and when making judgments about mental states from the eye region, healthy controls activate the amygdala in functional imaging studies (Baron-Cohen et al., 1999; Baron-Cohen et al., 2001). Bilateral damage to the amygdala has been shown to impair the recognition of negative basic emotions in facial expressions, notably fear (e.g. Adolphs et al., 1994; Calder et al., 1996; Broks et al., 1998; Anderson et al., 2000). Investigating the first patient reported to show this deficit (S.M.), Adolphs and colleagues (2005) demonstrated that her impairment stems from an inability to make normal use of information from the eye region of faces when judging emotions. They traced this deficit to a lack of spontaneous fixations on the eyes during free viewing of faces. Although SM fails to look normally at the eye region in all facial expressions, her selective impairment in recognizing fear is explained by the fact that the eyes are the most important feature for identifying this emotion. It is thus likely that inadequate evaluation of the eye region leads to impairments in the Approachability Task, and perhaps in some real life situations. While this mechanism may explain some of the impairments in social cognition seen in patients with amygdala damage, it would not explain others, such as detection of fear and anger from voices (Scott et al., 1997) impaired anthropomorphizing (Heberlein et al., 2004), or inferring internal mental states (Fine et al., 2001).

Performance on the Approachability Paradigm was not related to frontal dysfunction. While we cannot be certain, this suggests that the response pattern seen in the patients without frontal dysfunction was more likely to be due to amygdala involvement. Healthy volunteers judging the trustworthiness of faces activate the amygdala bilaterally for faces judged untrustworthy in an fMRI paradigm (Winston et al., 2002). Also, even in the presence of overt FTD, only half of the patients had abnormal performance on the Approachability Paradigm.

3. Phonemic and semantic verbal fluency in ALS

Verbal fluency tasks, which require an individual to generate words starting with a specified letter (phonemic fluency) or in a specified category (semantic fluency), have been shown to be sensitive tools for identifying cognitive dysfunction in neurologically impaired populations (Canning, Leach, Struss, Ngo, & Black, 2004; Ho et al., 2002; Fangundo et al., 2008; Libon et al., 2009). Phonemic fluency involves prefrontal and frontal functions because it requires strategic processes for searching the lexicon (Leggio, Silveri, Petrosini, & Molinari,, 2000; Martin, Wiggs, Lalonde, & Mack, 1994), while semantic fluency localizes more to the left anterior temporal lobe, where representations are categorized by meaning (Pihlajamki et al., 2000). Recent functional magnetic resonance imaging (fMRI) studies have verified the neuroanatomical locations involved in phonemic fluency in the left premotor and inferior frontal gyrus and for semantic fluency in the left fusiform and left middle temporal gyrus (Bim et al., 2009; Meinzer et al., 2009). Consequently, by evaluating ALS patient performances on phonemic and semantic fluencies, we were able to investigate frontal and temporal function in ALS patients.

The cognitive substrates underlying verbal fluency have been examined further in neuropsychological studies (Baldo, Schwartz Wilkins & Dronkers, 2006; Troyer, Moscovitch, & Winocur, 1997). Clustering and switching have been shown to be components that underlie verbal fluency performance (Troster et al., 1998; Troyer et al., 1997). Clusters are groups of related words, accessed through memory stores, in which intact performance is purported to rely on temporal lobe functioning. Switching refers to the process of changing from one cluster to another, which has been associated with frontal-lobe-mediated abilities (Troyer et al., 1998). We investigated differences in phonemic and semantic fluency between ALS patients, classified into neurocognitive subgroups, and healthy participants and whether these declines in verbal fluency were due predominantly to changes in clustering, switching, or a combination of the two component processes (Lepow et al., 2010).

3.1 Participants

A total of 49 ALS patients and 25 healthy control participants (HC) were recruited from the Baylor College of Medicine (BCM) ALS Association Clinic. The HC participants were caregivers or family members of the ALS patients who participated in this study. ALS patients' motor functioning was evaluated by the ALS Functional Rating Scale (ALS-FRS), and their site of onset (limb vs. bulbar) was recorded at their initial clinic visit.

A subset of these ALS patients (N = 36) underwent a comprehensive neuropsychological assessment, and these data were used to classify participants as cognitively intact (ALS-intact), mildly impaired (ALS-mild), or FTD (ALS-FTD). Patients were coded as ALS-FTD using Strong et al.'s (2009) criteria. Patients were coded as ALS-mild if their neuropsychological evaluation, excluding their performance on phonemic and semantic fluency measures, revealed cognitive deficits (<1.5 SDs below the mean for the appropriate normative sample) in one cognitive domain. The ALS cognitive impaired classification (ALSci) described by Strong et al. (2009) is based on impairments in executive functioning only; however, we excluded both phonemic and semantic fluency so as not to classify patients based on the measures under investigation. Hence, additional measures of executive functioning were limited. Consequently, patients were classified based on their entire comprehensive evaluation.

3.2 Methods
3.2.1 Neuropsychological evaluation

The comprehensive neuropsychological assessment examined basic orientation (Mini Mental Status Examination [Folstein Folstein & McHugh, 1975]), attention/ information-processing speed (Wechsler Adult Intelligence Scale-3rd Edition, [WAIS-III; The Psychological Corporation, 1997], Digit Span, Trail Making Test Part A, and Verbal Sustained Attention Test), verbal learning (Rey Auditory Verbal Learning Test [Schmidt, 1996], visual learning (Brief Visual Memory Test-Revised), language (Boston Naming Test [Kaplan, Goodglass, & Weintraub, 1983]), visual-spatial abilities (Rey-Osterrieth Complex Figure Test [Meyers, & Meyers 1995], WAIS-III Block Design), and executive function (Wisconsin Card Sorting Test [Heaton, 1981], Trail Making Test Part B).

3.2.2 Fluency scoring methods

Verbal fluency tests were administered to ALS patients and HC in the following manner: Patients were asked to generate a list of words that began with a specific letter (F, A, & S was used for phonemic fluency) or category (Animals was used for semantic fluency) in a 1-minute period. Prior to administering the test, patients were told that proper nouns and root words with different suffices were not allowed. Words generated (including repetitions and rule breaks) were recorded verbatim. The total number of words generated, excluding repetitions and rule breaks, was the standard measure of analysis and Troyer's (Troyer et al, 1997) scoring methods for clustering and switching were utilized.

3.2.3 Verbal fluency components

Phonemic fluency. Clusters are scored for groups of phonemic words, or words that are similar based on phonemic rules for each letter. Troyer and colleagues (1997) defined parameters for scoring clusters, including: (a) words beginning with the same first two letters, (b) rhyming words, and (c) words that are the same syllabic length and differ only by a vowel sound. For example, *follow, fog, fond, foster, forget* is a cluster of four because the words all begin with the same phoneme, and the cluster size begins with the second word of a cluster. Each word that is not classified in a group of related phonemic words is scored as a cluster of zero. The *number of clusters* is defined as the total sum of individual clusters, including clusters of zero. The *cluster value* is defined as the sum number of consecutive related words excluding the first word of each grouping, or the sum of the values assigned to the clusters. *Switches* are defined as any break between clusters, including clusters of zero.

Semantic fluency. In the semantic fluency task, clusters are composed of words that are semantically related. Troyer's method defines the categories for finding semantic clusters in "Animals" as living environments, zoological categories, and human use, with each supraordinate category containing specific exemplars. The *cluster size* begins with the second word of a cluster. For example the group, *cow, horse, chicken,* and *rooster,* is scored as a cluster of three because they are all farm animals. Number of clusters, cluster value, and switches were calculated as discussed above.

3.3 Results
3.3.1 Participant characteristics

The 49 ALS patients and the 25 HCs did not differ in age or education level (Table 1). There were significantly more female HCs than female ALS patients (p=0.006). Gender correlated significantly with Troyer's average number of switches for phonemic fluency; thus, gender was entered as a covariate in this analysis. There were no significant demographic differences between the three groups of ALS patients coded for degree of cognitive dysfunction (Table 1), including site of onset (p = 0.36) and total ALS-FRS scores (p = 0.34).

Phonemic fluency. ALS patients generated fewer numbers of clusters than did HCs (p = 0.04; Figure 1). ALS patients also generated fewer switches between clusters; however, once gender was entered as a covariate in the analysis, this difference was no longer significant (p =0.14). The number of clusters differed significantly between the ALS groups, with the ALS-intact group scoring higher than the ALS-mild and the ALS-FTD groups (p = 0.004; Table 2). The number of switches also differed between the ALS cognitive groups, with the ALS-

Overview of Cognitive Function in ALS, with Special Attention to the Temporal Lobe: Semantic Fluency and Rating
the Approachability of Faces
299

intact patients switching more often than both the ALS-mild and the ALS-FTD groups (p =0 .004; Table 2). The cluster value scores did not differ significantly between the ALS groups (p=0 .13).

Table 1	ALS				HC (n=25)	p-value
	Intact (n=13)	Mild (n=17)	FTD (n=7)	Total (n=49)		
Gender (M/F)	8/5	10/7	3/4	28/21	6/19	**0.006**
Age (yrs)	54.2 (8.96)	58.1 (12.1)	61.4 (14.2)	56.1 (11.3)	52.7 (13.0)	0.28
Education (yrs)	14.1 (2.95)	13.3 (1.32)	12.9 (3.44)	13.8 (2.71)	15.2 (2.99)	0.07

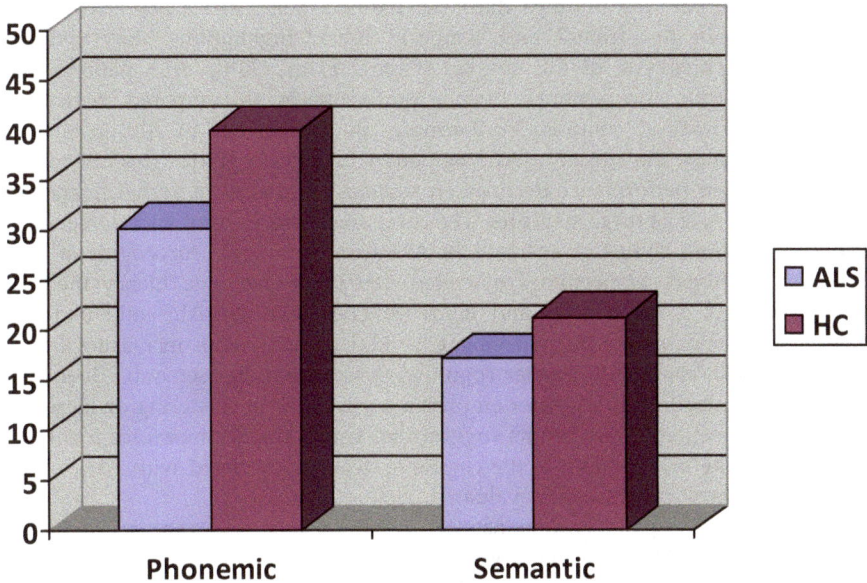

Fig. 1. Total Phonemic and Semantic Fluency Scores for ALS and HC groups

Semantic fluency. The total group of ALS patients generated fewer numbers of clusters (p = 0.01) and made significantly fewer switches between clusters (p =0.03) than did the HCs. The total groups did not differ significantly on the number of words within semantic clusters (cluster value=0.15). The ALS-FTD patients generated a smaller cluster value score than did ALS-intact and ALS-mild groups (p=0.03). The number of clusters and number of switches demonstrated trends toward significant differences between the groups (p=0.07, p= 0.06, respectively; Table 2).

Table 2	ALS intact Mean (SD)	ALS mild Mean (SD)	ALS FTD Mean (SD)	p-value
Total				
Phonemic	37.2 (10.9) [1,2]	30.1 (9.76) [1]	23.3 (6.54) [2]	**0.009**
Semantic	19.0 (5.29) [1,2]	18.3 (5.72) [1]	12.9 (4.05) [2]	**0.02**
Troyer				
Phonemic Fluency				
Number of Clusters	9.84 (2.34)[1,2]	7.15 (2.79)[1]	6.43 (2.17)[2]	**0.004**
Cluster Value	3.20 (1.77)	2.72 (1.62)	1.67 (1.12)	0.13
Switches	8.84 (2.34) [1,2]	6.15 (2.81) [1]	5.43 (2.17) [2]	**0.004**
Semantic Fluency				
Cluster Value	10.94 (3.78)[1]	8.85 (3.83)	6.43 (3.41)[1]	**0.03**
Number of clusters	10.59 (3.73)	8.54 (3.26)	7.29 (1.98)	0.07
Switches	9.59 (3.73)	7.46 (3.20)	6.29 (1.98)	0.06

3.4 Discussion

These results support the findings that ALS patients demonstrate cognitive impairment localizing to both the frontal and temporal lobes, highlighting the frontotemporal neurocognitive phenotype of this disease (Lepow et al., 2010). ALS patients exhibited decreased phonemic and semantic fluency performances as compared to healthy non-neurologically impaired controls. Furthermore, in comparison to ALS patients whose cognition was intact, the subset of ALS patients with mild cognitive dysfunction or ALS-FTD demonstrated performance declines on standard measures of verbal fluency and the component processes of these measures. The component processes of verbal fluency provide a unique opportunity to further evaluate the ALS frontotemporal neurocognitive phenotype from slightly different perspective (Troyer et al., 1997). For phonemic fluency, the intact ALS sample generated fewer clusters and more switches than the ALS-mild and ALS-FTD patients, suggesting temporal involvement in ALS patients, with increasing frontal lobe involvement in patients with greater cognitive dysfunction. For semantic fluency, similar results were obtained with a greater emphasis on declines in clustering or increased temporal lobe dysfunction. These results suggest that verbal fluency measures identify frontal and temporal lobe involvement in the cognitive decline associated with ALS, particularly when the component processes are evaluated.

As a group, the ALS patients demonstrated temporal lobe involvement as compared to individuals without ALS. However, when the ALS patients were stratified based on their level of cognitive dysfunction, the influence of the frontal lobe involvement became more pertinent to their ability to perform this task. In conclusion, the differences in phonemic and semantic fluency scores between ALS patients and HCs suggest temporal lobe involvement in ALS patients with increasing frontal lobe involvement across the neurocognitive spectrum of the disease. A frontotemporal neurocognitive phenotype is revealed in ALS patients who demonstrate cognitive changes.

4. General discussion

Up until the late 1980s, the prevalent view in the neurological literature was that ALS was a pure motor neuron disease only infrequently affecting cognitive function. This view has

Overview of Cognitive Function in ALS, with Special Attention to the Temporal Lobe: Semantic Fluency and Rating
the Approachability of Faces
301

changed in the last decade with several neuropsychological and functional imaging studies
confirming common involvement of cortex outside the motor strip. The concept of primarily
frontal lobe dysfunction in motor neuron disease was introduced by Montgomery and
Erickson (1987) as well as Iwasaki et al. (1990). Several studies have since confirmed the
association between FTLD, executive dysfunction, and ALS (eg. Massman et al., 1996; Strong
et al., 2009). The largest study examining cognitive function in ALS to date found that 51%
of patients had varying degrees of executive dysfunction (Ringholz et al., 2005; n = 279).
These numbers confirmed an earlier study by Lomen-Hoerth and colleagues (2003) who had
found evidence for frontal executive deficits in half of their patients, many of whom met
criteria for Frontotemporal Lobar Degeneration.

Whereas frontal pathology has become the focus of cognitive investigation in ALS patients,
the integrity of temporal structures (apart from the hippocampal formation) in ALS has not
received much attention. Temporal pathology is a hallmark of FTLD, and several behavioral
observations in ALS patients could suggest temporal pathology.

Several imaging studies and neuropathological investigations suggest that involvement of
the temporal cortex, as well as the amygdala and other limbic structures in the disease
process is very likely. Kew et al. (1993) showed reduced blood flow (rCBF) in the anterior
cingulate cortex, the medial prefrontal cortex (Brodmann area 9 and 10), parahippocampal
gyri and the anterior thalamic nuclear complex. Abrahams and colleagues (1995) observed
decreased activity across a wide area of the frontal lobes, which also included the insular
cortex and thalamic nuclear complex. In a small sample of clinically non-demented patients,
there was a decrease in cerebral blood flow of the frontal and temporal lobes, despite normal
MR imaging (Kokubo et al., 2003). Recently, a morphometric study of gray matter volume
on MR scans revealed significant differences between patients with ALS and normal
controls, predominantly in fronto-temporal areas, regardless of cognitive status; that is, the
differences in gray matter volume between the ALS group as a whole and the control group
were much more extensive than differences between cognitively normal and demented ALS
patients (Chang et al., 2005).

There have been a limited number of neuropathological studies looking at frontal and
temporal pathology in ALS. Wilson et al. (2001) found changes that where overall more
pronounced for cognitively affected patients (ubiquitin positive, alpha-synuclein-negative,
and tau-negative neuronal inclusions), most pronounced in the cingulate cortex. Cognitive
impairment was uniformly associated with superficial linear spongiosis, a pathologic
feature common to several forms of frontotemporal dementia. Wilson and colleagues did
not study temporal structures in more detail. In a group of ALS patients with cognitive
impairment, and decreased frontal blood flow on SPECT, neuropathologic examination
showed spongy degeneration and neuronal loss in the frontal lobe (Abe et al., 1997).

Pathologically, there is also a special tie between semantic dementia, or temporal variant
FTD, and ALS. Both FTD-MND (or FTD-ALS) and semantic dementia are characterized by
ubiquinated inclusions (FTD-U); the clinical spectrum of patients seen with this
histopathological finding varies from ALS, ALS with FTD and semantic dementia without
ALS (Davies & Xuereb, 2007). This suggests that patients with ALS caused by this
histopathological subtype would be expected to have overt or subtle features of temporal
involvement, especially impairments in semantic processing and amygdala function.

Some studies have specifically evaluated the limbic system in sporadic ALS. In the ALS-
Parkinson-dementia complex of Guam, tau and alpha-synuclein aggregates are a common

finding in the amygdala (e.g., Yamazaki et al., 2000). Case series of sporadic ALS patients with and without dementia have demonstrated ubiquitinated intraneuronal inclusions and spongiform changes in the neostriatum, the amygdala and the parahippocampal gyrus, as well as the temporal pole, anterior cingulate, orbitofrontal cortex and insula (Kawashima et al., 2001; Kato et al., 1994, also Tsuchiya et al., 2002).

We assume that the cognitive findings of decreased semantic fluency and abnormal approachability are the clinical correlate of the changes seen neuroradiologically and neuropathologically and suggest that many ALS patients may, in fact, have both clinically relevant amygdala dysfunction and difficulties with semantic processing.

Performance on the Approachability Paradigm was not related to frontal dysfunction. A similar lack of correlation between amygdala dysfunction and frontal cognitive changes was reported by Zimmerman and colleagues (2007). In their study, among the 8 patients with emotional perceptual impairment, one-half did not have depressive, or memory or cognitive symptoms on screening, whereas the remainder showed dementia symptoms alone or together with depressive symptoms. This finding is important in two ways: First, it suggests the response pattern seen in ALS patients in both studies was in fact due to amygdala involvement as hypothesized and was less likely to be the result of frontal dysfunction

Second, FTLD is known to have several subtypes with variable sites of onset, all of which can be seen in conjunction with ALS. Thus, it is not surprising to find that amygdala dysfunction and frontal dysfunction are not associated. It may be that there are groups of ALS patients that have predominantly temporal dysfunction at onset, while other groups have predominantly frontal onset. This also suggests that more ALS patients have clinical involvement outside the motor strip than the rough estimate of 50% percent from prior studies, which mainly concentrated on frontal cognitive dysfunction.

5. Conclusion

We have shown that more than half of patients with ALS have unusual response patterns on a paradigm asking participants to judge the approachability of unfamiliar faces, suggesting amygdala dysfunction. Performance on this task did not correlate with frontal-executive dysfunction on cognitive testing. Patients also had significantly reduced semantic fluency suggesting involvement of the temporal cortex. Disease involvement outside the motor cortex in ALS is common, and can manifest as frontal, temporal or frontal and temporal dysfunction. Further studies need to be done to clarify the relationship between histopathological subtypes and cognitive patterns.

6. References

Abe K, Fujimura H, Toyooka K, Sakoda S, Yorifuji S & Yanagihara T. (1997) Cognitive function in amyotrophic lateral sclerosis. *J Neurol Sci.* 1997 May 1;148(1):95-100.

Abrahams S, Leigh PN, Kew JJ, Goldstein LH, Lloyd CM & Brooks DJ. (1995) A positron emission tomography study of frontal lobe function (verbal fluency) in amyotrophic lateral sclerosis. *J Neurol Sci.* 1995 May;129 Suppl:44-6.

Abrahams S, Leigh PN, Harvey A, Vythelingum GN, Grise D, Goldstein LH. (2000) Verbal fluency and executive dysfunction in amyotrophic lateral sclerosis (ALS). *Neuropsychologia* 2000;38:734-747.

Adolphs R (2003) Cognitive Neuroscience of Human Social Behavior. *Nature Reviews Neuroscience* 4: 165 – 178

Adolphs R (2003) Is the human amygdala specialized for processing social information? *Ann NY Acad. Sci.* 985: 326 – 340

Adolphs R, Baron-Cohen S & Tranel D (2002) Impaired Recognition of social emotions following amygdala damage. *Journal of Cognitive Neuroscience* 14: 1264 - 1274

Adolphs R, Tranel D & Damasio AR (1998) The human amygdala in social judgment. *Nature.* 1998 Jun 4;393(6684):470-4.

Adolphs R, Gosselin F, Buchanan TW, Tranel D, Schyns P & Damasio AR (2005). A mechanism for impaired fear recognition after amygdala damage. *Nature.* 2005 Jan 6;433(7021):68-72.

Baldo J., Schwartz S., Wilkins D., & Dronkers N. (2006). Role of frontal versus temporal cortex in verbal fluency as revealed by voxel-based lesion symptom mapping. *Journal of the International Neuropsychological Society, 12,* 896-900.

Bim, R. M., Kenworthy, L., Case, L., Caravella, R., Jones, T. B., Bandettini, P. A., et al. (2010). Neural systems supporting phonemic search guided by letter and semantic category cues; A self-paced overt response fMRI study of verbal fluency. *NeuroImage, 49,* 1099-1107. doi:10.1016/j.neuroimage.2009.07.036

Blair KS, Geraci M, Krelitz K, OteroM, Ernst M, Leibenluft E, Blair RJ & Pine DS (2011) The pathology of social phobia is independent of developmental changes in faces processing. *American Journal of Psychiatry* Jun 1 Epub ahead of print

Canning, S. J., Leach, L., Struss, D., Ngo, L., & Black, S. E. (2004). Diagnostic utility of abbreviated fluency measures in Alzheimer disease and vascular dementia. *Neurology, 62,* 556-562.

Chang JL, Lomen-Hoerth C, Murphy J, Henry RG, Kramer JH, Miller BL, Gorno-Tempini ML. (2005) A voxel-based morphometry study of patterns of brain atrophy in ALS and ALS/FTLD. *Neurology* 2005;65:75-8

Davies RR & Xuereb JH (2007) The histopathology of frontotemporal dementia *in* Hodges JR (ed.) *Frontotemporal Dementia Syndromes,* Cambridge University Press, Cambridge pp. 161 - 207

Fagundo, A. B., Lopez, S., Romero, M., Guarch, J., Marcos, T., &. Salamero, M. (2008). Clustering and switching in semantic fluency: Predictors of the development of Alzheimer's disease. *International Journal of Geriatric Psychiatry, 23,* 1007-1013.

Flaherty-Craig, C., Brothers, A., yang, C., Svoboda, R., Simmons, Z. (2011). Decreases in problem solving and anosognosia in amyotrophic lateral sclerosis: Applications of Guilford's structure of intellect theory. *Cogn Behav Neurol;* 24(1): 26-34.

Folstein M. F., Folstein S. E., & McHugh P. R. (1975). Mini-mental state: A practical method for grading the cognitive state of patients for the clinician. *Journal of Psychiatric Research. 12,* 189-198.

Frank B, Haas J, Heinze HJ, Stark E & Munte TF (1997) Relation of neuropsychological and magnetic resonance findings in amyotrophic lateral sclerosis: evidence for subgroups. *Clin Neurol Neurosurg.* 1997 May;99(2):79-86.

Freitas-Ferrari MC, Hallak JE, Trzesniak C, Filho AS. Machado-de-Sousa JP, Chagas MH, Nardi AE, Crippa JA (2010) Neuroimaging in social anxiety disorder: a systematic review of the literature. *Prog Neuropsychopharmacol Biol Psychiatry* 34(4):565-80

Hamann S & Mao H. (2002) Positive and negative emotional verbal stimuli elicit activity in the left amygdala. *Neuroreport.* 2002 Jan 21;13(1):15-9.

Hamann S (2001). Cognitive and neural mechanisms of emotional memory. *Trends Cogn Sci.* 2001 Sep 1;5(9):394-400

Hamann SB, Cahill L, McGaugh JL & Squire LR (1997) Intact enhancement of declarative memory for emotional material in amnesia. *Learn Mem.* 1997 Sep-Oct;4(3):301-9.

Hanagasi HA, Gurvit IH, Ermutlu N, Kaptanoglu G, Karamursel S, Idrisoglu HA, Emre M & Demiralp T (2002) Cognitive impairment in amyotrophic lateral sclerosis: evidence from neuropsychological investigation and event-related potentials. *Brain Res Cogn Brain Res.* 2002 Aug;14(2):234-44.

Iwasaki Y, Kinoshita M, Ikeda K, Takamiya K & Shiojima T. (1990) Neuropsychological dysfunctions in amyotrophic lateral sclerosis: relation to motor disabilities. *Int J Neurosci.* 1990 Oct;54(3-4):191-5.

Heaton, R. K. (1981). *Wisconsin Card Sorting Test manual.* Odessa, FL: Psychological Assessment Resources.

Hecht MJ, Graesel E, Tigges S, et al. (2003) Burden of care in amyotrophic lateral sclerosis. *Palliat Med* 2003;17:327-333.

Ho, A. K., Sahakian, B. J., Robbins, T. W., Barker, R. A., Rosser, A. E., & Hodges, J. R. (2002). Verbal fluency in Huntington's disease: A longitudinal analysis of phonemics and semantic clustering and switching. *Neuropsychologia, 40,*1277-1284.

Hodges JR, Davies RR, Xuereb JH, et al. (2004) Clinicopathological correlates in frontotemporal dementia. *Ann Neurol* 2004;56:399-406.

Kaplan, E., Goodglass, H., &. Weintraub, S. (1983). *The Boston Naming Test.* Philadelphia: Lea & Febiger.

Kato S, Oda M, Hayashi H, Kawata A & Shimizu T. (1994) Participation of the limbic system and its associated areas in the dementia of amyotrophic lateral sclerosis. *J Neurol Sci.* 1994 Oct;126(1):62-9

Kawashima T, Doh-ura K, Kikuchi H & Iwaki T (2001). Cognitive dysfunction in patients with amyotrophic lateral sclerosis is associated with spherical or crescent-shaped ubiquitinated intraneuronal inclusions in the parahippocampal gyrus and amygdala, but not in the neostriatum. *Acta Neuropathol (Berl).* 2001 Nov;102(5):467-72.

Kertesz A, McMonagle P, Blair M, Davidson W, Munoz DG. (2005) The evolution and pathology of frontotemporal dementia. *Brain* 2005;128:1996-2005.

Kew JJ, Goldstein LH, Leigh PN, Abrahams S, Cosgrave N, Passingham RE, Frackowiak RS & Brooks DJ. (1993) The relationship between abnormalities of cognitive function and cerebral activation in amyotrophic lateral sclerosis. A neuropsychological and positron emission tomography study. *Brain.* 1993 Dec;116 (Pt 6):1399-423.

Kilani M, Micallef J, Soubrouillard C, et al. (2004) A longitudinal study of the evolution of cognitive function and affective state in patients with amyotrophic lateral sclerosis. *Amyotroph Lateral Scler Other Motor Neuron Disord* 2004;5:46-54.

Kokubo Y & Kuzuhara S. (2003) Neuroradiological study of patients with amyotrophic lateral sclerosis and parkinsonism-dementia complex on the Kii peninsula of Japan. *Arch Neurol.* 2003 Sep;60(9):1257-61

Leggio, M. G., Silveri, M. C, Petrosini, L., & Molinari, M. (2000). Phonological grouping is specifically affected in cerebellar patients: A verbal fluency study. *Journal of Neurology, Neurosurgery & Psychiatry*, 69, 444-A41.

Lepow, L., Van Sweringen, J., Strutt, A., Jawaid, A., MacAdam, C., Harati, Y., Schulz, P., York, M. (2010). Frontal and temporal lobe involvement on verbal fluency measures in amyotrophic lateral sclerosis. *Jour of Clin and Exp Neuropsych*, 39(9), 913-933.

Lezak M. Neuropsychological Assessment. New York: Oxford University Press, 1995.

Libon, D. J., McMillan, C, Gunawardena, D., Powers, C, Massimo, L., Kahn, A., et al. (2009). Neurocognitive contributions to verbal fluency deficits in frontotemporal lobar degeneration. *Neurology*, 73, 535-542.

Lomen-Hoerth C, Murphy J, Langmore S, Kramer JH, Olney RK & Miller B. (2003) Are amyotrophic lateral sclerosis patients cognitively normal? *Neurology*. 2003 Apr 8;60(7):1094-7.

Loman-Hoerth C, Anderson T, Miller B. (2002) The overlap of amyotrophic lateral sclerosis and frontotemporal dementia. *Neurology* 2002;59:1077-1079.

Martin, A., Wiggs, C. L., Lalonde, F., & Mack, C. (1994). Word retrieval to letter and semantic cues; A double dissociation in normal subjects using interference tasks. *Neuropsychologia, 32*, 1487-1494.

Massman PJ, Sims J, Cooke N, Haverkamp LJ, Appel V & Appel SH. (1996) Prevalence and correlates of neuropsychological deficits in amyotrophic lateral sclerosis. *J Neurol Neurosurg Psychiatry*. 1996 Nov;61(5):450-5

Meinzer, M., Flaisch, T., Wilser, L., Eulitz, C, Karsten, E., Rockstroh, B., et al. (2009). Neural signatures of semantic and phonemic fluency in young and old adults. *Journal of Cognitive Neuroscience, 21*, 2007-2018.

Meyers, J. E., & Meyers, K. R. (1995). *Rey Complex Figure Test and Recognition Trial: Professional Manual*. Odessa, FL: Psychological Assessment Resources.

Montgomery GK & Erickson LM. (1987) Neuropsychological perspectives in amyotrophic lateral sclerosis. *Neurol Clin*. 1987 Feb;5(1):61-81.

Poloni M, Capitani E, Mazzini L & Ceroni M. (1986) Neuropsychological measures in amyotrophic lateral sclerosis and their relationship with CT scan-assessed cerebral atrophy. *Acta Neurol Scand*. 1986 Oct;74(4):257-60.

Murphy, V., Felgoise, S., Walsh, S., Simmons, Z. (2009). Problem solving skills predict quality of life and psychological morbidity in ALS caregivers. *Amyotroph Lateral Scler*; 10(3): 147-153.

Pihlajamki, M., Tanila, H., Hannien, T., Kononen, M., Laakso, M., Partanen, K., et al. (2000). Verbal fluency activates the left medial temporal lobe: A functional magnetic resonance imaging study. *Annals of Neurology, 47*, 470-476.

Phukan J, Pender NP, Hardiman O. Cognitive impairment in amyotrophic lateral sclerosis. (2007) *Lancet Neurol*. 2007 Nov;6(11):994-1003.

Ringholz, G. M., Appel, S. H., Bradshaw, M., Cooke, N. A., Mosnik, D. M., & Schulz, P. E. (2005). Prevalence and patterns of cognitive impairment in sporadic ALS. *Neurology, 65*, 586-590.

Rippon, G. A., Scarmeas, N., Gordon, P., Murphy, P., Albert, S., Mitsumoto, H., Marden, K., Rowland, L., Stern Y. (2006). An observational study of cognitive impairment in amyotrophic lateral sclerosis. *Arch Neurol*, 63(3); 345-352.

Schmidt M. Rey Auditory and Verbal Learning Test. A handbook. Los Angeles: Western Psychological Services, 1996.

Schmolck, H., Mosnik, D., & Schulz, P. (2007). Rating the approachability of faces in ALS. *Neurology, 69,* 2232-2235.

Schmolck H & Squire LR (2001) Impaired perception of facial emotions following bilateral damage to the anterior temporal lobe. *Neuropsychology.* 2001 Jan;15(1):30-8.

Stark R, Schienle A, Walter B, Kirsch P, Sammer G, Ott U, Blecker C &Vaitl D (2003) Hemodynamic responses to fear and disgust-inducing pictures: an fMRI study. *Int J Psychophysiol.* 2003 Nov;50(3):225-34.

Strong MJ, Grace GM, Orange JB, Leeper HA, Menon RS &Aere C (1999) A prospective study of cognitive impairment in ALS. *Neurology.* 1999 Nov 10;53(8):1665-70.

Strong, M. J., Grace, G. M., Orange, J. B., & Leeper, H. A. (1996). Cognition, language, and speech in amyotrophic lateral sclerosis: A review. *Journal of Clinical and Experimental Neuropsychology 18,* 291-303

Strong MJ, Grace GM, Freedman M, Lomen-Hoerth C, Woolley S, Goldstein LH, et al., (2009) Consensus Criteria for the diagnosis of frontotemporal cognitive and behavioral syndromes in ALS. *Amyotrophic Lateral Sclerosis* 10(3), 131-146

The Psychological Corporation. (1997). *WAIS-III WMS-III technical manual.* San Antonio, TX; The Psychological Corporation.

Troster AI, Fields JA, Testa JA, et al. (1998). Cortical and subcortical influences on clustering and switching in the performance of verbal fluency tasks. *Neuropsychologia.* 36: 295-304.

Troyer, A. K., Moscovitch, M., Winocur, G., Alexander, M. P., & Struss, D. (1998). Clustering and switching on verbal fluency: The effects of focal frontal- and temporal-lobe lesions. *Neuropsychologia, 36,* 499-50.

Troyer, A. K., Moscovitch, M., & Winocur, G. (1997). Clustering and switching as two components of verbal fluency: Evidence from younger and older healthy adults. *Neuropsychology, 11,* 138-146.

Tsuchiya K, Takahashi M, Shiotsu H, Akiyama H, Haga C, Watabiki S, Taki K, Nakano I & Ikeda K. (2002) Sporadic amyotrophic lateral sclerosis with circumscribed temporal atrophy: a report of an autopsy case without dementia and with ubiquitinated intraneuronal inclusions. *Neuropathology.* 2002 Dec;22(4):308-16.

Wheaton, M. W., Salamone, A. R., Mosnik, D. M., McDonald, R. O., Appel, S. H., Schmolck, H. I., et al. (2007). Cognitive impairment in familial ALS. *Neurology, 16,* 1411-1417

Wilson CM, Grace GM, Munoz DG, He BP& Strong MJ (2001) Cognitive impairment in sporadic ALS: a pathologic continuum underlying a multisystem disorder. *Neurology.* 2001 Aug 28;57(4):651-7.

Winston JS, Strange BA, O'Doherty J, Dolan RJ (2002). Automatic and intentional brain responses during evaluation of trustworthiness of faces. *Nature Neuroscience* 5: 277-283

Woolley, S.C. and Katz, J. S. (2008). Cognitive and behavioral impairment in amyotrophic lateral sclerosis. *Phys Med Rehabil Clin N Am,* 19(3); 607-617

Yamazaki M, Arai Y, Baba M, Iwatsubo T, Mori O, Katayama Y & Oyanagi K (2000) Alpha-synuclein inclusions in amygdala in the brains of patients with the parkinsonism-dementia complex of Guam. *J Neuropathol Exp Neurol.* 2000 Jul;59(7):585-91.

Zimmerman EK, Eslinger PJ, Simmons Z, Barrett AM (2007) Emotional perception deficits in amyotrophic lateral sclerosis. *Cognitive and Behavioral Neurology* 20:79-82

15

Communication Impairment in ALS Patients Assessment and Treatment

Paolo Bongioanni

Neurological Rehabilitation Unit - Neuroscience Department,
University of Pisa/NeuroCare onlus
Italy

1. Introduction

Amyotrophic lateral sclerosis (ALS), also called *Lou Gehrig's disease*, is a rapidly progressive neuromuscular disease that attacks the neurons responsible for controlling voluntary muscles. It belongs to a group of disorders known as *Motor neuron diseases* (*MND*): all these syndromes share a common molecular and cellular pathology comprising degeneration of motor neurons (MNs) in cortex, brainstem and/or spinal cord, and the presence of characteristic ubiquitin and TDP-43-immunoreactive intraneuronal inclusions.

ALS prevalence in Western countries ranges from 2.7 to 7.4 per 100,000 (Worms, 2001). In 90 to 95 percent of all patients with ALS (PALS), the disease occurs sporadically (*sporadic ALS, sALS*); in 5 to 10 percent there is a family history of ALS (*familial ALS, fALS*). Most people developing ALS are between the ages of 40 and 70 years (Haverkamp et al., 1995). The disease is 20% more common in men than in women, although more recent data suggest that the gender ratio may be approaching equality (Logroscino et al., 2008).

The cause of ALS is not known, and it is not clear why ALS strikes some people and not others, but both genetic (Ticozzi et al., 2011) and environmental factors (Callaghan et al., 2011; Calvo et al., 2010; Ferrante et al., 1997) may play a role.

In PALS, both the brain upper MNs (UMNs) and the brainstem or spinal cord lower MNs (LMNs) degenerate or die: unable to function, the muscles gradually weaken, waste away, and twitch, leading to a wide range of disabilities. Patients lose their strength and the ability to move their body, but usually maintain control of eye muscles.

Approximately 70% of PALS have a *spinal form* of the disease: they present with symptoms which may start either distally or proximally in the upper or lower limbs. Some patients see the effects of the disease on a hand or arm, as they experience difficulty with simple tasks requiring manual dexterity, such as buttoning a shirt, writing, or turning a key in a lock; in other cases, symptoms initially affect one of the legs, and patients experience awkwardness when walking or running, or they notice that they are tripping or stumbling more often.

Patients with *bulbar-onset* ALS usually present with dysarthria leading to slow slurred speech or a nasal quality; they may also develop dysphagia for solid or liquids after noticing speech problems; almost all patients with bulbar symptoms complain of sialorrhoea with excessive drooling due to difficulty of swallowing saliva and UMN-type facial weakness, which affects the lower part of the face, causing difficulty with lip seal and blowing cheeks.

The gag reflex is preserved and often brisk, whereas the soft palate may be weak; patients show wasting and fasciculations of the tongue which moves slowly, also due to muscle hypertonia. The other cranial nerves remain intact, although in late stages of the disease patients may very rarely develop a supranuclear gaze palsy or oculomotor palsy (Kobayashi et al., 1999; Okuda et al., 1992).

2. Communication issues in ALS patients

Five functional domains have to be taken into account when communication is concerned: a) motivation to interact; b) cognitive skills (particularly - but not exclusively - those related to language); c) visual and auditory capacities; d) ability to utter sounds and words; and e) writing skills. As a matter of fact, affective disorders, anxiety and emotional discomfort, as well as cognitive impairment or sensory deficits, can compromise communication processes, by interfering directly and/or indirectly with speech and writing performances.

However, ALS does not usually either affect a person's ability to see, smell, taste, hear, or recognize touch; nor impair mind or intelligence - although a small percentage of patients may experience problems with memory or decision-making (Raaphorst et al., 2010; Ringholz et al., 2005), and there is growing evidence that some may even develop a form of dementia (Guedj et al., 2007). On the other hand, since the disease usually does not affect cognitive abilities, PALS are aware of their progressive loss of function and may become anxious and depressed (Patten et al., 2007).

The vast majority of PALS experience a motor speech disorder as the disease progresses: since ALS involves both UMNs and LMNs, it results in *mixed dysarthria* of the *flaccid-spastic* type characterized by effortful, slow productions with short phrases, inappropriate pauses, imprecise consonants, hypernasality, strain-strangled voice, as well as decreased pitch and loudness range (Duffy, 1995; Tomik & Guiloff, 2010).

In the early stages when dysarthria is mild, either spasticity or flaccidity is predominant: initial symptoms typically do not interfere with speech intelligibility and may be limited to a reduction in speaking rate, a change in phonatory quality, or imprecise articulation (Ball et al., 2004a; Nishio & Niimi, 2000; Yorkston et al., 1993; Yunusova et al., 2010).

Features of *spasmodic dysphonia* (or *focal laryngeal dystonia*) may also occur in PALS, sometimes as the initial clinical symptom (Roth et al., 1996). Typically, laryngeal structure is normal in appearance. When *corticobulbar* involvement prevails (*spastic* forms), there is often a pattern of hyperadduction of the vocal mechanism, and when *bulbar* involvement dominates (*flaccid* forms), there is usually a pattern of hypoadduction.

As disease progresses and dysarthria becomes severe, profound weakness resulting in reduced movement of the speech musculature and severe hypophonia become increasingly common (Yunusova et al., 2010).

Perceptual and acoustic features of dysarthria in ALS have been well studied (Tomik & Guiloff, 2010): the decrease in rate is often associated with increased pause time and enhanced segment durations, particularly for vowel sounds (Green et al., 2004; Tjaden & Turner, 2000; Turner & Weismer, 1993); spectral vowel and consonant properties (e.g., formant frequencies, transition extents and slopes) are also affected, with vowels becoming more centralized and the consonant frequency spectrum less distinct (Kent et al., 1989, 1992; Tjaden & Turner, 1997; Turner et al., 1995; Weismer et al., 1988, 1992, 2001).

Such acoustic findings have been presumed to be due to the disease-related reduction and slowing of articulatory movements (Weismer et al., 1992). Articulatory findings, although limited, support such an interpretation. An early study on articulatory kinematics in two PALS showed slowed articulatory movements, reduced displacement of the tongue and lip, together with exaggerated displacements of the jaw during diadokokinetic tasks (Hirose et al., 1982). A more recent study of articulatory movements in a group of 9 PALS reported an impairment of articulatory speed during vowels (Yunusova et al., 2008): aberrant displacements were found to be word- and vowel-dependent and were more consistently present in movements of the tongue than in those of other articulators, and occasionally in the jaw; the jaw displacements were smaller than normal in words requiring larger articulator movements (e.g., consonant plus low vowel), but were larger than normal in words that only required relatively small jaw movements (e.g., consonant plus high vowel), suggesting difficulty in scaling of the vowel-related movements.

Whereas initially, along a gradual slowing of *speaking rate*, *speech intelligibility* remains relatively high, it decreases overtime, when dysarthria becomes more and more apparent to PALS themselves and their listeners. Yorkston and co-workers (1993) suggested that speech intelligibility may vary across dysarthric patients depending on the subsystems that are preserved (e.g., relatively less impaired respiratory-phonatory subsystem and the jaw might be associated with better speech intelligibility); the rate of disease progression; and the patient's cognitive status.

Because a person's ability to communicate orally is typically assessed based on speech intelligibility, anticipating the decline in intelligibility in a sensitive way is critical for timely clinical management of bulbar PALS. In this regard, longitudinal studies are, indeed, necessary when the goal of research is to identify early predictors of future changes; additionally, longitudinal studies are advantageous when dealing with heterogeneous populations, as in the case of PALS, since each patient can serve as his own control. Investigations of such a type documented the decline in speech intelligibility and speaking rate (Kent et al., 1992; Mulligan et al, 1994; Nishio & Niimi, 2000; Yorkston et al., 1993); and some studies have also identified several acoustic-based speech markers of disease progression (Mulligan et al., 1994; Ramig et al., 1990).

In their retrospective study of more than a hundred clinical cases, Yorkston and co-workers (1993) reported that speaking rate was a reliable predictor of speech intelligibility decline, by observing a rapid deterioration in speech intelligibility shortly after a decline in speaking rate to 100-120 words per minute. Such a finding was replicated by Ball and co-workers (2002) in a large group of patients with bulbar symptoms of different severity: the authors suggested that speaking rate decline to 100-120 words per minute should serve as a clinical indicator for beginning to support communication by assistive technology.

Moreover, since ALS progresses so rapidly in many subjects, an important goal of clinical management is to anticipate functional changes in patients' performance in order to teach new communication strategies and compensatory skills before the patient's ability to learn these skills is impacted by the severity of their condition. Recently, Yunusova and co-workers (2010) in a longitudinal study on 3 PALS tested the feasibility of using kinematic measures as early predictors of intelligibility decline, trying to understand the relationship between physiologic changes in speech movements and clinical measures of speech performance (such as speaking rate and speech intelligibility). Lip and jaw movements were quantified with respect to their size, speed, and duration.

Results showed that, differently from oral strength measures, changes in lip and jaw movements were related to ALS progression: in two out of 3 PALS, the changes in measures of path distance and speed anticipated the drop in speech intelligibility by approximately 3 months, whereas speaking rate decline was more gradual; and increases in movement duration overtime closely mimicked the pattern of speech intelligibility decline. Overall, the kinematic measures seemed to be sensitive to disease progression: they might therefore be useful clinical markers for initiation of compensatory interventions.

Parallelly to decline in speech intelligibility, *communication effectiveness* is reduced at first in adverse speaking situations, such as noisy crowds, and then in all situations. Ball and co-workers (2004b) reported that perceptions of communication effectiveness for PALS were quite similar to those of their frequent listeners (spouse or family member) across 10 different social situations: a range of communication effectiveness was reported depending upon the adversity of specific social situations.

Significant dysarthria can lead to frustration on the part of the patient when others are unwilling to spend the time to carefully listen. Friends and healthcare workers may not listen to the patient; there is a temptation to anticipate answers and finish sentences for the patient.

Fatally, at some point in their disease progression, 80 to 95% of PALS are unable to meet their daily communication needs using their natural speech, and finally most become unable to speak at all.

Moreover, upper limb paralysis prevents them from using hands in writing (directly or through computer-linked keyboards or communication devices).

Ultimately, in the so-called "locked-in" cases, a diffuse somatic immobility takes them away any possibility to interact with the world, except by using eye movements - even more unfortunately lost in those PALS classified as having a "super locked-in" syndrome, who may rely only upon their brain electrical waves as a communication tool processed through complex *brain-computer interface (BCI)* devices.

3. Functional assessment

Many assessments have been proposed for patient's follow-up in order to analyze the state of motor function and their consequences on activities of everyday life (Couratier et al., 2006). Clinimetric scales must be validated and relatively simple to use, and generate ordinate results allowing statistical analysis: global scales - *Norris Scale* (Norris et al., 1974), *Appel ALS Rating Scale* (Appel et al., 1987), *ALS Severity Scale* (Hillel et al., 1989), and *ALS Functional Rating Scale (ALSFRS)* (Cedarbaum & Stambler, 1997) - can be employed to evaluate disability progression.

By using, for instance, ALSFRS - or its revised version, ALSFRS$_R$ (Cedarbaum et al., 1999) - , communication impairment can be assessed through scores on speech function together with those related to handwriting, since people communicate by speaking and/or writing: scores < 2 in both speech and handwriting items correspond to a substantial inability to communicate.

Dysarthric speech can be evaluated through the *Frenchay Dysarthria Assessment* (Enderby & Palmer, 2008) originally developed by Pamela Enderby in 1983, which represents a well-established clinical tool to quantitatively evaluate the organs involved in speech and provides a measurement of intelligibility.

Complete kit includes examiner's manual, 25 rating forms, and intelligibility cards: patient is rated on a number of simple performance tasks related to speech function.

Intelligibility can be measured also through another test developed by Yorkston and co-workers: the *Assessment of Intelligibility of Dysarthric Speech* (Yorkston et al., 1984), a tool for quantifying single-word intelligibility, sentence intelligibility, and speaking rate of adult and adolescent speakers with dysarthria. Standard protocols containing speaker tasks, recording techniques, and listener response formats are employed to obtain a variety of intelligibility and communication efficiency measures.

Yorkston and co-workers (1993) initially suggested that PALS speaking rate reduction precedes decreases in intelligibility; Ball and co-workers (2001, 2002) reported that speaking rate on the *Speech Intelligibility Test - Sentence Subtest* (Yorkston et al., 2007) is a relatively good predictor of PALS intelligibility deterioration. This computerized test supports the efficient measurement of speaking rate in clinical settings; it helps patients and their families monitor changes over time, and reinforces their understanding of speaking rate and intelligibility. Using this test, speaking rate can also be accurately monitored over the telephone if a patient lives at a distance, or is unable to travel (Ball et al., 2005$_a$): it should be noted, anyway, that speech intelligibility could not be objectively assessed over the telephone, as a clinical measure of understandability.

The *vocal impairment* can be difficult to assess because the voice disorder in dysarthria often occurs along with other impairments affecting articulation, resonance, and respiration: an effective assessment tool is the *Multi-Dimensional Voice Program*, a multi-parameter acoustic analysis (Kent et al., 2003).

4. Treatment

Differently from an acute, self-limited disease with expected recovery, the choice of appropriate therapeutic options for PALS raises more difficult concerns, since one must take into account many personal and ethical considerations. Several decisions by PALS and their families regarding treatment hinge on their concept of the quality of life that will result from such treatments.

At the present time, ALS therapy can be organized under the following multiple modalities: a **pathogenetic treatment** – to counteract MN degeneration; and a **symptomatic treatment** – to reduce impairments in motor abilities including those involved in communication. The appropriate implementation of each one of these types of therapy reflects the difficulties that we now have to face in ALS treatment. Supportive care is best provided by multidisciplinary teams of health care professionals, such as physicians; physical, occupational, and speech therapists; nutritionists; social workers; and home care and hospice nurses (Bede et al., 2011): working with patients and caregivers, these teams can design an individualized plan of medical and physical therapy and provide special equipment aimed at keeping patients as "functional" as possible.

Taking now into account such *a symptomatic approach*, two kinds of therapeutic strategies have to be implemented, those using drugs and those employing assistive/rehabilitative methods and techniques, aids and devices.

4.1 Pharmacological strategies

Physicians can prescribe medications to ameliorate fatigue, ease muscle cramps, control spasticity, and reduce excess saliva and phlegm; drugs also are available to help patients with pain, depression, anxiety, and sleep disturbances (Bede et al., 2011; Gordon, 2011; Guidubaldi et al., 2011; Guy et al., 2011; Miller et al., 1999; 2009$_{a,b}$).

It is almost obvious that a patient experiencing less fatigue, pain, anxiety and depression, and controlling better saliva and spasticity, also apart from specific speech and writing motor deficits (which, indeed, are improved by reduced sialorrhoea and muscle hypertonia), will be able to successfully manage his/her language impairment, being more committed to communicate and keep social contacts.

4.2 Non pharmacological strategies

The primary goal of an effective assistive rehabilitation for PALS is the management of disabilities, symptoms and complications arising from the progressive weakness of limb, trunk, and bulbar muscles. Further goals include keeping the patient functioning as independently as possible, and maintaining quality of life even into the terminal stage (Francis et al., 1999).

The rehabilitation program varies depending on whether the patient has a long clinical course or rapid progression of the disease: in the former case, PALS become able to compensate remarkably well for the motor unit loss and are able to continue with their daily activity for several years (Chen et al., 2008). The success of the rehabilitation approach depends on the active participation of the patient who should be a full partner in the therapeutic team even during the advanced stages of the disease. It may be difficult for the physician to discuss such a fatal illness: however, a direct approach allows the patient to deal most effectively with the disease and its physical limitations. This also helps in decisions about the intensity of the therapeutic effort (Bede et al., 2011; Gordon, 2011).

The family and other caregivers should be encouraged to participate in the patient's early rehabilitation program: the family role will then likely increase as weakness progresses, requirements for assistive devices change, and new problems arise in the management of activities of daily living.

4.2.1 Treatment of impaired communication

Loss of effective communication prevents patients from participating in many activities; may lead them to social isolation; and reduces their quality of life: the goal of clinical management of dysarthric PALS is to optimize communication effectiveness for as long as possible. Communication solutions, which may include no-technology, low-technology and high-technology options will be discussed, as well as the importance of psychosocial issues and the factors influencing the use of these systems.

Dysarthric PALS may benefit from working with a *speech therapist*: these health professionals can teach patients adaptive strategies, such as techniques to help them speak louder and more clearly. In early disease stages, patients can be taught to emphasize certain syllables and slow their speech patterns so that others can understand them better: lip and tongue exercises can sometimes help the patient to enunciate words more clearly on a regular basis.

A recent review on ALS communication research (Hanson et al., 2011) concluded that, due to ALS pathophysiology and the intrinsic degenerative nature of disease, speech treatment strategies designed to increase strength or mobility of the oral musculature are not recommended for PALS. Patients or their caregivers, on the contrary, often request oral exercises to improve strength and mobility for speech, as strengthening exercises seem intuitively to them as a way to increase performance: however, such exercise programs should be discouraged, and PALS should be informed that the speaking that they do each day provides a sufficient amount of speech mechanism activity and exercise.

Speech intervention should focus on learning to conserve energy for priority speaking tasks and to rest often to reduce fatigue, instead of increasing effort with speech exercises. PALS speakers should learn to avoid adverse speaking/listening situations by muting the television, inviting people to speak with them in a quiet place rather than in a crowded room, and using voice amplification when speaking in noisy environments to reduce the effort required (Ball et al., 2007; Yorkston et al., 2010).

On the basis of a retrospective study on 25 dysarthric PALS treated with a palatal lift and/or augmentation prosthesis, the use of such devices should be regarded as effective in improving speech: 84% of patients treated with a palatal lift reported reduction of hypernasality (76% benefiting, at least moderately, for 6 months), and 60 % of those treated with a combination of palatal lift and augmentation prosthesis demonstrated improvement in articulation (Esposito et al., 2000).

Writing may be used as a substitute for speech, and devices as simple as paper and pencil, alphabet cards, portable typewriter, and letter boards may be utilized by patients with adequate hand function. Becoming speech more and more difficult to understand, many PALS supplement their speech by identifying the first letter of each word on an alphabet board (*alphabet supplementation*), or by identifying the topic on a communication board (*topic supplementation*).

As ALS progresses, speech therapists can help patients develop ways for responding to yes-or-no questions with their eyes or by other nonverbal means, and can recommend aids such as speech synthesizers and computer-based communication systems: these methods and devices help patients communicate when they can no longer speak or produce vocal sounds.

The technological revolution has expanded communication options for PALS who cannot rely on natural speech and writing. The assistive technologies are categorized as *Augmentative and Alternative Communication (AAC)* devices. Four critical features need to be considered within clinical and research domains: language representation, output mode, motor access, and microprocessor units.

Language representation has got remarkable attention for speaking rate enhancement. Whereas most PALS spell and rely on typing as a form of input, they can never approach speech production rates: often the slowness of AAC devices reduces their utility. Nowadays devices are being designed that integrate natural language processing and prediction algorithms for word, utterance and even conversational level units as one tries to approach natural speaking rates.

The **output mode** has seen advances for the storage of digitized voice as well as qualitative improvements to synthetic speech.

Voice banking is often considered as an early treatment option: PALS with intact motor speech skills store their spoken sounds, words, sentences for future use in customized communication devices. The personalized voice and messages can be used along with standard text-to-speech output to retain the PALS' voice signature: engineering efforts to customize synthetic speech to the user's own voice through minimal speech sampling are going on. Scientists and technicians are pursuing the gold standard for a device: bad speech in and good speech out, with attention being paid to recognition of dysarthric speech and production of personalized voices.

Motor access problems are being addressed with visual evoked potentials, detection of alpha and theta waves, and eye gaze recognizers so that head, shoulders, knees and toes are no longer needed: most devices now offer a range of access methods, starting with keyboards, touch screens, a head mouse, and Morse code.

Finally, **microprocessor units** are available in every shape and size to meet user needs, from palmtops to laptops made of magnesium-alloy shells, to software that can be downloaded from the Internet and accessed through any home computer.

AAC has a remarkable importance in dysarthric PALS management. When a person has a severe verbal communication impairment, AAC can meet the overall goals of palliative care: AAC can improve quality of life by optimizing function, assisting with decision making, and providing opportunities for personal growth.

Clinical decision-making related to communication is quite complex as screening, referral, assessment, acquisition of technology, and training must occur in a timely manner, so that when residual speech is no longer effective, AAC strategies are in place to support communication related to personal care, healthcare, social interaction, community involvement. Many reports of use and frequency for the purposes of staying connected and discussing important issues point out that AAC technology can assist the patient-caregiver dyad in maintaining previous relationships. The face-to-face spontaneous conversation mode is used most frequently, despite the slow rate of production, the lack of permanence, and the demands on conversational partners during message generation (Fried-Oken et al., 2006).

PALS, their family members, and, at times, their medical team, usually do not wish to consider an AAC decision until the deteriorating speech intelligibility limits the communication effectiveness: unfortunately, once intelligibility begins to decrease, speech performance often deteriorates so rapidly that there is little time to implement an appropriate AAC intervention. Indeed, appropriate timing of referral for AAC assessment and intervention continues to be a relevant clinical decision-making issue. The speaking rate should be clinically monitored so that the referral for an AAC intervention is initiated in a timely manner: Ball and co-workers (2001, 2002) recommend that patients be referred for AAC assessment when their speaking rates reach 125 words/min (normal value: 190 words/min) on the *Speech Intelligibility Test - Sentence Subtest*) (Yorkston et al., 2007). With sufficient education and preparation, PALS and their caregivers are ready to examine their AAC options timely: nevertheless, speech deterioration can be so rapid anyway that individuals can be left with limited communication options, if they are not really prepared to act in an opportune manner.

Due to the extended AAC use with deteriorating levels of physical control, it is imperative that recommended technology has adjustable access options to meet the range of motor capability as the disease progresses (s. above).

PALS should be fitted with AAC technology that supports multiple access methods, such as allowing them to transition from hand access to scanning and/or head/eye-tracking. Many AAC devices now incorporate a variety of access options so that the technology can continue to meet the needs of the user despite a decline in physical capability: the sensitivity of dynamic touch screens can be adjusted to allow for lighter touch; the improved sensitivity of head-tracking technology has allowed many patients to use this access method with minimal head/neck movement control.

Perhaps the most significant advancement in access technology has occurred with the widespread availability of *eye-tracking systems* to allow cursor control with eye movement to access high-technology AAC devices. As the disease progresses, many PALS require the use of eye-tracking for several reasons. Firstly, compared to other access methods (such as switch-activated scanning), eye-tracking is often reported to be the least fatiguing method

(Gibbons & Beneteau, 2010) and its technology requires relatively little effort (Calvo et al., 2008; Harris & Goren, 2009): eye gaze is natural, and eye muscles generally do not fatigue with use. Secondly, eye gaze may be the only volitional movement that the individual continues to exhibit over time, particularly in cases where invasive ventilation has been chosen (Ball et al., 2010).

BCI technology has generated considerable interest for people who are physically "locked-in", such as PALS in the late stages of the disease. BCI devices translate into computer commands volitional modulation of brain signals which can be recorded from the scalp using electroencephalography (EEG) or magnetoencephalography; from the dura mater or cortical surface using electrocorticography; or from neurons within the cortex.

A common signal for BCI is the P300 event-related potential, a positive deflection in the EEG over parietal cortex, that occurs approximately 300 ms after an "oddball" stimulus: a rare but meaningful stimulus among a series of frequently occurring stimuli. Since the P300 occurs among other ongoing EEG activity, several P300 responses must usually be averaged for the response to be recognized (Polich, 2007). Farwell and Donchin (1988) introduced the first P300-based BCI paradigm: computer presents a 6×6 matrix of letters and commands on-screen and participants attend to the item they wish to select; groups of matrix items are flashed randomly: only flashes of groups containing the attended item should elicit a P300. Items are grouped for flashing as rows and columns: hence, the so-called "row-column paradigm" (RCP). The computer identifies the attended item as the intersection of the row and column that elicited the largest P300.

The RCP has been tested in various configurations to achieve efficient communication that is practical for in-home use (Krusienski et al., 2006; Lenhardt et al., 2008; Sellers et al., 2006); the paradigm itself has been modified (Guger et al., 2009; Hong et al., 2009; Martens et al., 2009; Salvaris & Sepulveda, 2009; Takano et al., 2009). Unfortunately, none of such alternative paradigms substantially improves P300-based BCI performance. The RCP remains subject to errors that slow communication, cause frustration and diminish attentional resources (Vaughan et al., 2006). Further RCP research could possibly help severely disabled BCI users, who desire speed, accuracy, and ease of use. Moreover, with the RCP, some people are not able to achieve accuracy high enough for practical BCI use (Sellers & Donchin, 2006).

In recognition of these issues, Townsend and co-workers (2010) sought to create an alternative stimulation paradigm that could be faster, more accurate and more reliable than the RCP: they designed the so-called "checkerboard paradigm" (CBP), using a standard 8×9 matrix of alphanumeric characters and keyboard commands. In the RCP, the 8 columns and 9 rows flash at random: in contrast, in the CBP, the standard matrix is virtually superimposed on a checkerboard which the subjects never actually see. The items in white cells of the standard matrix are segregated into a white 6×6 matrix and the items in the black cells are segregated into a black 6×6 matrix; before each sequence of flashes, the items randomly populate the white or black matrix, respectively. The end result is that the subjects see random groups of 6 items flashing (as opposed to rows and columns), because the virtual rows and columns flash. In other words, the standard matrix never changes: only the pattern of flashing items is changed. After all rows and columns in both matrices have flashed (i.e., 24 flashes, comprising one complete sequence), the program re-randomizes the positions of the items in each virtual matrix and the next sequence of flashes begins (Townsend et al., 2010). The CBP produced a significant increase in BCI performance and user acceptability over the RCP, thus providing a substantially more effective BCI, which is so important for PALS management. Experimental data showed that, whereas average PALS performances were much lower than those of the healthy controls using the RCP, upon switching to the CBP, PALS performed only slightly lower than the healthy controls: patients improved their classification accuracy rates by an average of about 25 % after switching from the RCP to the CBP, whereas accuracy rates of control group improved only of 14 %, thus suggesting that the CBP improvements may be more pronounced for PALS than for healthy controls. In particular, for two patients, the improvement brought them into an accuracy range sufficient for effective BCI control, while previously their accuracy was not consistently enough for effective control.

Non-invasive BCI methods have been utilized more extensively than invasive methods for people with disabilities (Birbaumer & Cohen, 2007; Birbaumer et al., 2008; Gerven et al., 2009): unfortunately, whereas PALS and other patients in "locked-in" conditions have motivated research in this area, very few systems have been successfully used - such as that reported by Townsend and co-workers (2010). It has been postulated that some forms of cognitive impairment and changes in EEG signatures in late ALS stages may contribute to the lack of success using BCI technology (Iversen et al., 2008), as the technology was introduced after the participants had become "locked-in" (Gerven et al., 2009; Münte et al., 1998): really, the most successful application for communication has occurred in people at the beginning stages of ALS (Birbaumer et al., 1999; Birbaumer, 2006; Kubler et al., 2001).

Nowadays, AAC acceptance and use represent two areas of interest for physicians and scientists. Both involve PALS and their caregivers.

In the Ball et al.'s review (2004b), those who rejected AAC had a co-occurring cognitive deficit or experienced a severe diseases, such as cancer, in addition to ALS.

Fried-Oken and co-workers (2006) reported very positive caregivers' attitudes toward AAC technology: those with greater AAC technology skills got greater rewards associated with caregiving.

In a follow-up study on 15 PALS, Ball and co-workers (2010) examined the acceptance, training, and extended use patterns of eye-tracking technology to support communication.

For 53% of the participants, eye-tracking technology was selected because eye movement was the only viable access option available. More than 90% of the participants reported successful implementation of the technology: the only one patient who was not able to successfully use eye-tracking technology had difficulty with eyelid control. The communicative functions served by eye-tracking devices were extensive: all of the participants used their device to support face-to-face communication, and other functions included group communication, phone, e-mail and internet. More than 40% of the participants also reported using the eye-tracking technology to support other computer-based functions (e.g., word processing, voice-related software programs).

Training and support are an essential component of AAC service delivery for PALS. The significant changes in movement abilities require that service providers not only be proactive in their AAC technology recommendations by fitting up technology options that can meet the changing physical needs over time, but also by supplying adequate training and support to ensure that PALS and their caregivers can successfully implement diachronically these access strategies. Reports of low AAC use often are related to descriptions of minimal training or follow-up (Murphy, 2004).

New advances in AAC technology may need a greater amount of training and intervention than other access options: for instance, implementation of eye-tracking systems often requires for successful technology use trouble-shooting in the form of physical or environmental compensations (Ball et al., 2010). Whereas AAC specialists are professionals who provide the AAC intervention services (such as assessment and initial instruction), AAC facilitators for PALS tend to be family members who typically provide ongoing support (including instruction of new communication partners and caregivers, programming new messages into the AAC device, maintaining the AAC system, and interacting with the technology manufacturer, if necessary) (Beukelman et al., 2008).

In a survey on 68 PALS using AAC technology Ball and co-workers (2005b) studied the AAC facilitators: almost all of them were family members, the majority with nontechnical backgrounds. They reported to prefer hands-on and detailed step-by-step instruction; and to have received an appropriate training amount (slightly over 2 hours of instruction).

5. Conclusion

Multifunctional impairments of PALS result from a relentlessly progressive muscle weakness, leading ultimately to a widespread body paralysis. In the late disease stages, patients eventually find themselves in a "locked-in" state, totally unable to move neck, trunk and limbs; autonomously breath and feed; and speak, although most of them retain their cognitive skills, thereby assisting impotent at their dreadful somatic decay.

As human beings, and therefore "persons", namely "individuals within a network of relationships", PALS particularly suffer from communication impairment.

Today, much more than in the past, we are able to give interdisciplinary assistance to them, enhancing their possibilities of keeping in touch with their caregivers, friends and other persons, with the aim to maintain their quality of life as high as possible.

Further research is needed to better implement AAC devices and services (trying to optimize communication aids and interfaces, and increase our understanding of acceptance and use of AAC approaches); and to develop new intervention strategies and document their effectiveness.

Anyway, besides scientific and clinical achievements, we look forward to building up in the near future more empathic care strategies for PALS and their families, with respect to them in their dignity of suffering persons.

6. References

Appel, V., Stewart, S., Smith, G. & Appel, S.H. (1987). A rating scale for amyotrophic lateral sclerosis: description and preliminary experience. *Annals of Neurology*, Vol. 22, pp. 328-333

Ball, L.J., Willis, A., Beukelman D.R. & Pattee, G.L. (2001). A protocol for identification of early bulbar signs in amyotrophic lateral sclerosis. *Journal of the Neurological Sciences*, Vol. 191, pp. 43-53

Ball, L.J., Beukelman, D.R. & Pattee, G.L. (2002). Timing of speech deterioration in people with amyotrophic lateral sclerosis. *Journal of Medical Speech-Language Pathology*, Vol. 10, pp. 231-235

Ball, L.J., Beukelman, D.R. & Pattee, G.L. (2004$_a$). Acceptance of augmentative and alternative communication technology by persons with amyotrophic lateral sclerosis. *Augmentative and Alternative Communication*, Vol. 20, pp. 113-122

Ball, L.J., Beukelman, D.R. & Pattee, G.L. (2004$_b$). Communication effectiveness of individuals with amyotrophic lateral sclerosis. *Journal of Communication Disorders*, Vol. 37, pp. 197-215

Ball, L.J., Beukelman, D.R., Ullman, C., Maassen, K. & Pattee, G.L. (2005$_a$). Monitoring speaking rate by telephone for persons with amyotrophic lateral sclerosis. *Journal of Medical Speech-Language Pathology*, Vol. 13, pp. 233-240

Ball, L.J., Schardt, K. & Beukelman, D.R. (2005$_b$) Primary communication facilitators. *Augmentative Communication News*, Vol. 17, pp. 6-7

Ball, L.J., Beukelman, D.R. & Bardach, L. (2007). AAC intervention for ALS, In: *Augmentative Communication Strategies for Adults with acute or chronic Medical Conditions*, D.R. Beukelman, K. Garrett & K. Yorkston (Eds.), pp. 287-316, Paul H. Brookes, Baltimore, Md, USA

Ball, L.J., Nordness, A., Fager, S.K., Kersch, K., Mohr, B., Pattee, G.L. & Beukelman, D.R. (2010). Eye-gaze access of AAC technology for persons with amyotrophic lateral sclerosis. *Journal of Medical Speech-Language Pathology*, Vol. 18, pp. 11-23

Bede, P., Oliver, D., Stodart, J., van den Berg, L., Simmons, Z., O Brannagáin, D., Borasio. G.D. & Hardiman, O. (2011). Palliative care in amyotrophic lateral sclerosis: a review of current international guidelines and initiatives. *Journal of Neurology, Neurosurgery & Psychiatry*, Vol. 82, pp. 413-418

Beukelman, D.R., Ball, L.J. & Fager, S. (2008). An AAC personnel framework: adults with acquired complex communication needs. *Augmentative and Alternative Communication*, Vol. 24, pp. 255-267

Birbaumer, N., Ghanayim, N., Hinterberger, T., Iversen, I., Kotchoubey, B., Kübler, A. & Perelmouter, J. (1999). A spelling device for the paralysed. *Nature*, Vol. 398, pp. 297-298

Birbaumer, N. (2006). Brain-computer-interface research: coming of age. *Clinical Neurophysiology*, Vol. 117, pp. 479-483

Birbaumer N. & Cohen, L.G. (2007). Brain-computer interfaces: communication and restoration of movement in paralysis. *Journal of Physiology*, Vol. 579, pp. 621-636

Birbaumer, N., Murguialday, A.R. & Cohen, L. (2008). Brain-computer interface in paralysis. *Current Opinion in Neurology*, Vol. 21, pp. 634-638

Callaghan, B., Feldman, D., Gruis, K. & Feldman, E. (2011). The association of exposure to lead, mercury, and selenium and the development of amyotrophic lateral sclerosis and the epigenetic implications. *Neurodegenerative Diseases*, Vol. 8, pp. 1-8

Calvo, A., Chiò, A. & Castellina, E. (2008). Eye tracking impact on quality-of-life of ALS patients, *Proceedings of the Conference on Computers Helping People with Special Needs*, 5101 (*Lecture Notes in Computer Science*), pp. 70-77

Calvo, A., Moglia, C., Balma, M. & Chiò, A. (2010). Involvement of immune response in the pathogenesis of amyotrophic lateral sclerosis: a therapeutic opportunity? *CNS Neurological Disorders Drug Targets*, Vol. 9, pp. 325-330

Cedarbaum, J.M. & Stambler, N. (1997). Performance of the ALS Functional Rating Scale (ALSFRS) in multicenter clinical trials. *Journal of the Neurological Sciences*, Vol. 152(S), pp. 1-9

Cedarbaum, J.M., Stambler, N., Malta, E., Fuller, C., Hilt, D., Thurmond, B. & Nakanishi, A. (1999). The ALSFRS-R: a revised ALS functional rating scale that incorporates assessments of respiratory function. BDNF ALS Study Group (Phase III). *Journal of the Neurological Sciences*, Vol. 169, pp. 13-21

Chen, A., Montes, J. & Mitsumoto, H. (2008). The role of exercise in amyotrophic lateral sclerosis. *Physical Medicine & Rehabilitation Clinics of North America*, Vol. 19, pp. 545-557

Couratier, P., Torny, F. & Lacoste, M. (2006). [Functional rating scales for amyotrophic lateral sclerosis]. *Revue Neurologie (Paris)*, Vol. 162, pp. 502-507

Duffy, J. (1995). *Motor Speech Disorders: Substrates, Differential Diagnosis, and Management*, Mosby, St. Louis, USA

Enderby, P. & Palmer, R. (2008). *FDA-2. The Frenchay Dysarthria Assessment. Examiner's Manual* (Second edition), Pro-Ed, Austin, Tex, USA

Esposito, S.J., Mitsumoto, H. & Shanks, M. (2000). Use of palatal lift and palatal augmentation prostheses to improve dysarthria in patients with amyotrophic lateral sclerosis: a case series. *Journal of Prosthetic Dentistry*, Vol. 83, pp. 90-98

Farwell, L.A. & Donchin, E. (1988). Talking off the top of your head: toward a mental prosthesis utilizing event-related brain potentials. *Electroencephalography and Clinical Neurophysiology*, Vol. 70, pp. 510-523

Ferrante, R.J., Browne, S.E., Shinobu, L.A., Bowling, A.C., Baik, M.J., MacGarvey, U., Kowall, N.W., Brown, R.H. Jr. & Beal, M.F. (1997). Evidence of increased oxidative damage in both sporadic and familial amyotrophic lateral sclerosis. *Journal of Neurochemistry*, Vol. 69, pp. 2064-2074

Francis, K., Bach, J.R. & DeLisa, J.A. (1999). Evaluation and rehabilitation of patients with adult motor neuron disease. *Archives of Physical Medicine and Rehabilitation*, Vol. 80, pp. 951-963

Fried-Oken, M., Fox, L., Rau, M.T., Tullman, J., Baker, G., Hindal, M., Wile, N. & Lou, J.S. (2006). Purposes of AAC device use for persons with ALS as reported by caregivers. *Augmentative Alternative Communication*, Vol. 20, pp. 209-221

Gerven, M.V., Farquhar, J. & Schaefer, R. (2009). The brain-computer interface cycle. *Journal of Neural Engineering*, Vol. 6, pp. 1-10

Gibbons, C. & Beneteau, E. (2010). Functional performance using eye control and single switch scanning by people with ALS. *Perspectives on Augmentative and Alternative Communication*, Vol. 19, pp. 64-69

Gordon, P.H. (2011). Amyotrophic lateral sclerosis: pathophysiology, diagnosis and management. *CNS Drugs*, Vol. 25, pp. 1-15

Green, J.R., Beukelman, D.R. & Ball, L.J. (2004). Algorithmic estimation of pauses in extended speech samples of dysarthric and typical speech. *Journal of Medical Speech-Language Pathology*, Vol. 12, pp. 149-154

Guedj, E., Ber, I., Lacomblez, L., Dubois, B., Verpillat, P., Didic, M., Salachas, F., Vera, P., Hannequin, D., Lotterie, J.A., Puel, M., Decousus, M., Thomas-Antérion, C., Magne, C., Vercelletto, M., Bernard, A.M., Golfier, V., Pasquier, J., Michel, B.F., Namer, I.,

Sellal, F., Bochet, J., Volteau, M., Brice, A., Meininger, V., French Research Network on FTD/FTD-MND & Habert, M.O. (2007). Brain SPECT perfusion of frontotemporal dementia associated with motor neuron disease. *Neurology*, Vol. 69, pp. 488-490

Guger, C., Daban, S., Sellers, E., Holzner, C., Krausz, G., Carabalona, R., Gramatica, F. & Edlinger, G. (2009). How many people are able to control a P300-based brain-computer interface (BCI)? *Neuroscience Letters*, Vol. 462, pp. 94-98

Guidubaldi, A., Fasano, A., Ialongo, T., Piano, C., Pompili, M., Mascianà, R., Siciliani, L., Sabatelli, M. & Bentivoglio, A.R. (2011). Botulinum toxin A versus B in sialorrhea: a prospective, randomized, double-blind, crossover pilot study in patients with amyotrophic lateral sclerosis or Parkinson's disease. *Movement Disorders*, Vol. 26, pp. 313-319

Guy, N., Bourry, N., Dallel, R., Dualé, C., Verrelle, P., Lapeyre, M. & Clavelou, P. (2011). Comparison of radiotherapy types in the treatment of sialorrhea in amyotrophic lateral sclerosis. *Journal of Palliative Medicine*, Vol. 14, pp. 391-395

Hanson, E., Yorkston, K. & Britton, D. (2011). Dysarthria in amyotrophic lateral sclerosis: a systematic review of characteristics, speech treatment, and AAC options. *Journal of Medical Speech-Language Pathology*. In press.

Harris, D. & Goren, M. (2009). The ERICA eye gaze system versus manual letter board to aid communication in ALS/MND. *British Journal of Neuroscience Nursing*, Vol. 5, pp. 227-230

Haverkamp, L.J., Appel, V. & Appel, S.H. (1995). Natural history of amyotrophic lateral sclerosis in a database population. Validation of a scoring system and a model for survival prediction. *Brain*, Vol. 118, pp. 707-719

Hillel, A.D., Miller, R.M., Yorkston, K., McDonald, E., Norris, F.H. & Konikow, N. (1989). Amyotrophic lateral sclerosis severity scale. *Neuroepidemiology*, Vol. 8, pp. 142-150

Hirose, H., Kiritani, S. & Sawashima, M. (1982). Patterns of dysarthric movement in patients with Amyotrophic Lateral Sclerosis and Pseudobulbar Palsy. *Folia Phoniatrica et Logopaedica*, Vol. 34, pp. 106-112

Hong, B., Guo, F., Liu, T., Gao, X. & Gao, S. (2009). N200-speller using motion-onset visual response. *Clinical Neurophysiology*, Vol. 120, pp. 1658-1666

Iversen, I.H., Ghanayim, N., Kübler, A., Neumann, N., Birbaumer, N. & Kaiser, J. (2008). A brain-computer interface tool to assess cognitive functions in completely paralyzed patients with amyotrophic lateral sclerosis. *Clinical Neurophysiology*, Vol. 119, pp. 2214-2223

Kent, R.D., Kent, J.F., Weismer, G., Martin, R.E., Sufit, R.L. & Rosenbek, J.C. (1989). Relationships between speech intelligibility and the slope of second-formant transitions in dysarthric subjects. *Clinical Linguistics and Phonetics*, Vol. 3, pp. 347-358

Kent, J.F., Kent, R.D., Rosenbek, J.C., Weismer, G., Martin, R. & Sufit, R. (1992). Quantitative description of the dysarthria in women with amyotrophic lateral sclerosis. *Journal of Speech and Hearing Research*, Vol. 35, pp. 723-733

Kent, R.D., Vorperian, H.K., Kent, J.F. & Duffy, J.R. (2003). Voice dysfunction in dysarthria: application of the Multi-Dimensional Voice Program. *Journal of Communication Disorders*, Vol. 36, pp. 281-306

Kobayashi, M., Ikeda, K., Kinoshita, M. & Iwasaki Y. (1999). Amyotrophic lateral sclerosis with supranuclear ophthalmoplegia and rigidity. *Neurological Research*, Vol. 21, pp. 661-664

Krusienski, D.J., Sellers, E.W., Cabestaing, F., Bayoudh, S., McFarland, D.J., Vaughan, T.M. & Wolpaw, J.R. (2006). A comparison of classification techniques for the P300 Speller. *Journal of Neural Engineering*, Vol. 3, pp. 299-305

Kubler, A., Neumann, N., Kaiser, J., Kotchoubey, B., Hinterberger, T. & Birbaumer, N. (2001). Brain-computer communication: self-regulation of slow cortical potentials for verbal communication. *Archives of Physical Medicine and Rehabilitation*, Vol. 82, pp. 1533-1539

Lenhardt, A., Kaper, M. & Ritter, H.J. (2008). An adaptive P300-based online brain-computer interface. *IEEE Transactions on Neural Systems and Rehabilitation Engineering*, Vol. 16, pp. 121-130

Logroscino, G., Traynor, B.J., Hardiman, O., Chiò, A., Couratier, P., Mitchell, J.D., Swingler, R.J. & Beghi, E. for EURALS. (2008). Descriptive epidemiology of amyotrophic lateral sclerosis: new evidence and unsolved issues. *Journal of Neurology, Neurosurgery & Psychiatry*, Vol. 79, pp. 6-11

Martens, S.M., Hill, N.J., Farquhar, J. & Scholkopf, B. (2009). Overlap and refractory effects in a brain-computer interface speller based on the visual P300 event-related potential. *Journal of Neural Engineering*, Vol. 6, pp. 026003

Miller, R.G., Rosenberg, J.A., Gelinas, D.F., Mitsumoto, H., Newman, D., Sufit, R., Borasio, G.D., Bradley, W.G., Bromberg, M.B., Brooks, B.R., Kasarskis, E.J., Munsat, T.L. & Oppenheimer, E.A. (1999). Practice parameter: the care of the patient with amyotrophic lateral sclerosis (an evidence-based review): report of the Quality Standards Subcommittee of the American Academy of Neurology: ALS Practice Parameters Task Force. *Neurology*, Vol. 52, pp. 1311-1323

Miller, R.G., Jackson, C.E., Kasarskis, E.J., England, J.D., Forshew, D., Johnston, W., Kalra, S., Katz, J.S., Mitsumoto, H., Rosenfeld, J., Shoesmith, C., Strong, M.J. & Woolley, S.C., Quality Standards Subcommittee of the American Academy of Neurology. (2009a). Practice parameter update: The care of the patient with amyotrophic lateral sclerosis: drug, nutritional, and respiratory therapies (an evidence-based review): report of the Quality Standards Subcommittee of the American Academy of Neurology. *Neurology*, Vol. 73, pp. 1218-1226

Miller, R.G., Jackson, C.E., Kasarskis, E.J., England, J.D., Forshew, D., Johnston, W., Kalra, S., Katz, J.S., Mitsumoto, H., Rosenfeld, J., Shoesmith, C., Strong, M.J. & Woolley, S.C., Quality Standards Subcommittee of the American Academy of Neurology. (2009b). Practice parameter update: The care of the patient with amyotrophic lateral sclerosis: multidisciplinary care, symptom management, and cognitive/behavioral impairment (an evidence-based review): report of the Quality Standards Subcommittee of the American Academy of Neurology. *Neurology*, Vol. 73, pp. 1227-1233

Mulligan, M., Carpenter, J., Riddel, J., Delaney, M.K., Badger, G. & Krusinski, P. (1994). Intelligibility and the acoustic characteristics of speech in amyotrophic lateral sclerosis (ALS). *Journal of Speech and Hearing Research*, Vol. 37, pp. 496-503

Münte, T.F., Tröger, M.C., Nusser, I., Wieringa, B.M., Johannes, S., Matzke, M. & Dengler, R. (1998). Alteration of early components of the visual evoked potential in amyotrophic lateral sclerosis. *Journal of Neurology*, Vol. 245, pp. 206-210

Murphy, J. (2004). "I prefer contact this close": perceptions of AAC by people with motor neurone disease and their communication partners. *Augmentative and Alternative Communication*, Vol. 20, pp. 259-271

Nishio, M. & Niimi, S. (2000). Changes over time in dysarthric patients with amyotrophic lateral sclerosis (ALS): a study of changes in speaking rate and maximum repetition rate (MRR). *Clinical Linguistics and Phonetics*, Vol. 14, pp. 485-497

Norris, F.H., Calanchini, P.R., Fallat, R.J., Pancharis, S. & Jewett, B. (1974). Administration of guanidine in amyotrophic lateral sclerosis. *Neurology*, Vol. 24, pp. 721-728

Okuda, B., Yamamoto, T., Yamasaki, M., Maya, K. & Imai, T. (1992). Motor neuron disease with slow eye movements and vertical gaze palsy. *Acta Neurologica Scandinavica*, Vol. 85, pp. 71-76

Patten, S.B., Svenson, L.W, White, C.M., Khaled, S.M. & Metz, L.M. (2007). Affective disorders in motor neuron disease: a population-based study. *Neuroepidemiology*, Vol. 28, pp. 1-7

Polich, J. (2007). Updating P300: an integrative theory of P3a and P3b. *Clinical Neurophysiology*, Vol. 118, pp. 2128-2148

Raaphorst, J., De Visser, M., Linssen, W.H., De Haan, R.J. & Schmand, B. (2010). The cognitive profile of amyotrophic lateral sclerosis: A meta-analysis. *Amyotrophic Lateral Sclerosis*, Vol. 11, pp. 27-37

Ramig, L.O., Scherer, R.C., Klasner, E.R., Titze, I.R. & Horii, Y. (1990). Acoustic analysis of voice in amyotrophic lateral sclerosis: A longitudinal case study. *Journal of Speech and Hearing Disorders*, Vol. 55, pp. 2-14

Ringholz, G.M., Appel, S.H., Bradshaw, M., Cooke, N.A., Mosnik, D.M. & Schulz, P.E. (2005). Prevalence and patterns of cognitive impairment in sporadic ALS. *Neurology*, Vol. 65, pp. 586-590

Roth, C., Glaze, L., Goding, G. & David, W. (1996). Spasmodic dysphonia symptoms as initial presentation of amyotrophic lateral sclerosis. *Journal of Voice*, Vol. 10, pp. 362-367

Salvaris, M. & Sepulveda, F. (2009). Visual modifications on the P300 speller BCI paradigm. *Journal of Neural Engineering*, Vol. 6, pp. 046011

Sellers, E.W. & Donchin, E. (2006). A P300-based brain-computer interface: initial tests by ALS patients. *Clinical Neurophysiology*, Vol. 117, pp. 538-548

Sellers, E.W., Krusienski, D.J., McFarland, D.J., Vaughan, T.M. & Wolpaw, J.R. (2006). A P300 event-related potential brain-computer interface (BCI): the effects of matrix size and inter stimulus interval on performance. *Biological Psychology*, Vol. 73, pp. 242-252

Takano, K., Komatsu, T., Hata, N., Nakajima, Y. & Kansaku, K. (2009). Visual stimuli for the P300 brain-computer interface: a comparison of white/gray and green/blue flicker matrices. *Clinical Neurophysiology*, Vol. 20, pp. 1562-1566

Ticozzi, N., Tiloca, C., Morelli, C., Colombrita, C., Poletti, B., Doretti, A., Maderna, L., Messina, S., Ratti, A. & Silani, V. (2011). Genetics of familial Amyotrophic Lateral Sclerosis. *Archives Italiennes de Biologie*, Vol. 149, pp. 65-82

Tjaden, K. & Turner, G.S. (1997). Spectral properties of fricative in amyotrophic lateral sclerosis. *Journal of Speech, Language and Hearing Research*, Vol. 40, pp. 1358-1372

Tjaden, K. & Turner, G.S. (2000). Segmental timing in amyotrophic lateral sclerosis. *Journal of Speech, Language and Hearing Research*, Vol. 43, pp. 683-696

Tomik, B. & Guiloff, R.J. (2010). Dysarthria in amyotrophic lateral sclerosis: A review. *Amyotrophic Lateral Sclerosis*, Vol. 11, pp. 4-15

Townsend, G., La Pallo, B.K., Boulay, C.B., Krusienski, D.J., Frye, G.E., Hauser, C.K., Schwartz, N.E., Vaughan, T.M., Wolpaw, J.R. & Sellers, E.W. (2010). A novel P300-based brain-computer interface stimulus presentation paradigm: moving beyond rows and columns. *Clinical Neurophysiology*, Vol. 121, pp. 1109-1120

Turner, G.S., Tjaden, K. & Weismer, G. (1995). The influence of speaking rate on vowel space and speech intelligibility for individuals with ALS. *Journal of Speech and Hearing Research*, Vol. 38, pp. 1001-1013

Turner, G.S. & Weismer, G. (1993). Characteristics of speaking rate in the dysarthria associated with amyotrophic lateral sclerosis. *Journal of Speech and Hearing Research*, Vol. 36, pp. 1134-1144

Vaughan, T.M., McFarland, D.J., Schalk, G., Sarnacki, W.A., Krusienski, D.J., Sellers, E.W. & Wolpaw, J.R. (2006). The Wadsworth BCI Research and Development Program: at home with BCI. *IEEE Transactions on Neural Systems and Rehabilitation Engineering*, Vol. 14, pp. 229-233

Weismer, G., Kent, R.D., Hodge, M. & Martin, R. (1988). The acoustic signatures for intelligibility test words. *Journal of the Acoustical Society of America*, Vol. 84, pp. 1281-1291

Weismer, G., Martin, R., Kent, J.F, & Kent, R.D. (1992). Formant trajectory characteristics of males with amyotrophic lateral sclerosis. *Journal of the Acoustical Society of America*, Vol. 91, pp. 1085-1097

Weismer, G., Jeng, J.Y., Laures, J.S., Kent, R.D. & Kent, J.F. (2001). Acoustic and intelligibility characteristics of sentence production in neurogenic speech disorders. *Folia Phoniatrica et Logopaedica*, Vol. 53, pp. 1-18

Worms, P.M. (2001). The epidemiology of motor neuron diseases: a review of recent studies. *Journal of the Neurological Sciences*, Vol. 191, pp. 3-9

Yorkston, K., Beukelman, D.R. & Traynor, C. (1984). *Assessment of Intelligibility of Dysarthric Speech*, Pro-Ed, Austin, Tex, USA

Yorkston K., Strand, E., Miller, R., Hillel, A. & Smith, K. (1993). Speech deterioration in amyotrophic lateral sclerosis: implications for the timing of intervention. *Journal of Medical Speech-Language Pathology*, Vol. 1, pp. 35-46

Yorkston, K., Beukelman, D.R., Hakel, M. & Dorsey, M. (2007). *Sentence Intelligibility Test, Speech Intelligibility Test*, Madonna Rehabilitation Hospital, Lincoln, Neb, USA

Yorkston, K., Beukelman, D.R., Strand, E. & Hakel, M. (2010). *Management of Motor Speech Disorders in Children and Adults*, Pro-Ed, Austin, Tex, USA

Yunusova, Y., Weismer, G., Westbury, J.R. & Lindstrom, M.J. (2008). Articulatory movements during vowels in speakers with dysarthria and normal controls. *Journal of Speech, Language and Hearing Research*, Vol. 51, pp. 596-611

Yunusova, Y., Green, J.R., Lindstrom, M.J., Ball, L.J., Pattee, G.L. & Zinman, L. (2010). Kinematics of disease progression in bulbar ALS. *Journal of Communication Disorders*, Vol. 43, pp. 6–20.

16

Human Computer Interactions for Amyotrophic Lateral Sclerosis Patients

Ali Bülent Uşaklı
The NCO Academy
Turkey

1. Introduction

In this chapter, alternative communication and device control channels, which are helpful for Amyotrophic lateral sclerosis (ALS) patients, are introduced. In this context, human computer interactions (HCIs) will be discussed in three respects; electrical brain activities, eye movements and hemoglobin level in the blood.

With technological advances, fighting or minimization side effects of the diseases is the main purpose of biomedical research. Under this motto, this chapter focuses on HCIs for individuals suffering from motor neuron diseases. ALS is a progressive neurodegenerative disease caused by the degeneration of motor neurons. ALS or other tetraplegic clinical conditions, otherwise known as the locked-in syndrome, have severe disabilities in controlling muscles and consequently have problems in moving the entire body. Some of these patients can only move their eyes. In severe conditions of the progressive motor neuron diseases, patients cannot move their eyes nor can they speak. Establishing an efficient communication channel without overt speaking and hand motions makes the patient's life a bit easier and increases their quality of life.

ALS occurs in between 4 and 8 out of every 100,000 individuals and only a small percentage of cases arise from a known genetic cause (Parker & Parker, 2007). Concerning other motor neuron diseases or speaking and muscular disabilities, there are more than 100 million potential users in need of alternative channels such as brain computer interface (BCI) for communicating with their environment or for controlling devices (Guger, 2008). Considering life span extension and increasing causes of injuries including traffic accidents and explosions, which may result in spinal cord injuries in serious cases, the need for an efficient communication or control channel has been drastically increasing.

HCIs are a research field which includes interactions such as communication and device/machine control between a user and a computer. The aim of the HCI is to improve performance of the interaction, meaning a minimization of the barrier between the human and the computer. Accurate and fast interpretation of what the user wants to do as well as a correct understanding by the computer of the user's intentions or demand is the aim of this research field.

Man-machine interface (MMI), brain-machine interface (BMI) and BCI can be thought of as applications of HCIs. If communication or control is established directly from the brain, it is called BCI and it is the only method of interaction for the individuals with complete paralysis. Because these research fields are new, there is a need for development in terms of efficiency; meaning accuracy, reliability and quick responses are necessary. Many research groups from all over the world are focusing on HCI applications in order to improve alternative communication channels for the disabled. An efficient alternative channel for communication and control device without overt speaking and muscular movements is important to make life easier for individuals who are suffering from ALS or other illnesses that prevent proper limb and muscular responses. Because of this, the area of study related with HCIs has high expectations and are important for improving quality of life.

In this chapter, ALS related HCI in particular, is discussed. The very common field electroencephalogram (EEG) based BCI and other approaches in this field are presented. With interdisciplinary studies, developing new interfaces and interaction techniques are opening new research fields for investigation. Especially for the paralysis patients, the classical communication or control ways, such as overt speaking or hand motions cannot be used. Using bio-signals such as EEG and its various methodologies (i.e. P300, slow cortical potentials, etc), electrooculogram (EOG), hearth rate (HR) or galvanic skin response (GSR) as well as the hemoglobin level which is related to oxygenation, are the only ways to send messages or control signals to devices regarding user's demands, intentions or expectations. This does not only give the patients the potential ability to give messages on computer screens and control a powered wheelchair or robot arm without muscular movements, but also can be potentially useful for the elderly as well.

The aim of this chapter is to present the state of the art of the technology on HCIs. This chapter also addresses the use of different bio-signals individually or the integrated hybrid/integrated multi-modal system approach for communication and control with high performance. In order to increase performance, processing combined bio-signals and multi-modal integrated systems will be discussed. For this purpose, several bio-signals such as EEG, EOG, and functional near infrared (fNIR) spectroscopy based system research are introduced.

2. Human computer interactions

In general, HCIs are related to the adaptation of a human and a computer. HMIs adapt human demands to the machine. Human computer interface operation requires the effective interaction of two sides; user and system. Here, a system can be an integrated system of computers and a word speller, a robot arm, a powered wheelchair, house appliances such as door locks, TVs or musical instruments, etc. In order to reflect intent/demands, instead of overt speaking or muscular movements, other bio-signals can be used. Effective BCIs may serve as assessment tools and adaptive systems for HCI for able-bodied people and be proven for people with severe motor neuron diseases.

Research in this field is typically focused on several areas of improvement for HCIs in order to increase its usefulness and effectiveness. These areas are:

i.   High performance
    a.   Accuracy
    b.   Reliability
    c.   Fast
    d.   Robustness
ii. User friendliness (including user training)
iii. Ease of application
iv. Cost effectiveness.

In short, HCI should reflect user demands and expectations accurately and quickly. The next sections of this chapter will introduce the EEG, EOG, NIRS based systems, as they are technologies that show much promise. In addition to these technologies, electrocorticography (ECoG), functional magnetic resonance imaging (fMRI), galvanic skin response (GSR) and heart rate (HR) based systems; and multi-modal integrated design rationale are introduced briefly.

2.1 Brain computer interfaces

From a broad perspective, BMI refers to the interface between a brain and a machine (for review Lebedev & Nicolelis, 2006). In this section, the common term - brain computer interface (BCI) will be presented. BCI can be described as a translation of human intentions into a control signal without using the muscles. The aim of BCI is to provide communication and control for people with severe motor disabilities.

The BCI system translates the signals that are encoded by the user's intentions into messages and control commands. Research in this field has been rapidly growing in neuroscience and bioengineering. Specifically, this technology is promising for users with motor neuron diseases. Table 1 shows the estimated potential users of BCI. According to this table, there are more than 100 million potential users in the world.

Type of the Disease	Number of Patients
Amyotrophic Lateral Sclerosis	400,000/3,000,000
Multiple Sclerosis	2,000,000
Muscular Dystrophy	1,000,000
Brainstem Stroke	10,000,000
Cerebral Palsy	16,000,000
Spinal Cord Injury	5,000,000
Postpolio Syndrome	7,000,000
Guillain-Barre Syndrome	70,000
Other types of Stroke	60,000,000

Table 1. Potential users of BCI in the world (Guger, 2008).

Electrical brain activities (electroencephalography, EEG) related to human intentions can be monitored using electrodes attached to the scalp surface, non-invasively. EEG signals are gross potential of the thousands of neurons, roughly reflecting bodily functions. Because the skull and scalp play the role of a barrier for the electrical signals, EEG signals have low amplitudes (in micro-volts scale) and exist in the 0.5–30 Hz frequency band. Figure 1 shows the ongoing time series EEG signal and its power spectral density. As it is shown from this figure, 8-12 Hz (α band) and 26 Hz (β band) components are dominant.

In order to increase efficiency, brain electrical signals can be recorded by subdural electrodes (electrocorticogram, ECoG), invasively. ECoGs are neuronal activity that is acquired from smaller cortical areas when compared to EEGs. Epidural or subdural recording is less invasive than intra-cortical recording. While their applications are difficult, the resolution of these recordings can be significantly higher than conventional EEG. The BCI usefulness of intra-cortical signals is promising (Wolpaw, 2003).

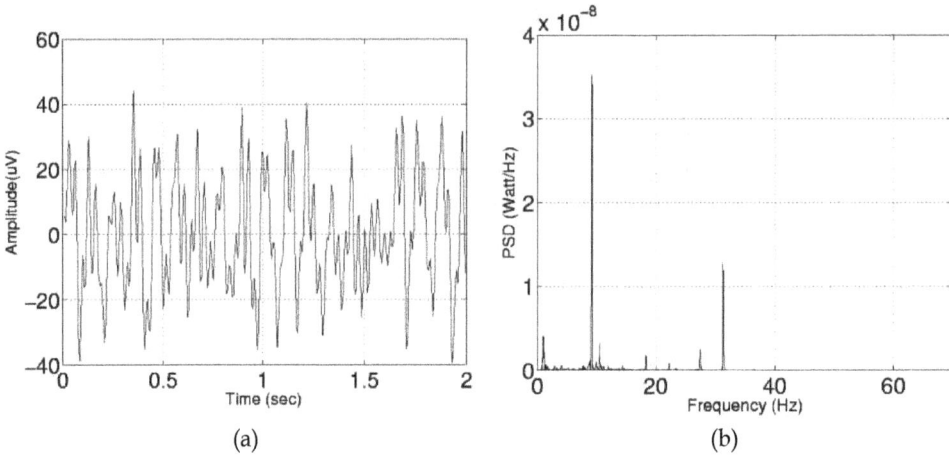

(a)   (b)

Fig. 1. Ongoing EEG recording from 27-year old male subject's occipital lobe: (a) the time series signal, and (b) power spectral density.

BCI systems can provide a communication and control channel, which bypasses conventional neuromuscular pathways involved in speaking or movement activity made to manipulate objects (Wolpaw et al., 2002). The command for device control can be generated by self-regulated μ rhythms (Wolpaw et al., 2000), motor imagery (Pfurtscheller et al., 2000) or a visual evoked potential (Sutter, 1992).

An EEG based BCI system can use the signals listed below.

- P300 response,
- steady state visual evoked potential (SSVEP),
- event related desynchronisation (ERD),
- slow cortical potential (SCP) and
- sensorimotor rhythm (SMR).

P300 and SSVEP methods require external stimulation that the user has to focus attention on or gaze into flickering lights, which the other methods do not need (self-paced systems). Because of this, the user is not free to decide on performing an action; the user depends on computer software for the synchronization. Each of these methods is advantageous or disadvantageous with respect to performance, information transfer rate and user training time. The BCI systems may not use just one of these approaches, but may use a combination of two or more signals as a hybrid approached system.

As an event related potential (ERP), the common method is using the P300 response (Farwell & Donchin, 1988). The P300 response is elicited between 300 msec and 400 msec after stimulation, as it is shown in figure 2. Because ERPs are so small, for clarity, signal (epoch) averaging is necessary. The latency and amplitude may change from user to user, however the shape of the signal is roughly the same. In addition to using P300 response, SSVEPs (Gao et al, 2003) and SCPs, μ (8-12 Hz) and high β (18-26 Hz) rhythms (sensorimotor applications) are used in BCI applications.

The SSVEP is a brain response evoked mainly in the visual and parietal cortices as a response to flickering visual stimuli. The SSVEP has gained popularity in the BCI research because it provides advantages in terms of speed and robustness. ERD and Event-related synchronization was quantified by the most reactive frequency bands were chosen then band-pass filtered within those bands. SCPs are slow shifts of the EEG with duration from 300 msec to several seconds. The group of SCPs includes the contingent negative variation, premovement potentials, the Bereitschaftspotential and expectancy waves (Pfurtscheller et al., 2005).

While these approaches are important for the detection of imagery motor activities, the approach of the P300 waveform is very common in BCI applications. As it is shown figure 2, the P300 response is a large, positive potential (conventionally opposite polarization) that has been studied extensively within the context of the oddball paradigm. Donchin and colleagues first reported the use of the P300 for BCI communication (Donchin et al., 2000). International approaches for the detection of P300 speller, a matrix of grey symbols on a dark background (virtual keyboard) are shown in figure 3.

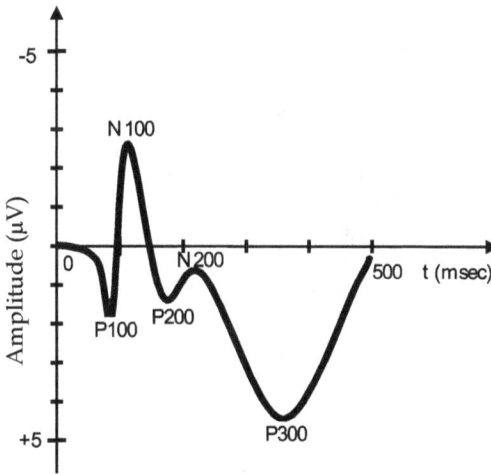

Fig. 2. Typical averaged event related potentials after stimulation. In BCI applications P300 component is extensively used.

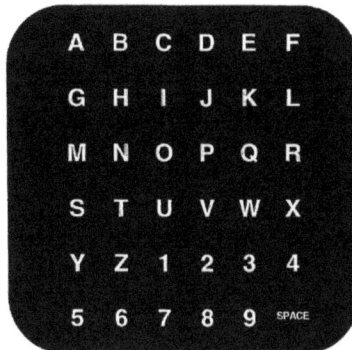

Fig. 3. The matrix for P300 speller. The stimulus matrix monitored by the subject. Typically, one of the rows or columns of the matrix was intensified every 125 ms (The matrix is proposed first by Donchin and colleagues 1988).

The P300 speller paradigm has been common as a promising communication tool. Using the P300, a virtual keyboard without using or requiring any activation of skeletal muscles can be realized (Farwell & Donchin, 1988; Donchin et al., 2000; Sellers & Donchin, 2006). In the virtual keyboard, rows and columns of the matrix were randomly intensified typically every 125 ms. A P300 was produced after attended character is flashed. The attended symbol was selected by averaging responses for rows and columns. Accurate performance is obtained in users with and without motor impairments. Users with ALS are able to use the P300 based, single-stimulus system using either auditory or visual presentations. The Oddball paradigm to implement using the commands: Yes, No, Pass, and End with three presentation modes: auditory, visual, and both auditory and visual were used (Sellers et al., 2006). Detecting P300 signals the mind spelled characters (words, sentences, stories), enable the communication-disabled via internet (van Kokswijk & van Hulle, 2010) were realized.

People can learn to control EEG features consisting of SMR amplitudes and can use this control to move a cursor to a target on a screen. EEG recordings during right and left motor imagery allow users to establish a new communication channel. Such an EEG-based BCI can be used to develop a simple binary response for the control of a device (Guger et al., 2000). To control cursor movement 8-12 Hz (μ) or 18-26 Hz (β) frequency bands over sensorimotor cortex can be used (Fabiani et al., 2004). In the standard one-dimensional application, the cursor moves horizontally from left to right at a fixed rate while vertical cursor movement is continuously controlled by SMR (μ and β rhythms) amplitude over left and/or right sensorimotor cortex (McFarland & Wolpaw, 2005). Intention of movement of left or right index finger, or right foot is recognized in EEG signals (Peters et al., 2001).

The model usually employed in many BCI systems is presented in Figure 4. Here, messages can be word speller output and commands can be for the powered wheelchair, robot hand or domotic (house) appliances control commands.

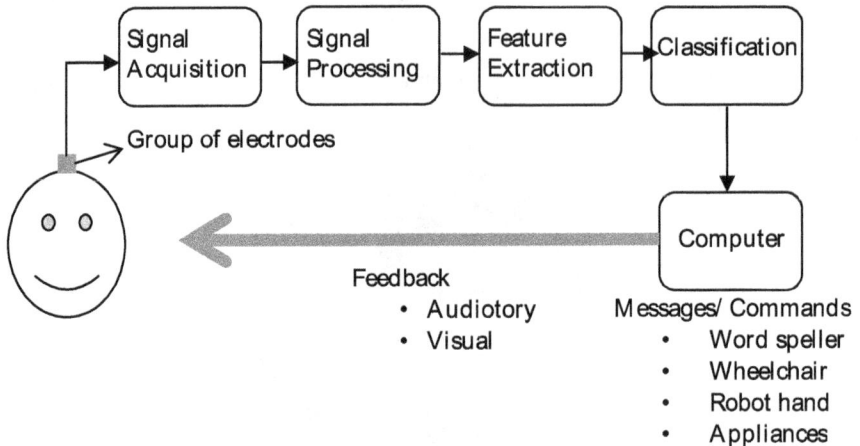

Fig. 4. A Typical BCI system.

To increase usefulness, BCI research groups are focusing several respects. In order to evaluate the usefulness of approaches for user intention, it is important to recognize that intention is normally formatted as a goal (Wolpaw, 2003). This goal may be "Write letter 'A' (On the screen)", "Move forward (powered wheelchair)" "Hit target (cursor)", "Grasp the glass", "Turn on the TV" or "Unlock the door", etc. After real time processing regarding the goal, the next step is goal-directed feedback generation.

The BCI systems may be self-paced. This means that the system allows communication or control whenever the user wishes. These systems' performance determined the true positive rate and the false positive rate. The true positive rate is the percentage of intentional control commands that are correctly detected by the BCI system. False positive rate are false positives generated by the system during the periods for which the user does not intend control.

A synchronous BCI uses external stimulation whereas in asynchronous BCI the subject makes self-paced decisions on when to switch from one mental task to the next. A virtual keyboard and a mobile robot which respond every 0.5 s were developed (Millan & Mourino, 2003). Additionally, an asynchronous BCI analyzes and classifies EEG data continuously (Townsend et al., 2004). These systems are designed to process only one brain state in the ongoing EEG. For this purpose, only one channel may be sufficient. To control a powered wheelchair using a delayed response task a binary classification of left and right movement intentions were classified with a classification rate of over 80% from single trial EEG (Kaneswaran et al., 2010).

In order to improve the BCI system's performance, a rapid transition of various types of parameter estimation and classification algorithms to real-time implementation and testing (Guger, et al., 2001), classification accuracy and communication rate (Turnip et al., 2010) were realized. Identifying errors through the brain's reaction to mistakes is used to improve the robustness, flexibility, and reliability of BCIs (Buttfield et al., 2006). In addition to algorithmic improvement to increase performance, or in other words - high-resolution, multi-channel EEG systems have been developed to enhance the spatial information content of EEG activity. All these factors help to increasing the efficiency of BCI systems.

For standardization of BCI research, there is a documented general-purpose BCI research and development platform known as BCI2000. This platform can incorporate independent or a combination of any brain signals, signal processing methods, output devices and operating protocols (Wolpaw et al., 2003; Schalk, et al., 2004).

As a new approach to drive BCIs, functional magnetic resonance imaging (fMRI), have been used. The temporal resolution of the hemodynamic deoxyhemoglobin changes in the range of 1-2 seconds, while its spatial resolution is generally observable with the current imaging techniques at a few millimeters scale. Local hemodynamic response can be measured by fMRI. Hence, fMRI responses and cortical sources of EEG data are spatially related. It is possible to estimate the cortical activity with a spatial resolution of few millimeters and with a temporal resolution of milliseconds from noninvasive EEG measurements (Astolfi et al., 2010).

Although an fMRI based BCIs noninvasively records activity of the entire brain with a high spatial resolution, they are not suitable for everyday use. They have temporal delays of several seconds. However, they have good spatial resolution and they can sample the activity of deep brain structures (Lebedev & Nicolelis, 2006). An fMRI-based BCI platform which performs data processing and feedback of the hemodynamic brain activity within 1.3 s (Weiskopf et al., 2004), psychophysiological markers (Nijboer et al., 2009), and communication using real-time fMRI (Eklund et al., 2010) were developed. In the later system, the subject in the MR scanner sees a virtual keyboard and steers a cursor to select different letters that can be combined to create words. The cursor is moved to the left by activating the left hand, to the right by activating the right hand, down by activating the left toes and up by activating the right toes (Eklund et al., 2010).

It can be concluded that as an alternative method for communication through speaking and muscular movements, BCIs are allowing communication and control for individuals with motor neuron disease such as ALS. A BCI system consists of recognition by a computation of the patterns of brain electrical activity on the scalp acquired from an array of electrodes. Although this technology is quite useful, it still needs to be developed in terms of efficiency.

2.2 Electrooculography based systems

Paralyzed patients are unable to communicate normally with their environment. For these patients, the only part of their body that is under their control, in terms of muscular movement, is their eyes. Some research in this area has been focused on investigating new efficient communication tools for paralyzed patients to translate their eye movements into appropriate communication messages or control signals.

With eye movements, a potential across the cornea and retina exists. This potential is called the cornea-retinal potential and it is the source of the electrooculogram (EOG). Communicating and controlling with EOG can be used for the disabled. An EOG based HCI device is able to recognize the subject's eye movements by using the electrical activity generated by the eye movements. EOG signals have certain patterns for each kind of eye movement (left, right, up, down, blink or wink). These signal patterns can be acquired and then recognized as signals which can be used for controlling external devices like a virtual keyboard, a powered wheelchair, a robot arm or a movable robot. As a very common application, the EOG-based virtual keyboard provides a means for paralyzed patients to write letters on a screen with eye movements without using a conventional keyboard. An EOG-based system for HCI application is presented in figure 5 and EOG signal samples are shown in figure 6.

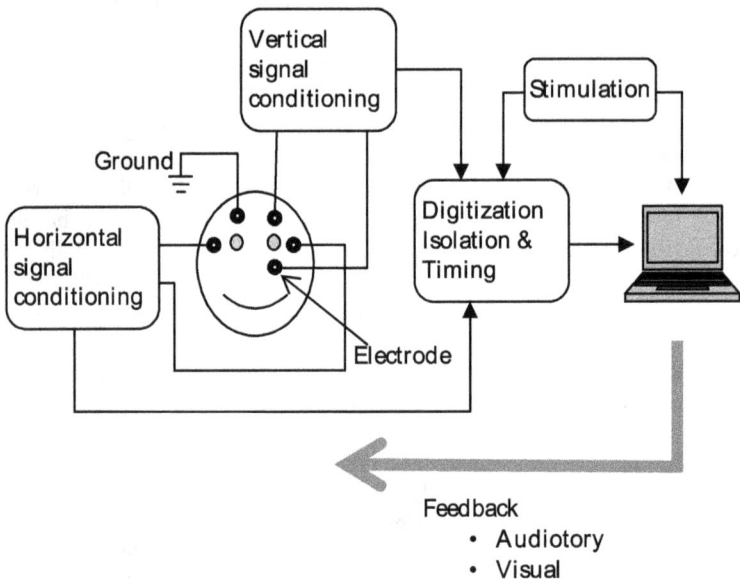

Fig. 5. Typical EOG-based interface.

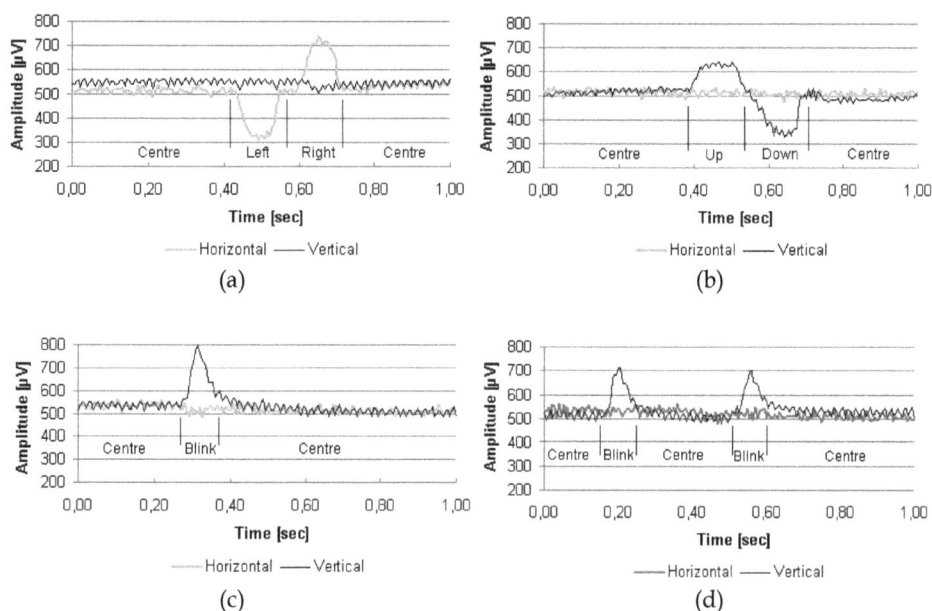

Fig. 6. Voluntary EOG signals: a) Horizontal, b) Vertical, c) Eye blink and d) double blink (Usakli & Gurkan, 2010).

Many studies exist in the literature concerning the application of eye movements to the HCI (Bahill, 1982; Yoshiaki, 1997; Juhola, 1985; Allison et al., 1996; Hutchinson et al., 1989; Norris & Wilson, 1997; Kuno, et al., 1998; Chen et al., 1999; Ihara et al., 2009). The research focused mainly on the word speller. Recognizing eye movements; such as left, right, up and down, and eye blinks to select characters from the virtual keyboard on the screen can use giving a message (Kherlopian et al., 2006; Akan & Argunsah, 2007; Usakli et al, 2009). With the EOG based word speller, it is reported that 5 letter-word such as "Water" can be written in 25 seconds (Usakli & Gurkan, 2010). The menus of this system are shown in figure 7. EOG-controlled cursor interfaces, where the cursor can be controlled by eye movement (Tomita et al., 2006; Tamura et al., 2010) are realized, successfully.

As a communication device, a prototype of a head-mounted display with the eye-gaze detection function was developed which a user can operate by eye movements (Handa & Ebisawa, 2008). With this device, the eye-gaze point was determined from the relative position between the pupil center and the corneal reflection of the light source which were detected by the camera. An eye-gaze controlled navigation and electromyography (EMG) enter (confirm) the selection of letter (Dhillon et al. 2009), and an eye-movement tracking system (Krueger & Stieglitz, 2007; Deng et al., 2009; Septanto et al., 2009) were developed. Another promising EOG based method is a Morse code generator (Wu et al., 2007). Additionally, an EOG-based a powered wheelchair (Barea et al., 2002; Chung-Hsien et al., 2009) and a portable wireless device (Zheng et al., 2009) were realized. The EOG based device allows the patients to generate decisions on a screen by means of simple eye movement signals. These signals can be measured with EMG/EEG electrodes, without the need of complex systems or infra-red cameras. Then, patients are able to select letters on the screen or even communicate basic needs (food drinks, etc.) to the caregiver with a simple movement of their eyes (Usakli et al, 2009). All these studies show that EOG signals can be used as an input for efficient HCI applications. Since the EOG signals are larger, measurement of these signals are easy compared to EEG. This property makes EOG applications much more efficient.

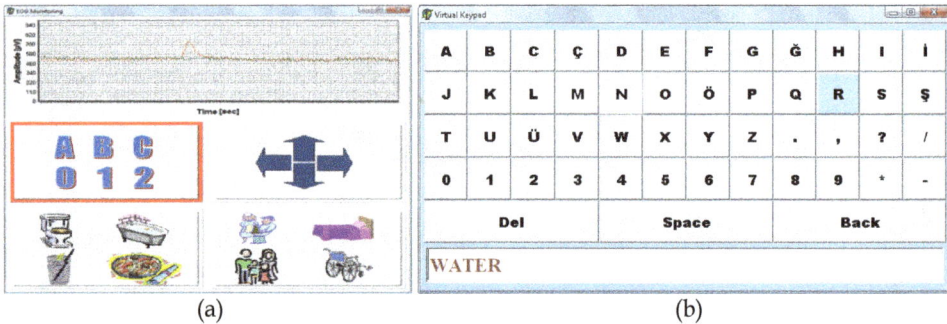

	(a)										(b)

Fig. 7. The EOG-based user interface (Usakli & Gurkan, 2010): a) Main menu, on the top, vertical and horizontal EOG signals are shown. b) Virtual keyboard: A 5-letter word can be written in 25 seconds.

2.3 Near-infrared spectroscopy based systems

Another approach for noninvasive BCI is based on optical means that measure brain activity by monitoring the hemodynamic response. Near Infrared Spectroscopy (NIRS) optical recording technology measures changes in the brain's oxygen absorption based on the optical properties of hemoglobin. Optical imaging spectroscopy can provide high spatial temporal resolution information about fractional changes in the hemodynamic response to increased neural activity (Mayhev et al, 2000). Human performance and cognitive activities such as attention, working memory, problem solving, etc., can be assessed by fNIR technology (Izzetoglu et al, 2007). NIRS technology usage is growing throughout the world for better understanding cortical activity during cognitive tasks.

NIRS is a spectroscopic method that uses about 800 nm wavelengths in the electromagnetic spectrum. The absorption spectrum in the near-infrared window is presented in figure 8. The level of light absorption related to the amount of oxy-hemoglobin can be measured with detectors. While concentrating, brain uses much more oxygen than normal state. This demand meets with clean blood, then the number of oxy-hemoglobin increases. Therefore, it causes more absorption of the light (Chance et al., 1998). This method gives an idea of oxygenation (changes of (de)oxy-hemoglobin) of blood in cortical capillary vessels.

The primary application of NIRS in the human body is seen through the measurement of the transmission and absorption of NIR light in human body tissues containing information about the changes in hemoglobin concentration. When a specific area of the brain is activated, the localized blood volume in that area changes quickly. Maximum response is observed between the 5th – 9th seconds (Malonek et al. 1997). Optical imaging can measure the location and activity of specific regions of the brain by continuously monitoring blood hemoglobin levels through the determination of optical absorption coefficients.

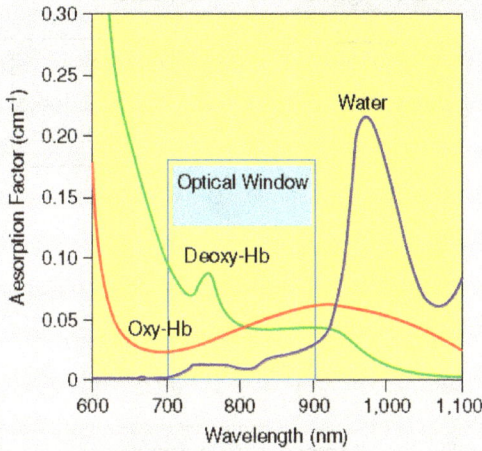

Fig. 8. Absorbtion spectrum in near-infrared window (Izzetoglu et al., 2007).

Figure 9 and 10 show measurement principles of oxygen level in a general NIR system. Photons transmitted with capillary vessels detected by detectors and measured photon intensity related to the oxygen level. fNIR spectroscopy can be used for BCI for the patients with ALS diseases (Bunce et al., 2006); to detect cognitive activity from prefrontal cortex elicited voluntarily (Ayaz et al., 2007).

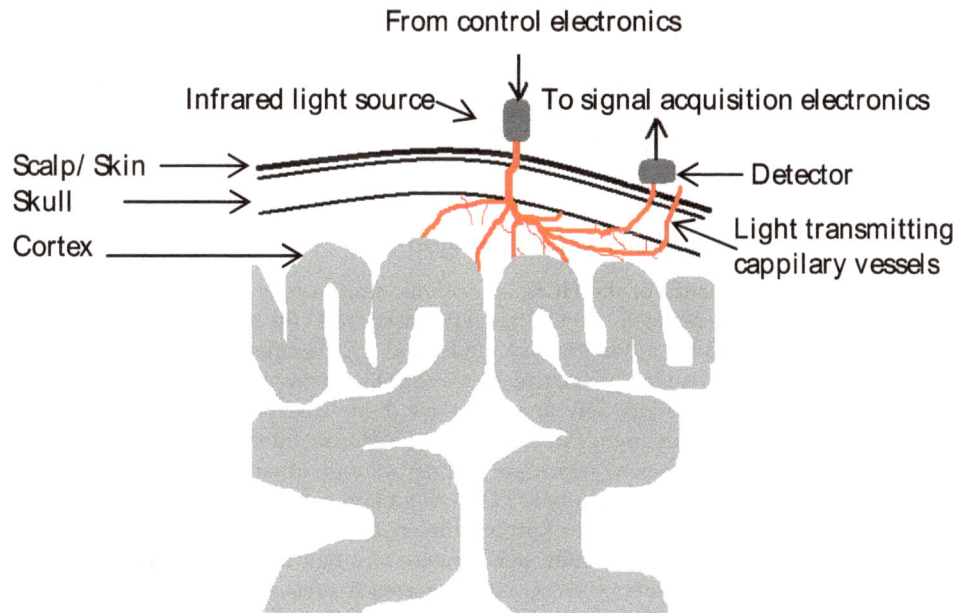

Fig. 9. Measurement of oxygen level in a NIR system. More light absorption means more hemoglobin, and consequently, more oxygenation.

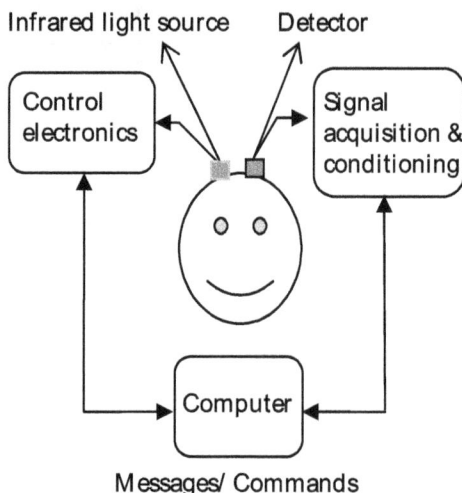

Fig. 10. The block diagram of a NIR system.

2.4 Other approaches

The behavior of active motor units identified via analysis of EMG signals recorded from the first dorsal interosseous muscle using a quadrifilar needle electrode is investigated. According to this study, the motor unit action potential waveforms recorded from patients were more complex than those recorded from control subjects as often observed in motor neuron diseases (Kasi et al., 2009). An eating assistant robot used to assist in eating independence was developed. This assistant robot is useful for people with severe disabilities. A spoon and a camera are attached on the tip of the robotic arm (Takahashi et al., 2001). Additionally, detecting the stress level of the computer user could possibly develop the computers' ability to respond intelligently and help calm negative emotional states of the user during HCI.

3. Feature extraction and classification algorithms

To increase the performance of the HCIs, algorithmic studies related to feature extraction and classification were realized. Motor imagery based BCI, the feature extraction, was performed with an adaptive autoregressive model and the classifier used was an adaptive quadratic discriminant analysis (Vidaurre et al., 2006). A new algorithm for single-trial online classification of imagery left and right hand movements was developed. This algorithm is based on time-frequency information derived from filtering EEG wideband raw data with causal Morlet wavelets, which are adapted to individual EEG spectra (Lemm et al., 2004). For motor imagery EEG, a new EEG recognition algorithm which combined the discrete wavelet transform with the backpropagation neural network was developed (Ming-Ai et al., 2009). According to the results, performance of motor imagery based BCI using a single recording session of EEG or ECoG signals for each subject, is not sufficient. It was relatively easy to obtain classifiable signals quickly from most of the non-paralyzed subjects. However, it was proved that it is impossible to classify the signals obtained from the paralyzed patients by the same methods (Hill, et al., 2006). To detect the ERPs, EEG recordings are transformed into a Haar-wavelet series (Kawakami et al., 1996) and variational Kalman filtering (Sykacek et al., 2004) for adaptive classification in the BCI system was used. The later algorithm translates EEG segments adaptively into probabilities of cognitive states. It allows for nonstationarities in the joint process over cognitive states and generated EEG which may occur during a consecutive number of trials. The wavelet features are used to determine the characteristic of eye movement waveform (Daud & Sudirman, 2010).

A new two-stage approach to extract the µ rhythm component was developed. The first stage uses second-order blind identification with stationary wavelet transform to automatically remove the artifacts. In the second stage, second-order blind identification is applied again to find the µ rhythm component. In this method artifact removal enhances the extraction of the µ rhythm component (Ng & Raveendran, 2009). For classification of motor execution signals, fractal approach provides promising results (Usakli, 2010). An EEG based BCI for users to control a cursor on a computer display is one of the common study area. The developed system uses an adaptive algorithm, based on kernel partial least squares classification, to associate patterns in multichannel EEG frequency spectra with cursor controls (Trejo et al., 2006). For the BCI related classification review can be found in (Lotte et al., 2007).

4. Hybrid approach of human computer interaction

To increase HCI efficiency, hybrid approaches offer good results. Three physiological signals: blood volume pulse, galvanic skin response and pupil diameter, to automatically monitor stress were used, successfully (Zhai et al., 2005). A vision-based multimodal human computer interface system using eye and hand motion tracking was developed. This vision-based virtual interface integrates the function of the motion tracking of eye blinking and hand gestures with the function of their recognition as a virtual interface (Shin & Chun, 2007). EEG error-related signals present a hybrid approach for HCI. This approach uses human gestures to send commands to a computer and exploits brain activity to provide implicit feedback about the recognition of such commands (Chavarriaga et al., 2010).

4.1 Progressing study for hybrid multi-modal human computer interaction

In order to contribute to the HCI field, a novel multi-modal integrated design is completed and establishing an efficient communication and control channel for individuals with motor neuron diseases such as ALS has been continuing. The preliminary results are promising. Using experience in relevant fields such as EEG (Usakli & Gencer, 2007a; Usakli & Gencer, 2007b), EOG (Usakli & Gurkan, 2010; Usakli et al., 2009), BCI prototyping (Erdogan et al, 2009), feature extraction (Usakli, 2010), this novel system attempts to increase usefulness and performance. HR and GSR signals are to be processed with the bio-signals mentioned above, simultaneously. Evaluation of these signals is whether individually or combined, depends on the user. The situation of the severity of the disease also determines the mode of the hybrid multi-mode operation. Through focusing on one of the tasks and sending correct or wrong messages, the bio signals of the subjects will be acquired and processed. Detecting these changes can be used to send data without speaking or control the device.

4.2 Design rationale

The novel system is microcontroller based and battery powered. Data is transferred via optic fiber. To remove the dc level and 50-Hz power line noise, differentiating approach is used. This approach is more successful and practical than the classical methods in the application. After signal conditioning; including filtering and amplification, the analog signal is digitized (at least 12 effective bits) at variable sampling rates and then transferred to the PC via optic fiber. To classify bio-signals, feature extraction with the fractal approach (Usakli, 2010) and wavelet transformed data is applied to artificial neural networks for classification. By using a user-friendly interface, the virtual keyboard and controlling pad allows messages to be given, and some other needs such as cleanup or medical assistance can be selected.

The integrated HCI system provides with high 1) efficiency, 2) usefulness, 3) robustness 4) accurate and reliable output, 5) fast response, 6) user friendly, 7) flexibility, 8) cheap, and 9) designed available components.

5. Conclusions and discussions

ALS is a progressive disease that affects the control of muscle movement by damaging motor neurons. ALS kills the pyramidal neurons of the motor cortex as a corollary muscular functions deteriorate rapidly. For the present, there is no known cure for ALS. Because of these movement and muscular disabilities, these patients need an efficient alternative channel to communicate with their environment or to control devices. In this chapter, HCIs especially BCI technology focused on ALS patients, are presented.

The EEG-based BCI systems represent the only technology for severely paralyzed patients to increase or maintain their communication and control needs. The P300 paradigm for the EEG-based BCI systems is due to the fact that such waveform occurs spontaneously for many of the subjects without need of particular training, which is be useful for increasing the quality of life for the patients. EEG is still the most attractive and popular technology for clinical BCI.

The EOG-based side of the system seems more accurate and fast when compared to the EEG-based systems. It must be noted that the solution for the EOG system is cheaper when compared to the EEG solution and can be used as a first step for the hybrid device for all users. The general idea of a hybrid device is to familiarize the patient with a unique interface, while the user can switch the bioelectric signal for the communication/control of the external devices.

NIRS is a non-invasive optical technique, suitable to assess functional activity by measuring cortical oxygenation (HbO$_2$) and deoxygenation (Hb). This technology is also a promising and cheap technology for establishing efficient alternative channel, however needs more study on this field to prove ability of efficiency.

In order to increase the usefulness and improve performance, hybrid approaches and multi-modal designs should be investigated. For EEG based BCI systems two or more signal of: P300 response, steady state visual evoked potential, event related desynchronisation, slow cortical potential, sensorimotor rhythms and error-related potentials can be used for an efficient hybrid system. There is no sufficient study in the literature concerning multi-modal system designs. Combination of several bio-signals such as: EEG, EOG, NIRS, HR and GSR, etc offer an improved performance results. The usage of this two or several signals combination may be used depends on the situation of the disability.

6. References

Akan, B. & Argunsah, A.O. (2007). A Human-Computer Interface (HCI) Based on Electrooculogram (EOG) for Handicapped, *Signal Processing and Communications Applications SIU 2007 IEEE 15th*, Eskisehir, Turkey, 11-13 June 2007.

Allison, R.S.; Eizenman, M. & Cheung, B. (1996). Combined Head and Eye Tracking System for Dynamic Testing of the Vestibular System, *IEEE Trans. on Biomedical Engineering*, vol.43, no.11, pp.1073-1082.

Astolfi, L.; Gonzalez Andino, S.; De Vico Fallani, F. & Babiloni, F. (2010). Processing of Brain Signals by Using Hemodynamic and Neuroelectromagnetic Modalities, *Computational Intelligence and Neuroscience*, 2010, ID 934180, pp.1-2.

Ayaz, H.; Izzetoglu, M.; Bunce, S.; Heiman-Patterson & T. Onaral, B. (2007). Detecting Cognitive Activity Related Hemodynamic Signal for Brain Computer Interface Using Functional Near Infrared Spectroscopy, *Neural Engineering, 2007. CNE'07. 3rd International IEEE/EMBS Conference on*, 342, Kohala Coast, HI, USA, 2-5 May 2007.

Bahill, A.T. (1982). Prediction Final Eye Position Halfway Through a Saccade, *IEEE Trans. on Biomedical Engineering*, vol.30, no.12, pp.781-786.

Barea, R.; Boquete, L.; Mazo, M. & Lopez, E. (2002). System for Assisted Mobility Using Eye Movements Based on Electrooculography, *Neural Systems and Rehabilitation Engineering, IEEE Transactions on*, Vol. 10 4, pp. 209 – 218, ISSN: 1534-4320

Bunce, S.; İzzetoglu, M.; İzzetoglu, K.; Onaral, B. & Pourrezaei, K. (2006). Functional Near Infrared Spectroscopy: An Emerging Neuroimaging Modality, *IEEE Engineering in Medicine and Biology Magazine, Special Issue on Clinical Neuroengineering*, 25(4): pp. 54-62.

Buttfield, A.; Ferrez, P.W. & Millan, Jd.R. (2006). Towards a Robust BCI: Error Potentials and Online Learning, *Neural Systems and Rehabilitation Engineering, IEEE Transactions on*, Vol. 14 2, pp. 164 - 168ISSN: 1534-4320

Chance, B.; Anday, E.; Nioka, S.; Zhou, S.; Hong, L.; Worden, .K.; Li, C.; Murray, T.; Ovetsky, Y.; Pidikiti, D. & Thomas, R. (1998). A Novel Method for Fast Imaging of Brain Function, Non-invasively, With Light. *Optics Express*, 2, 10.

Chavarriaga, R.; Biasiucci, A.; Forster, K.; Roggen, D.; Troster, G. & Millan Jdel, R. (2010). Adaptation of Hybrid Human-computer Interaction Systems Using EEG Error-related Potentials, *Conference Proceedings IEEE Eng Med Biol Soc.* pp. 4226-4229, Argentina, Aug. 31-Sept. 4 2010.

Chen, S.; Tsai T. & Luo, C. (1999). Portable Clinical EOG Instrument System, *Proc. of the First Joint BMES/EMBS Conference*, pp.858-859, Atlanta, USA, 13-16 Oct. 1999.

Chung-Hsien, K.; Yi-Chang, C.; Hung-Chyun, C. & Jia-Wun S. (2009). Eyeglasses based electrooculography human-wheelchair interface Systems, *Man and Cybernetics, 2009. SMC 2009. IEEE International Conference on*, San Antonio, TX, USA, pp. 4746 – 4751, ISSN: 1062-922X, 11-14 Oct. 2009.

Daud, W.M.B.W. & Sudirman, R. (2010). A Wavelet Approach on Energy Distribution of Eye Movement Potential Towards Direction, *Industrial Electronics & Applications (ISIEA), 2010 IEEE Symposium on*, Penang, Malaysia, 3-5 Oct. 2010.

Deng, L.Y.; Chun-Liang Hsu Tzu-Ching Lin Jui-Sen Tuan Yung-Hui Chen, (2009). EOG-Based Signal Detection and Verification for HCI, *Machine Learning and Cybernetics, 2009 International Conference on*, 12-15 July 2009, Vol. 6, 3342, Baoding, Hebei, China, ISBN: 978-1-4244-3702-3, 2009

Dhillon, H.S.; Singla, R.; Rekhi, N.S. & Jha, R. (2009). EOG and EMG Based Virtual Keyboard: A Brain-Computer Interface, Computer Science and Information Technology, *ICCSIT 2009. 2nd IEEE International Conference on*, 8-11 Aug. 2009, Beijing, China.

Donchin, E.; Spencer, K.M. & Wijesinghe, R. (2000). The Mental Prosthesis: Assessing the Speed of a P300-Based Brain–Computer Interface, *IEEE Transactions on Rehabilitation Engineering*, Vol. 8, No. 2, pp. 174-178.

Eklund, A.; Andersson, M.; Ohlsson, H.; Ynnerman, A. & Knutsson, H. (2010). A Brain Computer Interface for Communication Using Real-Time fMRI, *Pattern Recognition (ICPR), 2010 20th International Conference on*, Istanbul, Turkey, pp. 3665, ISSN : 1051-4651, 23-26 Aug. 2010.

Erdoğan, B.; Akıncı, B.; Acar, E.; Uşaklı, A. B. & Gençer, N. G. (2009). Prototype Hardware Design for Brain Computer Interface Applications, *14. Biyomedikal Mühendisliği Ulusal Toplantısı*, Izmir, Turkey, 20-22 Mayıs 2009.

Fabiani, G.E.; McFarland, D.J.; Wolpaw, J.R. & Pfurtscheller, G. (2004). Conversion of EEG Activity into Cursor Movement by a Brain-Computer Interface (BCI), *Neural Systems and Rehabilitation Engineering, IEEE Transactions on*, Vol. 12 3, pp. 331 – 338, ISSN: 1534-4320.

Farwell L.A. & Donchin, E. (1988). Talking off the Top of Your Head: A Mental Prosthesis Utilizing Event-Related Brain Potentials, *Electroencephalogr.Clin. Neurophysiol.*, Vol. 70, pp. 510–523.

Gao, X.; Xu, D.; Cheng, M. & Gao, S. (2003). A BCI-Based Environmental Controller for the Motion-Disabled, *Neural Systems and Rehabilitation Engineering, IEEE Transactions on*, Vol. 11, 2, pp. 137 – 140, ISSN: 1534-4320

Gevins, A.; Brickett, P.; Costales, B.; Le, J. & Reutter, B. (1990). Beyond Topographic Mapping: Towards Functional-Anatomical Imaging with 124-Channel EEGs and 3-D MRIs, *Brain Topogr.* 3, pp. 53–64.

Guger C. (2008). Brain Computer Interface, *Lecture notes in The 4th International Summer School on Emerging Technologies in Biomedicine: Advanced Methods for the Estimation of Human Brain Activity and Connectivity, Applications to Rehabilitation Engineering*, Patras, Greece, 29 June – 4 July 2008.

Guger, C. Schlogl, A. Neuper, C. Walterspacher, D. Strein, T. Pfurtscheller, G. (2001). Rapid Prototyping of an EEG-Based Brain-Computer Interface (BCI), *Neural Systems and Rehabilitation Engineerin,g IEEE Transactions on*, Vol. 9 , 1, 49, ISSN : 1534-4320.

Guger, C.; Ramoser, H. & Pfurtscheller, G. (2000). Real-Time EEG Analysis with Subject-Specific Spatial Patterns for a Brain-Computer Interface (BCI), *Rehabilitation Engineering, IEEE Transactions on*, (Dec 2000), Vol. 8 4 , pp. 447 – 456, ISSN: 1063-6528

Handa, S. & Ebisawa, Y. (2008). Development of Head-Mounted Display with Eye-Gaze Detection Function for the Severely Disabled, *Virtual Environments, Human-Computer Interfaces and Measurement Systems, VECIMS 2008 IEEE Conference on*, İstanbul, Turkey, 14-16 July 2008.

Hill, N.J.; Lal, T.N.; Schroder, M.; Hinterberger, T.; Wilhelm, B.; Nijboer, F.; Mochty, U.; Widman, G.; Elger, C.; Scholkopf, B.; Kubler, A. & Birbaumer, N. (2006). Classifying EEG and ECoG Signals Without Subject Training for Fast BCI Implementation: Comparison of Nonparalyzed and Completely Paralyzed Subjects, *Neural Systems and Rehabilitation Engineering, IEEE Transactions on*, Vol. 14, 2 183.

Hutchinson, T.E.; White, K.P.; Martin, W.N.; Reichert K.C. & Frey, L.A. (1989). Human-Computer Interaction Using Eye-Gaze Input, *IEEE Trans. on Systems, Man and Cybernetics*, vol.19, issue 6, pp.1527-1534.

Ihara, T.; Sugi, T.; Eriguchi, M.; Asami, T. & Nakamura, M. (2009). Construction of Simple Communication Method by Use of Neuro-Biological Signals, *ICCAS-SICE, 2009*, pp. 3152, Fukuoka, Japan, 18-21 Aug. 2009.

Izzetoglu, M.; Bunce, S. C.; Izzetoglu, K.; Onaral, B. & Pourrezaei, K. (2007). Functional Brain Imaging, Using Near-Infrared Technology Assessing Cognitive Activity in Real-Life Situations, *IEEE Engineering in Medicine and Biology Magazine*, pp. 38-46.

Juhola, M. (1985). Detection of Saccadic Eye Movements Using a Non-Recursive Adaptive Digital Filter, *Computer Methods and Programs in Biomedicine*, vol.21, pp.81-88.

Kaneswaran, K.; Arshak, K.; Burke, E. & Condron, J. (2010). Towards a Brain Controlled Assistive Technology for Powered Mobility, *Engineering in Medicine and Biology Society (EMBC), 2010 Annual International Conference of the IEEE*, Aug. 31 2010-Sept. 4 2010, Buenos Aires, Argentina, 4176, ISSN : 1557-170X

Kasi, P.K.; Krivickas, L.S.; Meister, M.; Chew, E.; Bonato, P. ; Schmid, M.; Kamen, G. & Pu Liu Clancy, E.A. (2009). Characterization of Motor Unit Behavior in Patients with Amyotrophic Lateral Sclerosis, *Conference on Neural Engineering NER'09 4th International IEEE/EMBS*, Antalya, Turkey, 2009.

Kawakami, T.; Inoue, M.; Kobayashi, Y. & Nakashima, K. (1996). Application of Event Related Brain Potentials to Communication Aids, *Engineering in Medicine and Biology Society, 1996. Bridging Disciplines for Biomedicine, Proceedings of the 18th Annual International Conference of the IEEE*, Vol.: 5, 2229, Amsterdam, Holland, 31 Oct -03 Nov 1996.

Kherlopian, A.R.; Gerrein, J.P.; Yue, M.; Kim, K.E.; Kim, J.W.; Sukumaran, M. & Sajda, P. (2006). Electrooculogram Based System for Computer Control Using a Multiple Feature Classification Model, *Engineering in Medicine and Biology Society, EMBS'06. 28th Annual International Conference of the IEEE*, New York, USA, 2006.

Kuno, Y.; Yagi, T. & Uchikawa, Y. (1998). Development of Eye Pointer with Free Head-Motion, Proc. of the 20th Annual International Conference of the IEEE Engineering in Medicine and Biology Society, Vol. 20, No 4, pp. 1750-1752.

Lebedev, M. A. & Nicolelis, M. A. L. (2006). Brain–machine Interfaces: Past, Present and Future, *Trends in Neurosciences*, Vol. 29 No.9, pp. 536-546.

Lemm, S.; Schafer, C. & Curio, G. (2004). BCI competition 2003-Data Set III: Probabilistic Modeling of Sensorimotor μ Rhythms for Classification of Imaginary Hand Movements, *Biomedical Engineering, IEEE Transactions o,n* Vol. 51 6, pp. 1077 – 1080, ISSN: 0018-9294.

Li, M. A.; Wang, R.; Hao, D. M. & Yang, J.F. (2009). Feature Extraction and Classification of Mental EEG for Motor Imagery, *Natural Computation, 2009 ICNC '09 Fifth International Conference on*, Vol. 2, pp. 139., Tianjin, China, 14-16 Aug. 2009.

Lotte, F.; Congedo, M.; Lécuyer,; A. Lamarche, F. & Arnaldi, B. (2007). A Review of Classification Algorithms for EEG-based Brain-Computer Interfaces, *Journal of Neural Engineering*, Vol.: 4, 2, pp. 1-24, ISSN: 17412560.

Malonek, D.; Dirnagl, U.; Lindauer, U.; Yamada, K.; Kanno, I. & Grinvald, A. (1997). Vascular Imprints of Neuronal Activity: Relationships Between the Dynamics of Cortical Blood Flow, Oxygenation and Volume Changes Following Sensory Stimulation, *Proc. Natl. Acad. Sci.* Vol. 94, pp 14826–14831, USA, December 1997.

Mayhew, J.; Johnston, D.; Berwick, J.; Jones, M.; Coffey, P. & Zheng, Y. (2000). Spectroscopic Analysis of Neural Activity in Brain: Increased Oxygen Consumption Following Activation of Barrel Cortex, *NeuroImage*, 12, pp. 664–675.

McFarland, D.J. & Wolpaw, J.R. (2005). Sensorimotor Rhythm-Based Brain-Computer Interface (BCI): Feature Selection by Regression Improves Performance, *Neural Systems and Rehabilitation Engineering, IEEE Transactions on*, (Sept. 2005), Vol. 13 3, pp. 372 – 379, ISSN: 1534-4320

Millan, J.R.; & Mourino, J. (2003). Asynchronous BCI and Local Neural Classifiers: An Overview of the Adaptive Brain Interface Project, *Neural Systems and Rehabilitation Engineering, IEEE Transactions on*, (June 2003), Vol. 11 2, pp. 159 – 161

Ng, S.C. & Raveendran, P. (2009). Enhanced Rhythm Extraction Using Blind Source Separation and Wavelet Transform, *Biomedical Engineering, IEEE Transactions on*, Vol. 56 , 8, pp. 2024.

Nijboer, F.; Carmien, S.P. ; Leon, E.; Morin, F.O.; Koene, R.A. & Hoffmann, U. (2009). Affective Brain-Computer Interfaces: Psychophysiological Markers of Emotion in Healthy Persons and in Persons with Amyotrophic Lateral Sclerosis, *Affective Computing and Intelligent Interaction and Workshops, ACII 2009. 3rd International Conference on*, Amsterdam, Holland, 10-12 September 2009

Norris, G. & Wilson, E. (1997). The Eye Mouse, an Eye Communication Device, *IEEE Proc. of Bioengineering Conference*, pp.66-67, Durham, N. Carolina , USA, 21-22 May 1997.

Nunez, P. L. (1995). *Neocortical Dynamics and Human EEG Rhythms*, Oxford University Press: New York, 1995, pp. 200-250.

Parker, J.N. & Parker, P.M. (2007). *Amyotrophic Lateral Sclerosis: A Bibliography and Dictionary for Physicians, Patients, and Genome Researchers*, ICON Health Publications, USA, ISBN: 0-497-11327-9, pp. 4.

Peters, B.O.; Pfurtscheller, G. & Flyvbjerg, H. (2001). Automatic Differentiation of Multichannel EEG Signals, (Jan. 2001), Vol. 48 1, pp. 111, ISSN : 0018-9294.

Pfurtscheller, G.; Neuper, C.; Guger, C.; Harkam, W.; Ramoser, H.; Schlögl, A.; Obermaier, B. & Pregenzer, M. (2000). Current Trends in Graz Brain-Computer Interface (BCI) Research, *IEEE Trans. Rehab. Eng.*, vol. 8, pp. 216–219.

Pfurtscheller, G.; Neuper, C. & Birbaumer, N. (2005). Human Brain–Computer Interface, *Motor Cortex In Voluntary Movements, A Distributed System For Distributed Functions*, Alexa Riehle and Eilon Vaadia , (Ed), CRC Press, USA, Chapter 14, pp.1-35.

Schalk, G.;   McFarland, D.J.;   Hinterberger, T.;   Birbaumer, N.;   Wolpaw, J.R. (2004). BCI2000: a General-Purpose Brain-Computer Interface (BCI) System, *Biomedical Engineering, IEEE Transactions on* (June 2004), Vol.: 51 6, pp. 1034 – 1043, ISSN: 0018-9294.

Sellers, E. W. & Donchin, E. (2006). A P300-Based Brain-Computer Interface: Initial Tests by ALS Patients, *Clinical Neurophysiology*, 117, pp.538-548.

Sellers, E.W.; Kubler, A. & Donchin, E. (2006). Brain-Computer Interface Research at the University of South Florida Cognitive Psychophysiology Laboratory: The P300 Speller. *Neural Systems and Rehabilitation Engineering, IEEE Transactions on*, Vol.14, No.2, (June 2006) , ISSN : 1534-4320.

Septanto, H.;   Prihatmanto, A.S.;   Indrayanto, A. (2009). A Computer Cursor Controlled by Eye Movements and Voluntary Eye Winks Using a Single Channel EOG, *Electrical Engineering and Informatics, Selangor, 2009. ICEEI'09. International Conference on*, Issue Date: 5-7 Aug. 2009, pp. 117 – 120.

Shin, G. & Chun J. (2007). Vision-Based Multimodal Human Computer Interface Based on Parallel Tracking of Eye and Hand Motion, *Convergence Information Technology International Conference on*, 21-23 Nov. 2007, pp. 2443, Gyeongju, S. Korea.

Sutter, E. E. (1992). The Brain Response Interface: Communication Through Visually-induced Electrical Brain Response, *J. Microcomput. Appl.*, vol. 15, pp. 31–45.

Sykacek, P.; Roberts, S.J. & Stokes, M. (2004). Adaptive BCI based on Variational Bayesian Kalman Filtering: an Empirical Evaluation, *Biomedical Engineering, IEEE Transactions on*, (May 2004), Vol. 51 5, pp. 719 – 727, ISSN: 0018-9294.

Takahashi, Y.; Hasegawa, N.; Takahashi, K. & Hatakeyama, T. (2001). Human Interface Using PC Display with Head Pointing Device for Eating Assist Robot and Emotional Evaluation by GSR Sensor, *Robotics and Automation, 2001, Proceedings 2001 ICRA IEEE International Conference on*, Vol. 4, pp. 3674, ISSN:1050-4729, Seoul, S. Korea, May 21-26 2001.

Tamura, H.; Miyashita, M.; Tanno, K. & Fuse, Y. (2010). Mouse Cursor Control System Using Electrooculogram Signals, *World Automation Congress WAC 2010*, ISSN : 2154-4824, Kobe, Japan, 19-23 Sept. 2010.

Tomita, Y.; Igarashi, Y.; Honda, S. & Matsuo, N. (1996). Electro-Oculography Mouse for Amyotrophic Lateral Sclerosis Patients, *Bridging Engineering in Medicine and Biology Society Disciplines for Biomedicine Proceedings of the 18th Annual International Conference of the IEEE*, Vol. 5, pp. 1780 – 1781, Amsterdam, Holland, 31 Oct-3 Nov 1996.

Townsend, G.; Graimann, B. & Pfurtscheller, G. (2004). Continuous EEG Classification During Motor Imagery-Simulation of an Asynchronous BCI, *Neural Systems and Rehabilitation Engineering, IEEE Transactions on*, Vol. 12 2, pp. 258 – 265, ISSN: 1534-4320.

Trejo, L.J.; Rosipal, R. & Matthews, B. (2006). Brain-Computer Interfaces for 1-D and 2-D Cursor Control: Designs Using Volitional Control of the EEG Spectrum or Steady-state Visual Evoked Potentials, *Neural Systems and Rehabilitation Engineering, IEEE Transactions on*, Vol. 14 2, pp. 225, ISSN : 1534-4320.

Turnip, A.; Hong, K.S.; Ge, S.S. & Jeong, M. Y. (2010). Neural Networks Training Based on Sequential Extended Kalman Filtering for Single Trial EEG Classification, *Knowledge and Systems Engineering KSE 2010 Second International Conference on*, p. 85, Hanoi, Vietnam, 7-9 October 2010.

Usakli, A. B.; Gurkan, S.; Aloise, F.; Vecchiato, G. & Babiloni, F.(2009). A Hybrid Platform Based on EOG and EEG Signals to Restore Communication for Patients Afflicted with Progressive Motor Neuron Diseases, *31st Annual International Conference of the IEEE EMBS*, pp.543-546, Minneapolis, Minnesota, USA, September 2-6, 2009.

Usakli, A.B. & Gencer N.G., (2007). A USB-Based 256-Channel Electroencephalographic Data-Acquisition System for Electrical Source Imaging of the Human Brain, *Instrumentation Science and Technology*, Vol. 35, pp.255-273.

Usakli, A.B. & Gencer, N.G. (2007). Performance Tests of A Novel Electroencephalographic Data-Acquisition System, *The Fifth International Conference on Biomedical Engineering IASTED BIOMED 2007*, pp. 253-257, Innsbruck, Austria, February 14–16, 2007.

Usakli, A.B. & Gurkan S. (2010). Design of a Novel Efficient Human Computer Interface: An Electrooculagram Based Virtual Keyboard, *IEEE Transaction on Instrumentation and Measurement*, Vol. 59, No.8, pp. 2099-2108.

Usakli, A.B. (2010). Modeling of Movement-Related Potentials Using a Fractal Approach, *Journal of Computational Neuroscience*, Vol.28, No. 3, pp. 595-603.

Van Kokswijk, J. & Van Hulle, M. (2010). Self Adaptive BCI as Service-Oriented Information System for Patients with Communication Disabilities, *New Trends in Information Science and Service Science NISS 2010 4th International Conference on*, pp. 264-269, Gyeongju, S. Korea, 11-13 May 2010.

Vidaurre, C.; Schlogl, A.; Cabeza, R.; Scherer, R. & Pfurtscheller, G. (2006). A Fully On-Line Adaptive BCI, *Biomedical Engineering, IEEE Transactions on*, (June 2006), Vol. 53 6, pp. 1214 – 1219, ISSN: 0018-9294.

Weiskopf, N.; Mathiak, K.; Bock, S.W.; Scharnowski, F.; Veit, R.; Grodd, W.; Goebel, R. & Birbaumer, N. (2004). Principles of a Brain-Computer Interface (BCI) Based on Real-Time Functional Magnetic Resonance Imaging (fMRI), *Biomedical Engineering, IEEE Transactions on*, (June 2004), Vol. 51 6, pp. 966 – 970, ISSN: 0018-9294.

Wolpaw, J. R (2003). Brain-Computer Interfaces: Signals, Methods, and Goals, *Proceedings of the 1st International IEEE EMBS Conference on Neural Engineering*, pp. 584-585, Capri Island, Italy, March 20-22, 2003.

Wolpaw, J.; Birbaumer, N.; McFarland, D.; Pfurtscheller, G. & Vaughan, T. (2002). Brain-Computer Interfaces for Communication and Control, *Electroencephalography and Clinical Neurophysiology*, vol. 113 6, pp. 767-791.

Wolpaw, J.R.; McFarland, D. J. & Vaughan, T. M. (2000). Brain-Computer Interface Research at the Wadsworth center, *IEEE Trans. Rehab. Eng.*, vol. 8, pp. 222–226.

Wolpaw, J.R.; McFarland, D.J.; Vaughan, T.M. & Schalk, G. (2003). The Wadsworth Center Brain-Computer Interface (BCI) Research and Development Program, *Neural Systems and Rehabilitation Engineering, IEEE Transactions on*, (June 2003), Vol.: 11 2 pp. 1 – 4, ISSN: 1534-4320.

Wu, C.M.; Huang, K.G.; Chang, S.H.; Hsu, S.C. & Lin, C.L. (2007). EOG Single Switch Morse Code Translate Input Device for Individuals with the Motor Neuron Disease, *TENCON 2007 - 2007 IEEE Region 10 Conference*, Taipei, Oct. 30-Nov. 2 2007.

Wu, C.M.; Huang, K.G.; Chang, S.H.; Hsu, S.C. & Lin, C.L. (2007). EOG Single Switch Morse Code Translate Input Device for Individuals with the Motor Neuron disease, *ENCON 2007 - 2007 IEEE Region 10 Conference*, Taipei, Taiwan, Oct. 30 2007-Nov. 2 2007.

Yoshiaki, K. (1997). Development of Eye-Gaze Input Interface, *Proc. of 7th International conference on Human Computer Interaction*, pp.44-49.

Zhai, J.; Barreto, A.; Chin, C. & Chao, L. (2005). Realization of Stress Detection Using Psychophysiological Signals for Improvement of Human-computer Interactions, *Southeast Conference Proceedings, IEEE*, pp.415-420, Fort Lauderdale, Florida, USA, 8-10 April 2005.

Zheng, X.; Liu, X. L. J.; Chen, W. & Hao, Y. (2009). A Portable Wireless Eye Movement-Controlled Human-Computer Interface for the Disabled, *Complex Medical Engineering, 2009. CME. ICME International Conference on*, Tempe, Arizona, USA, 9-11 April 2009.

Permissions

The contributors of this book come from diverse backgrounds, making this book a truly international effort. This book will bring forth new frontiers with its revolutionizing research information and detailed analysis of the nascent developments around the world.

We would like to thank Martin H. Maurer, for lending his expertise to make the book truly unique. He has played a crucial role in the development of this book. Without his invaluable contribution this book wouldn't have been possible. He has made vital efforts to compile up to date information on the varied aspects of this subject to make this book a valuable addition to the collection of many professionals and students.

This book was conceptualized with the vision of imparting up-to-date information and advanced data in this field. To ensure the same, a matchless editorial board was set up. Every individual on the board went through rigorous rounds of assessment to prove their worth. After which they invested a large part of their time researching and compiling the most relevant data for our readers. Conferences and sessions were held from time to time between the editorial board and the contributing authors to present the data in the most comprehensible form. The editorial team has worked tirelessly to provide valuable and valid information to help people across the globe.

Every chapter published in this book has been scrutinized by our experts. Their significance has been extensively debated. The topics covered herein carry significant findings which will fuel the growth of the discipline. They may even be implemented as practical applications or may be referred to as a beginning point for another development. Chapters in this book were first published by InTech; hereby published with permission under the Creative Commons Attribution License or equivalent.

The editorial board has been involved in producing this book since its inception. They have spent rigorous hours researching and exploring the diverse topics which have resulted in the successful publishing of this book. They have passed on their knowledge of decades through this book. To expedite this challenging task, the publisher supported the team at every step. A small team of assistant editors was also appointed to further simplify the editing procedure and attain best results for the readers.

Our editorial team has been hand-picked from every corner of the world. Their multi-ethnicity adds dynamic inputs to the discussions which result in innovative outcomes. These outcomes are then further discussed with the researchers and contributors who give their valuable feedback and opinion regarding the same. The feedback is then collaborated with the researches and they are edited in a comprehensive manner to aid the understanding of the subject.

Apart from the editorial board, the designing team has also invested a significant amount of their time in understanding the subject and creating the most relevant covers. They scrutinized every image to scout for the most suitable representation of the subject and create an appropriate cover for the book.

The publishing team has been involved in this book since its early stages. They were actively engaged in every process, be it collecting the data, connecting with the contributors or procuring relevant information. The team has been an ardent support to the editorial, designing and production team. Their endless efforts to recruit the best for this project, has resulted in the accomplishment of this book. They are a veteran in the field of academics and their pool of knowledge is as vast as their experience in printing. Their expertise and guidance has proved useful at every step. Their uncompromising quality standards have made this book an exceptional effort. Their encouragement from time to time has been an inspiration for everyone.

The publisher and the editorial board hope that this book will prove to be a valuable piece of knowledge for researchers, students, practitioners and scholars across the globe.

List of Contributors

John D. Lee, Jia Y. Lee, Stephen M. Taylor, and Trent M. Woodruff
School of Biomedical Sciences, Australia

Peter G. Noakes
School of Biomedical Sciences, Australia Queensland Brain Institute, University of Queensland, Australia

Kim Staats and Ludo Van Den Bosch
University of Leuven, Belgium VIB Vesalius Research Center, Belgium

Cristina Cereda, Stella Gagliardi, Emanuela Cova
Laboratory of Experimental Neurobiology, IRCCS, National Neurological Institute "C. Mondino", Pavia, Italy

Luca Diamanti and Mauro Ceroni
General Neurology Department, IRCCS, National Neurological Institute "C. Mondino", Pavia, Department of Neurological Sciences, University of Pavia, Pavia, Italy

Amanda M. Haidet-Phillips and Nicholas J. Maragakis
Department of Neurology, Johns Hopkins University, Baltimore, Maryland, USA

Masatoshi Suzuki, Chak Foon Tso and Michael G. Meyer
University of Wisconsin-Madison, U. S. A.

Emily F. Goodall, Joanna J. Bury, Johnathan Cooper-Knock, Pamela J. Shaw and Janine Kirby
Sheffield Institute for Translational Neuroscience, University of Sheffield, Sheffield, United Kingdom

R. Jeroen Pasterkamp and Max Koppers
Departments of Neurology, University Medical Center Utrecht, The Netherlands

Michael van Es, Leonard H. van den Berg and Jan H. Veldink
Department of Neuroscience and Pharmacology, University Medical Center Utrecht, The Netherlands

Ilse Gijselinck, Kristel Sleegers, Christine Van Broeckhoven and Marc Cruts
Department of Molecular Genetics, VIB, Antwerpen, Belgium University of Antwerp, Antwerpen, Belgium

Daniele Lo Coco
ALS Clinical Research Center, Dipartimento di Biomedicina Sperimentale e Neuroscienze Cliniche (BioNeC), University of Palermo, Palermo, Italy

Alfonsa Claudia Taiello, Rossella Spataro and Vincenzo La Bella
ALS Clinical Research Center, Dipartimento di Biomedicina Sperimentale e Neuroscienze Cliniche (BioNeC), University of Palermo, Palermo, Italy

Paolo Volanti, Domenico De Cicco and Gianluca Battaglia
Neurorehabilitation Unit, Fondazione Salvatore Maugeri, Mistretta (ME), Italy

Antonio Spanevello
Università Degli Studi dell'Insubria, Varese, Italy

Santino Marchese
Respiratory Intensive Care Unit, Ospedale Civico ARNAS, Palermo, Italy

Louisa Ng and Fary Khan
Royal Melbourne Hospital and University of Melbourne, Australia

Luciano Bruno de Carvalho-Silva
Federal University of Alfenas- MG (UNIFAL-MG); Center for Food Security Studies (NEPA), State University of Campinas (UNICAMP), Brazil

Lucia Briscese and Chiara Rossi
Department of Neuroscience, Unit of Neurology, Pisa University Medical School, Italy Institute of Neuroscience, CNR, Pisa, Italy Department of Neuroscience, Unit Outpatients Neurological Activity, Pisa University Medical School, Pisa, Italy Department of Neurological Neurosurgical and Behavioural Sciences, Siena University Medical School, Siena, Italy

Ferdinando Sartucci
Department of Neuroscience, Unit of Neurology, Pisa University Medical School, Italy Institute of Neuroscience, CNR, Pisa, Italy Department of Neuroscience, Unit Outpatients Neurological Activity, Pisa University Medical School, Pisa, Italy Department of Neurological Neurosurgical and Behavioural Sciences, Siena University Medical School, Siena, Italy

Tommaso Bocci
Department of Neuroscience, Unit of Neurology, Pisa University Medical School, Italy Department of Neurological Neurosurgical and Behavioural Sciences, Siena University Medical School, Siena, Italy

Fabio Giannini
Department of Neurological Neurosurgical and Behavioural Sciences, Siena University Medical School, Siena, Italy

Chiara Pecori
Department of Neuroscience, Unit of Neurology, Pisa University Medical School, Italy Department of Neuroscience, Unit Outpatients Neurological Activity, Pisa University Medical School, Pisa, Italy

Arun Aggarwal
University of Sydney, Australia

Michele York
Baylor, USA Veterans Hospital, USA

Heike Schmolck
Baylor, USA Ruan Neuroscience Center, USA

Paul Schulz
Baylor, USA Veterans Hospital, USA University of Texas, USA

Paolo Bongioanni
Neurological Rehabilitation Unit - Neuroscience Department, University of Pisa/NeuroCare onlus, Italy

Ali Bülent Uşaklı
The NCO Academy, Turkey